Differentiating Surgical Instruments

D0205101

Differentiating Surgical Instruments

Colleen Rutherford, RN, MS, CNOR
Surgical Technology, Program Coordinator
Concord Hospital
Concord, New Hampshire

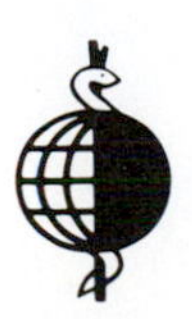

F. A. Davis Company • Philadelphia

F. A. Davis Company
1915 Arch Street
Philadelphia, PA 19103
www.fadavis.com

Copyright © 2005 by F. A. Davis Company

Copyright © 2005 by F. A. Davis Company. All rights reserved. This book is protected by copyright.No part of it may be reproduced, stored in a retrieval system, or transmitted in any form or by any means, electronic, mechanical, photocopying, recording, or otherwise, without written permission from the publisher.

Printed in the United States of America

Last digit indicates print number: 10 9 8 7

Acquisitions Editor: Christa Fratantoro
Developmental Editor: Melissa Reed
Design Manager and Illustrator: Joan Wendt

As new scientific information becomes available through basic and clinical research, recommended treatments and drug therapies undergo changes. The author(s) and publisher have done everything possible to make this book accurate, up to date, and in accord with accepted standards at the time of publication. The author(s), editors, and publisher are not responsible for errors or omissions or for consequences from application of the book, and make no warranty, expressed or implied, in regard to the contents of the book. Any practice described in this book should be applied by the reader in accordance with professional standards of care used in regard to the unique circumstances that may apply in each situation. The reader is advised always to check product information (package inserts) for changes and new information regarding dose and contraindications before administering any drug. Caution is especially urged when using new or infrequently ordered drugs.

ISBN 10: 0-8036-1224-9
ISBN 13: 978-0-8036-1224-2

Authorization to photocopy items for internal or personal use, or the internal or personal use of specific clients, is granted by F. A. Davis Company for users registered with the Copyright Clearance Center (CCC) Transactional Reporting Service, provided that the fee of $.25 per copy is paid directly to CCC, 222 Rosewood Drive, Danvers, MA 01923.For those organizations that have been granted a photocopy license by CCC, a separate system of payment has been arranged. The fee code for users of the Transactional Reporting Service is: 8036-1224/05 0+$.25.

Dedication

To the staff, anesthesia personnel, and surgeons who work in

Concord Hospital's Main OR, DSC OR,

and

Orthopedic Surgery Center

—your dedication and hard work make the "miracle of modern surgery" a reality for our patients every day.

To the staff of

Concord Hospital's Central Sterile Supply

—you provide an often unheralded but critically important service.

PREFACE

"Crile, Pean, Mosquito, Mixter" ... To those who are new to the operating room environment, the number of instruments one has to learn can seem overwhelming. Learning is further complicated by the fact that many of the instruments look similar. The purpose of this text is to help you differentiate among the common surgical instruments. As an instructor for a Surgical Technology program, I have seen students struggle to learn the surgical instruments. The students (and I) felt the books that were available did not do an adequate job of showing the tips of the instruments, which is often the only way to differentiate between them. That inadequacy is the reason I decided to photograph and write this book. My goal was to show the whole instrument as well as a close-up of the tips to aid students and new operating room staff in identifying instruments. A description is included with each instrument to further aid in identification and classification.

One of the most important methods used to identify an instrument is to look at the tip. Is the jaw smooth or serrated? If it is serrated, do the serrations run horizontally or longitudinally? Does the jaw have teeth and what do the teeth look like? In this text, you will find close-up pictures of the jaws as well as a description and picture of the whole instrument that will help you to differentiate one instrument from another. I photographed each instrument's tip at the angle that I thought best showed what made it different from other similar instruments. This should help those new to the operating room environment decide which instrument they are looking at. As an instructor, I felt it was important to place instruments that look alike on the same page so that students will be able to see the sometimes subtle differences in size or jaw serrations.

It would be impossible to include in any text *all* of the surgical instruments used in every type of surgical procedure. In this text, I have chosen to include the most commonly used instruments and instrument types that operating room personnel should be familiar with.

Instrument nicknames can vary from institution to institution, even from surgeon to surgeon. I have endeavored to include the instrument nickname ("alias") only if it is referred to this way on a large regional or national basis. This text has been critiqued by reviewers from different parts of the country to get feedback on whether an "alias" was common enough to be included. Instrument websites and catalogs were also consulted for nickname information (see Acknowledgements).

This text is divided into chapters covering each common specialty service, beginning with general surgery instrumentation. You may see many of the general surgery instruments used in specialty surgical procedures. In the interest of space, I have not repeated those instruments in the specialty chapter unless I felt they were used so frequently that they warranted being included.

At the end of each section is a short "quiz" referred to as a "Surgical Session." These quizzes can be used to reinforce your own learning or if you are an instructor, you may wish to assign these as in-class work or homework and discuss the answers in class.

To assist educators in preparing their course materials, I have developed an electronic test bank and a searchable, digital image bank to accompany this text. These ancillaries are provided on CD-ROM and are made available to educators who adopt this book.

Whether you are a student, a new employee of the operating room or central sterile supply area, or are a seasoned veteran wishing to review instrument names, I hope you will find this text a useful and valuable resource.

Acknowledgments

No one writes a book alone. I would like to acknowledge the following people and resources for their contributions to this project:

First, to Christa Fratantoro, Acquisitions Editor, and Melissa Reed, Assistant Editor, Development, of F.A. Davis Publishing Company. You took a first-time author and helped me through the process. Your unwavering support and belief in me and in this book helped motivate me and kept me going. I could not have done it without the two of you. I have come to think of you as not only business associates but as friends.

To my parents—I would like to say thank you for all the love and support you have given me throughout the years. You raised me to not be afraid of new challenges and to believe in what I could accomplish. It is one of the greatest gifts you could ever have given me.

To my friends—your support, caring, and advice mean more than I can say. You truly bring joy into my life on a daily basis.

I would also like to acknowledge the use of the following surgical instrument company catalogs and websites in aiding me to identify and differentiate some of the instruments: Boss, Codman, Innomed, Jarit, Pilling, Skylar, Snowden, Synthes spine, Stortz, and V. Mueller.

Reviewers

The author would like to thank the following educators for their careful review:

Kevin R. Craycraft, CST
Surgical Technology
Central Kentucky Technical College
Lexington, Kentucky

Diona Davis, CST
Surgical Technology
Montana State University
Great Falls, Montana

Diane May, CST
Surgical Technology
Santa Fe Community College
Gainesville, Florida

Judith Schatte, RN, CNOR, CRNFA
Department of Health Sciences
Brevard Community College
Cocoa, Florida

Pauline Sielski, RN, PhD
Surgical Technology
Triton College
River Grove, Illinois

Steve Wherrey, CST, NREMTB
Surgical Technology
Career Centers of Texas, El Paso
El Paso, Texas

Contents

A Few Words About Surgical Instruments

Although there are hundreds of different surgical instruments, the one thing that most of them have in common is that they are made partially or wholly of metal. In the past, instruments where made from a variety of metals but most surgical instruments today are made of stainless steel. Stainless steel is the choice for most manufacturers because it is a combination of several metals. Two important components of stainless steel are carbon, which adds strength to the instrument, and chromium, which makes it more resistant to the corrosion that can occur with repeated cleaning and sterilization.

A word of caution about metal. Although stainless steel is the most common metal used in the manufacture of surgical instruments, other metals (or alloys) such as aluminum, brass, or copper are sometimes used. It is important to know what metal your instrument is made of when you are using an ultrasonic cleaner or washer decontaminator. Dissimilar metals (such as stainless and bronze) coming in contact with each other in a hot, wet environment can cause one metal to plate to the other, resulting in permanent damage to the instruments.

As the instruments are made, manufacturers place a coating on them. The coating can be shiny (polished), dull (satin), or black (made to use with lasers). The shiny finish looks nice and helps to resist corrosion but can reflect surgical lighting, causing glare and making it difficult for the operating team to see. The dull (satin) finish reduces the glare. Both the shiny and dull finish could potentially deflect laser beams so caution needs to be used if they are to be employed during a laser procedure. The black finish all but eliminates glare and reflection making it useful for laser procedures because the laser beam cannot be deflected off of it.

Parts of the Surgical Instrument

When discussing surgical instruments, people often refer to the various parts of the instrument. Many ringed surgical instruments consists of six parts—the finger rings, the ratchet, the shanks, the boxlock, the jaws, and the tips. In the next picture, the parts of the instrument are labeled. The text that follows the picture describes the functions of the various parts.

Functions of the instrument parts:

- Finger Rings: Provides a place for the user to place his/her fingers and grip the instrument securely.
- Ratchet: Allows the instrument to be locked in place.

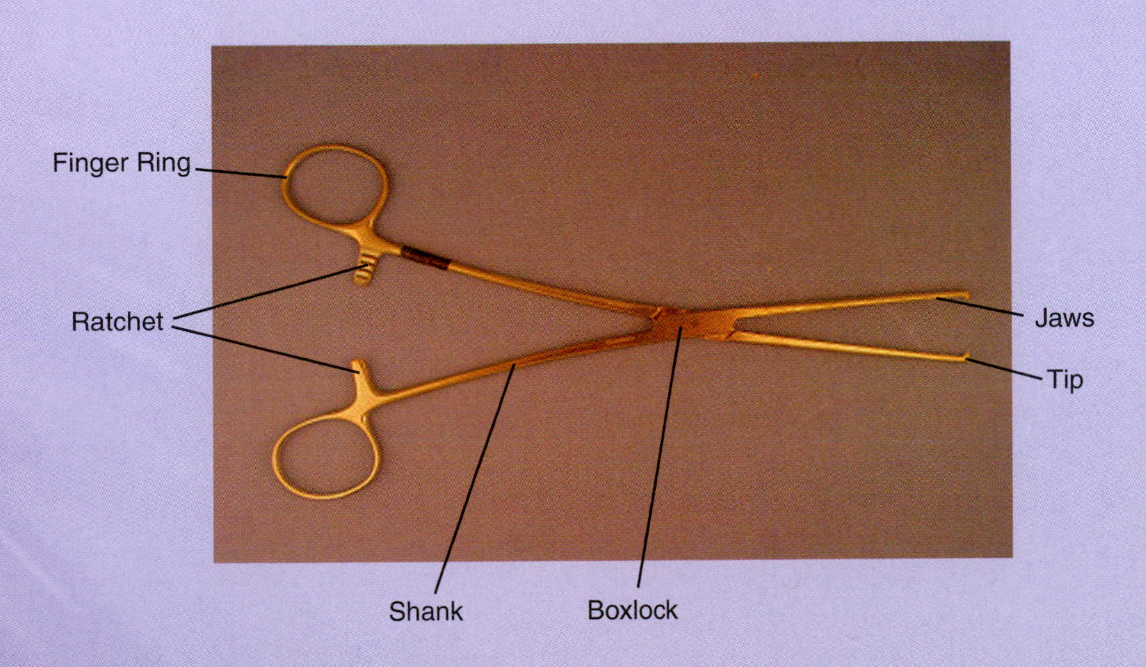

- Shank: Connects the boxlock to the finger rings.
- Boxlock: Controls the jaws of the instrument (also known as a hinge joint).
- Jaws: Along with the tip is the "working" part of the instrument. The jaws may be smooth, serrated, or cross-hatched for grasping tissue or suture. Jaws can be straight or curved to various degrees, depending on the intended use of the instrument.
- Tips: The tips can be pointed or round and have teeth or no teeth (atraumatic). The intended use of the instrument determines the number of teeth a tip has (if any) and how the tip is designed.

General Instruments 1

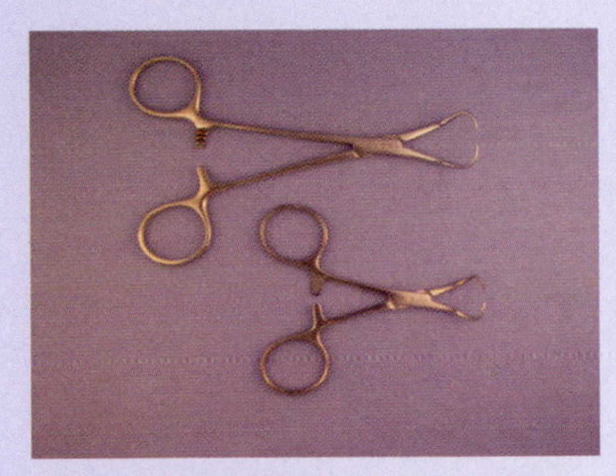

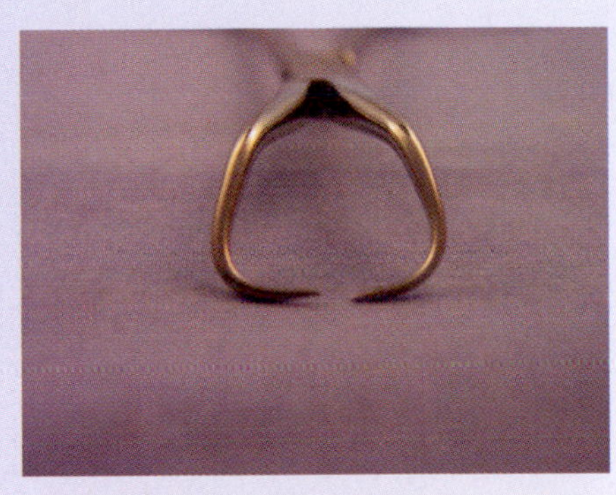

Name: Backhaus towel clip

Alias: towel clip

Category: accessory

Use: grasping tissue; securing towels or drapes; holding or reducing small bone fractures

Length: 3.5" or 5"

Additional information: perforating

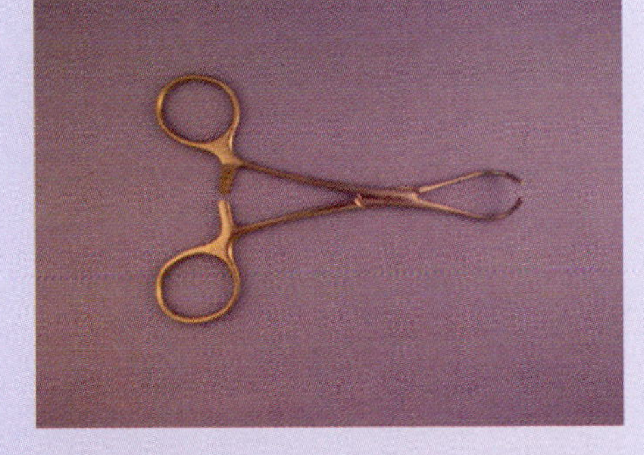

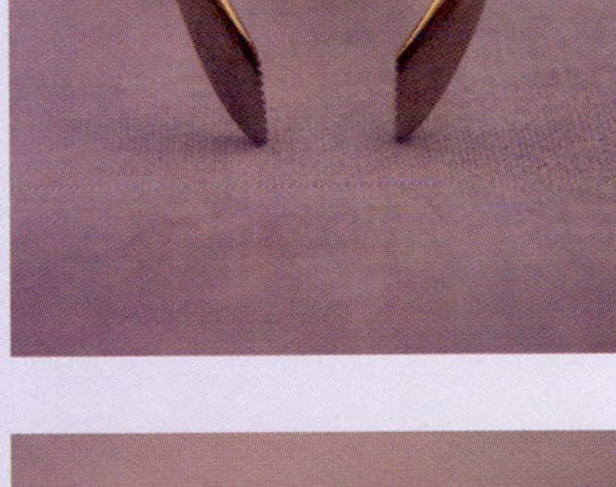

Name: Edna towel clip

Alias: Lorna

Category: accessory

Use: securing drapes; securing suction, ESU, camera cords to the drape

Length: 3.5" or 5"

Additional Information: non-perforating

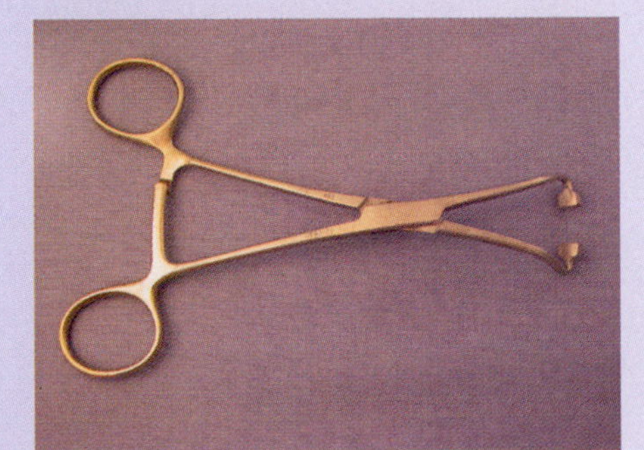

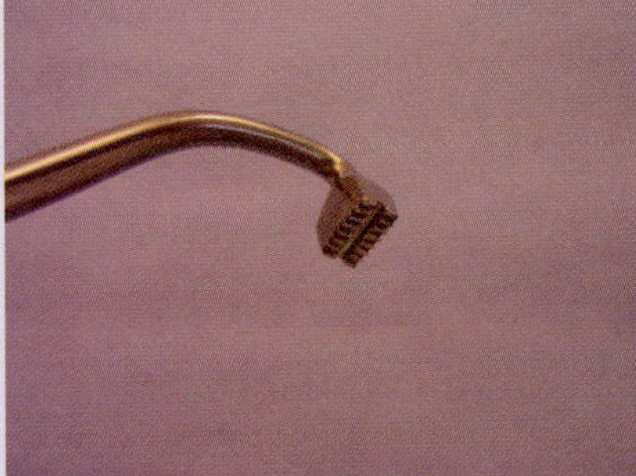

Name: Peers towel clip

Alias: none

Category: accessory

Use: holding cords to the drapes; holding towels in place

Length: 5"

Additional Information: non-perforating jaws

Name: Roeder towel clip

Alias: Roeder towel clip
Category: accessory
Use: holding towels in place; grasping tissue to be removed
Length: 5.5"
Additional Information: perforating tips; ball stops on tips

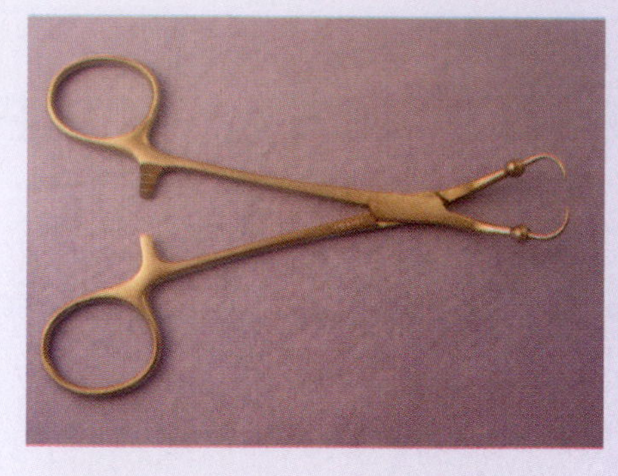

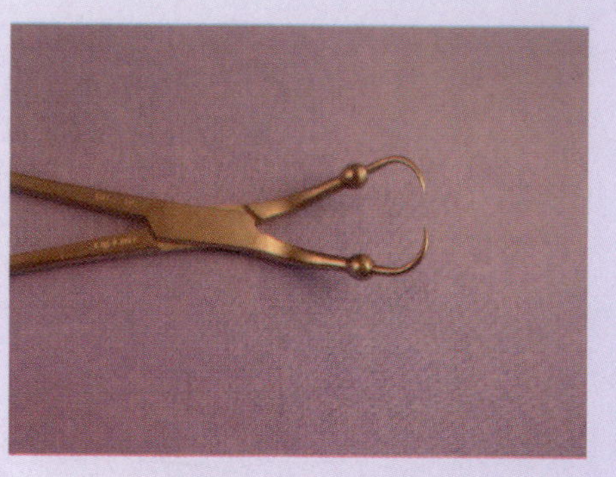

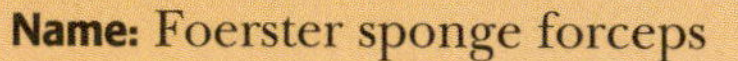

Name: Foerster sponge forceps

Alias: sponge stick
Category: grasping
Use: grasping tissue or holding Raytec sponges
Length: 9.5"
Additional Information: jaws can be smooth or serrated

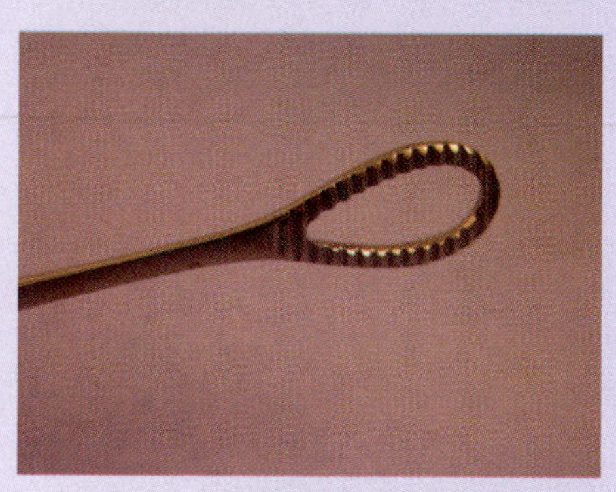

Name: Ballenger sponge forceps

Alias: sponge stick
Category: grasping
Use: grasping tissue or holding Raytec sponges
Length: 7"
Additional Information: jaws can be smooth or serrated; looks like a Foerster sponge stick but is shorter in length

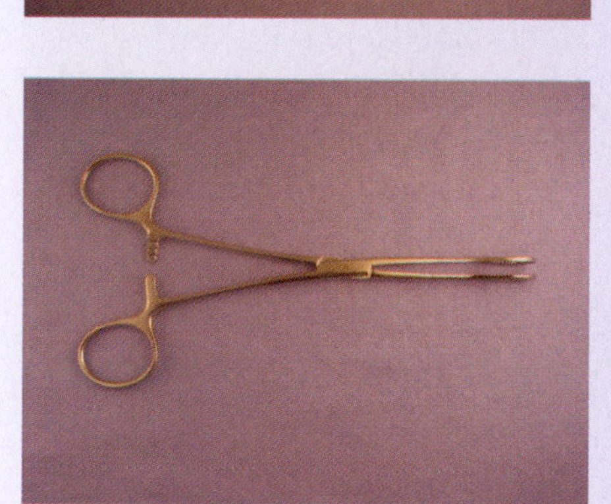

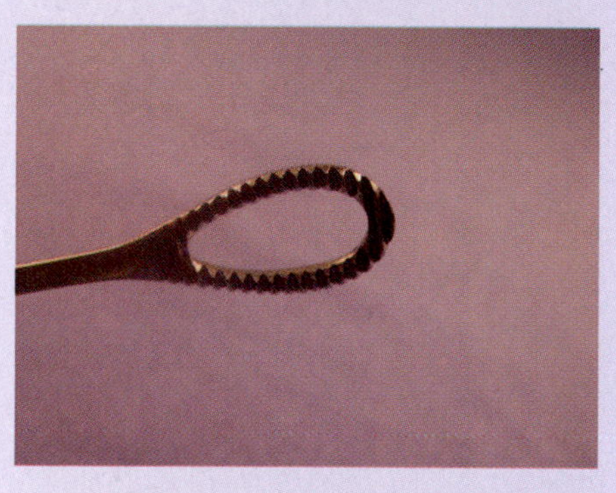

Name: Frazier suction

Alias: nasal suction; ENT suction; neuro suction
Category: suctioning
Use: suctioning small quantities of fluid/blood; suctioning in small areas
Length: 6.5"
Additional Information: short or long tips; 6 Fr to 16 Fr diameter; can be metal or disposable; angled

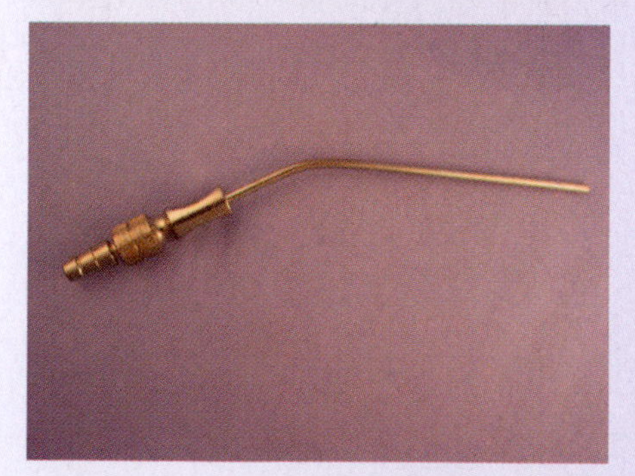

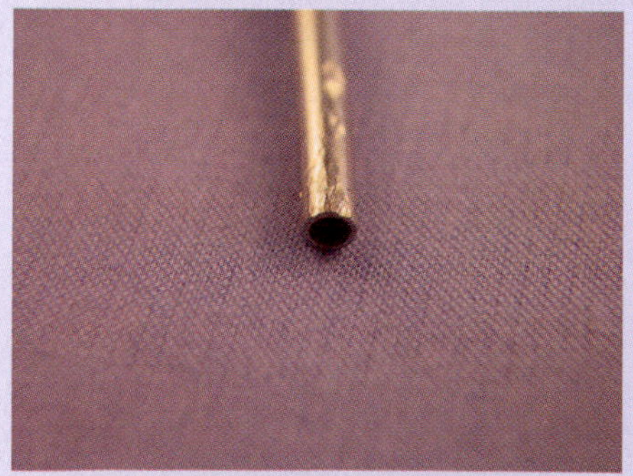

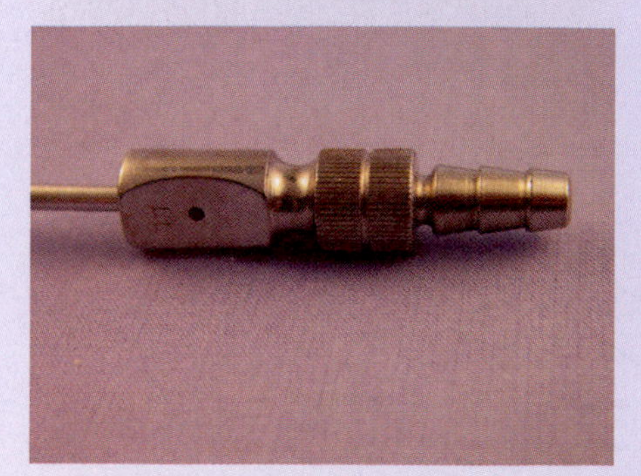

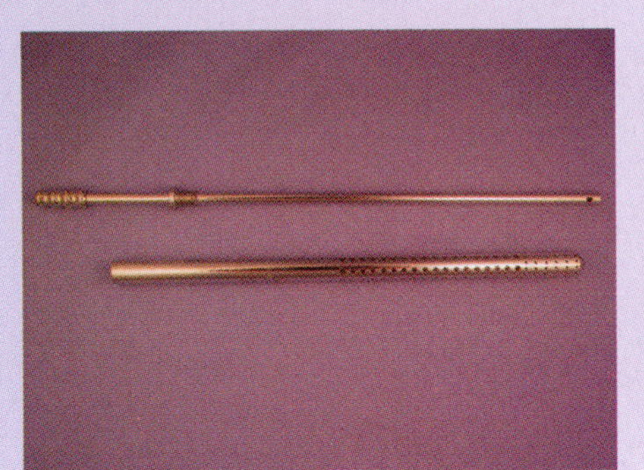

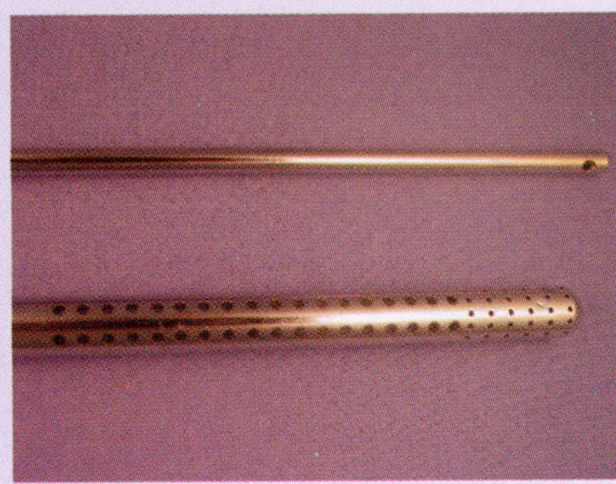

Name: Poole suction (also may be spelled Pool)

Alias: abdominal suction
Category: suctioning

Use: suctioning large quantities of fluid/blood

Length: 8.25”

Additional Information: sheath may be removed and suction cannula used alone to suction small areas; both pieces must be accounted for in an instrument count

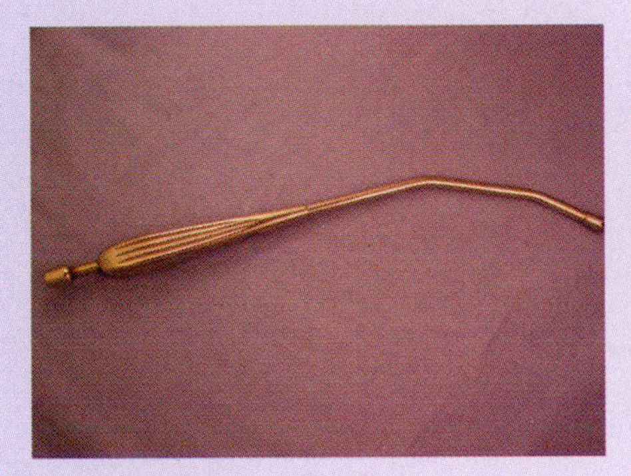

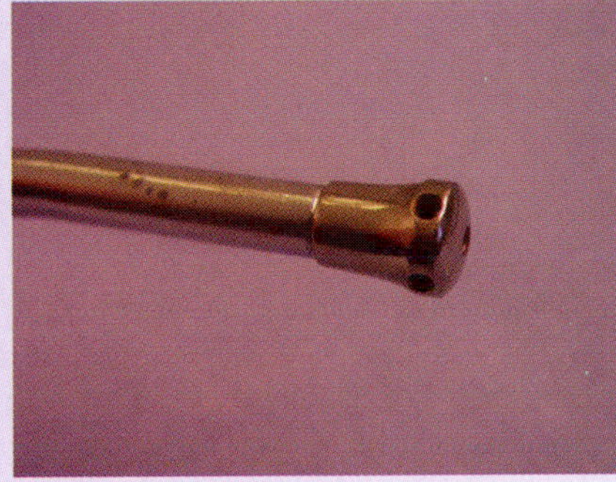

Name: Yankauer suction

Alias: tonsil suction
Category: suctioning

Use: suctioning fluid or blood; may be used to suction smoke

Length: 11” or 12”

Additional Information: Most commonly used suction; comes in metal or plastic (single-patient use) versions; if using the two piece metal suction with removable tip, both pieces must be accounted for in the instrument count

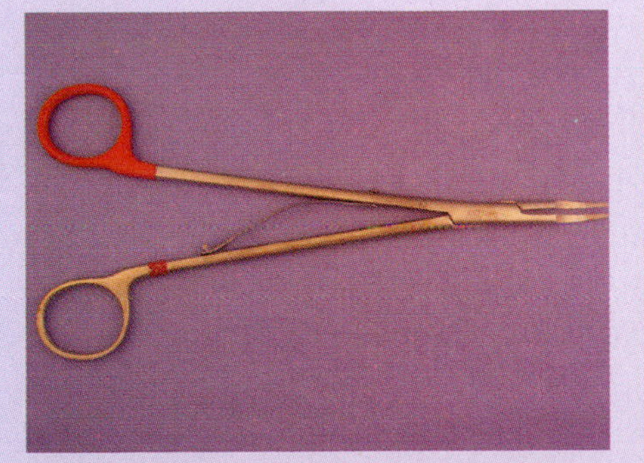

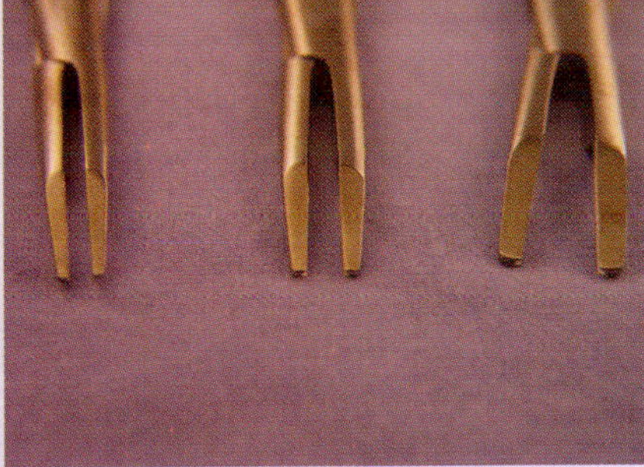

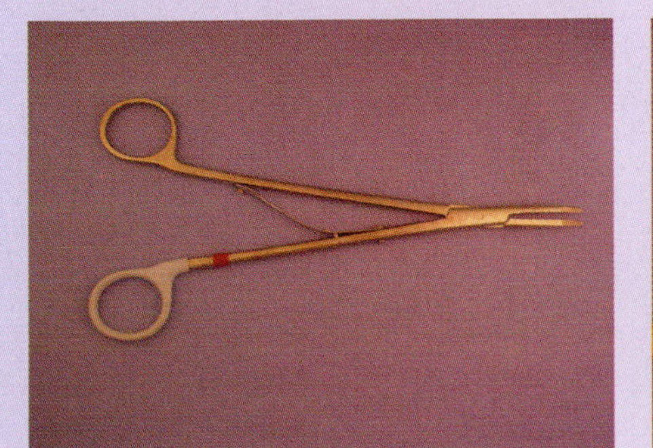

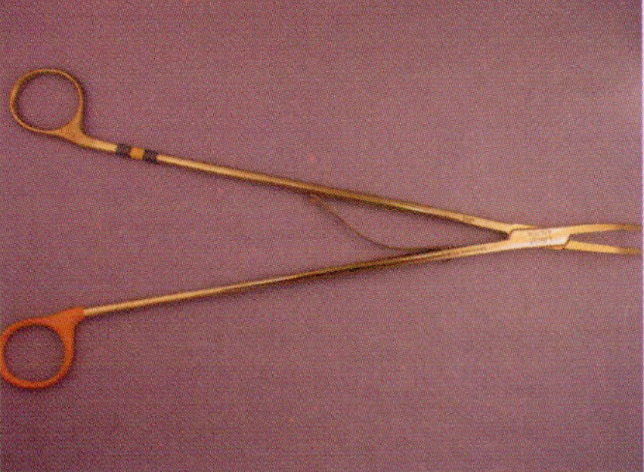

Name: Hemoclip appliers

Alias: clip appliers
Category: accessory

Use: holding and applying hemoclips used for hemostasis

Length: 6.5”, 7.75”, or 9”

Additional Information: available in small, medium, and large sizes; jaws can be straight or angled; finger rings are color coded to match clip cartridges

Name: Williams splinter forceps
Alias: Steiglitz splinter forceps
Category: grasping
Use: removing splinters
Length: 5.5”

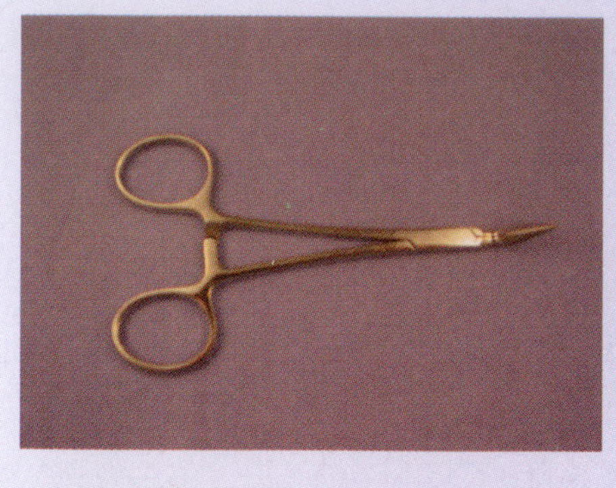

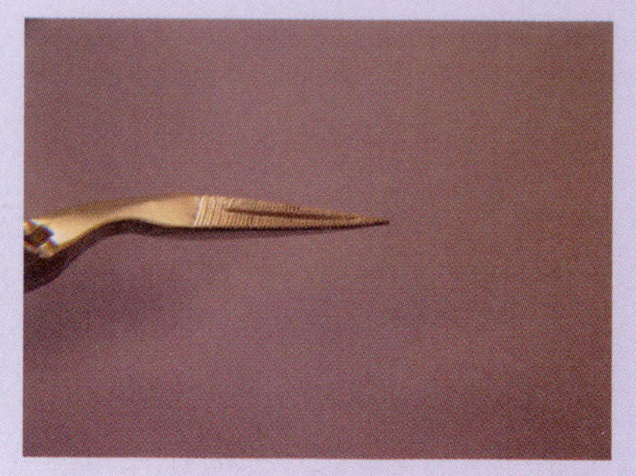

Name: Crile-Wood needle holder
Alias: fine needle driver
Category: suturing
Use: holding small or medium size suture needles
Length: 5.5”, 6”, 7”, 8”, 9”
Additional Information: used in delicate surgery

Name: Mayo-Hegar needle holder
Alias: needle driver
Category: suturing
Use: holding heavy (large) suture needles
Length: 6”, 7”, 8”, 9”, 10”
Other: widely used in general surgery

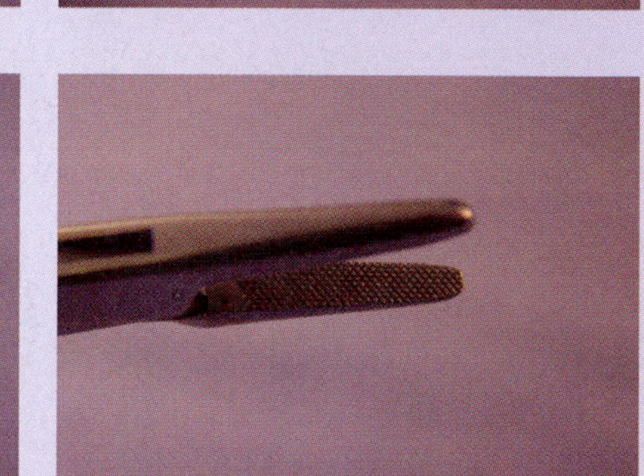

Name: Baumgartner needle holder
Alias: none
Category: suturing
Use: holding suture needles
Length: 5”
Additional Information: jaws shorter than in Crile-Wood or Mayo-Hegar

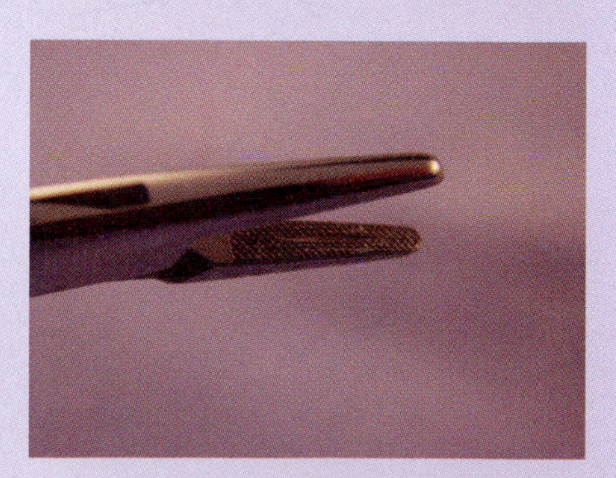

Name: Ryder needle holder
Alias: Ryder needle driver; french eye needle holder; neurosurgical needle holder
Category: suturing
Use: holding small suture needles; used mostly in vascular, neurosurgery, or intestinal surgery
Length: 5”to 9”
Additional Information: narrow jaws; smooth or carbide jaws

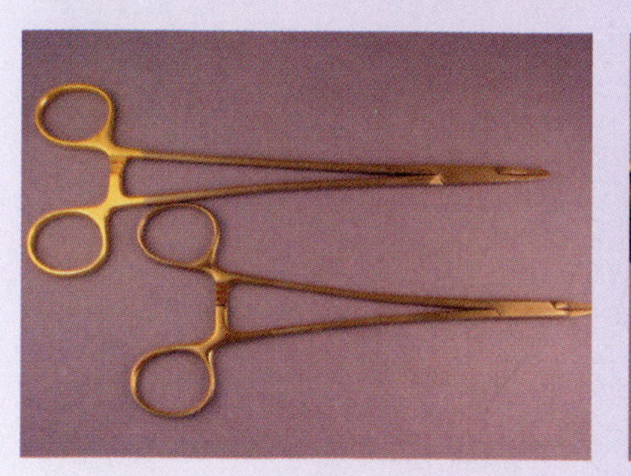

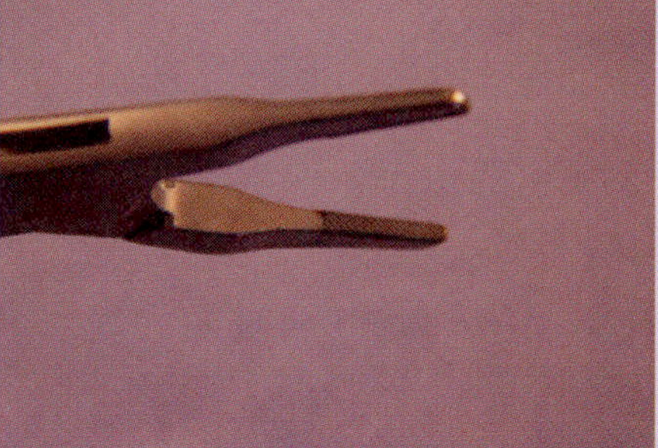

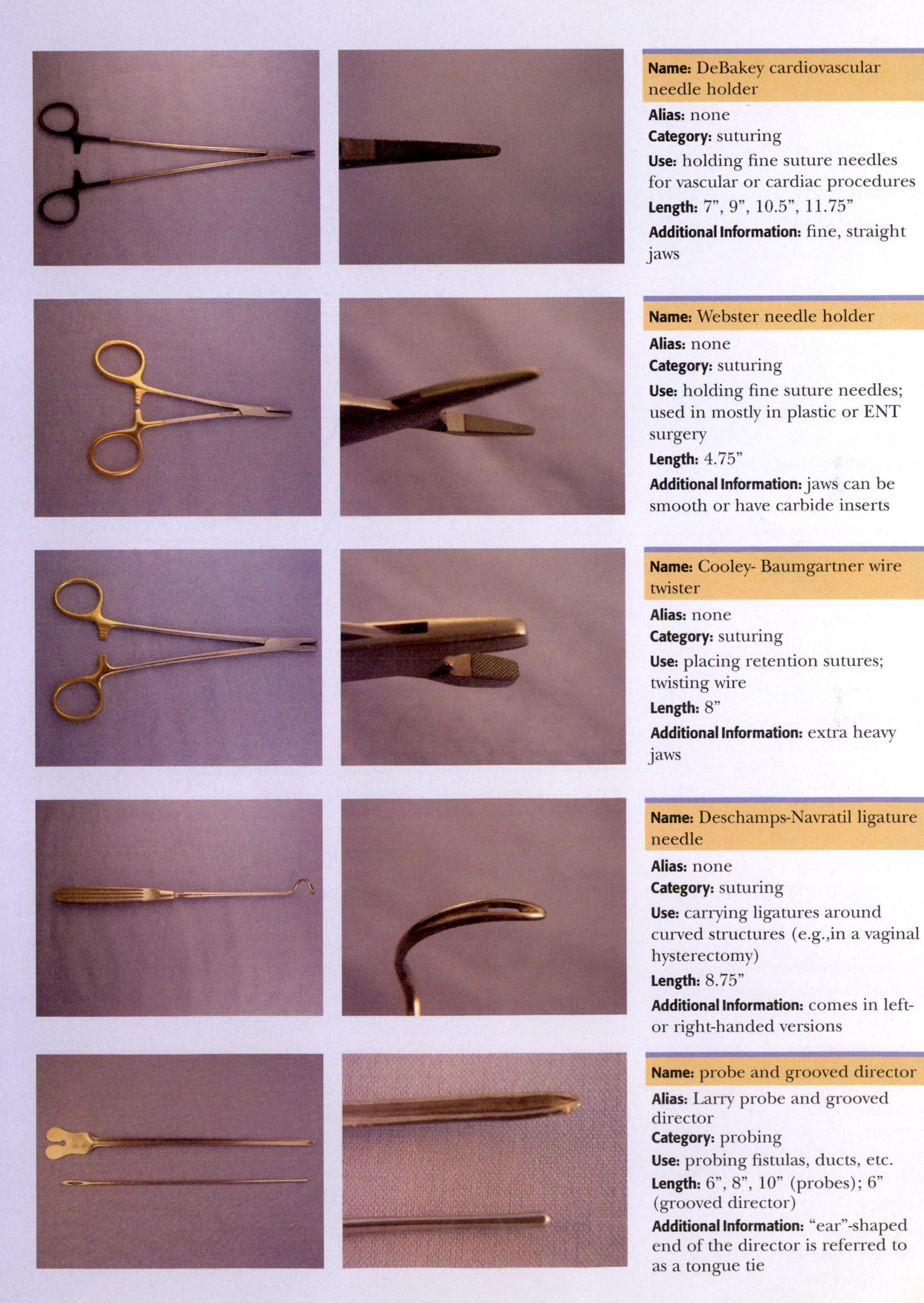

Name: DeBakey cardiovascular needle holder
Alias: none
Category: suturing
Use: holding fine suture needles for vascular or cardiac procedures
Length: 7”, 9”, 10.5”, 11.75”
Additional Information: fine, straight jaws

Name: Webster needle holder
Alias: none
Category: suturing
Use: holding fine suture needles; used in mostly in plastic or ENT surgery
Length: 4.75”
Additional Information: jaws can be smooth or have carbide inserts

Name: Cooley- Baumgartner wire twister
Alias: none
Category: suturing
Use: placing retention sutures; twisting wire
Length: 8”
Additional Information: extra heavy jaws

Name: Deschamps-Navratil ligature needle
Alias: none
Category: suturing
Use: carrying ligatures around curved structures (e.g.,in a vaginal hysterectomy)
Length: 8.75”
Additional Information: comes in left- or right-handed versions

Name: probe and grooved director
Alias: Larry probe and grooved director
Category: probing
Use: probing fistulas, ducts, etc.
Length: 6”, 8”, 10” (probes); 6” (grooved director)
Additional Information: “ear”-shaped end of the director is referred to as a tongue tie

Name: ruler
Alias: none
Category: accessory
Use: measuring
Length: 6"
Additional Information: measurements marked in inches and centimeters

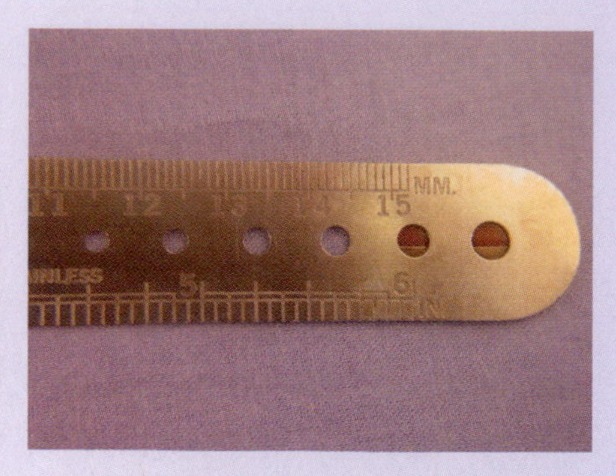

Name: electrosurgical pencil
Alias: active electrode; Bovie pencil
Category: cutting
Use: coagulating blood vessels and/or cutting tissue
Length: n/a
Additional Information: a variety of tips are available to use with the pencil; tip types include blades (spatulas), points, extensions, and balls

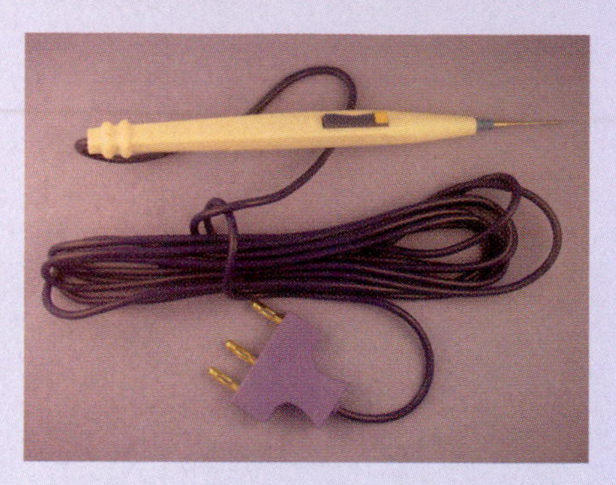

Name: hand-held cautery
Alias: none
Category: accessory
Use: cauterizing fine vessels or tissue (such as in hand surgery)
Length: n/a
Additional Information: single-patient use

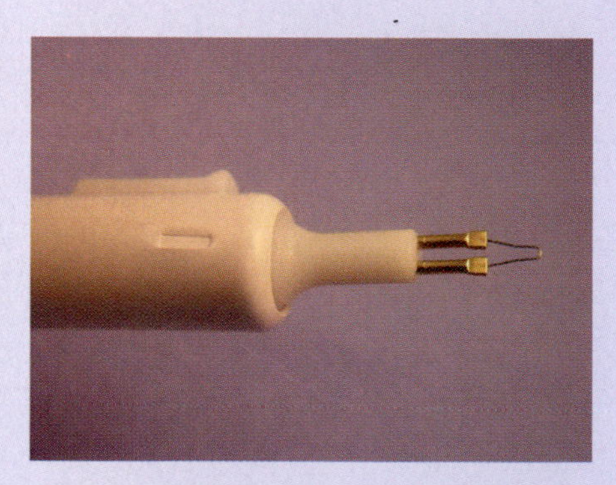

Name: Gerald bipolar forceps
Alias: none
Category: accessory
Use: coagulating small blood vessels
Length: 5.75"
Additional Information: delicate, narrow tips; bayonet-shaped handle

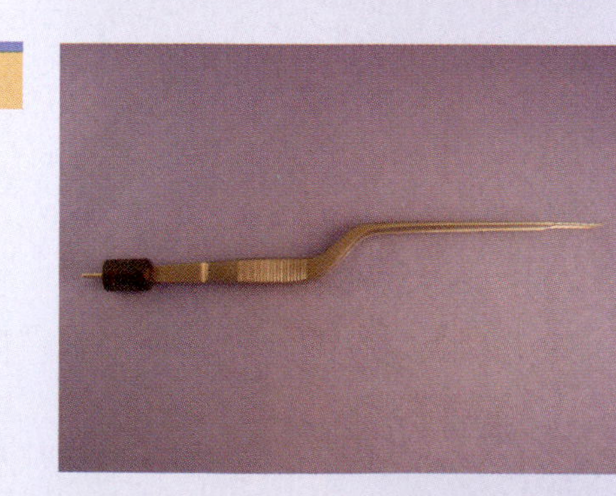
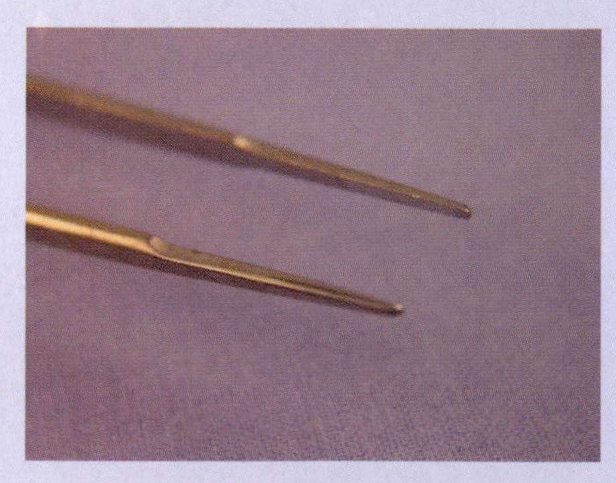

Name: Malis mirror finish bipolar cautery forceps
Alias: none
Category: accessory
Use: cauterizing small blood vessels or delicate tissue
Length: 7"
Additional Information: can have sharp or blunt tips

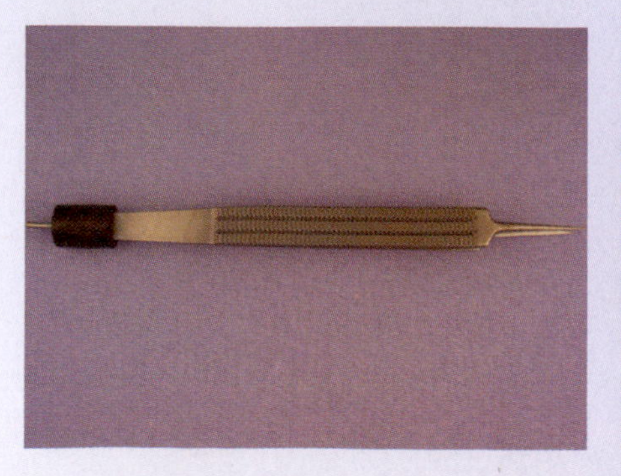
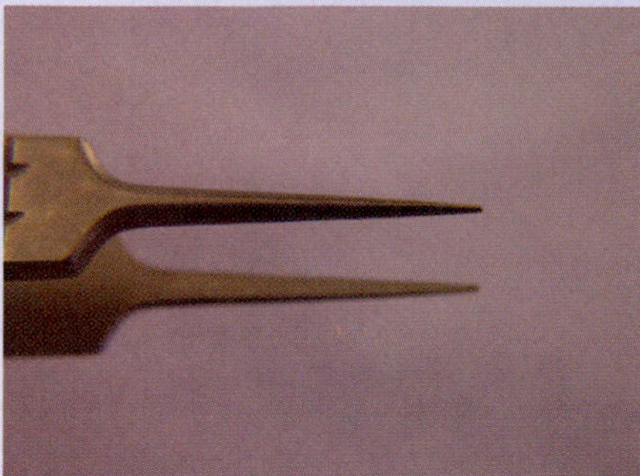

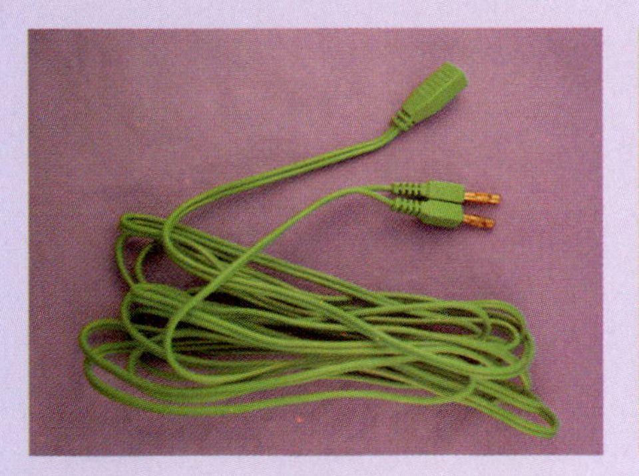

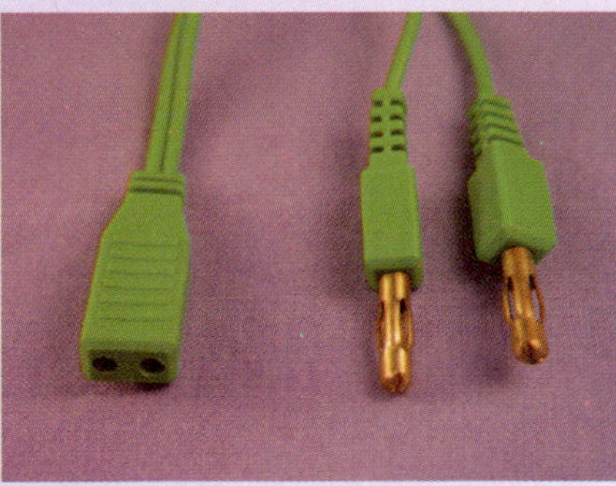

Name: bipolar cautery cord

Alias: none

Category: accessory

Use: attaching bipolar cautery forceps to electrosurgical power unit

Length: 12' long

Additional Information: use with bipolar cautery forceps only

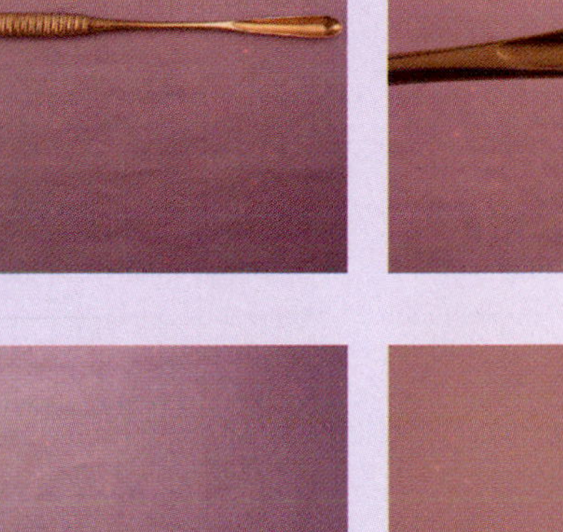

Name: Mayo gallstone scoop

Alias: none

Category: accessory

Use: retrieving gallstones

Length: 10.75"

Additional Information: double ended

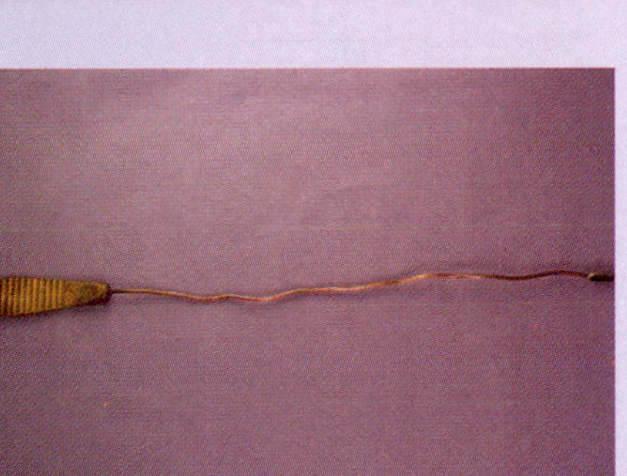

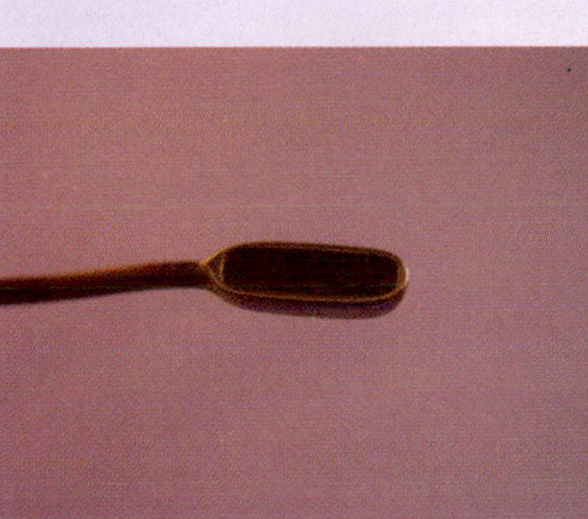

Name: Mayo common duct scoop

Alias: none

Category: accessory

Use: removing stones from the common duct

Length: 11"

Additional Information: comes in small, medium, or large size

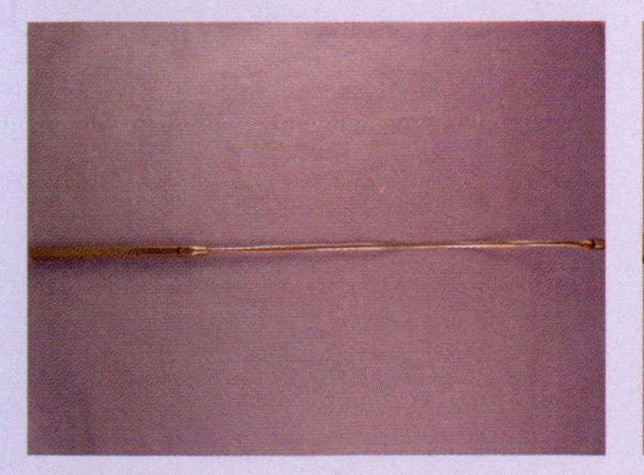

Name: Desjardin gallstone scoop

Alias: none

Category: accessory

Use: removing gallstones

Length: 11"

Additional Information: comes in 6-mm, 7-mm, 8-mm, and 9-mm sizes

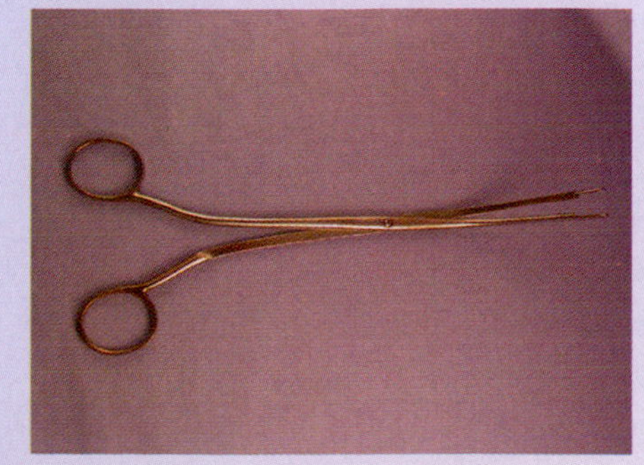

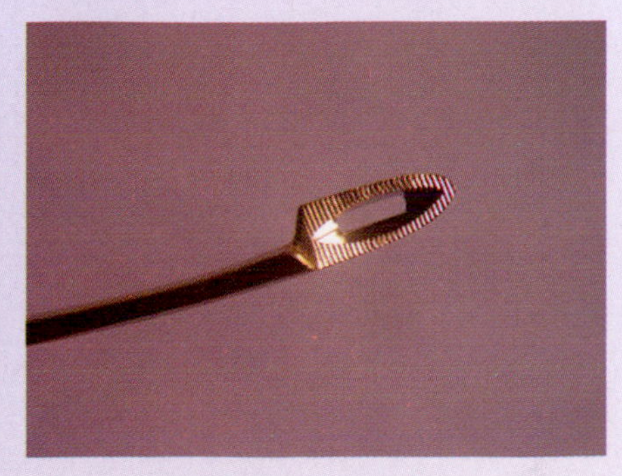

Name: Best common duct stone forceps

Alias: none

Category: grasping

Use: removing stones from the common duct

Length: 8.5"

Additional Information: jaws are cupped and serrated for better grasping of stones

Name: Bakes common bile duct dilators
Alias: none
Category: dilating
Use: dilating the common bile duct
Length: 9"
Additional Information: comes in tip sizes 3 mm to 11 mm

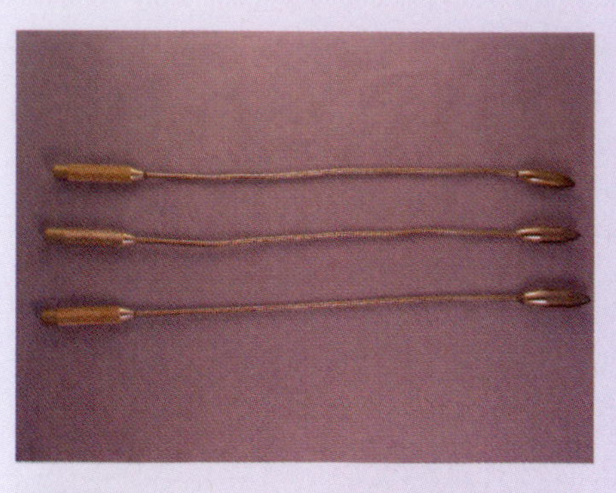
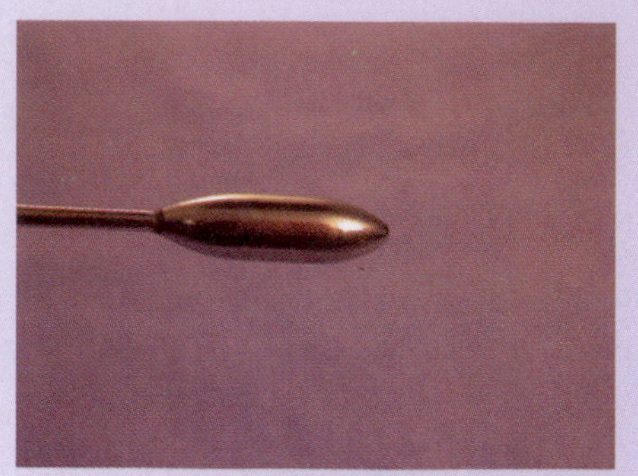

Name: esophageal dilators
Alias: bougies
Category: dilating
Use: dilating esophagus for treatment of esophageal stenosis
Length: 29.5"
Additional Information: tips tapered; come in sizes 20 to 60 Fr

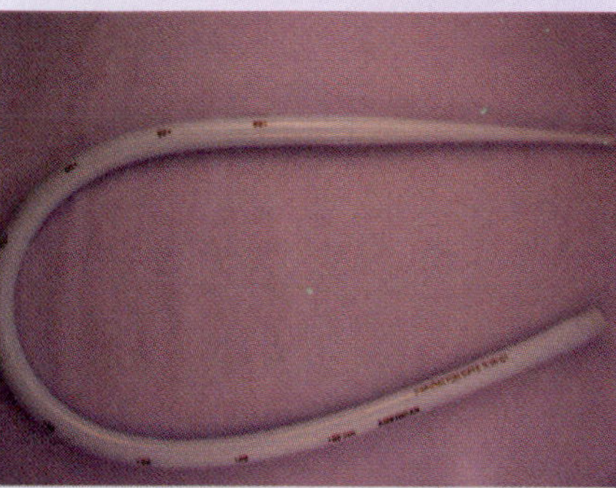
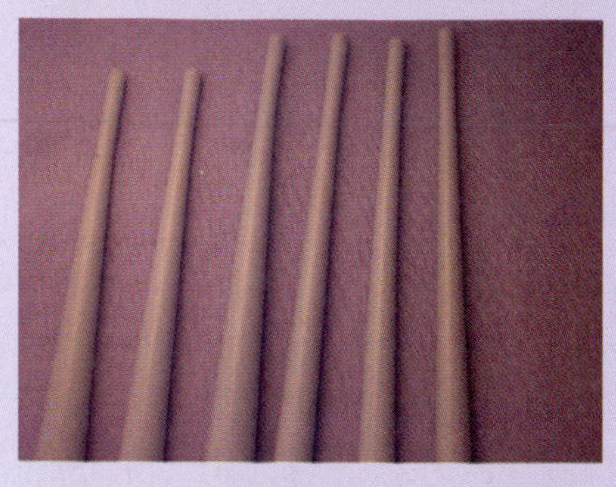

Name: sigmoidoscope; proctoscope
Alias: none
Category: accessory
Use: viewing the inside of the anal canal and sigmoid colon
Length: n/a
Additional Information: single-patient use scope tip is attached to the scope head

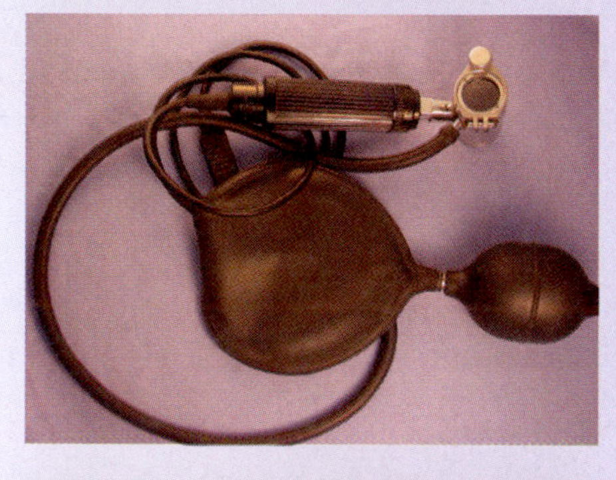
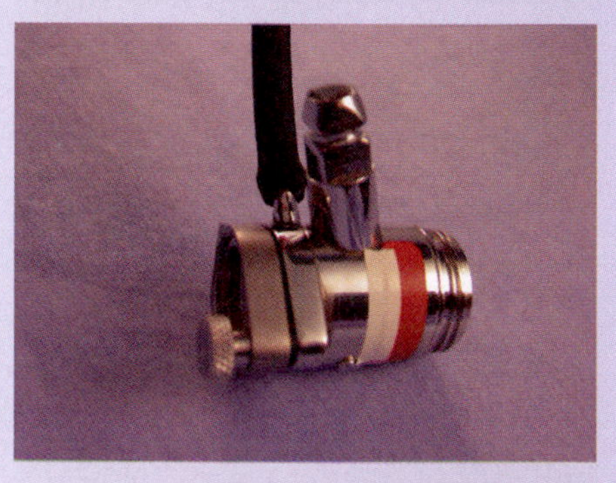

Name: anoscope with obturator
Alias: none
Category: retracting
Use: retracting/viewing of the anus
Length: n/a
Additional Information: rounded obturator is used for insertion then removed

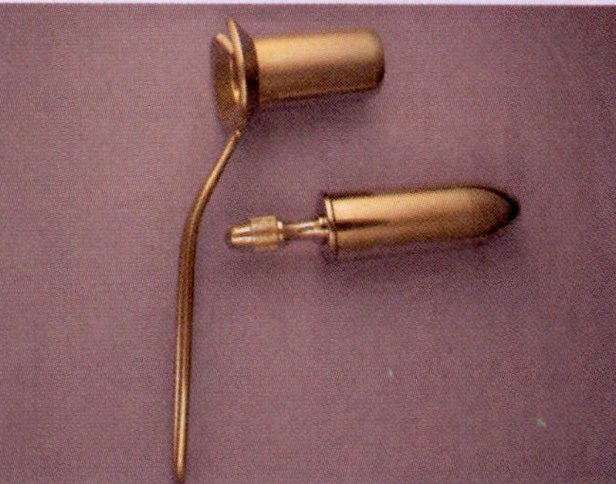
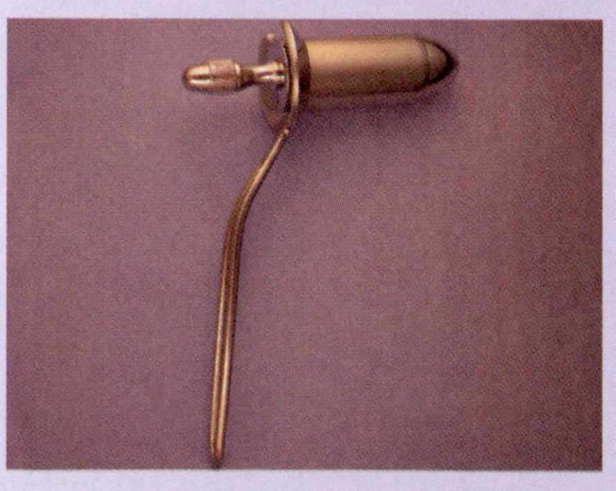

GENERAL GRASPING

Name: Adson dressing forceps
Alias: none
Category: grasping
Use: grasping tissue
Length: 4.75"
Additional Information: serrated tips

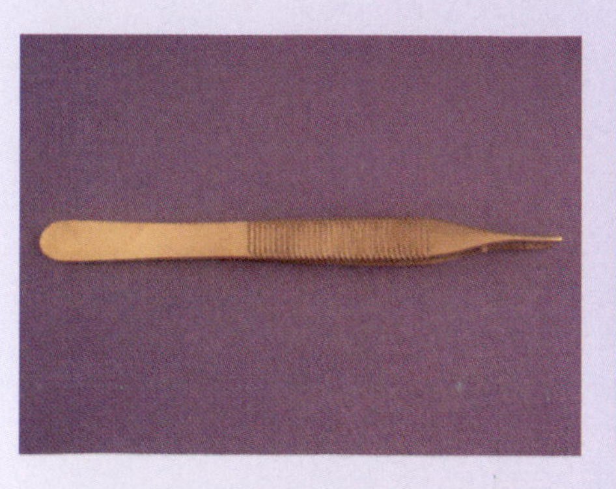
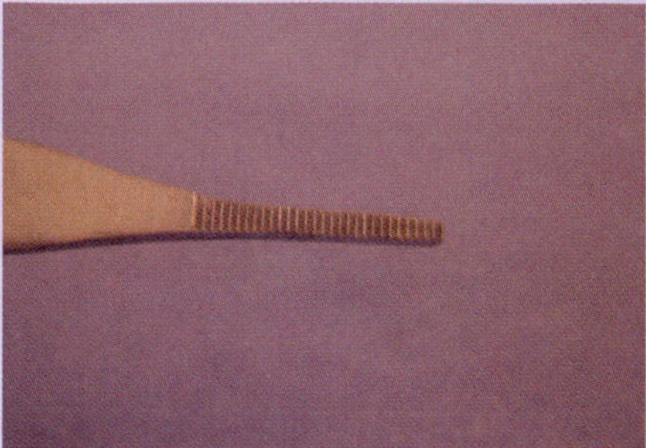

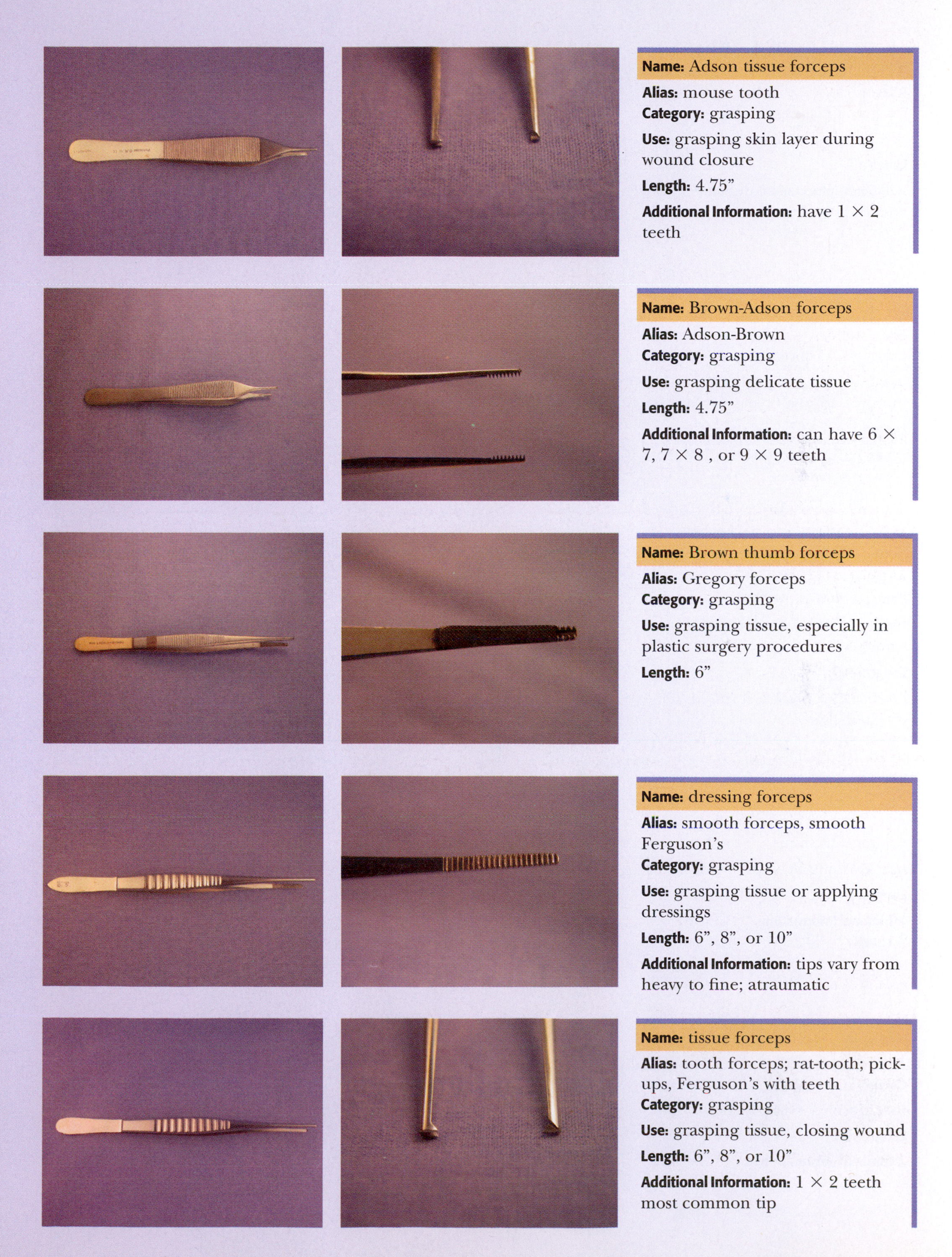

Name: Adson tissue forceps

Alias: mouse tooth
Category: grasping

Use: grasping skin layer during wound closure

Length: 4.75"

Additional Information: have 1 × 2 teeth

Name: Brown-Adson forceps

Alias: Adson-Brown
Category: grasping

Use: grasping delicate tissue

Length: 4.75"

Additional Information: can have 6 × 7, 7 × 8 , or 9 × 9 teeth

Name: Brown thumb forceps

Alias: Gregory forceps
Category: grasping

Use: grasping tissue, especially in plastic surgery procedures

Length: 6"

Name: dressing forceps

Alias: smooth forceps, smooth Ferguson's
Category: grasping

Use: grasping tissue or applying dressings

Length: 6", 8", or 10"

Additional Information: tips vary from heavy to fine; atraumatic

Name: tissue forceps

Alias: tooth forceps; rat-tooth; pick-ups, Ferguson's with teeth
Category: grasping

Use: grasping tissue, closing wound

Length: 6", 8", or 10"

Additional Information: 1 × 2 teeth most common tip

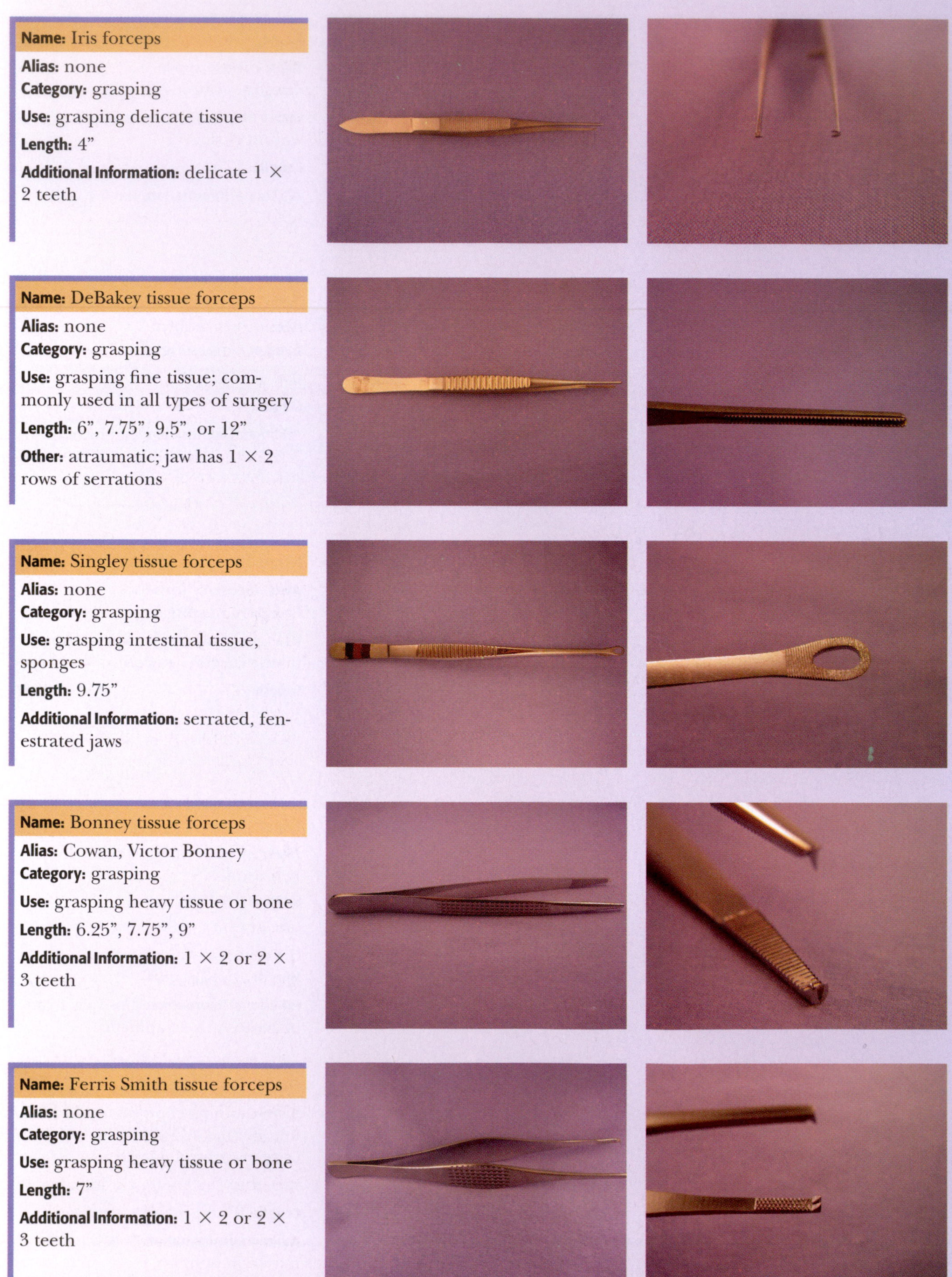

Name: Iris forceps
Alias: none
Category: grasping
Use: grasping delicate tissue
Length: 4"
Additional Information: delicate 1 × 2 teeth

Name: DeBakey tissue forceps
Alias: none
Category: grasping
Use: grasping fine tissue; commonly used in all types of surgery
Length: 6", 7.75", 9.5", or 12"
Other: atraumatic; jaw has 1 × 2 rows of serrations

Name: Singley tissue forceps
Alias: none
Category: grasping
Use: grasping intestinal tissue, sponges
Length: 9.75"
Additional Information: serrated, fenestrated jaws

Name: Bonney tissue forceps
Alias: Cowan, Victor Bonney
Category: grasping
Use: grasping heavy tissue or bone
Length: 6.25", 7.75", 9"
Additional Information: 1 × 2 or 2 × 3 teeth

Name: Ferris Smith tissue forceps
Alias: none
Category: grasping
Use: grasping heavy tissue or bone
Length: 7"
Additional Information: 1 × 2 or 2 × 3 teeth

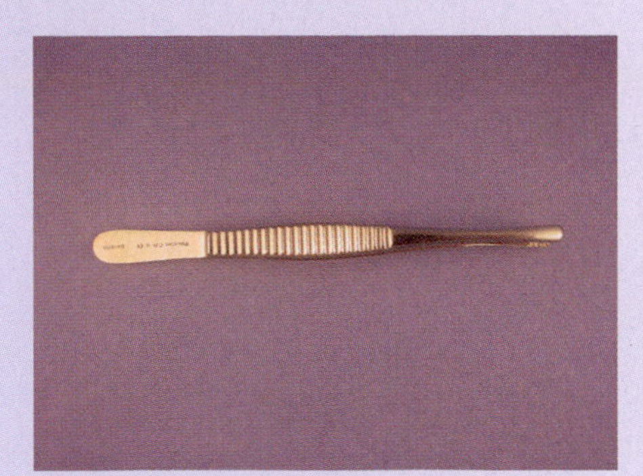

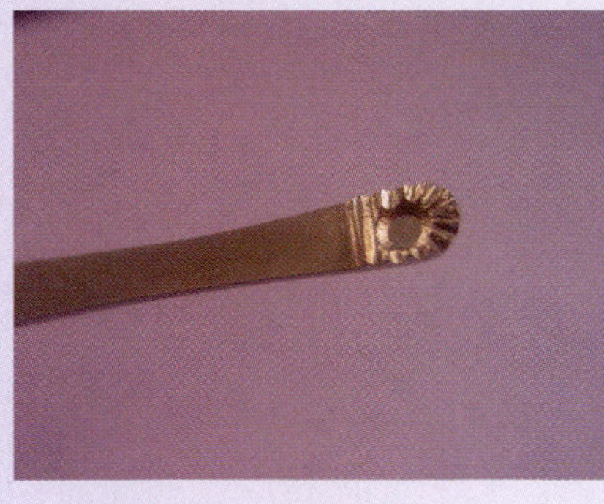

Name: Russian forceps

Alias: none

Category: grasping

Use: grasping tissue, aortic aneurysm plaque

Length: 6", 8", 10"

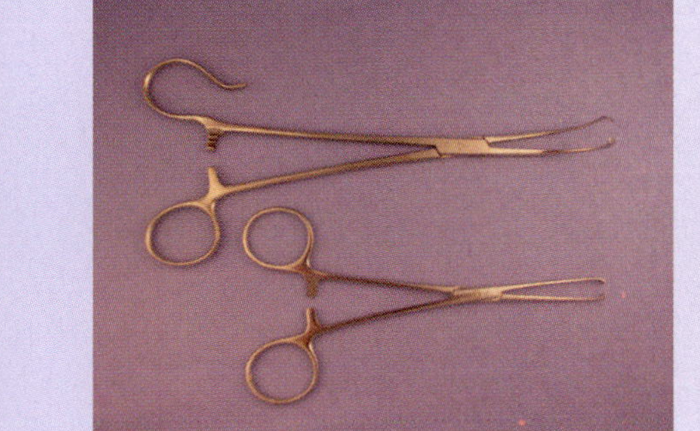

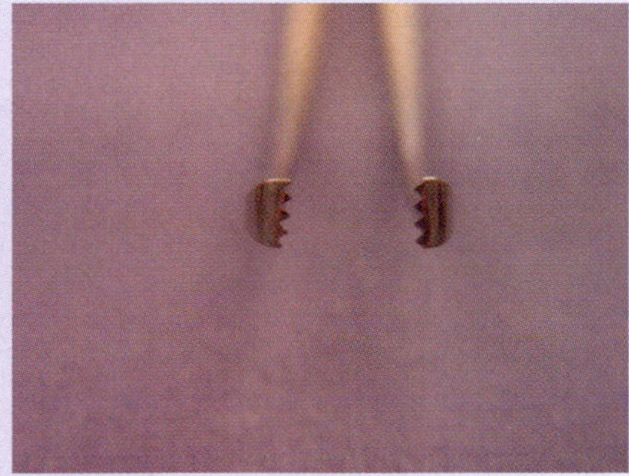

Name: Allis

Alias: none

Category: grasping

Use: grasping organ or tissue that is being removed

Length: 6", 7.5", or 10"

Additional Information 2 × 3, 3 × 4, 4 × 5, 5 × 6 teeth; tips can be straight or angled

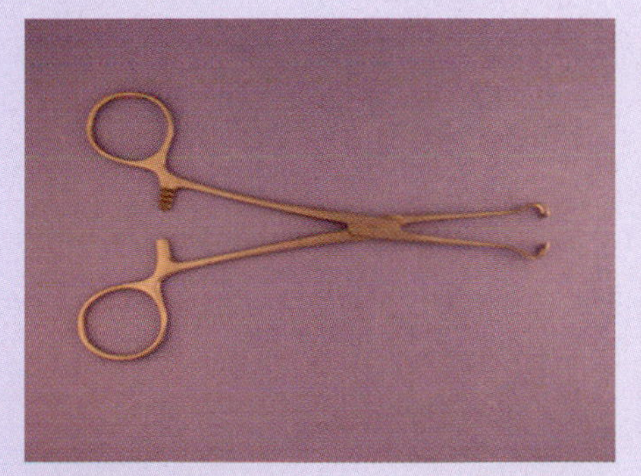

Name: Babcock

Alias: none

Category: grasping

Use: grasping delicate tissue (e.g., fallopian tube, bowel, vas deferens)

Length: 6", 7.5", or 9"

Additional Information: no teeth—atraumatic

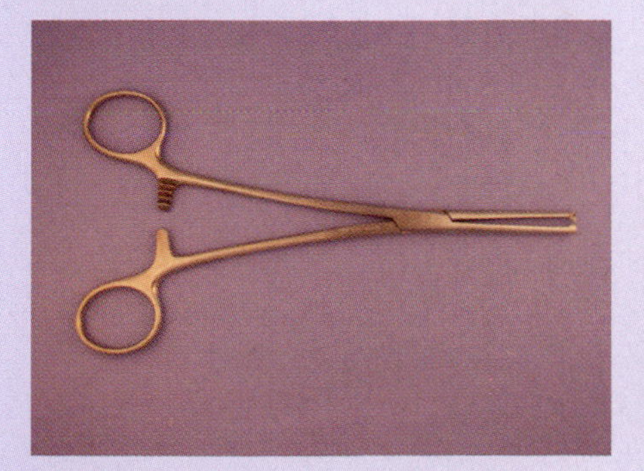

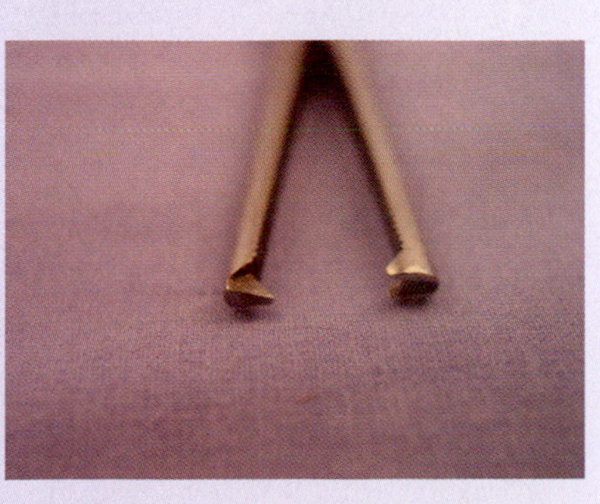

Name: Kocher

Alias: Ochsner; Rochester-Ochsner

Category: grasping

Use: grasping heavy tissue (e.g., fascia)

Length: 5.5", 6.25", 7", 8", 9",10"

Additional Information: 1 × 2 teeth

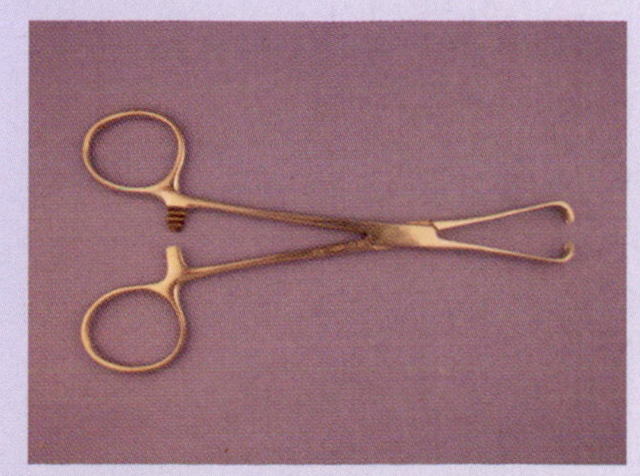

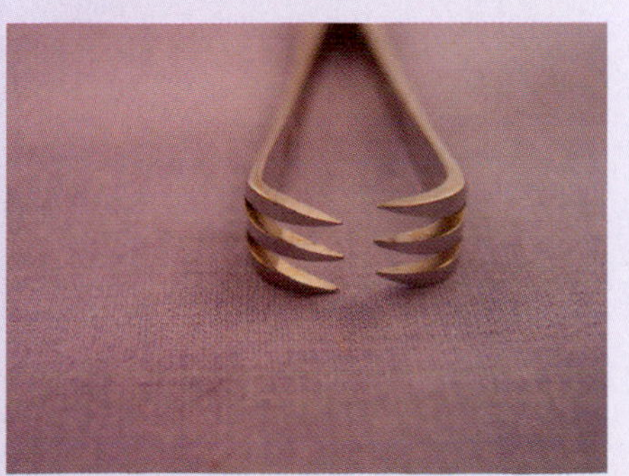

Name: Lahey traction forceps

Alias: tenaculum

Category: grasping

Use: grasping tissue that is being removed

Length: 6"

Additional Information: 3 × 3 teeth

Name: Pennington forceps

Alias: none

Category: grasping

Use: grasping tissue, especially in intestinal or rectal surgeries and cesarean section

Length: 6", 7.5"

Additional Information: triangular jaws

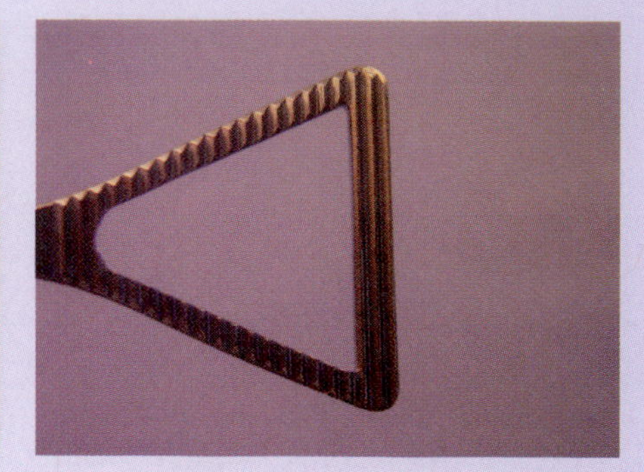

Name: Magill catheter forceps

Alias: intubating forceps

Category: grasping

Use: grasping endotracheal tube during intubation

Length: 7.75" (child) or 9.75" (adult)

Additional Information: can be used to grasp other types of catheters during insertion

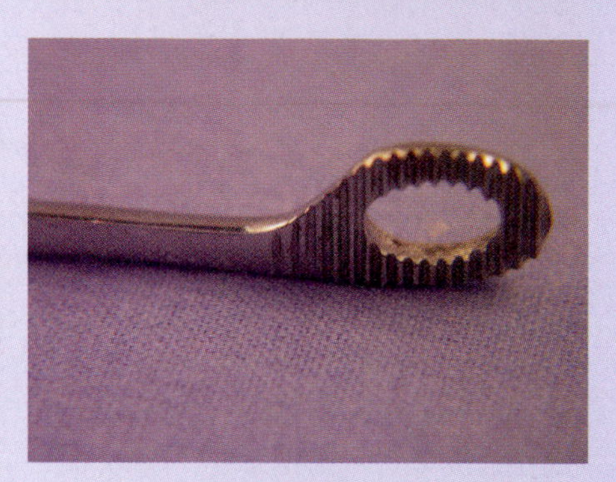

Name: Randall forceps

Alias: kidney stone forceps

Category: grasping

Use: grasping stones or polyps

Length: 9"

Additional Information: curved jaws

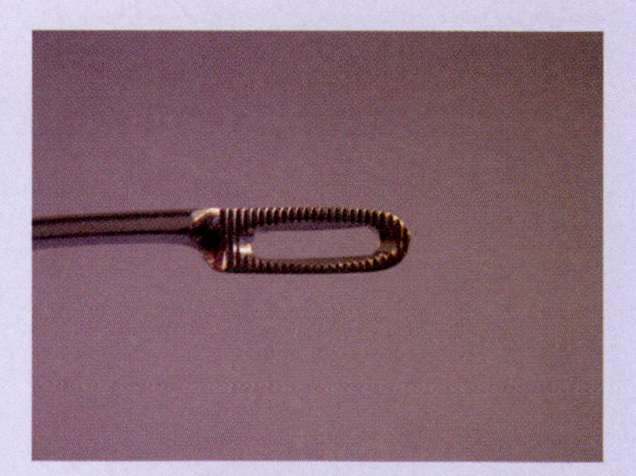

Name: Fletcher-Van Doren uterine polyp and sponge-holding forceps

Alias: Kitner holder; peanut holder

Category: grasping

Use: grasping uterine polyps; holding Kitner sponges for blunt dissection

Length: 9.5"

Additional Information: double curved; serrated tips

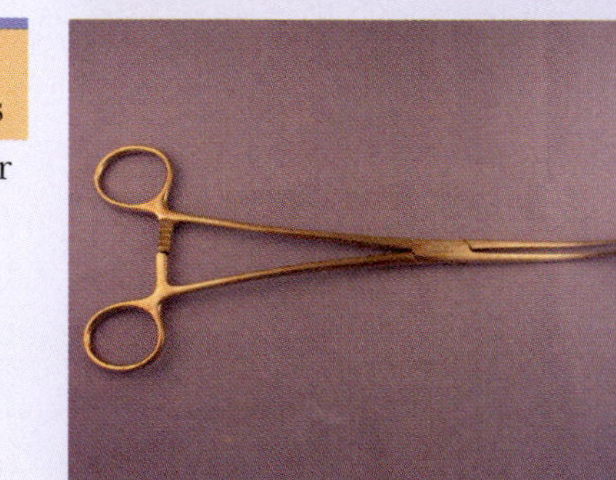

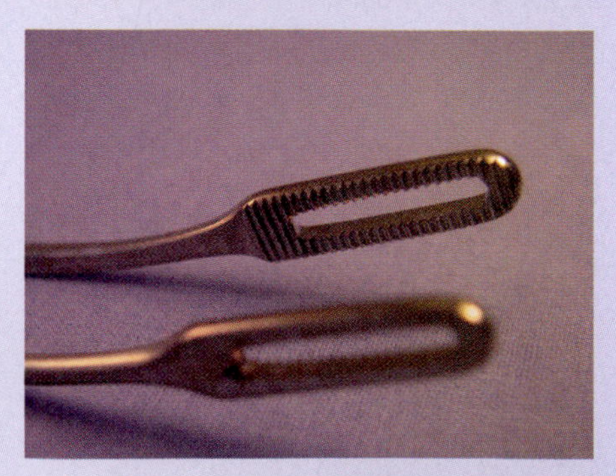

Name: Blake gallstone forceps

Alias: none

Category: grasping

Use: removing gallstones from gallbladder

Length: 8.75"

Additional Information: jaws can be straight or curved

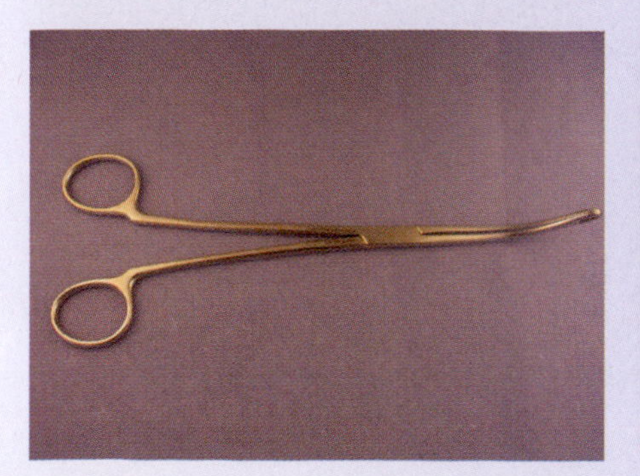

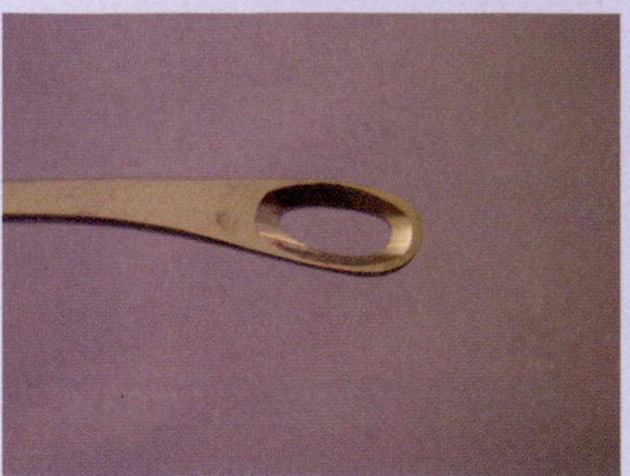

GENERAL CLAMPS

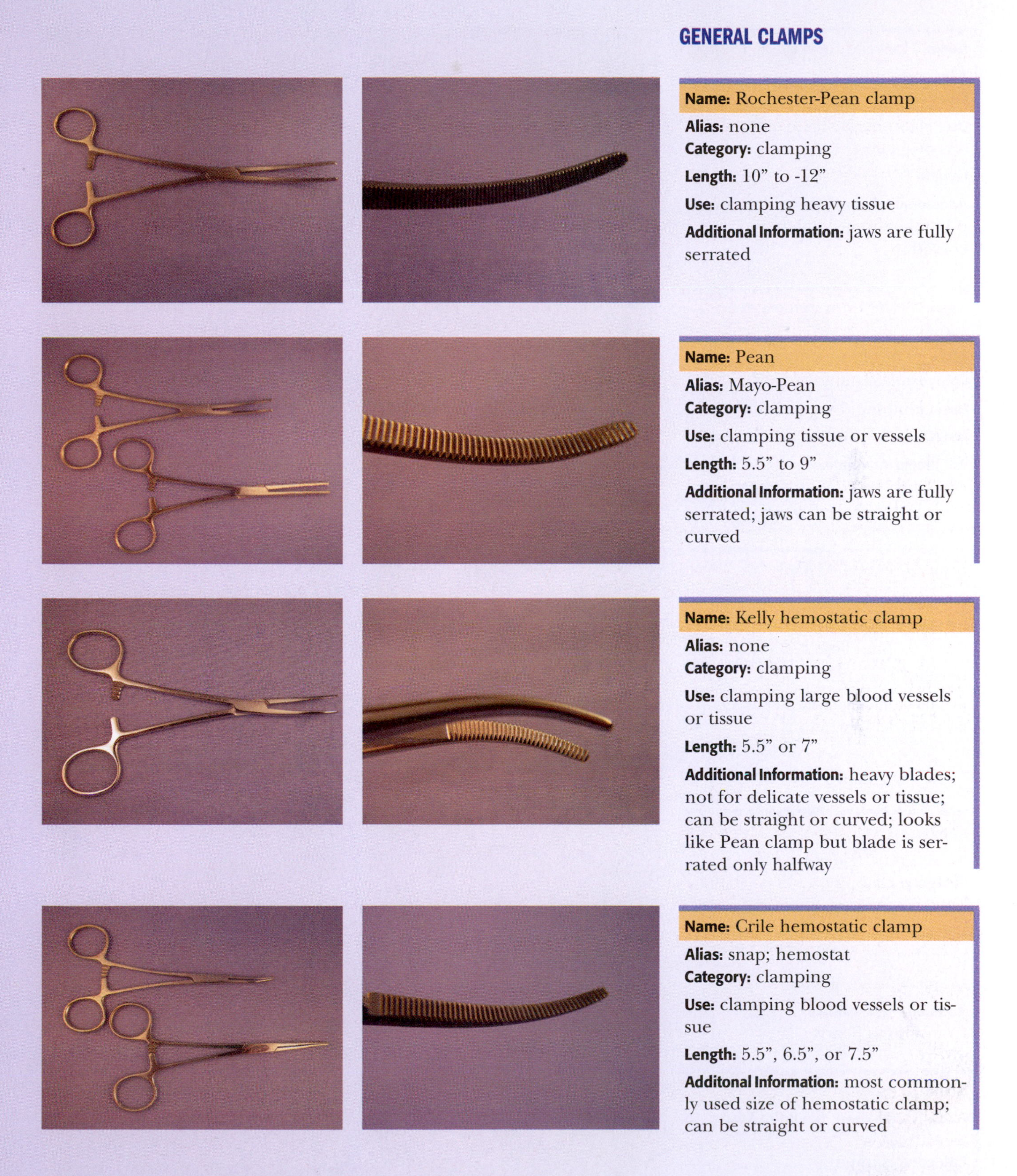

Name: Rochester-Pean clamp
Alias: none
Category: clamping
Length: 10” to -12”
Use: clamping heavy tissue
Additional Information: jaws are fully serrated

Name: Pean
Alias: Mayo-Pean
Category: clamping
Use: clamping tissue or vessels
Length: 5.5” to 9”
Additional Information: jaws are fully serrated; jaws can be straight or curved

Name: Kelly hemostatic clamp
Alias: none
Category: clamping
Use: clamping large blood vessels or tissue
Length: 5.5” or 7”
Additional Information: heavy blades; not for delicate vessels or tissue; can be straight or curved; looks like Pean clamp but blade is serrated only halfway

Name: Crile hemostatic clamp
Alias: snap; hemostat
Category: clamping
Use: clamping blood vessels or tissue
Length: 5.5”, 6.5”, or 7.5”
Additonal Information: most commonly used size of hemostatic clamp; can be straight or curved

Name: Halstead hemostatic clamp

Alias: mosquito; stat
Category: clamping

Use: clamping delicate blood vessels or tissue

Length: 5”

Additional Information: for delicate use only; can be straight or curved

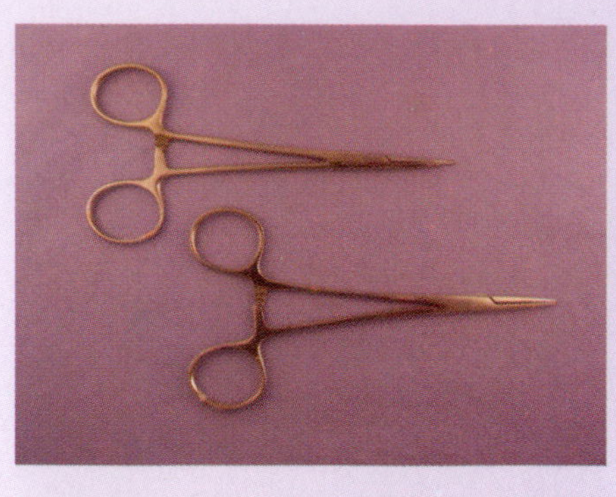

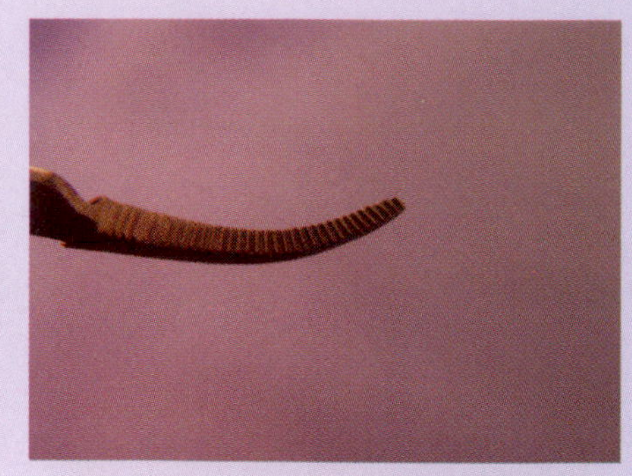

Name: Pratt-Smith hemostatic forceps

Alias: Pratt “T” forceps
Category: clamping

Use: clamping delicate tissue

Length: 6”

Additional Information: t-shaped, concave jaws; jaws delicately serrated

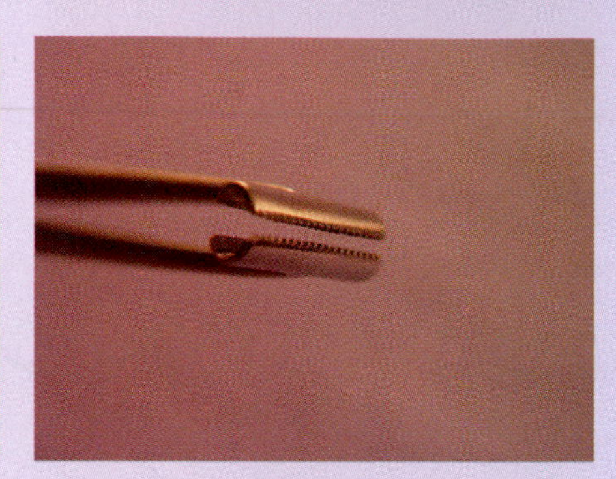

Name: Rochester mixter

Alias: none
Category: clamping

Use: clamping bowel

Length: 10” to 12”

Additional Information: full curved jaws; vertical serrations

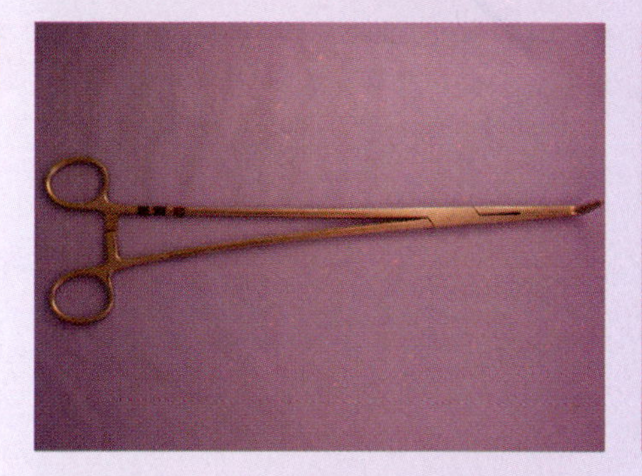

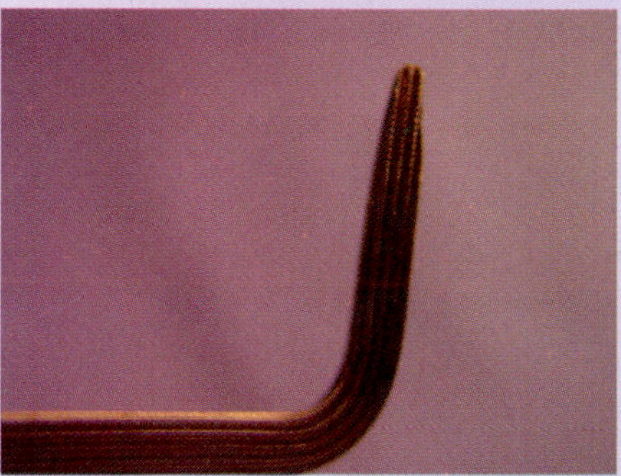

Name: mixter

Alias: right angle; Gemini
Category: clamping

Use: clamping tissue or grasping a ligature around a curve (such as a pedicle or blood vessel)

Length: 5.5”, 7”, 9”, 10.5”, 12”

Additional Information: jaws vary from fine to heavy

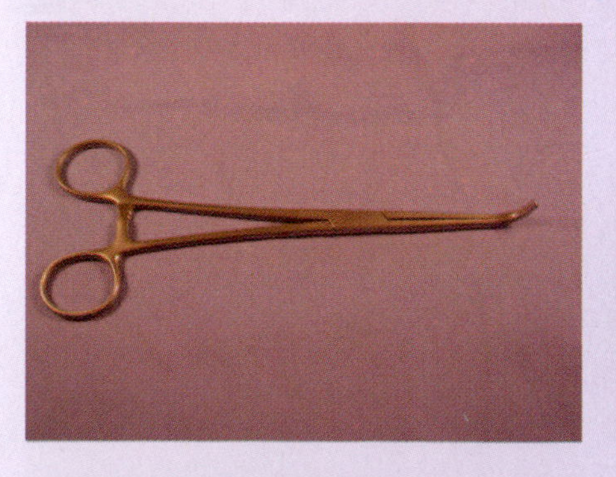

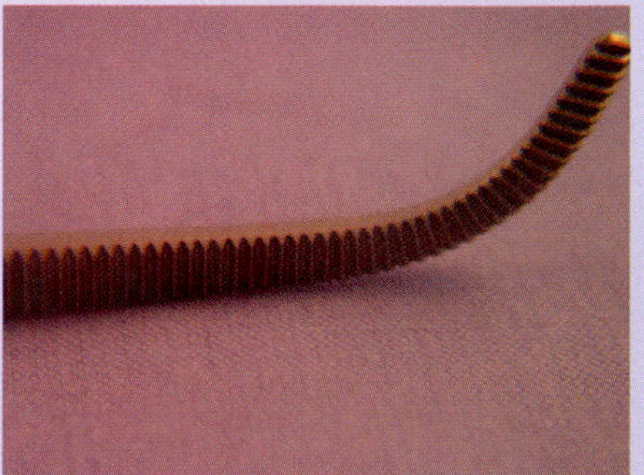

Name: Schnidt hemostat

Alias: tonsil snap; Sawtell; Adson tonsil
Category: clamping

Use: clamping tissue; holding tonsil sponge

Length: 7.25”

Additional Information: serrated only about halfway up the jaw

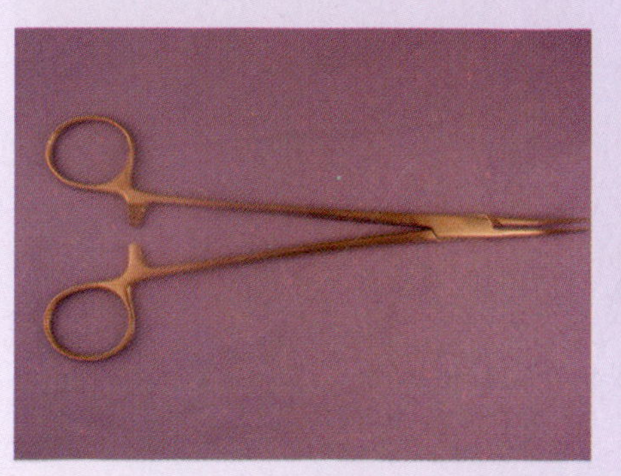

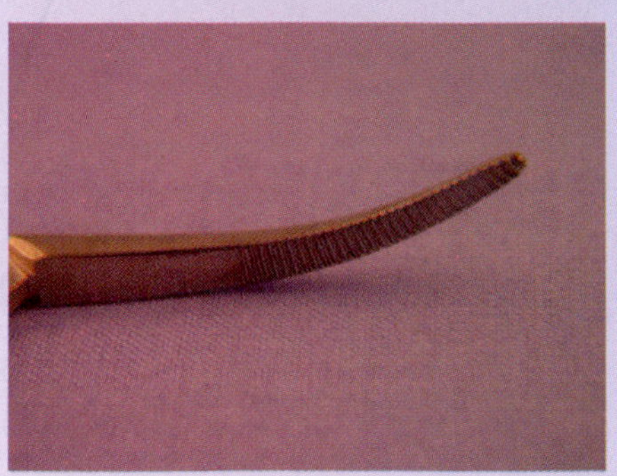

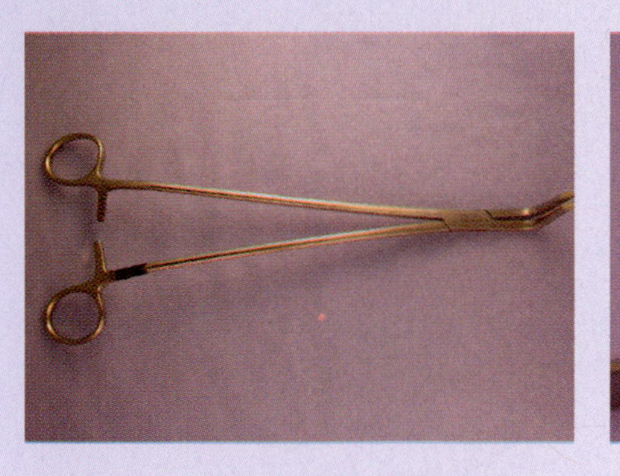
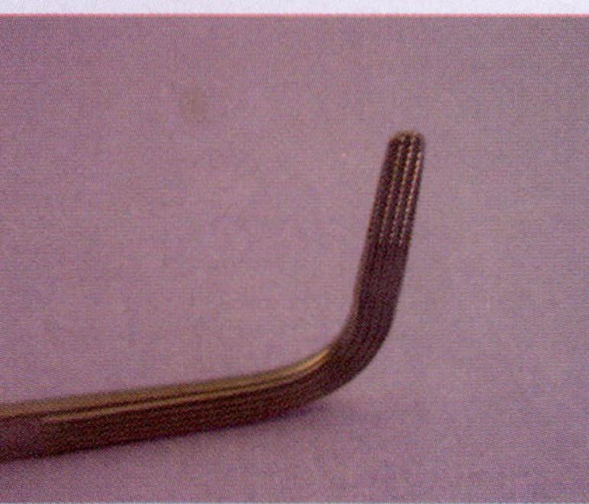

Name: Best right-angle colon clamp
Alias: none
Category: clamping
Use: clamping the colon
Length: 11"
Additional Information: jaws are a 90-degree angle; jaw length can be 1 3/8" to 3"

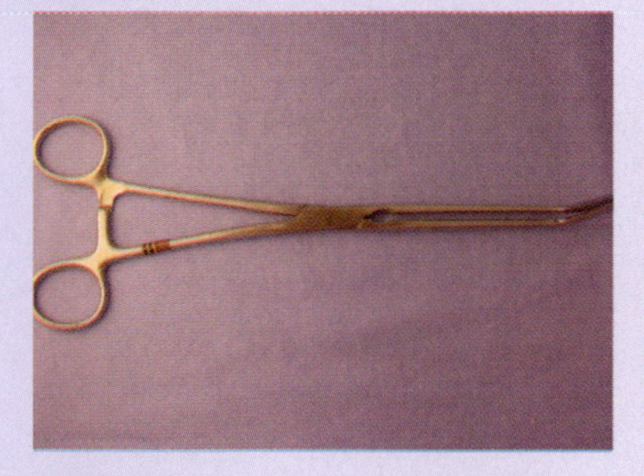
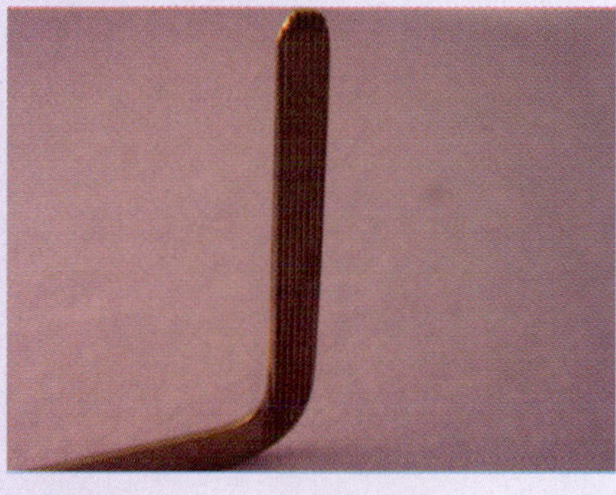

Name: Fehland right-angle colon clamp
Alias: none
Category: clamping
Use: clamping colon tissue
Length: 9.75"
Additional Information: horizontal serrations on jaws; jaw length 3.25"

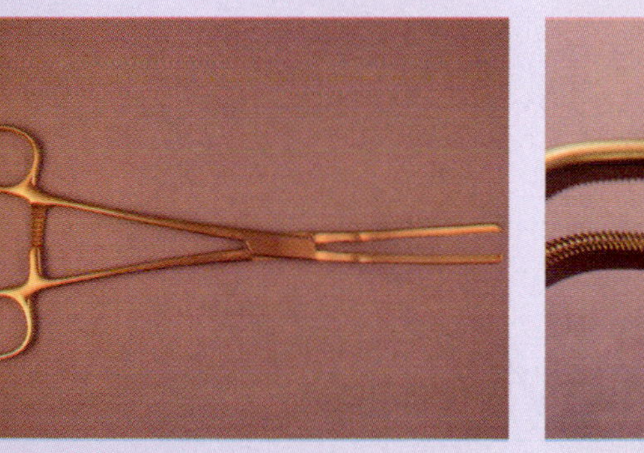

Name: Carter-Glassman resection clamp
Alias: none
Category: clamping
Use: clamping bowel during resection
Length: 10"
Additional Information: jaws angled 45 degrees

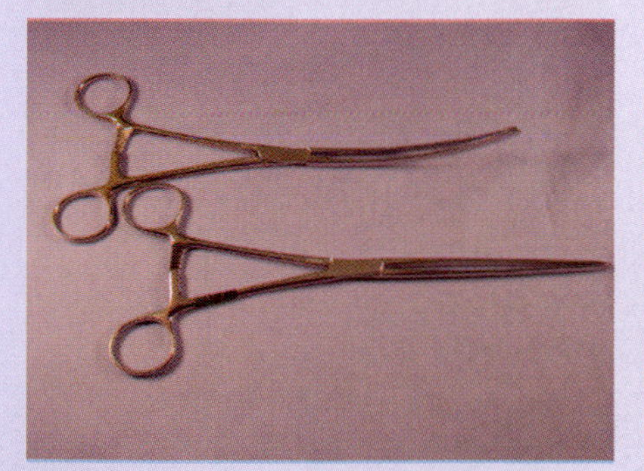
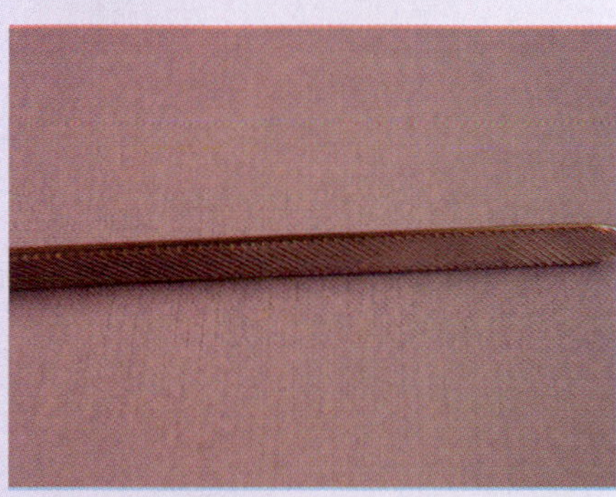

Name: Doyen intestinal forceps
Alias: Mayo-Robson
Category: clamping
Use: clamping bowel tissue
Length: 9" to 10"
Additional Information: straight or curved jaws; longitudinal serrations; may cover jaws with clamp covers (pants, linen shods)

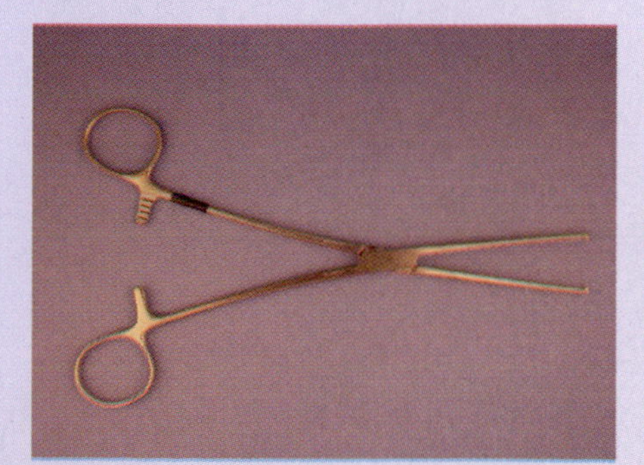
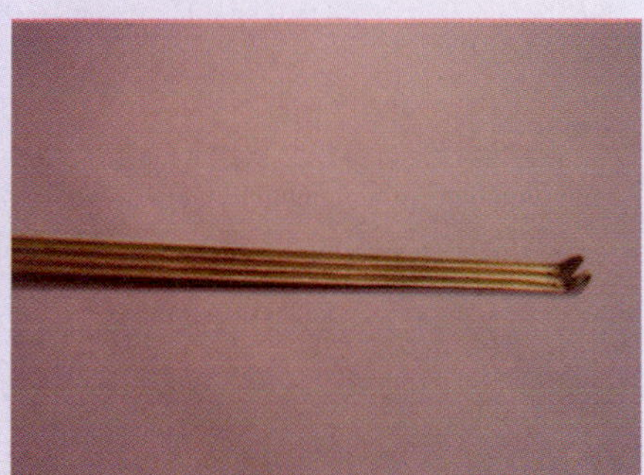

Name: Allen intestinal clamp
Alias: none
Category: clamping
Use: clamping bowel
Length: 8"
Additional Information: 1 × 2 teeth; vertical serrations

Name: Bainbridge intestinal clamp

Alias: none

Category: clamping

Use: clamping bowel

Length: 6" or 7.25"

Additional Information: longitudinal serrations; jaws can be straight or curved

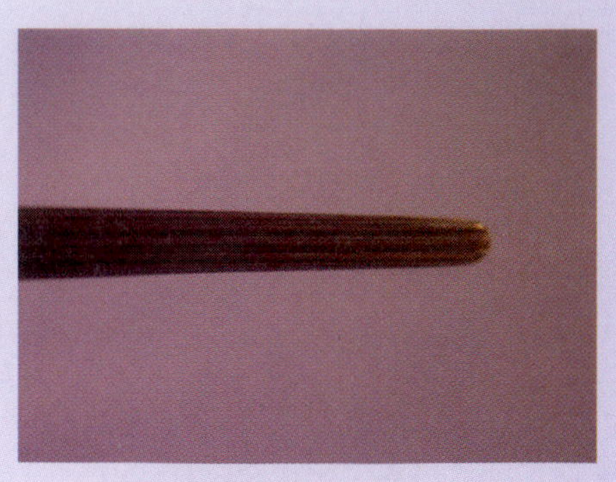

GENERAL CUTTING

Name: straight Mayo scissors

Alias: suture scissors

Category: cutting

Use: cutting sutures, dressings, drains

Length: 5.5", 6.75", 9"

Additional Information: heavy blades

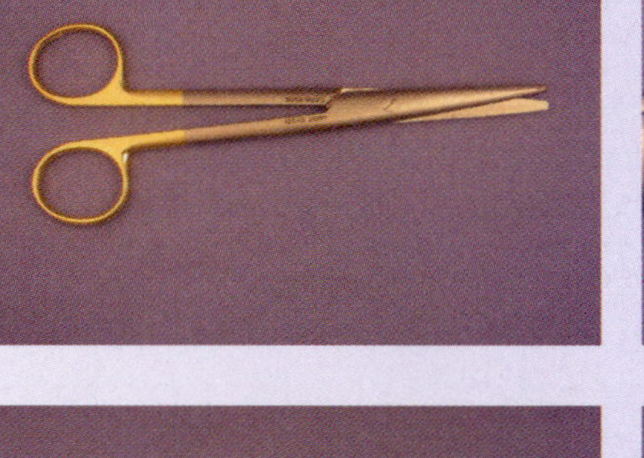

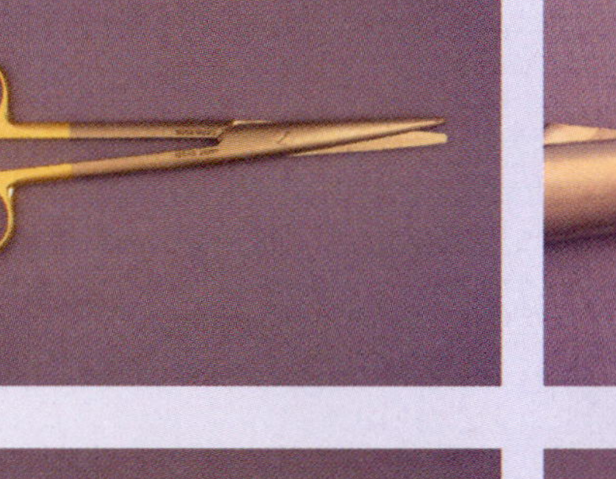

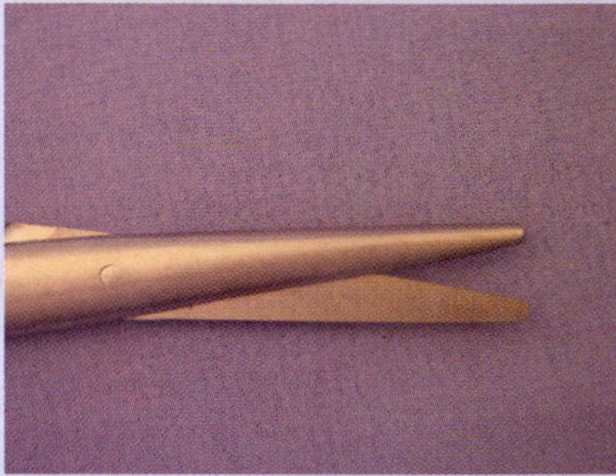

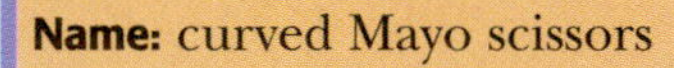

Name: curved Mayo scissors

Alias: dissecting scissors

Category: cutting

Use: cutting or dissecting heavy tissue or muscle

Length: 5.5", 6.75", 9"

Additional Information: heavy blades

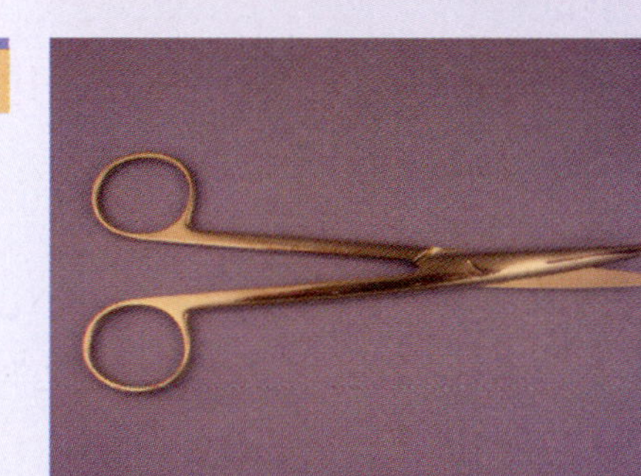

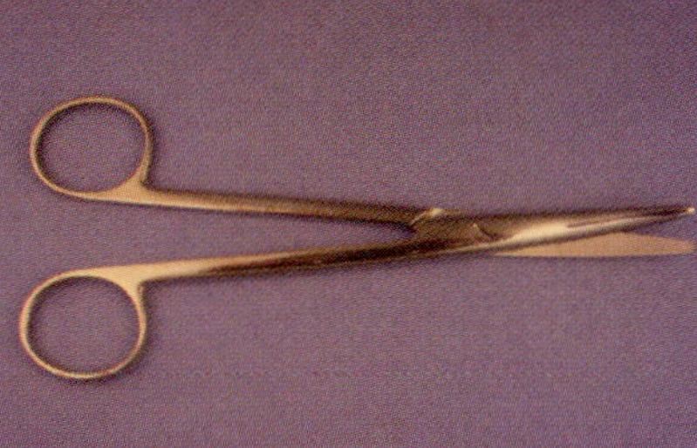

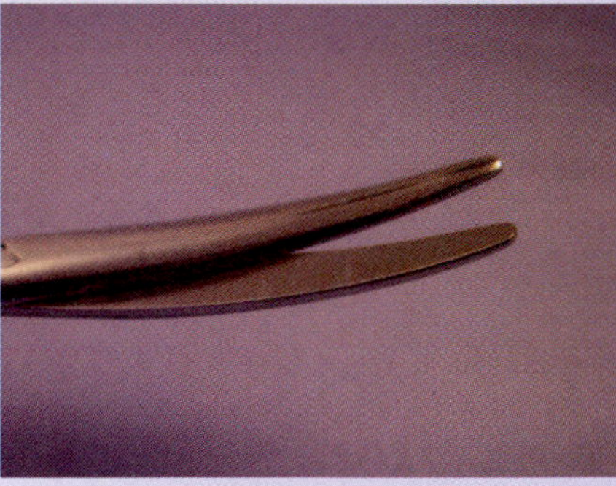

Name: Metzenbaum scissors

Alias: Metz

Category: cutting

Use: cutting or dissecting delicate tissue

Length: 5.75", 7", 9" or 10"

Additional Information: blades are delicate—DO NOT use for cutting sutures, drains, heavy tissue

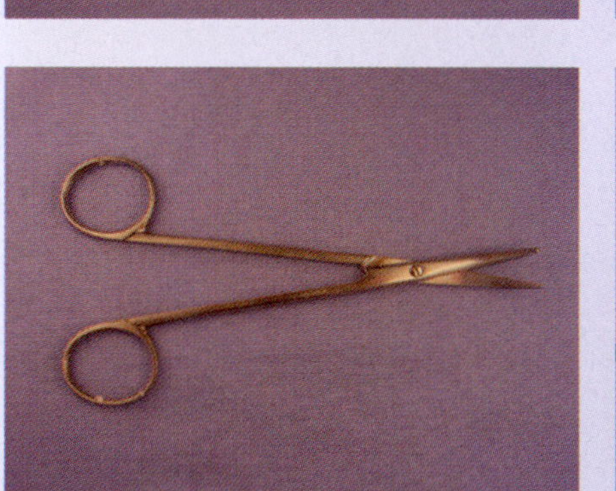

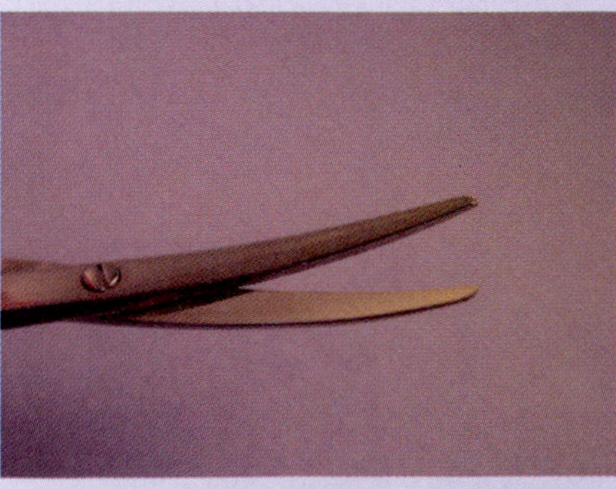

Name: operating scissors

Alias: none

Category: cutting

Length: 4.5" to 6.5"

Use: cutting tissue or dressings

Additional Information: can have 2 sharp tips or 1 sharp and 1 blunt tip; tips can be delicate to heavy

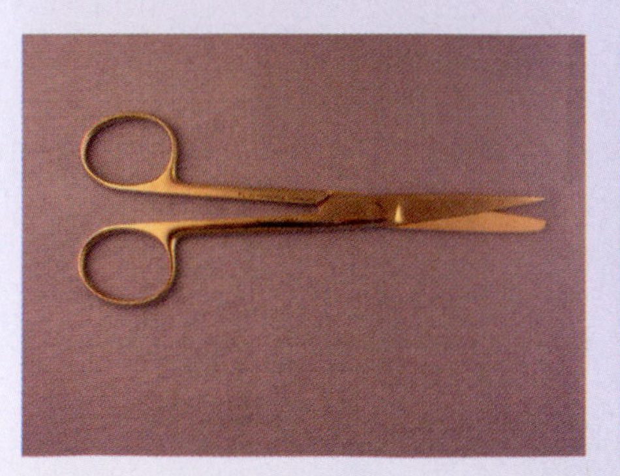

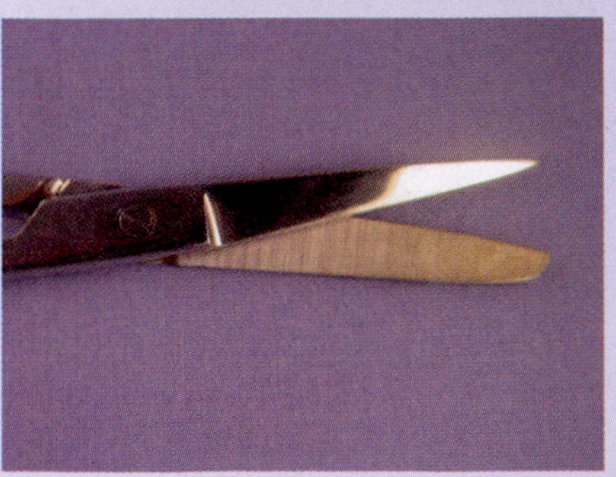

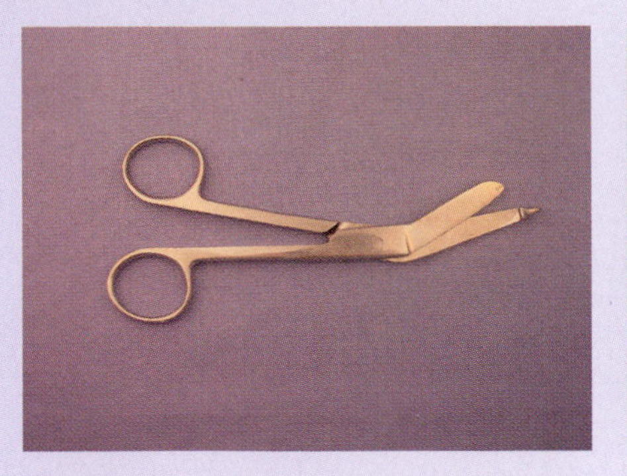
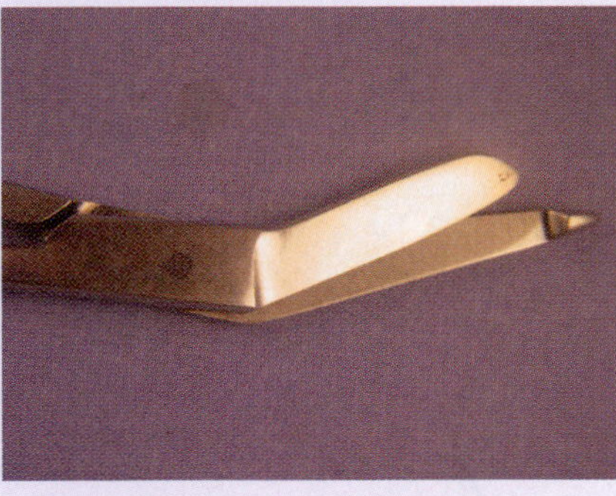

Name: Lister scissors
Alias: bandage scissors
Category: cutting
Use: cutting dressings and bandag-es
Length: 3.5", 4.5" 5.5", 7.5"or 8"
Additional Information: guarded blade

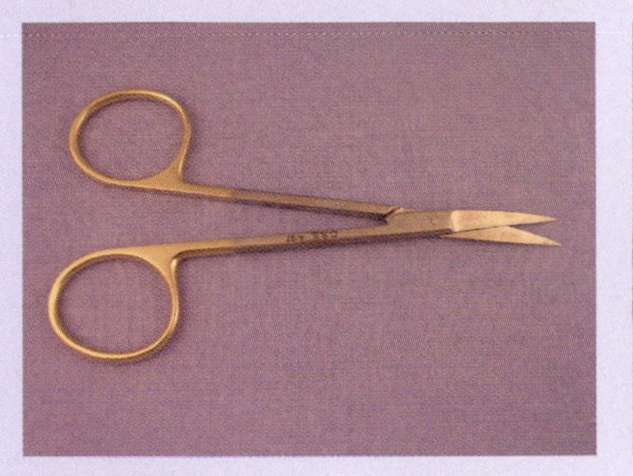
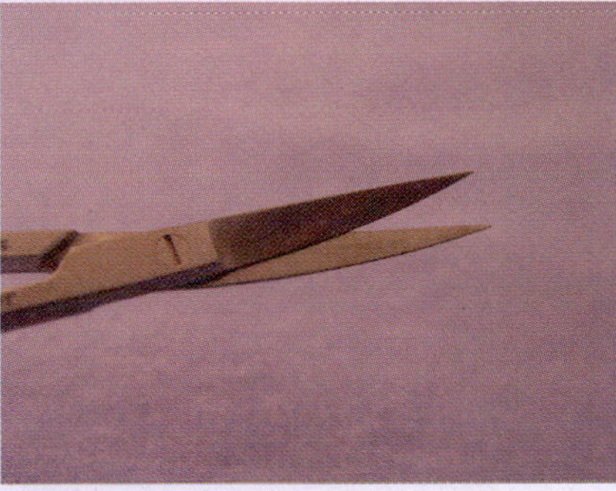

Name: Iris scissors
Alias: none
Category: cutting
Use: cutting and dissecting fine tis-sue
Length: 3.5" or 4.5"
Additional Information: blades can be curved or straight; sharp points

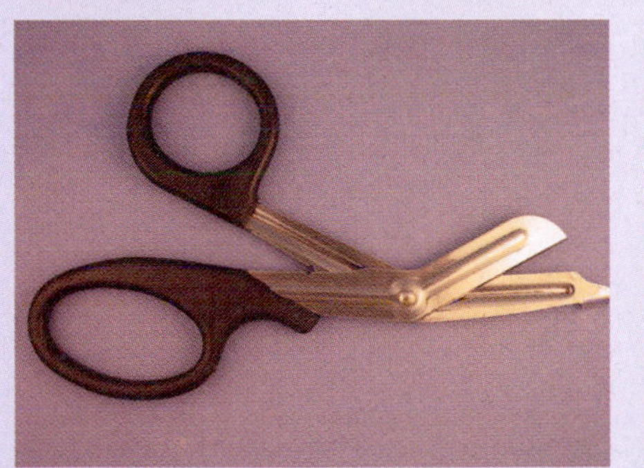
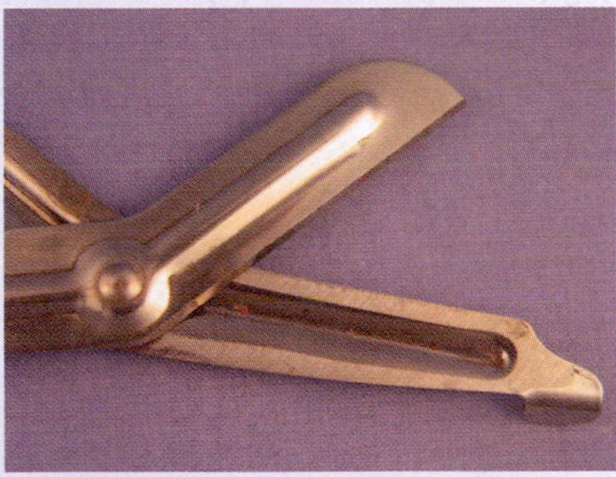

Name: utility scissors
Alias: trauma scissors; trauma shears
Category: cutting
Use: heavy duty cutting (clothes, bandages); *not used on tissue*
Length: 6" or 7.5"
Additional Information: serrated blades

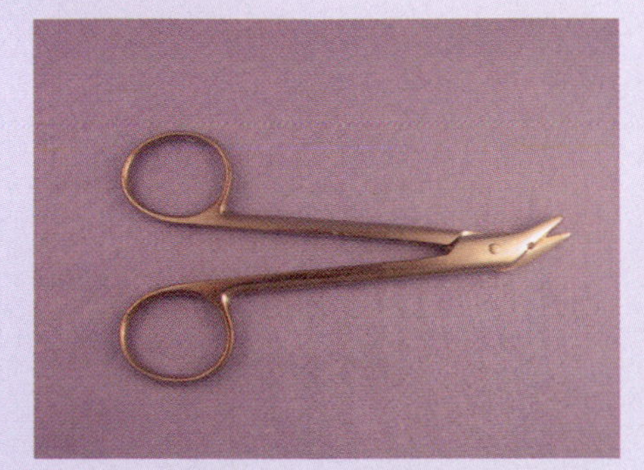
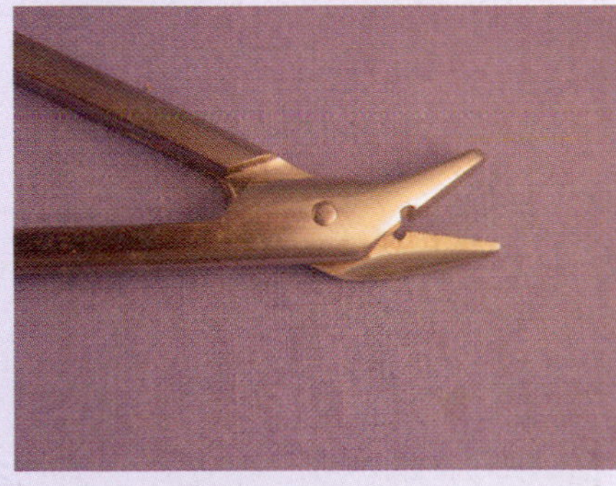

Name: wire cutting scissors (angled blade)
Alias: wire cutter
Category: cutting
Use: cutting wire sutures, wire, or wire mesh
Length: 4.75"
Additional Information: has one ser-rated blade to keep the wire from slipping

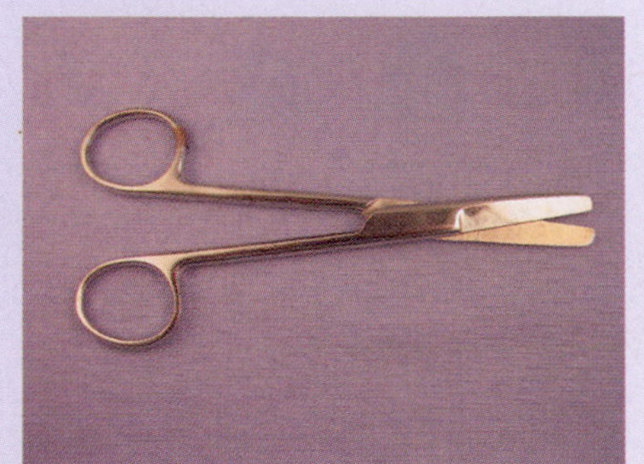
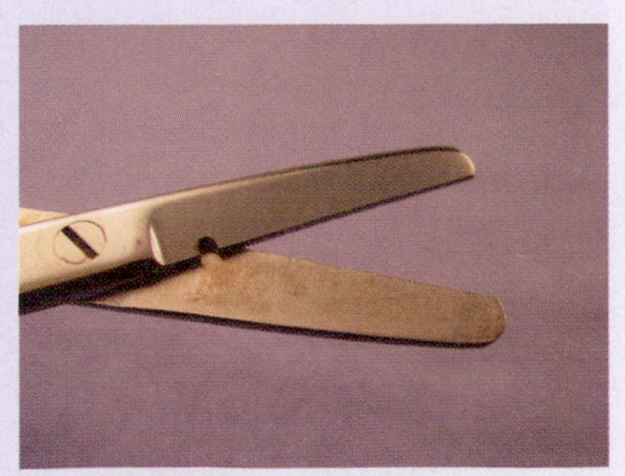

Name: wire-cutting scissors
Alias: wire cutter
Category: cutting
Use: cutting wire sutures, wire, or wire mesh
Length: 5.5"
Additional Information: blades can be straight or curved

Name: #3 scalpel handle

Alias: knife handle

Category: cutting

Use: holding scalpel blade

Length: 5.5" or 8.5"

Additional Information: use with # 10, #11, #12, or #15 blade

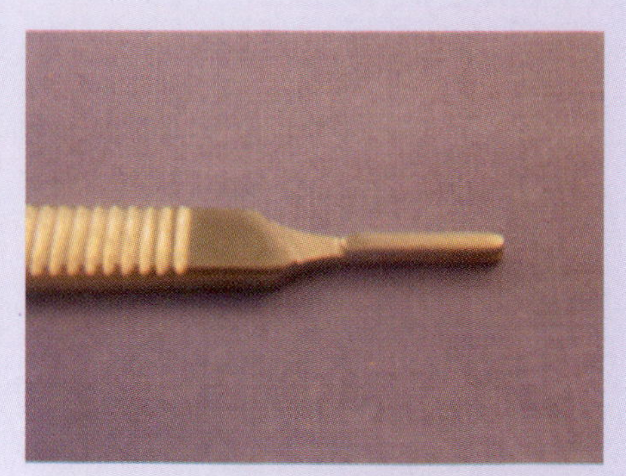

Name: #7 scalpel handle

Alias: knife handle

Category: cutting

Use: holding scalpel blade; thinner handle—fits in smaller areas

Length: 6.5"

Additional Information: use with #10, #11, #12, or #15 blade

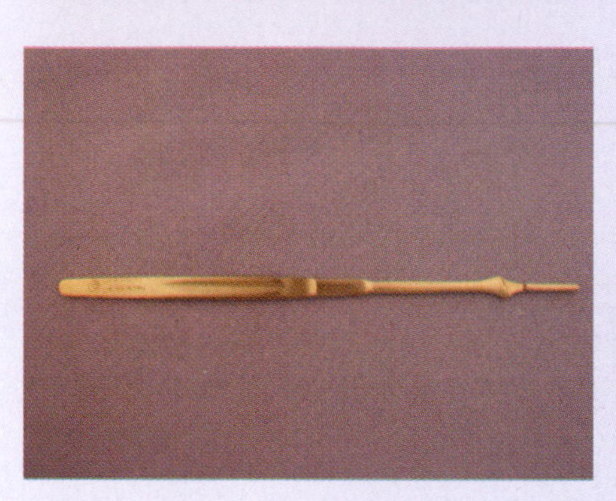

Name: #10 Blade: generally used for skin incisions

#11 Blade: for small "puncture" incisions (such as in a hook phlebectomy, arthroscopic or endoscopic procedures)

#12 Blade: curved with a cutting surface on the inside; used in oropharyngeal surgery (tonsils, UPPP)

#15 Blade: used for cutting small vessels and tissue, plastic surgery skin incisions and hand procedures

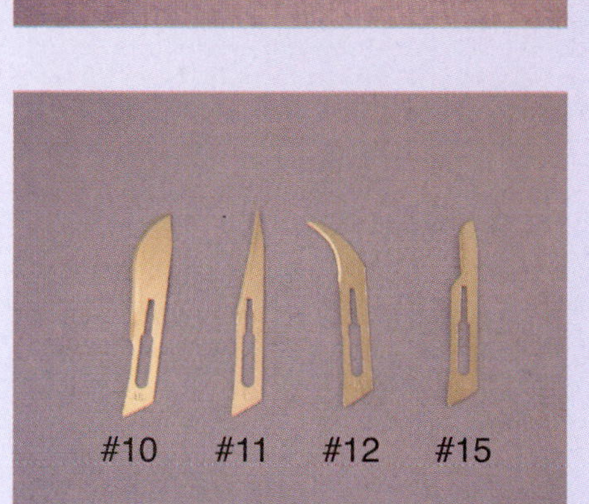

Name: #4 scalpel handle

Alias: knife handle

Category: cutting

Use: holding large-size scalpel blade for cutting heavy tissue or bone

Length: 5.5"

Additional Information: use with #20, 21, 22, 23 blades

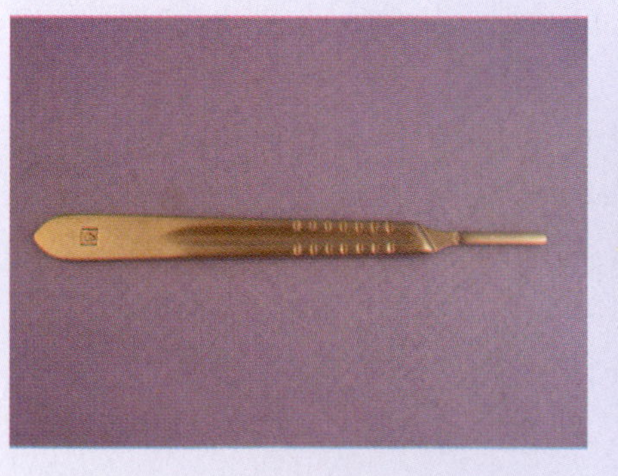

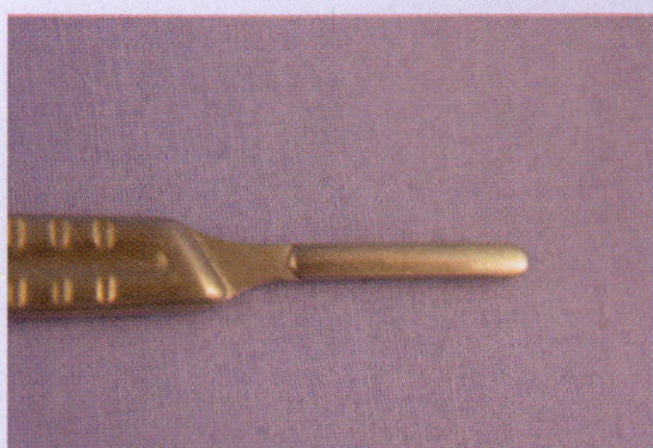

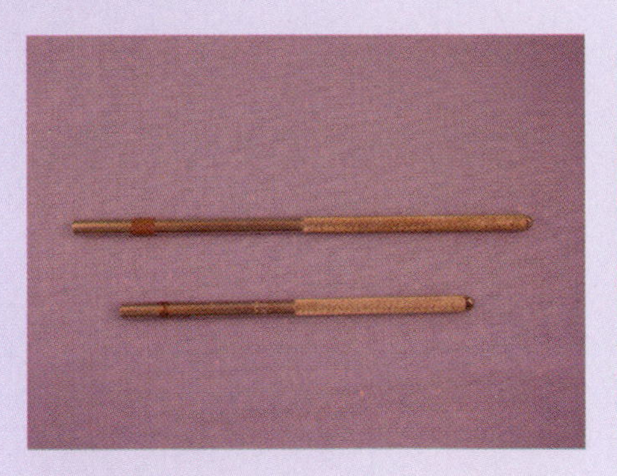

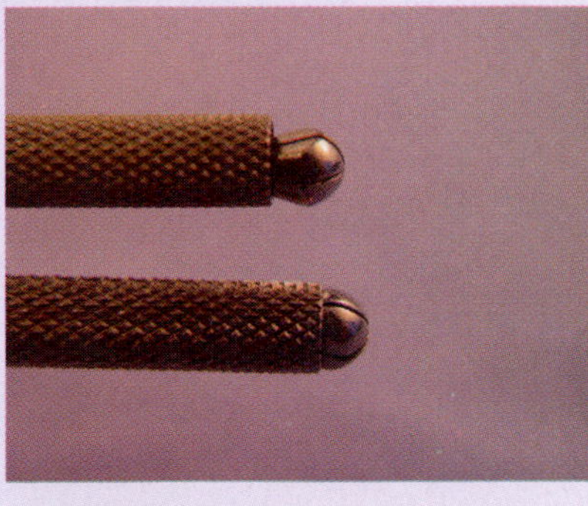

Name: blade knife handle

Alias: beaver blade handle
Category: cutting

Use: holding knife blades

Length: 3" to 5.5"

Additional Information: for use with series 50, 60, 70 blades

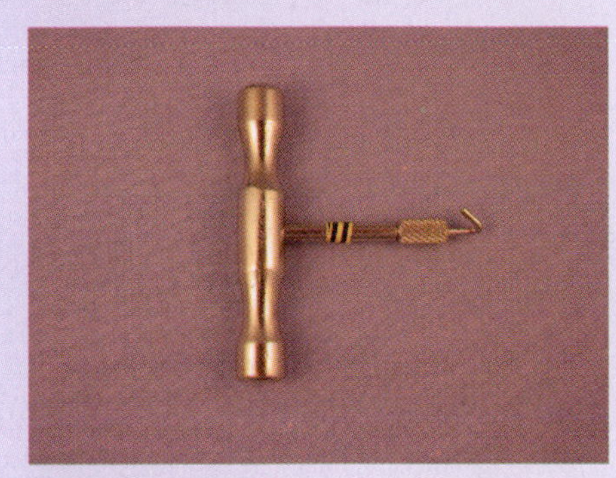

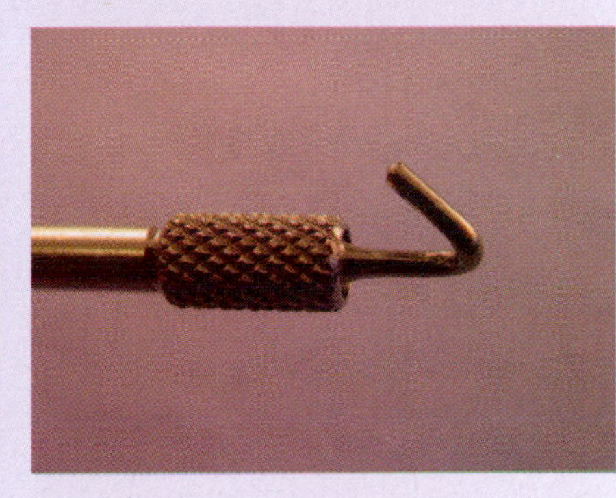

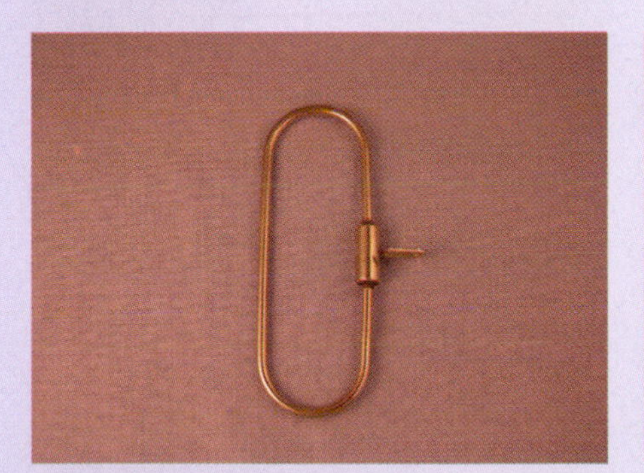

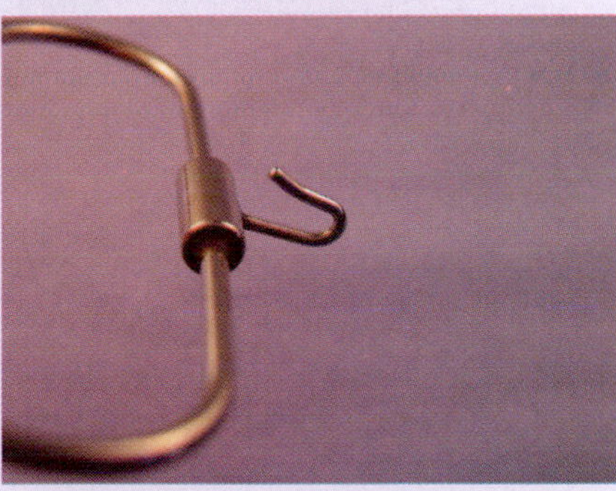

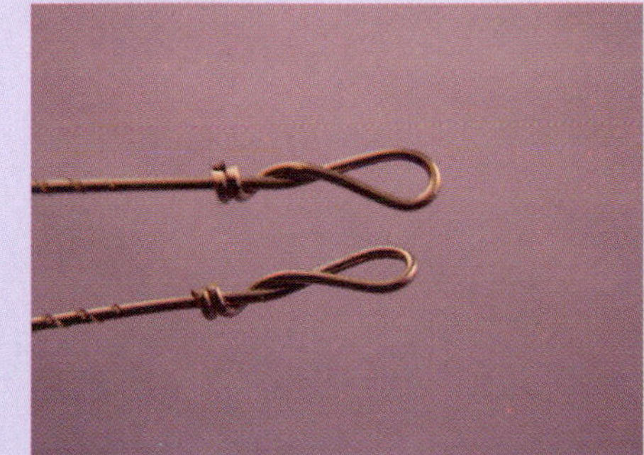

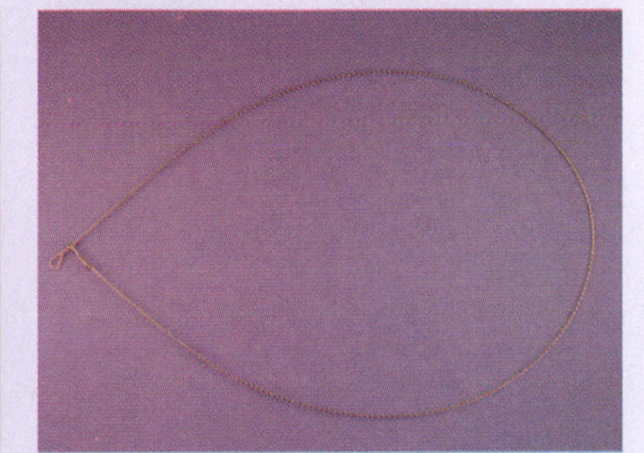

Name: Gigli saw handle

Alias: none
Category: cutting

Use: sawing bone

Length: wires can be 12" or 20" in length

Additional Information: wire can be used with either type of handle

GENERAL RETRACTORS

Name: Balfour retractor

Alias: abdominal self-retracting
Category: retracting

Use: deep abdominal retraction

Length: 8" or 10" blades

Additional Information: have moistened lap pads available to hand to the surgeon (used as padding between the blades and tissue); newer versions have interchangeable blades

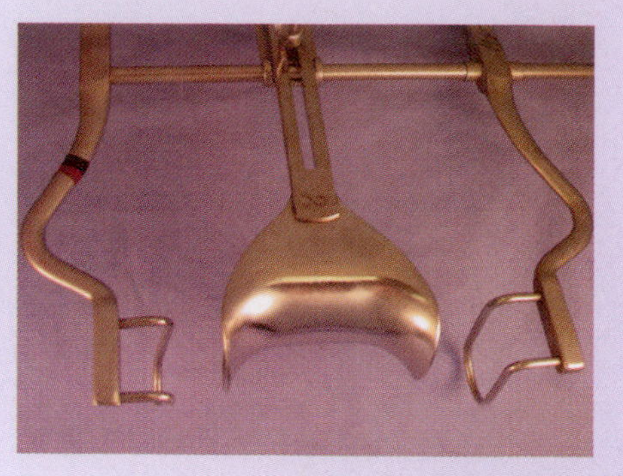

Name: Bookwalter system

Alias: universal ring retractor system
Category: retracting

Use: deep retraction in the abdomen and pelvis

Length: n/a

Additional Information: have moistened lap pads available to hand to the surgeon (to use as padding between the blades and tissue); comes with oval and round rings and various sizes/types of retractor blades

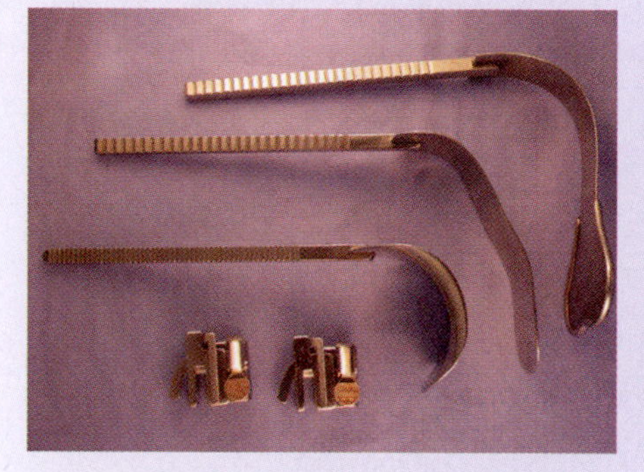

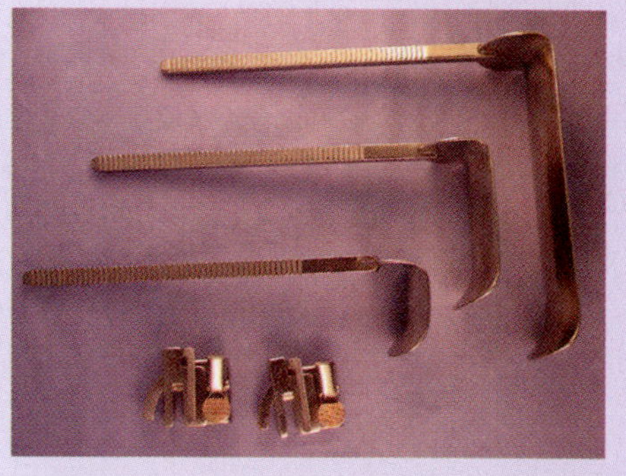

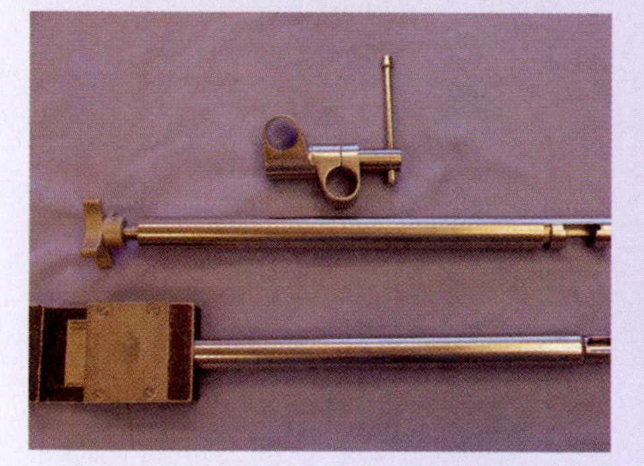

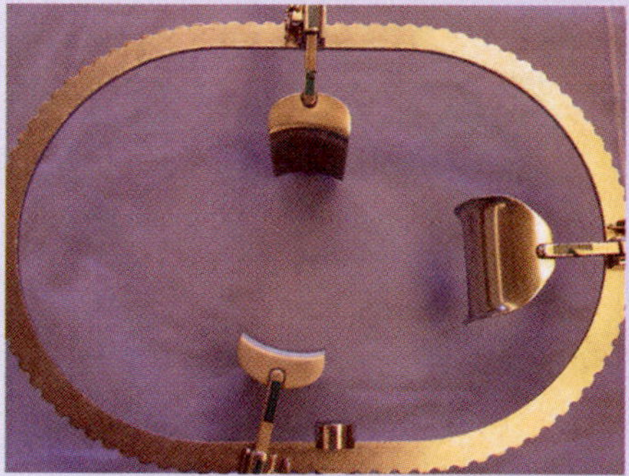

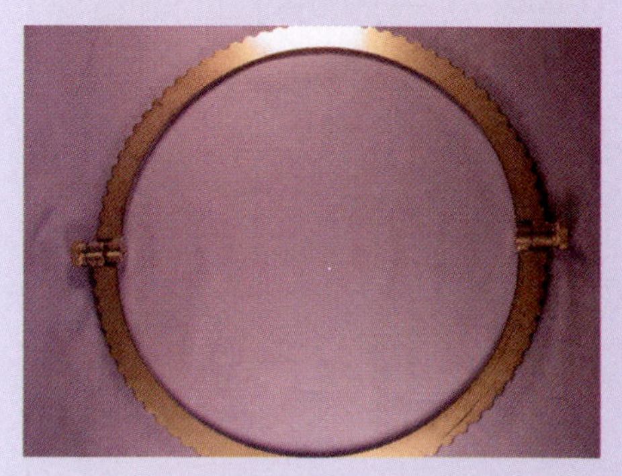

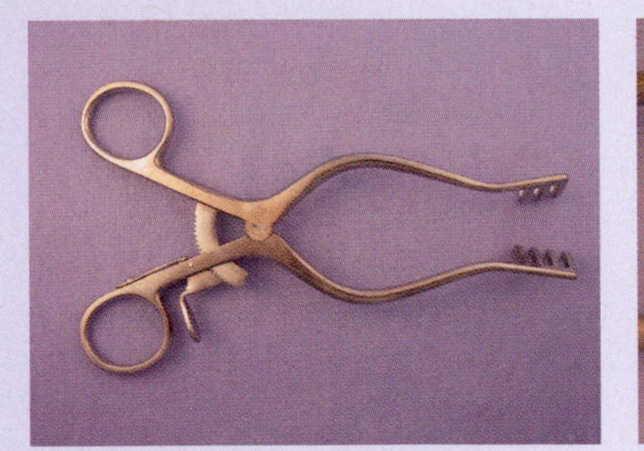

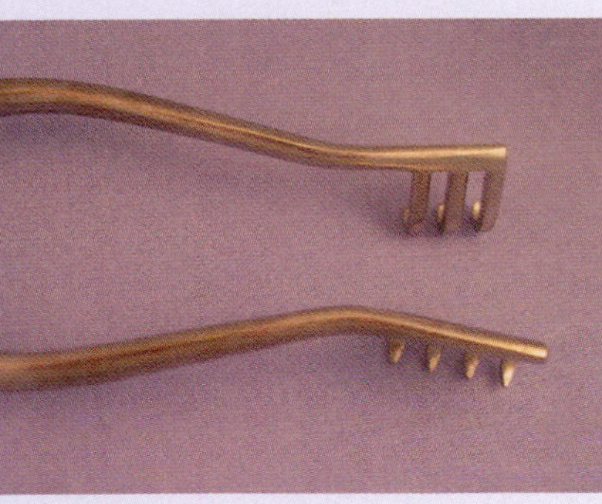

Name: Weitlaner retractor

Alias: none

Category: retracting

Use: exposing superficial wound

Length: 4", 5.5", 6.5", 8" or 9.5 "

Additional Information: self-retaining; prongs can be sharp or dull; 2 × 3 prongs (4"), 3 × 4 prongs (all other sizes)

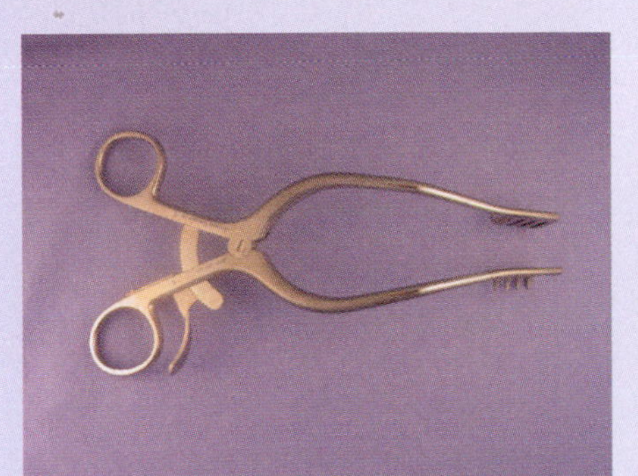

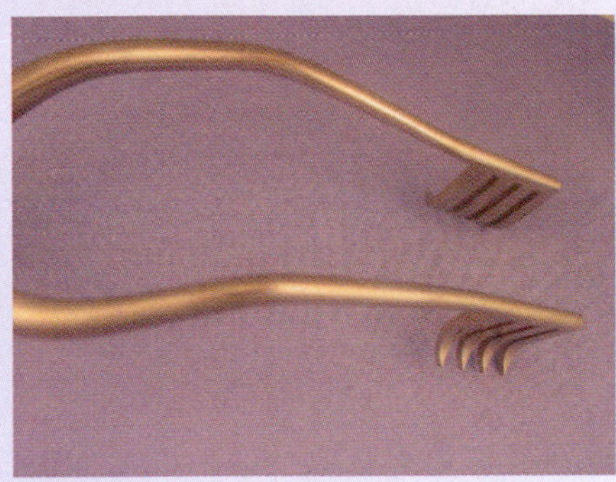

Name: Cerebellar retractor

Alias: Adson retractor

Category: retracting

Use: exposing wound

Length: 8"

Additional Information: self-retaining; 4 × 4 prongs; shanks are angled

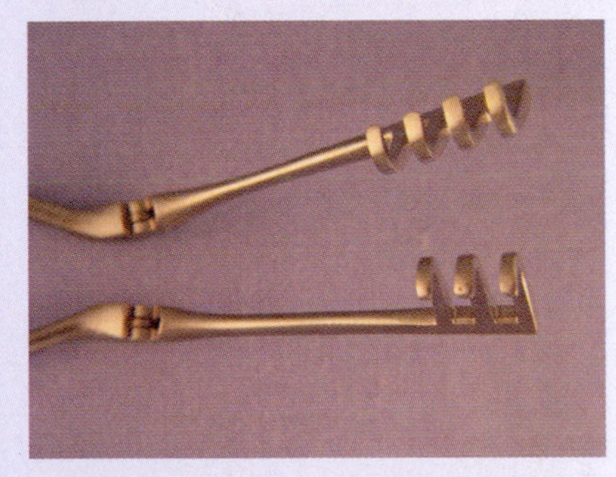

Name: Beckmann retractor

Alias: none

Category: retracting

Use: retracting soft tissue

Length: 5.5" or 6.5"

Additional Information: self-retaining; 3 × 4 prongs; prongs can be sharp or blunt; hinged arms

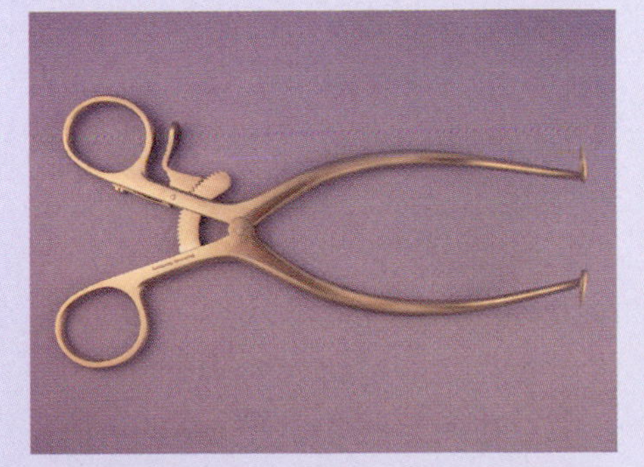

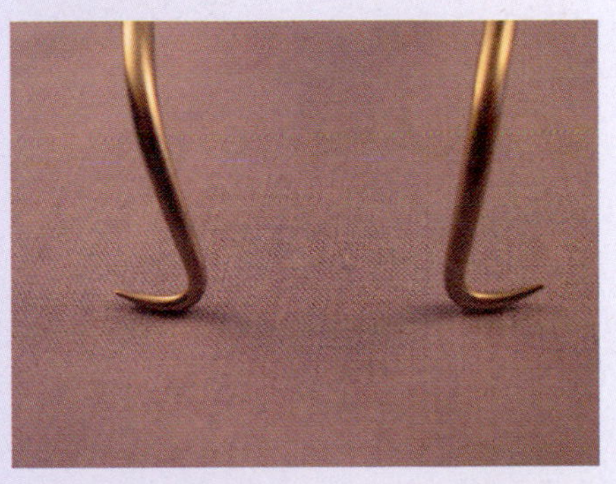

Name: Gelpi retractor

Alias: none

Category: retracting

Use: superficial wound exposure

Length: 4.5", 5.5", 7.5", or 10"

Additional Information: self-retaining; single sharp tines

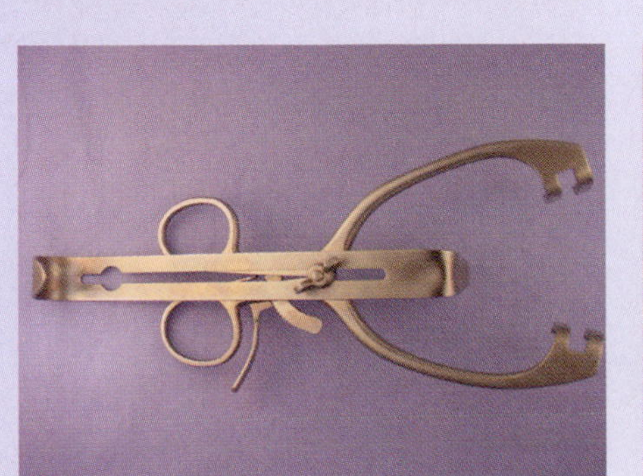

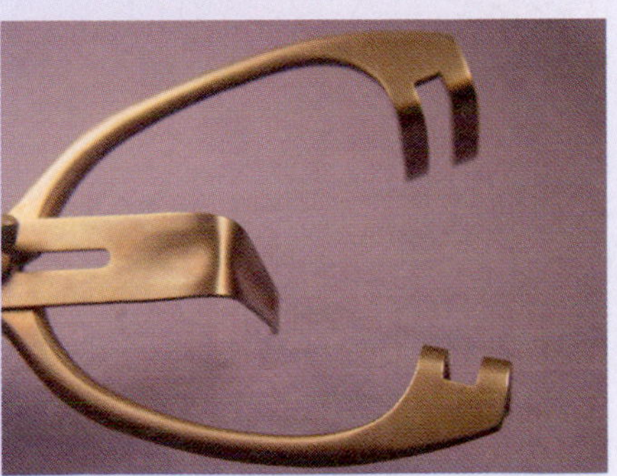

Name: Mayo-Collins appendectomy retractor

Alias: none

Category: retracting

Use: retracting McBurney incision

Length: 6.75"

Additional Information: self-retaining

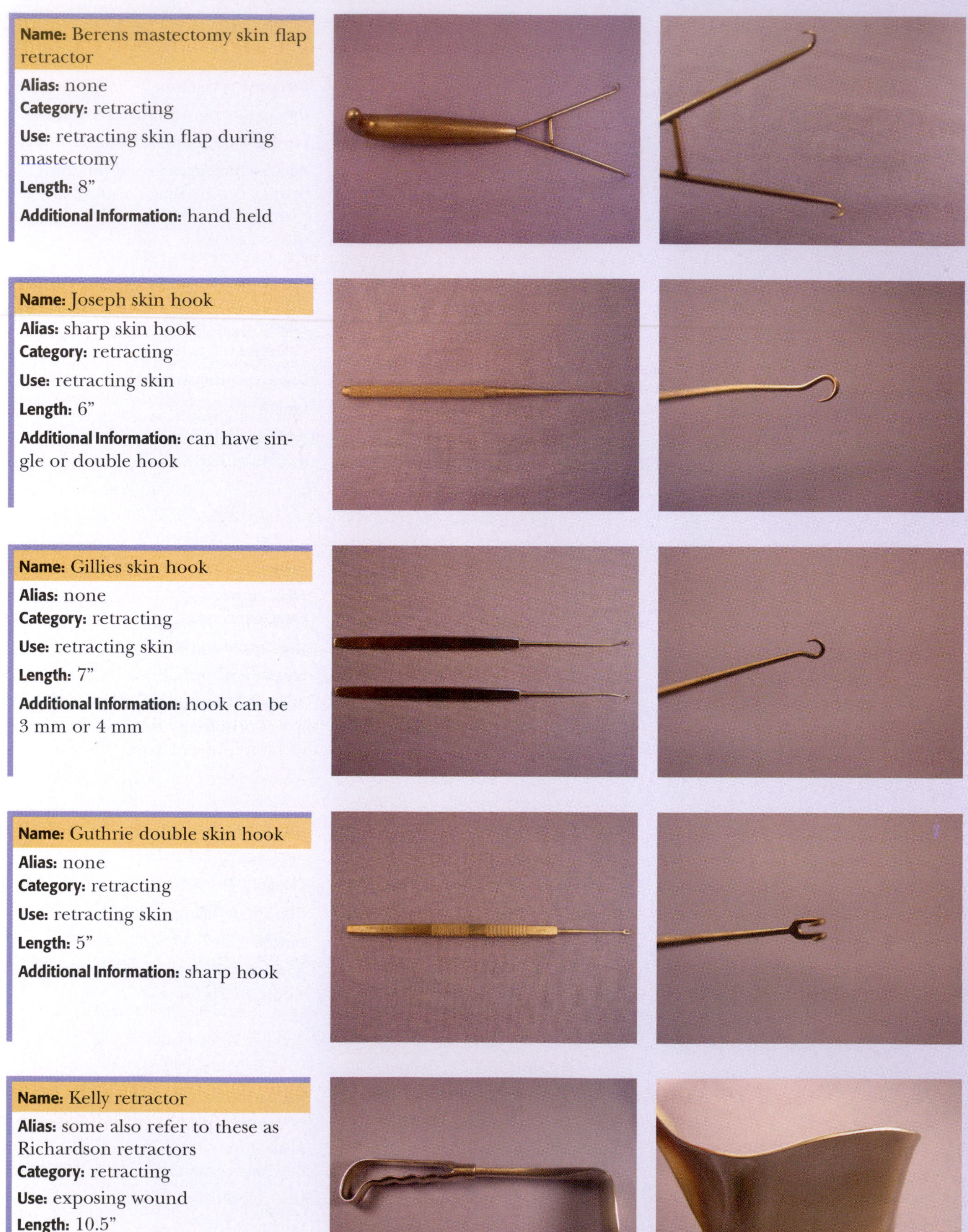

Name: Berens mastectomy skin flap retractor
Alias: none
Category: retracting
Use: retracting skin flap during mastectomy
Length: 8”
Additional Information: hand held

Name: Joseph skin hook
Alias: sharp skin hook
Category: retracting
Use: retracting skin
Length: 6”
Additional Information: can have single or double hook

Name: Gillies skin hook
Alias: none
Category: retracting
Use: retracting skin
Length: 7”
Additional Information: hook can be 3 mm or 4 mm

Name: Guthrie double skin hook
Alias: none
Category: retracting
Use: retracting skin
Length: 5”
Additional Information: sharp hook

Name: Kelly retractor
Alias: some also refer to these as Richardson retractors
Category: retracting
Use: exposing wound
Length: 10.5”
Additional Information: hand held; smooth edge (no lip); blades vary in width from 2.5” to 4”

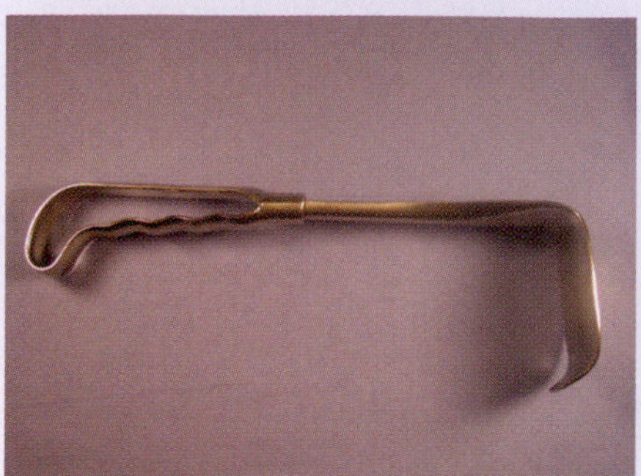

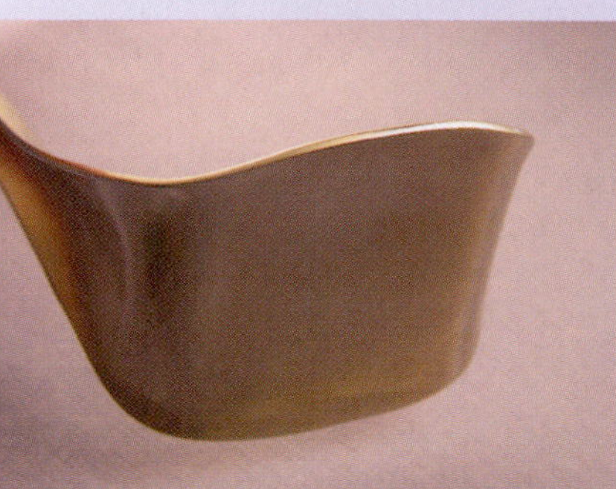

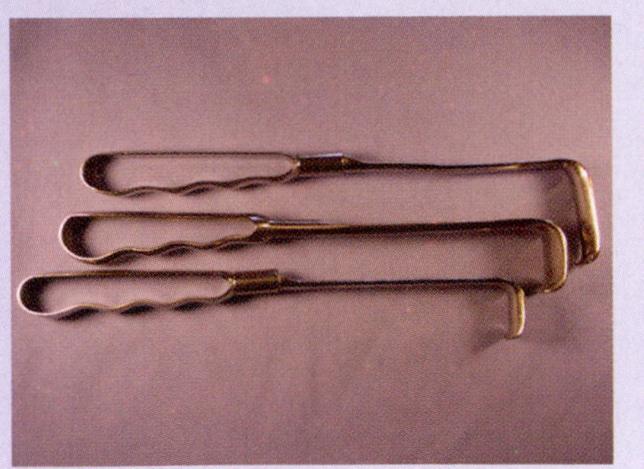

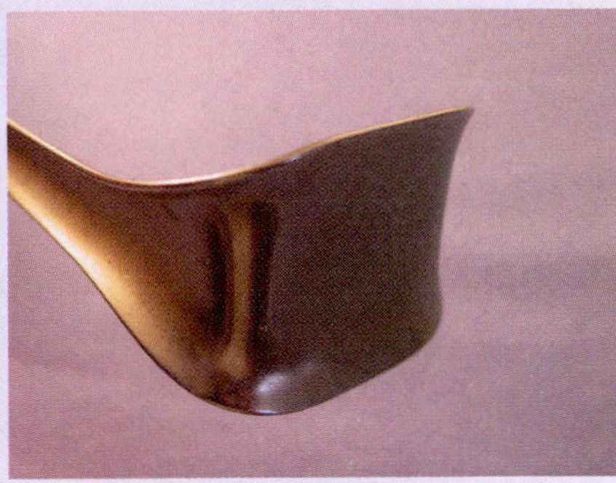

Name: Richardson retractor

Alias: Richie: #1, #2, or #3

Category: retracting

Use: exposing wound

Length: 9.5”

Additional Information: hand held; has “lip” around the edge of blade; blades vary in width from 7/8” to 1.5”; long thin one may be known as a “thyroid”

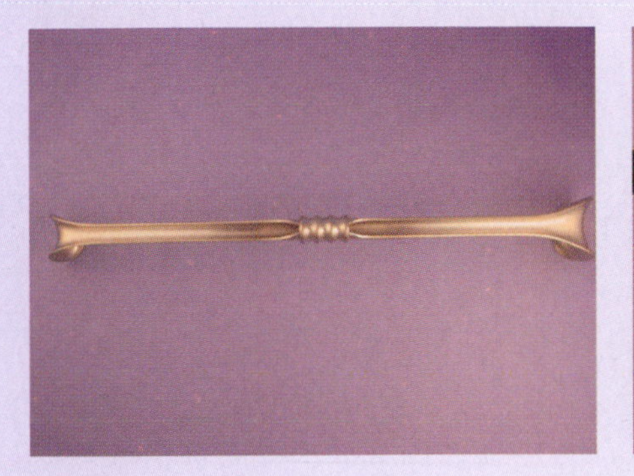

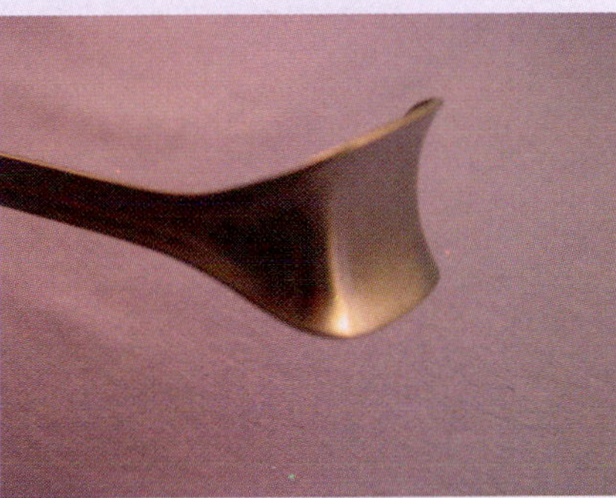

Name: Richardson-Eastman retractor

Alias: none

Category: retracting

Use: exposing wound

Additional Information: hand held; double ended; comes in blade widths of $\frac{3}{4}$” × 1.13”, 1.13” × 1.5”, 1.5” × 1.75” or 1 5/8” × 2.5”

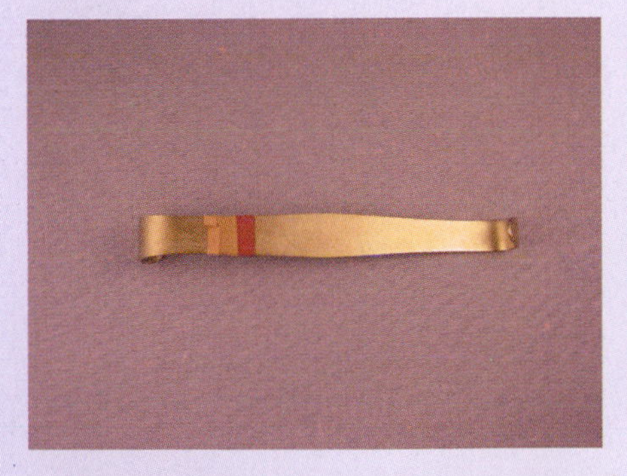

Name: Roux retractor

Alias: none

Category: retracting

Use: exposing wound

Length: 6” to 6.75”

Additional Information: hand held; double ended- one end wider than the other; can have ends facing the same way or can be “s” shaped (ends facing opposite ways)

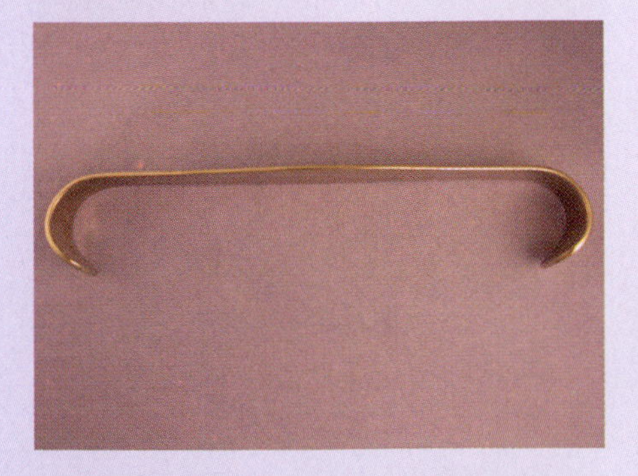

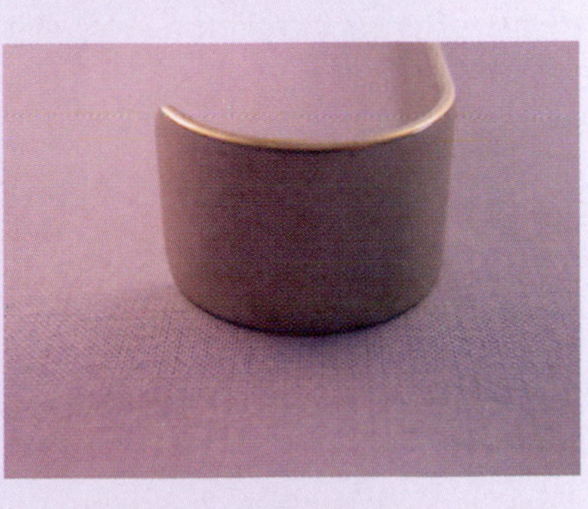

Name: Parker retractor

Alias: Bard-Parker

Category: retracting

Use: exposing superficial wound

Length: 5” or 7”

Other Information: hand held; double ended; usually used in pairs

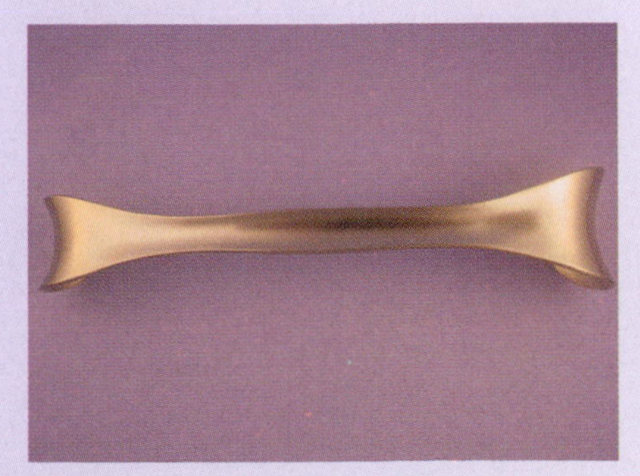

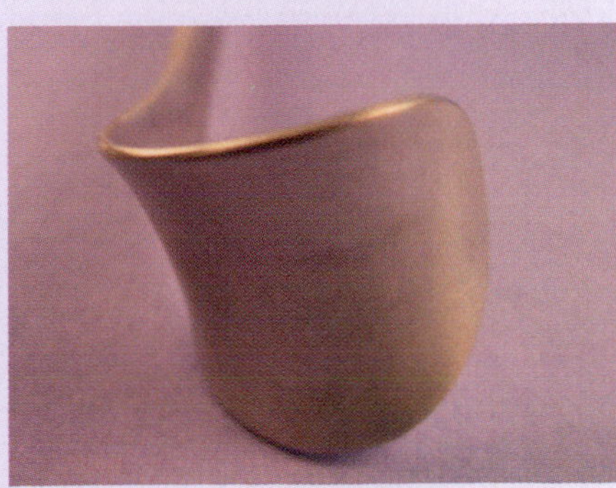

Name: Goelet retractor

Alias: none

Category: retracting

Use: retracting superficial tissue

Length: 7.5”

Additional Information: hand held; double ended; usually used in pairs

Name: U.S. Army retractor
Alias: Army-Navy
Category: retracting
Use: exposing superficial wound
Length: 8.5”
Additional Information: hand held; double ended; usually used in pairs

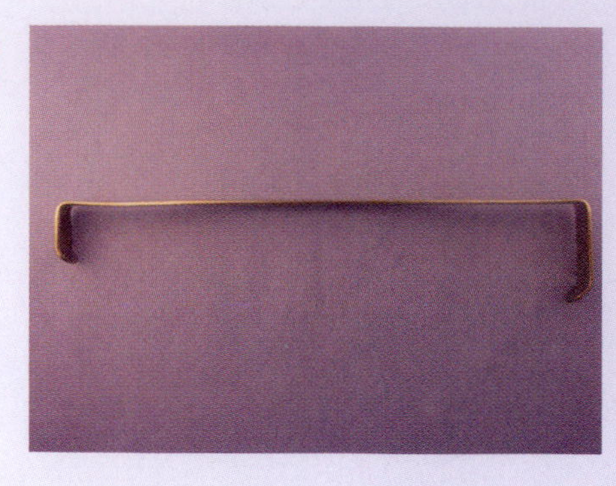

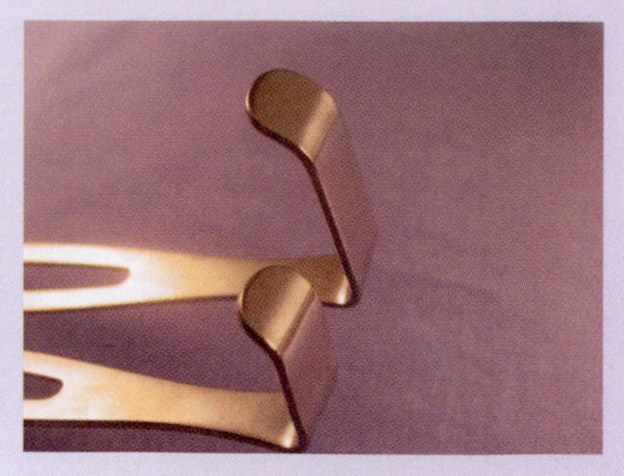

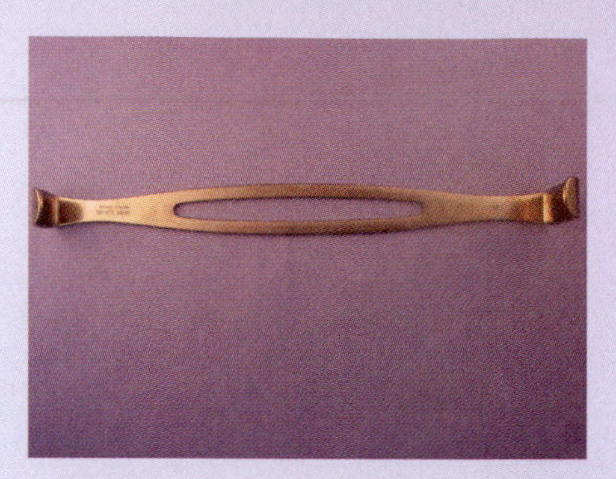

Name: Senn retractor
Alias: none
Category: retracting
Use: exposing superficial wound
Length: 6”
Additional Information: hand held; double ended; prongs can be sharp or dull; usually used in pairs

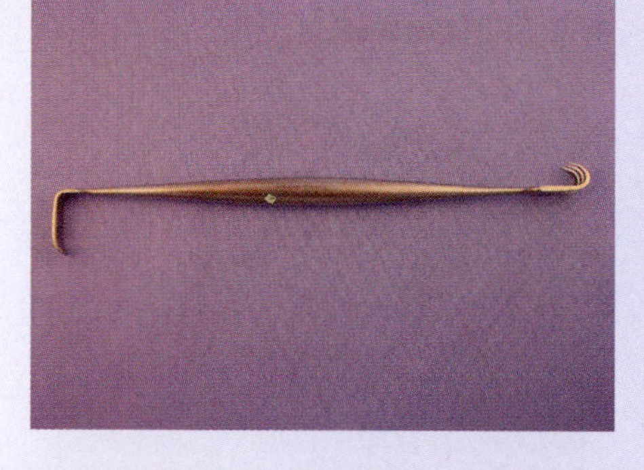

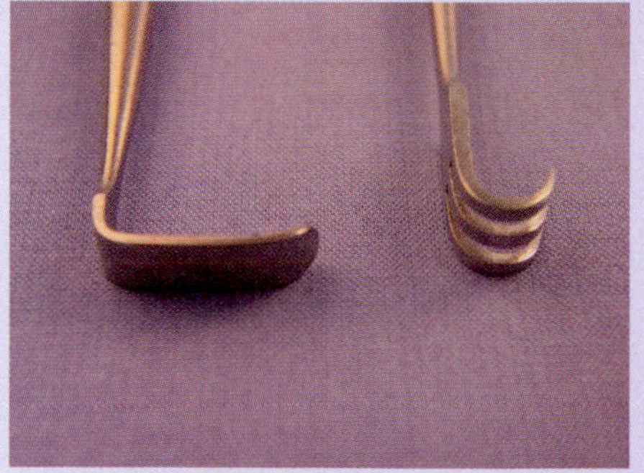

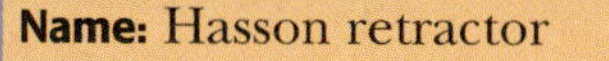

Name: Hasson retractor
Alias: S retractor
Category: retracting
Use: exposing laparoscopic wound incisions
Length: n/a
Additional Information: hand held

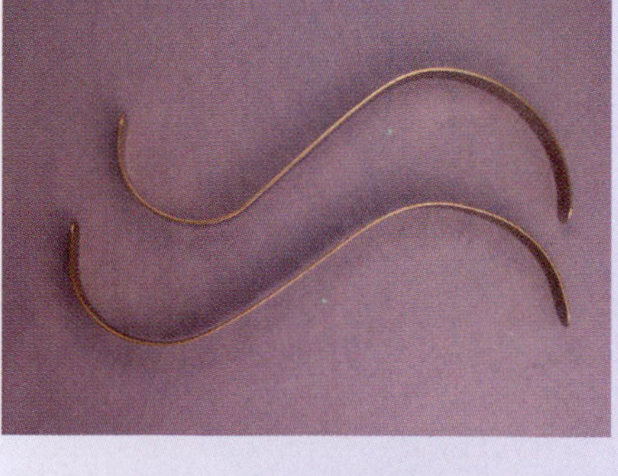

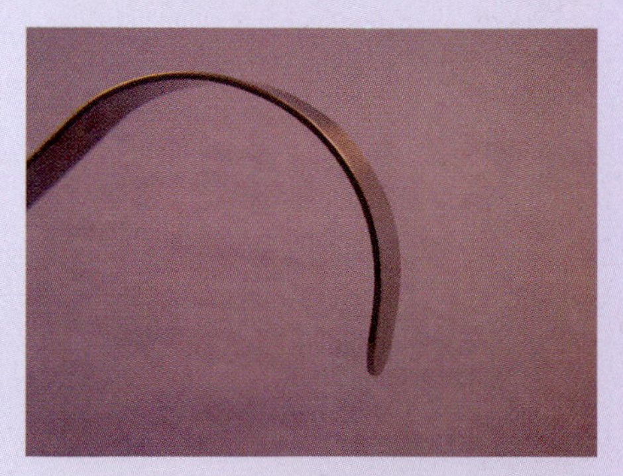

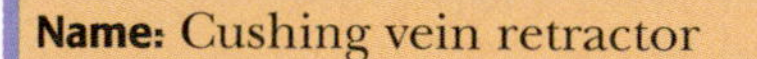

Name: Cushing vein retractor
Alias: none
Category: retracting
Use: retracting blood vessels
Length: 8” or 12”
Additional Information: hand held; open handle

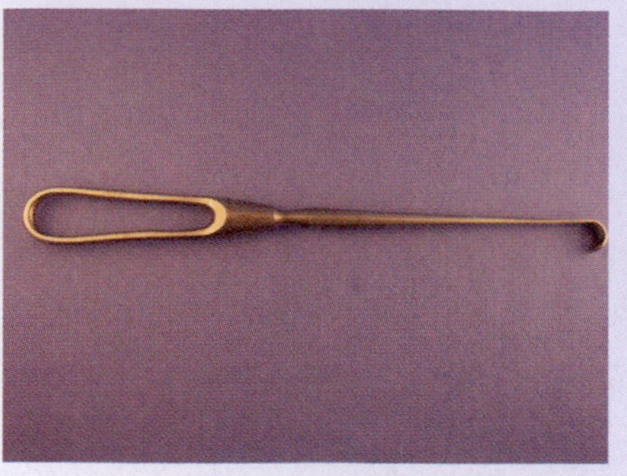

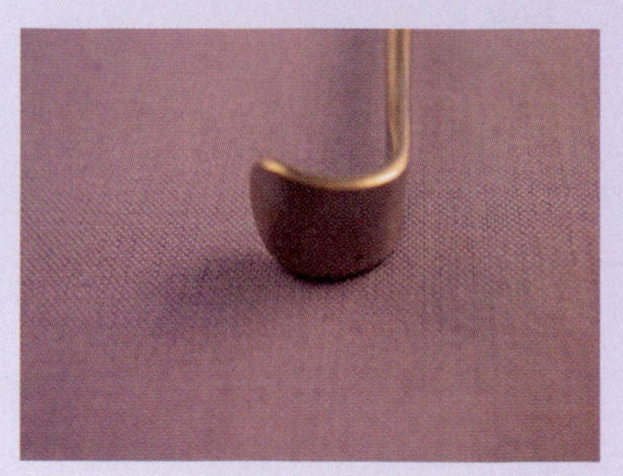

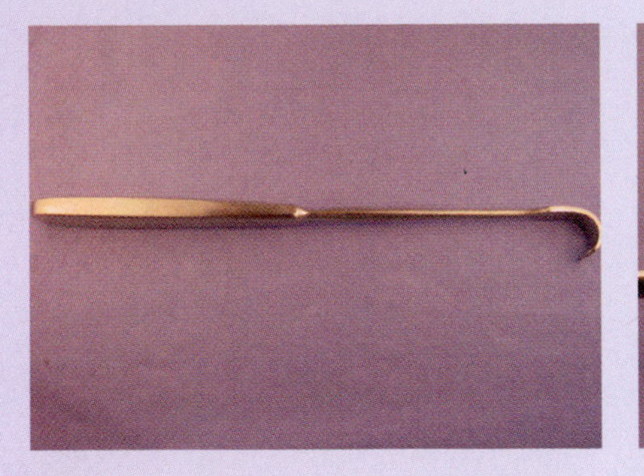

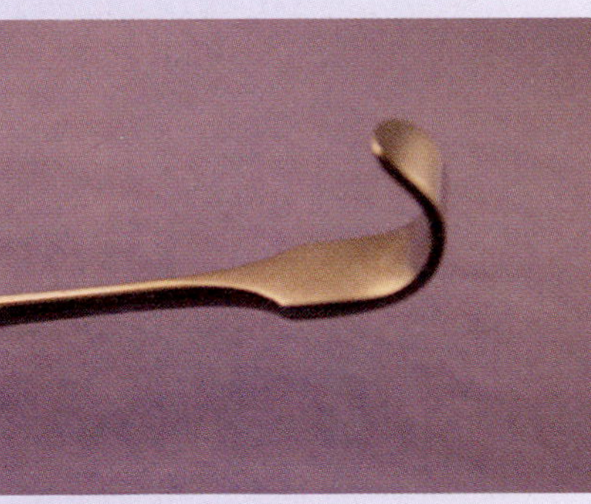

Name: Little retractor

Alias: none

Category: retracting

Use: exposing superficial wound

Length: 7.5"

Additional Information: hand held

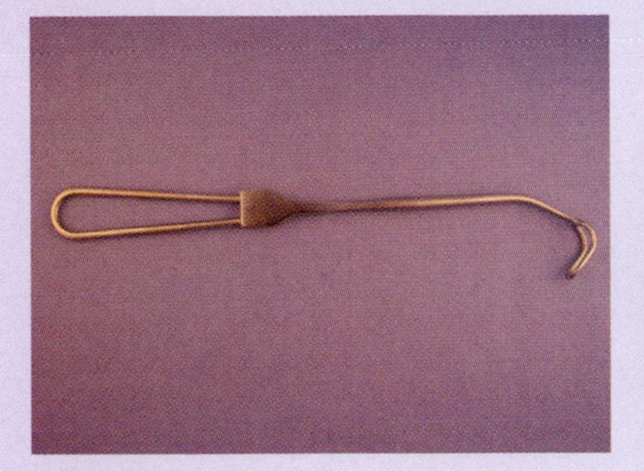

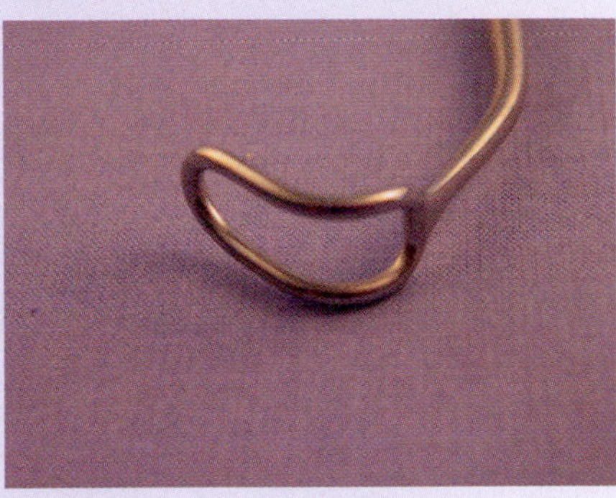

Name: Green retractor

Alias: goiter retractor; loop retractor

Category: retracting

Use: retracting soft tissue

Length: 8.5"

Additional Information: hand held; fenestrated blade

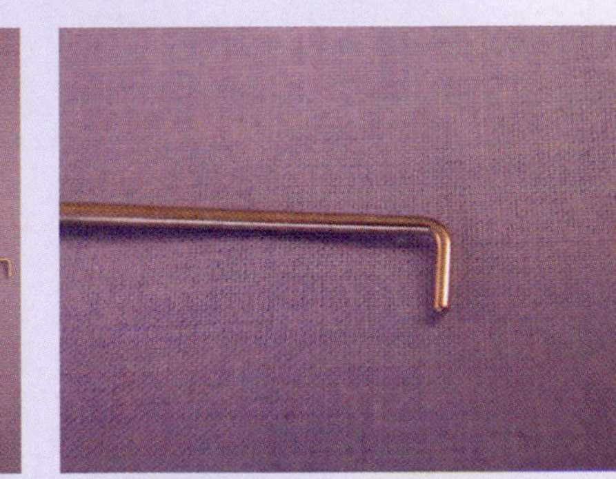

Name: Dandy nerve hook

Alias: none

Category: retracting

Use: retracting nerves

Length: 8.5"

Additional Information: blunt tip; tip can be pointed straight, left, or right

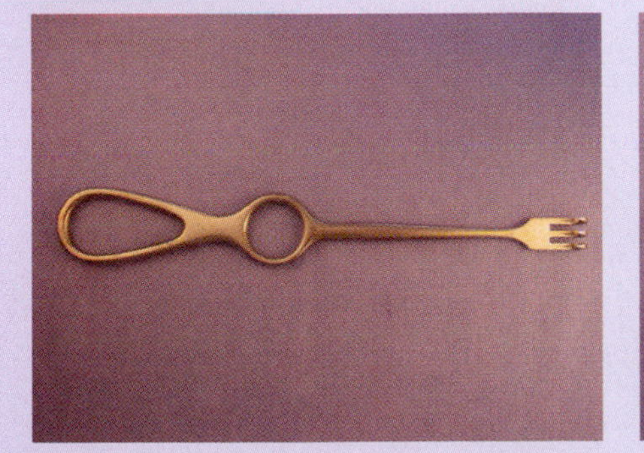

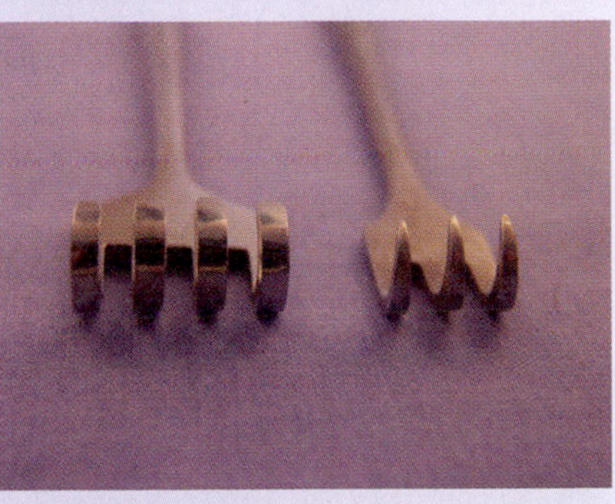

Name: Volkmann retractor

Alias: rake

Category: retracting

Use: exposing superficial wound

Length: 8.5"

Other: hand held; sharp or blunt tips; can have 2 to 6 teeth

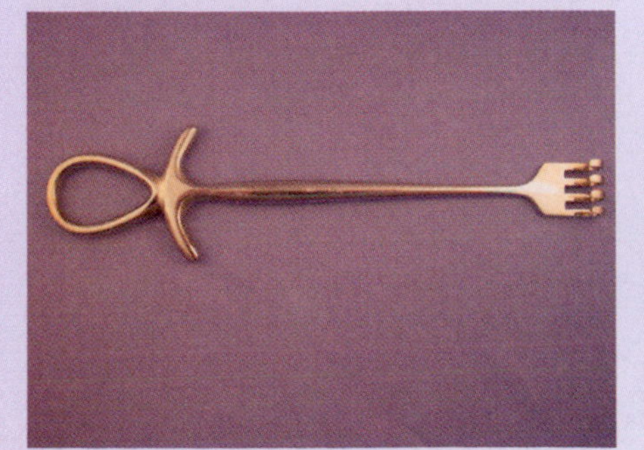

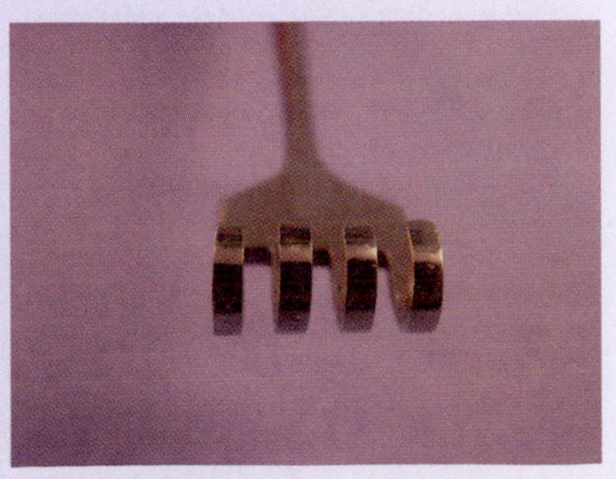

Name: Murphy retractor

Alias: rake

Category: retracting

Use: exposing superficial wound

Length: 7.5"

Additional Information: hand held; similar to Volkmann retractor but has finger grips (prongs) on the handle

Name: Ollier retractor
Alias: none
Category: retracting
Use: retracting heavy tissue
Length: 9"
Additional Information: hand held; blades are 2.25" × 1.75"

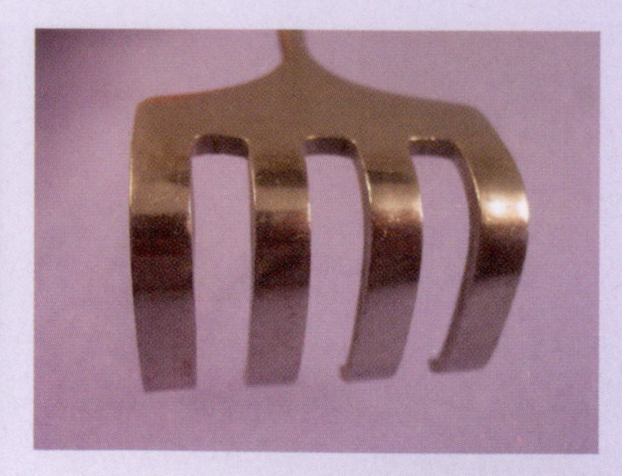

Name: Israel retractor
Alias: Israel rake
Category: retracting
Use: retracting heavy tissue
Length: 8"
Additional Information: hand held; rake can have 4 or 5 prongs; blades are 1.75" × 1.75"; used mostly in orthopedic surgery (shown here for comparison to Ollier retractor)

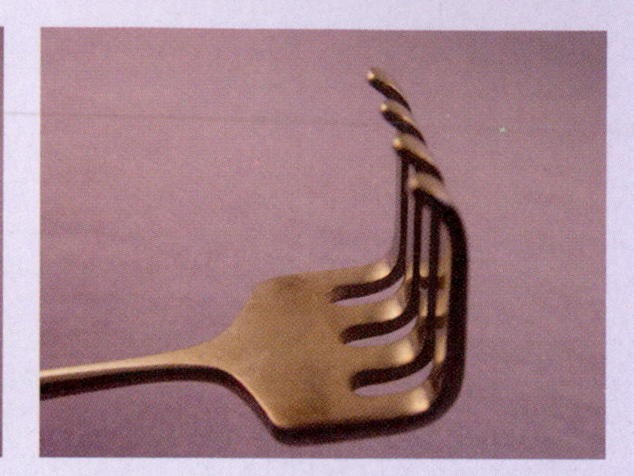

Name: Lahey goiter retractor
Alias: none
Category: retracting
Use: exposing wound; retracting small tissue masses
Length: 8"
Additional Information: hand held; right angle blade; blade length 1"

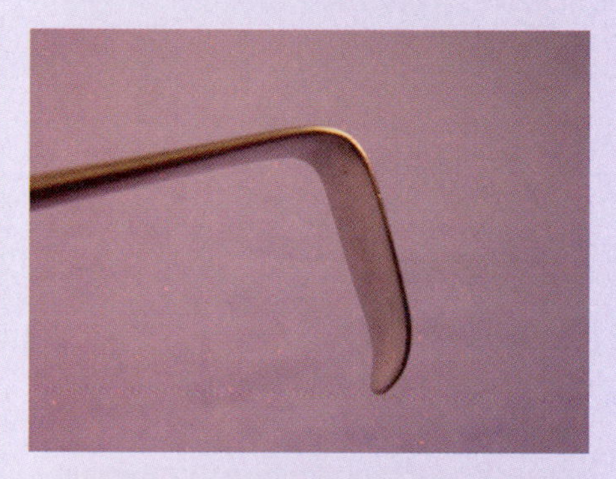

Name: Deaver retractor
Alias: none
Category: retracting
Use: deep retraction
Length: 10" 12" or 14"
Additional Information: hand held; blade width can vary from 1" to 4"

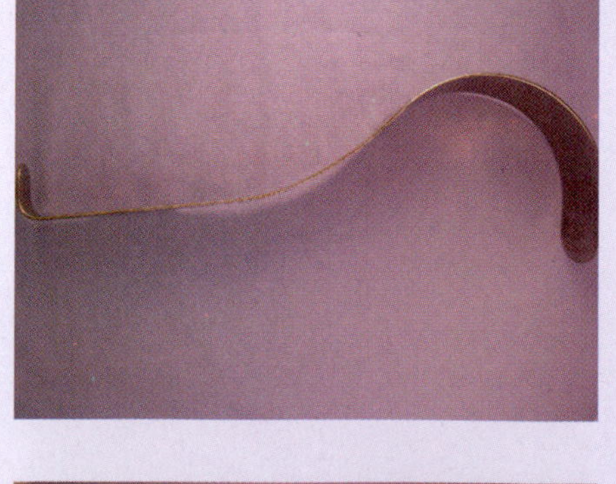

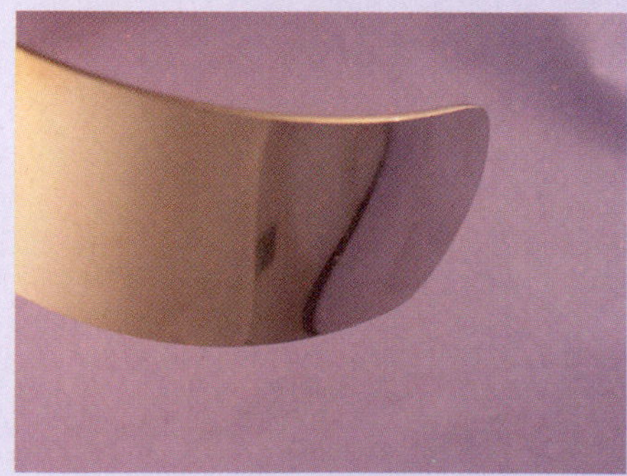

Name: Harrington retractor
Alias: sweetheart; valentine
Category: retracting
Use: exposing deep wound
Length: 12"
Other: hand held; blade can be 1.5" to 2.5" wide

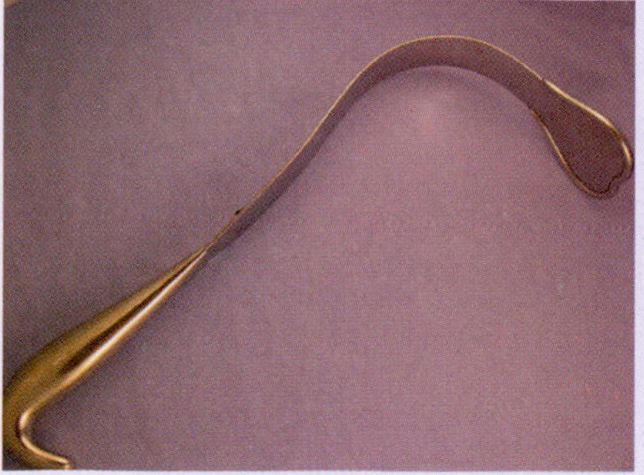

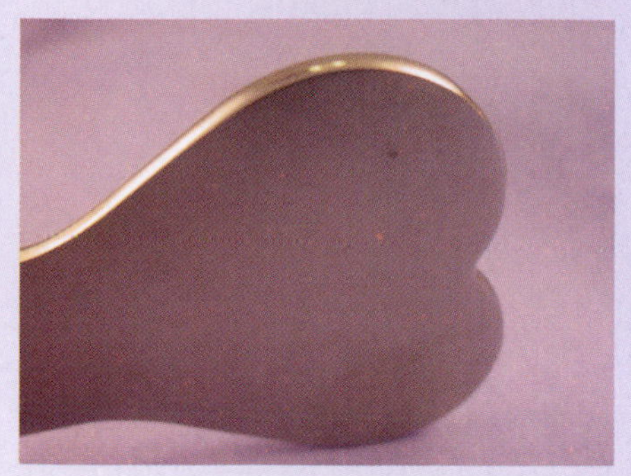

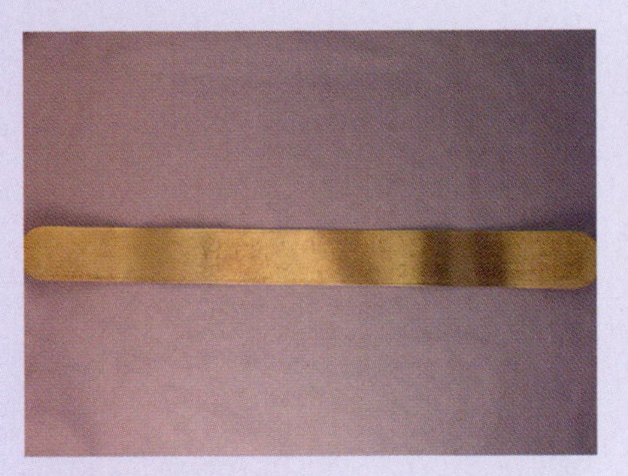

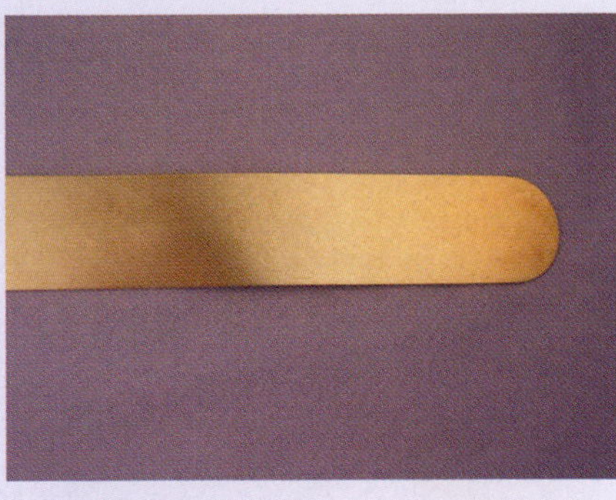

Name: Malleable retractor

Alias: ribbon

Category: retracting

Use: exposing wound

Length: 10" or 13"

Additional Information: hand held; straight—may be bent to desired shape; varies in width from 1" to 3"

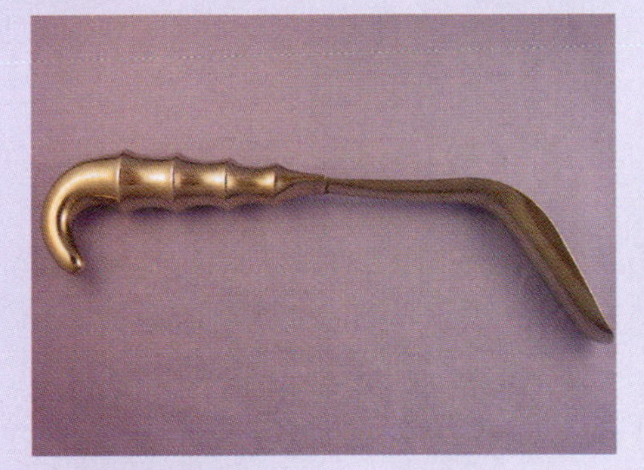

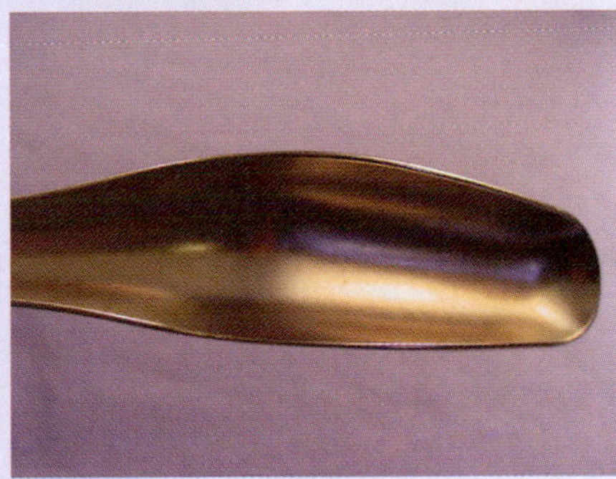

Name: Sawyer rectal retractor

Alias: none

Category: retracting

Use: retracting anal and/or rectal wall

Length: blade length 2.25" or 3.25"

Additional Information: hand held

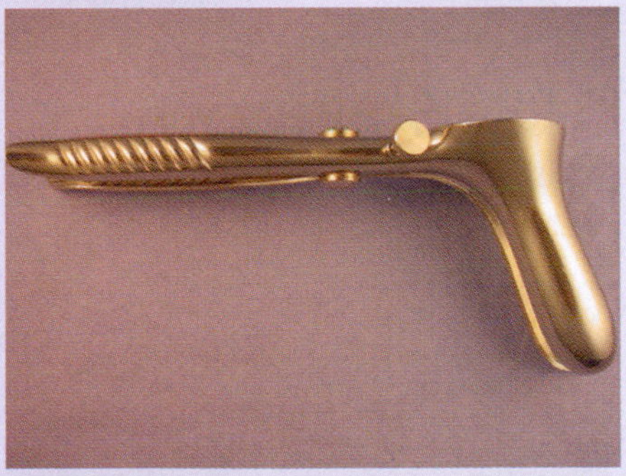

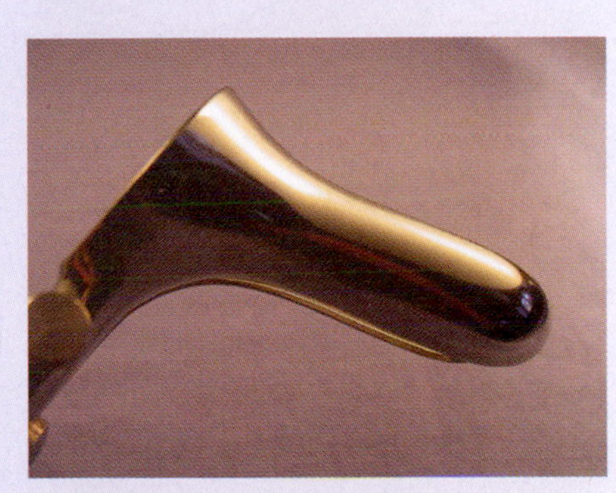

Name: Pratt speculum

Alias: none

Category: retracting

Use: retracting and viewing anus and rectum

Length: blade length 3.5"

Additional Information: comes in large diameter (2.5 cm) or small diameter (1.7 cm)

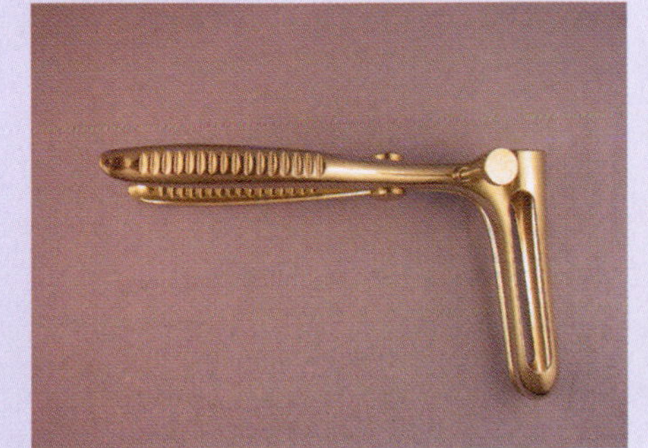

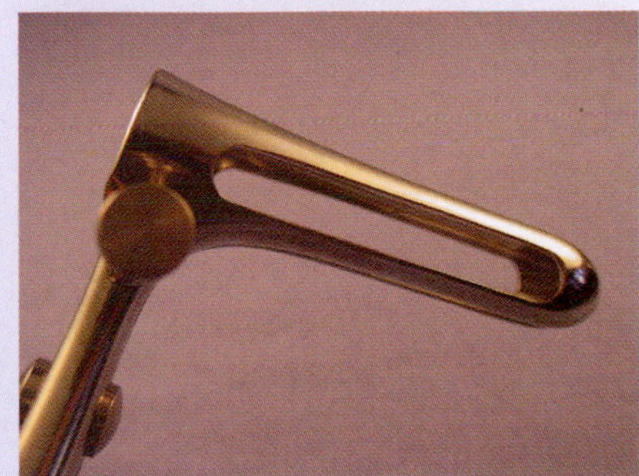

Name: Sims speculum

Alias: none

Category: retracting

Use: retracting and viewing anus and rectum

Length: blades 3.5" long

Additional Information: fenestrated blades

LAPAROSCOPIC INSTRUMENTS

Name: camera

Alias: none

Category: accessory

Use: viewing inside the body during endoscopic procedures

Length: n/a

Additional Information: many different systems available; need a compatible light cord and light source

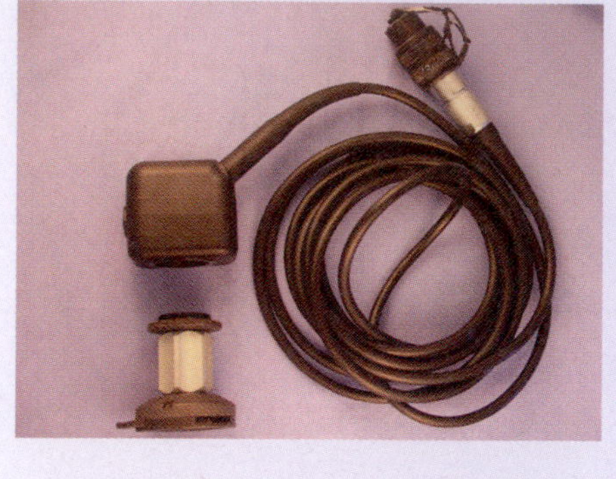

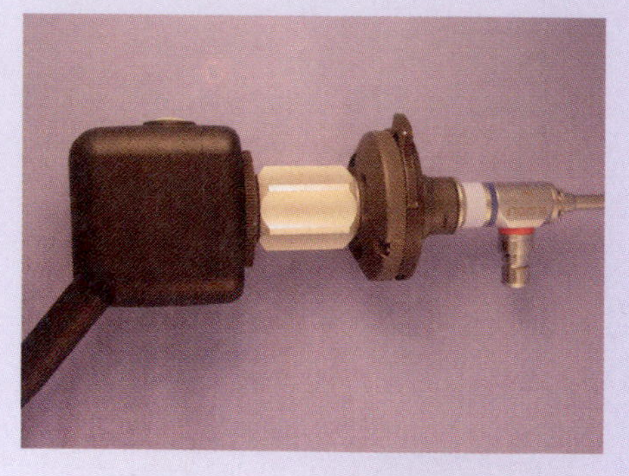

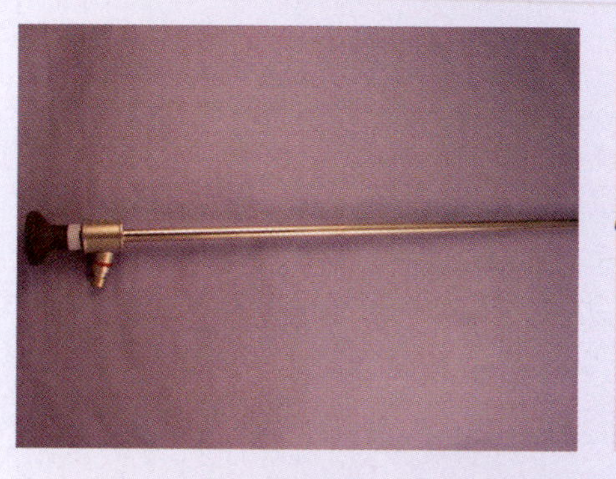

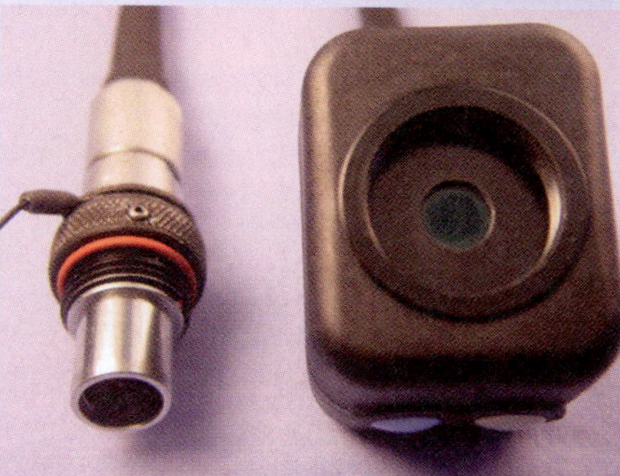

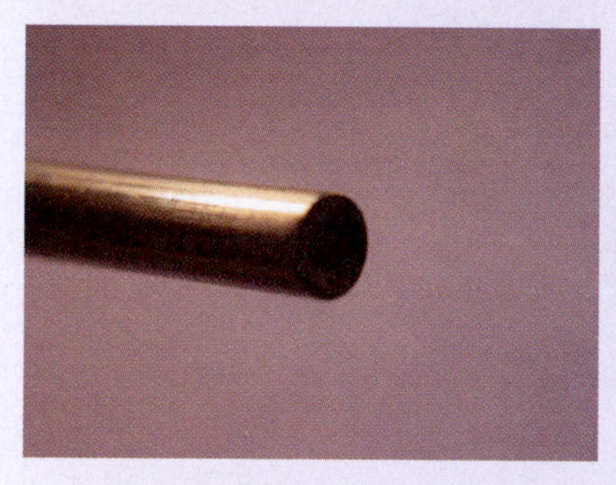

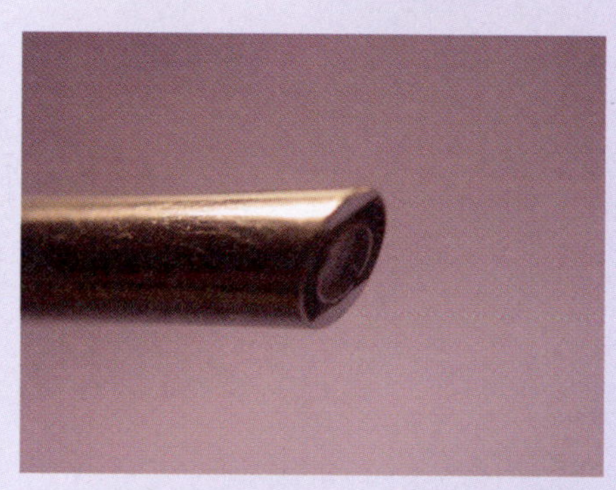

Name: Veress needle

Alias: Verres needle

Category: accessory

Use: puncturing the peritoneum and introducing carbon dioxide to create a pneumoperitoneum for laparoscopic surgery

Length: 10 cm, 12 cm, or 15 cm

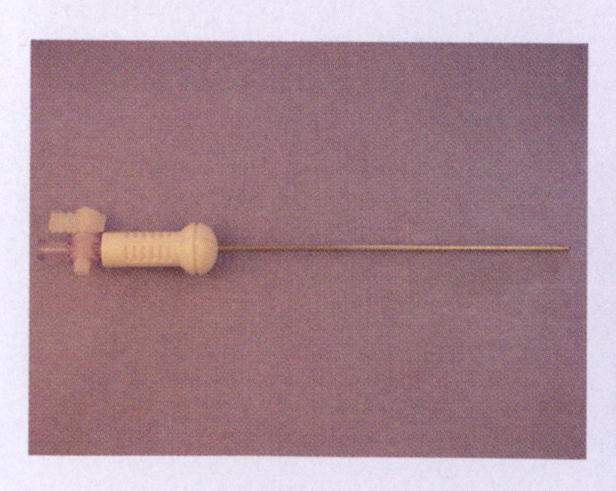

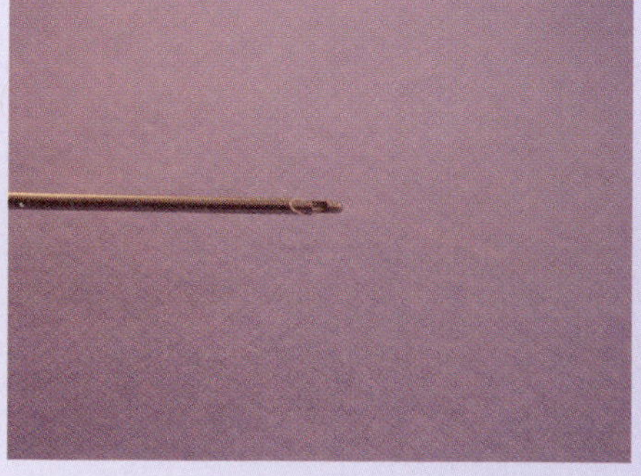

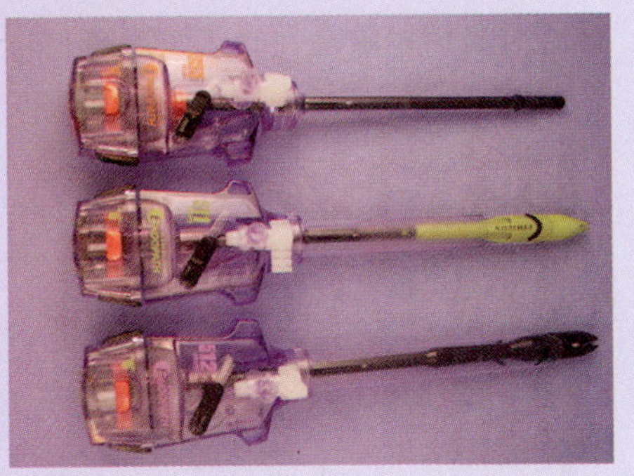

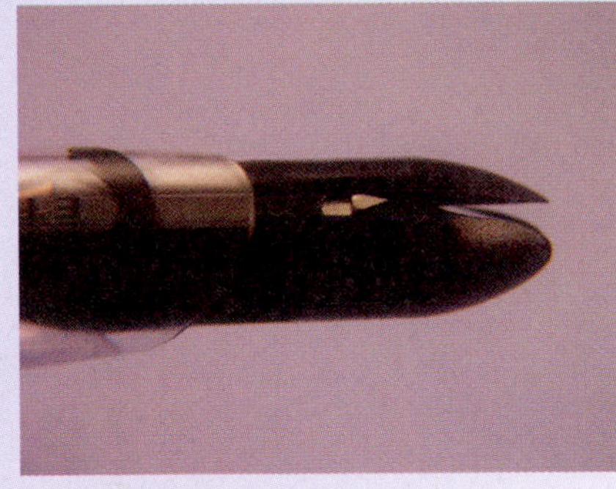

Name: disposable trocars and ports

Alias: none

Category: accessory

Use: allowing introduction of instruments and camera to the inside of body cavities for endoscopic surgery

Other: single-patient use only

Name: reusable trocars and ports

Alias: none

Category: accessory

Use: allowing introduction of instruments and camera into the inside of body cavities for endoscopic surgery

Length: 16.5 cm or 18.5 cm

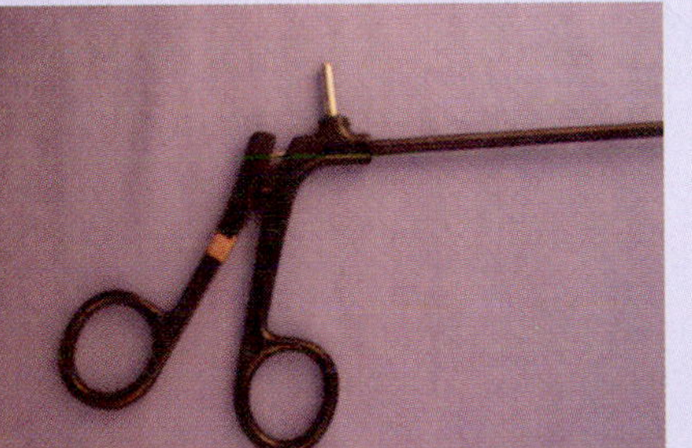

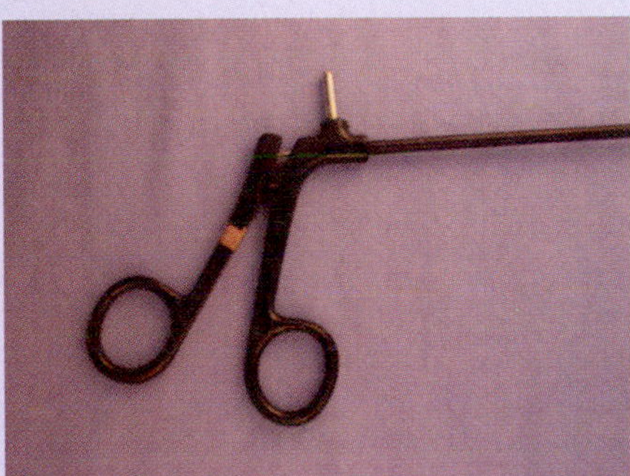

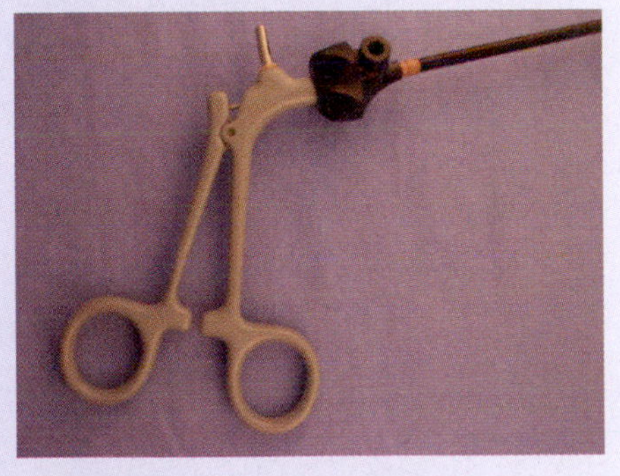

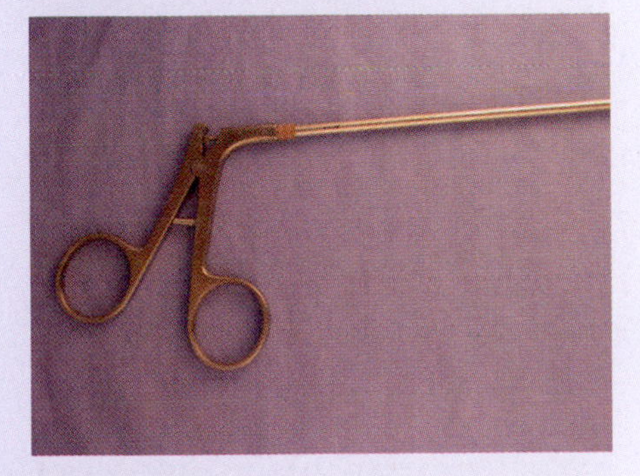

Name: laparoscopic instrument handles

Alias: none

Category: n/a

Use: manipulating laparoscopic instruments

Length: n/a

Additional Information: handle 1: rotating handle with cautery connection; handle 2: insulated handle with cautery connection; handle 3: handle with rachet

Please note: The tips shown on the following pages will usually operate with one of these three types of handles.

Name: 10 mm suction

Alias: none

Category: suction

Use: suctioning large amounts fluids/blood

Length: 32 cm or 45 cm

Other: laparoscopic suctions available in other diameters

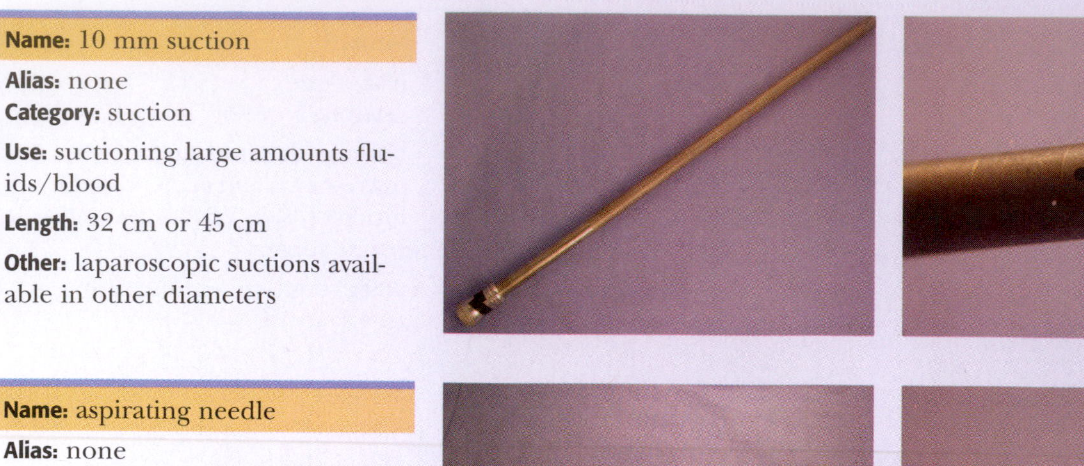

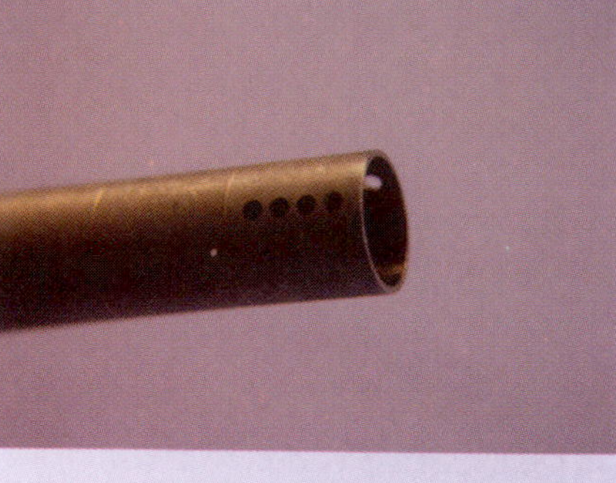

Name: aspirating needle

Alias: none

Category: accessory

Use: aspirating fluid from a cyst, organ, or tissue

Length: n/a

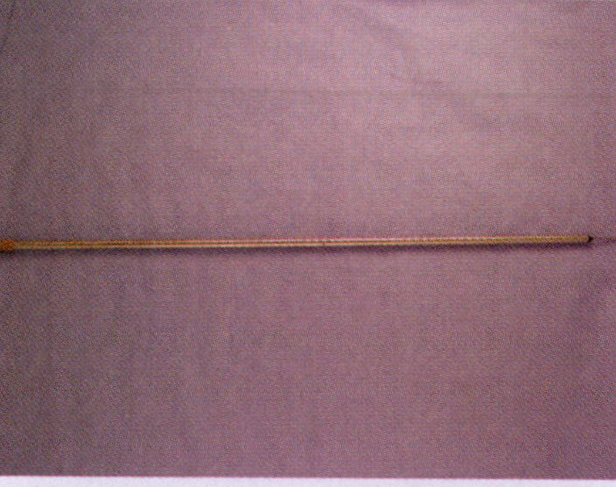

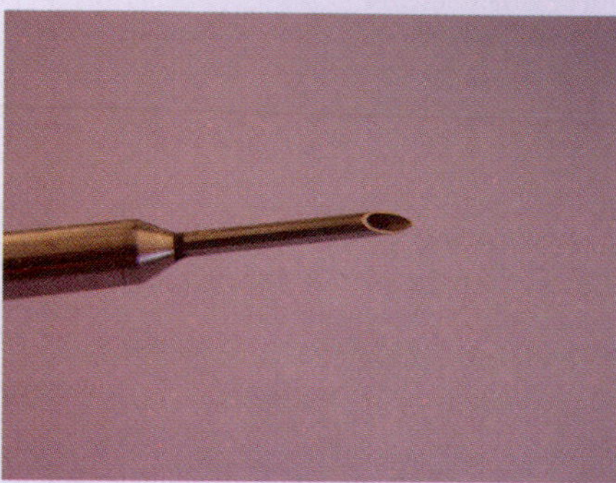

Name: blunt probe

Alias: none

Category: probing

Use: probing in a wound, duct, or tissue

Length: 32 cm or 45 cm

Other: can be graduated or plain

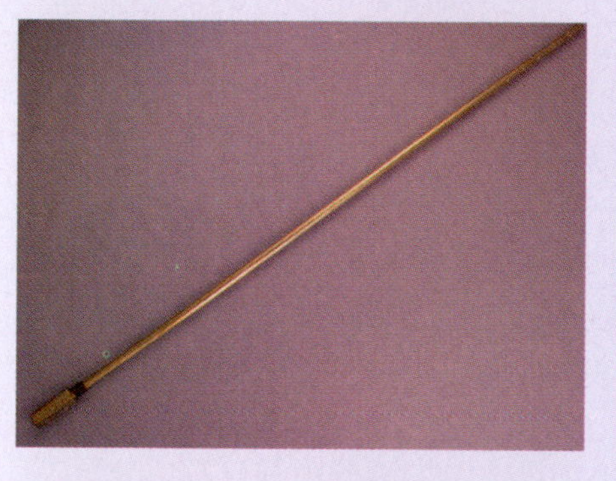

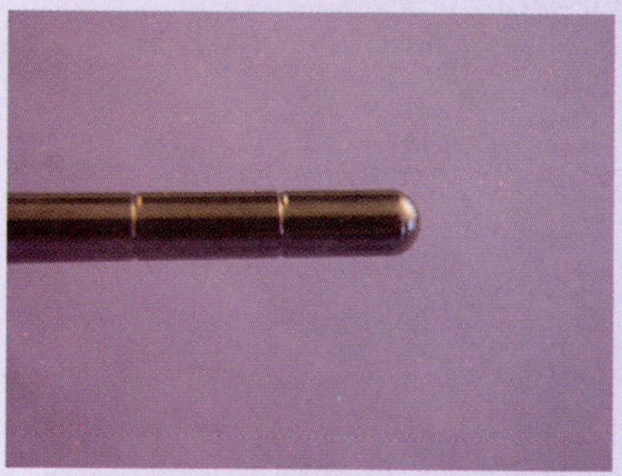

Name: Gore suture passer

Alias: none

Category: suturing

Use: passing suture through laparoscopic incision

Length: n/a

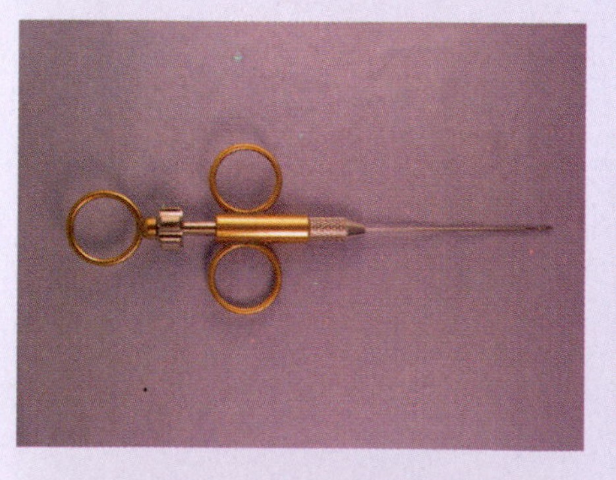

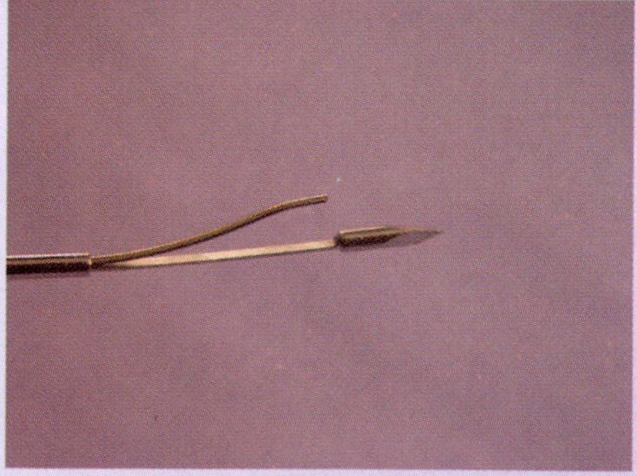

Name: suture hook

Alias: none

Category: suturing

Use: grasping sutures

Length: 32 cm

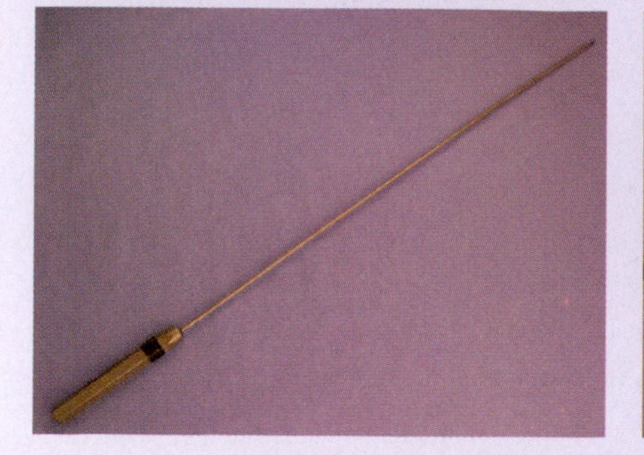

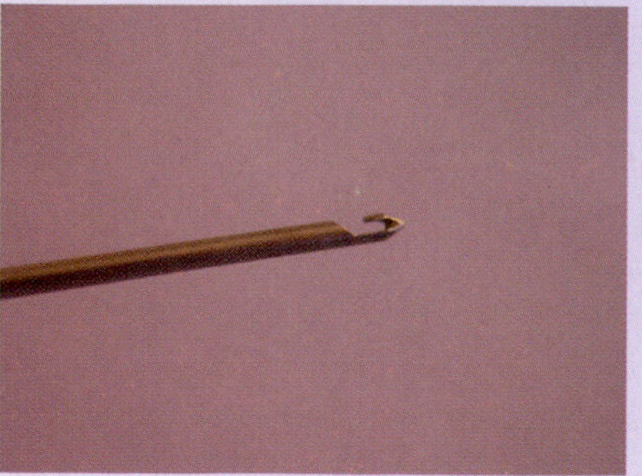

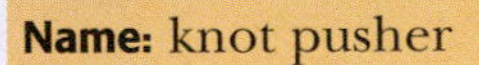

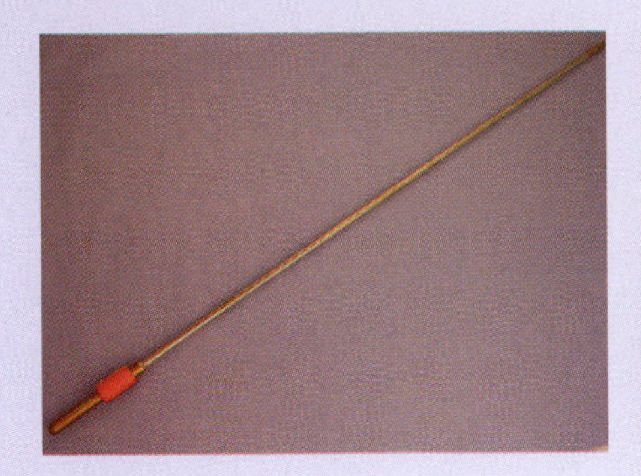

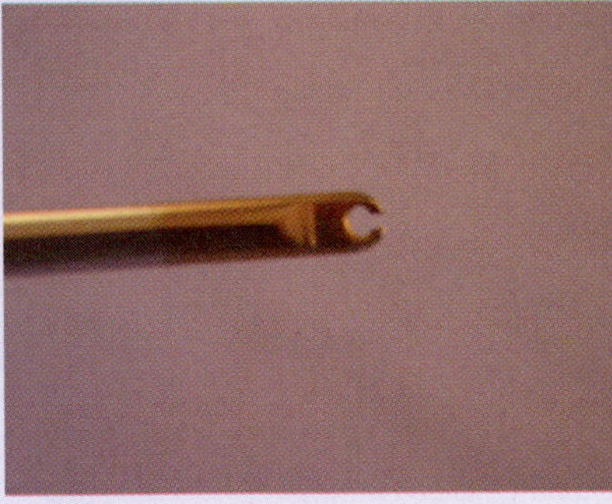

Name: knot pusher

Alias: none

Category: suturing

Use: pushing suture knots into place

Length: n/a

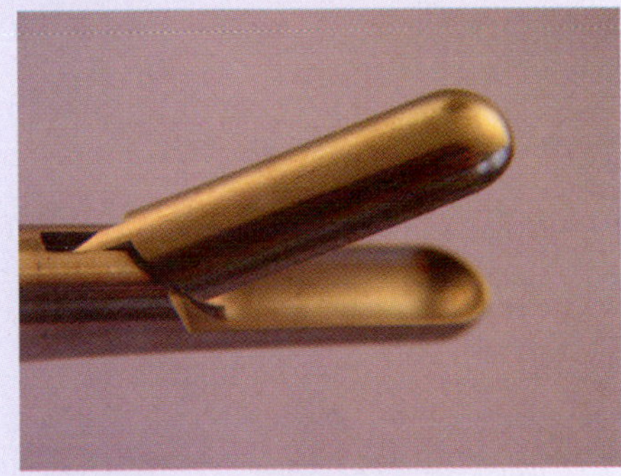

Name: 10 mm spoon

Alias: none

Category: grasping

Use: removing tissue

Length: 32 cm

Other: laparoscopic spoons available in 5 mm size

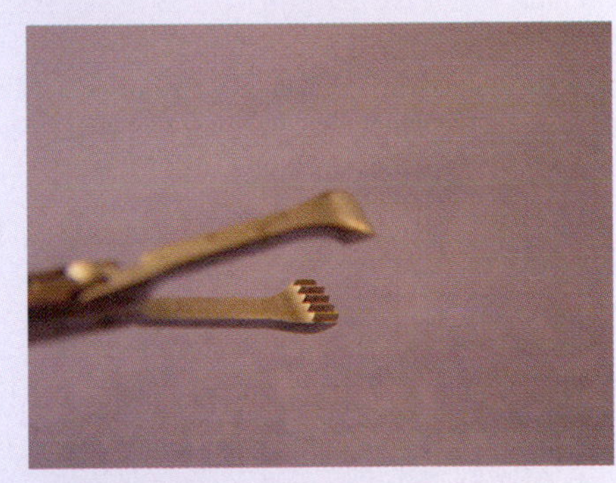

Name: Allis forceps

Alias: none

Category: grasping

Use: grasping tissue to be removed

Length: 32 cm

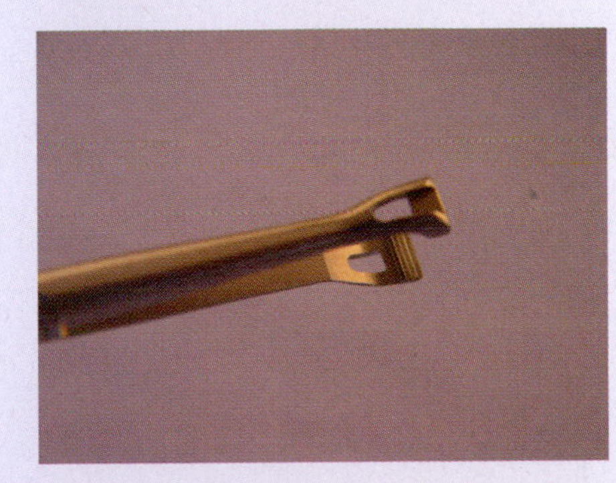

Name: Babcock

Alias: none

Category: grasping

Use: grasping/holding delicate tissue

Length: 32 cm

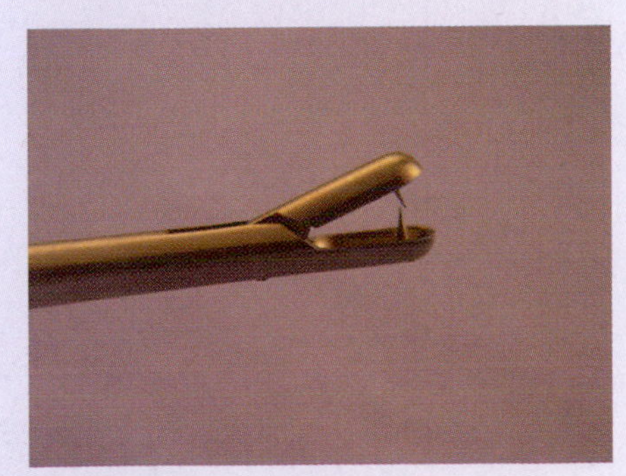

Name: biopsy forceps

Alias: none

Category: grasping

Use: obtaining small pieces of tissue for biopsy specimens

Length: 32 cm

Other: available in several sizes

Name: curved grasper
Alias: none
Category: grasping
Use: grasping tissue or organs
Length: 32 cm

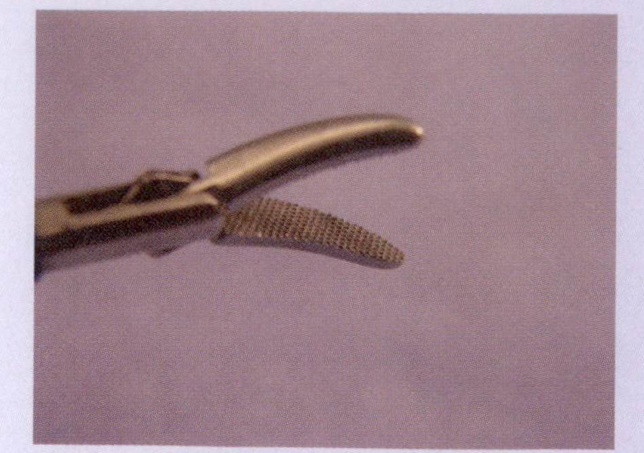

Name: bowel clamp
Alias: none
Category: clamping
Use: clamping or grasping bowel
Length: 32 cm

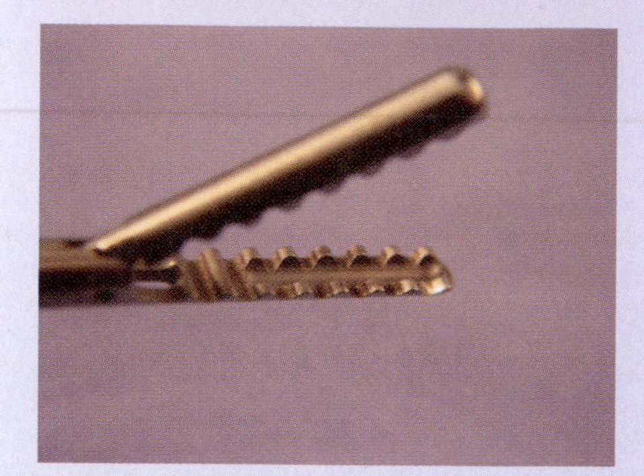

Name: Kocher
Alias: none
Category: grasping
Use: grasping tissue to be removed
Length: 32 cm

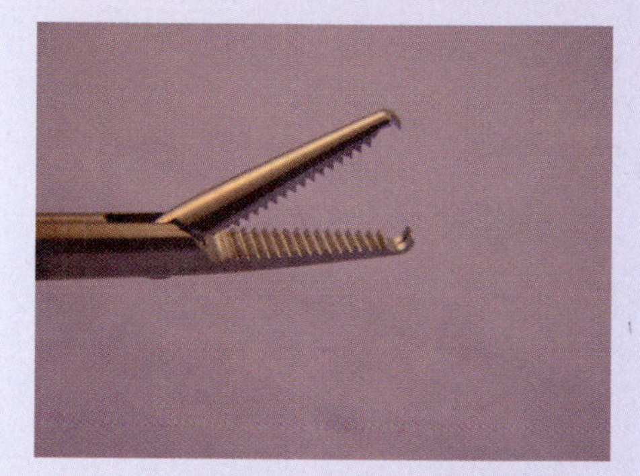

Name: dissector
Alias: Maryland dissector (curved)
Category: grasping
Use: grasping tissue or tissue dissection
Length: 32 cm
Other: tips can be straight or curved; fully serrated blades

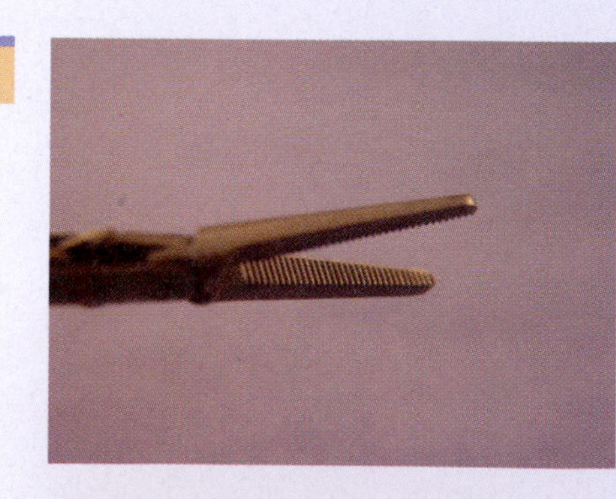

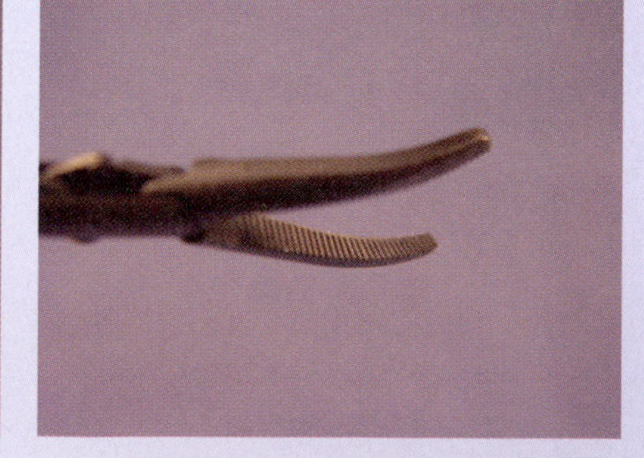

Name: alligator forceps
Alias: none
Category: grasping
Use: grasping tissue
Length: 32 cm
Other: tip can be square or rectangular; fully serrated tip

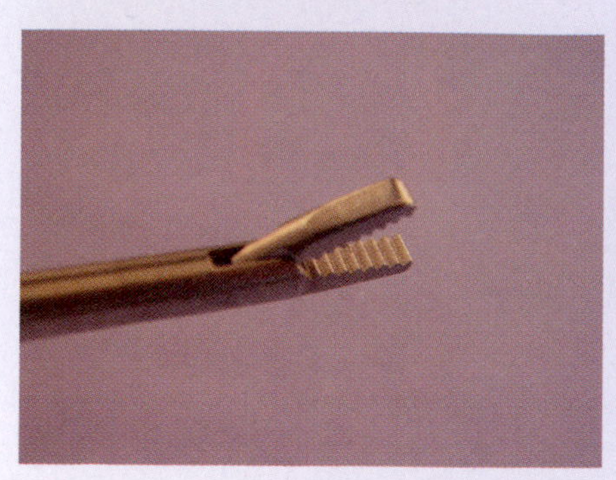

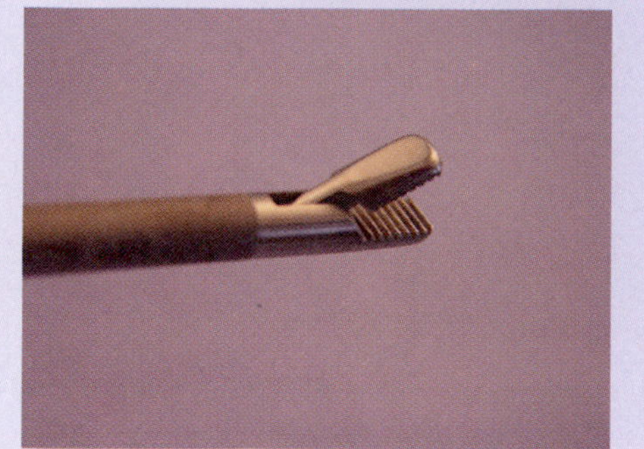

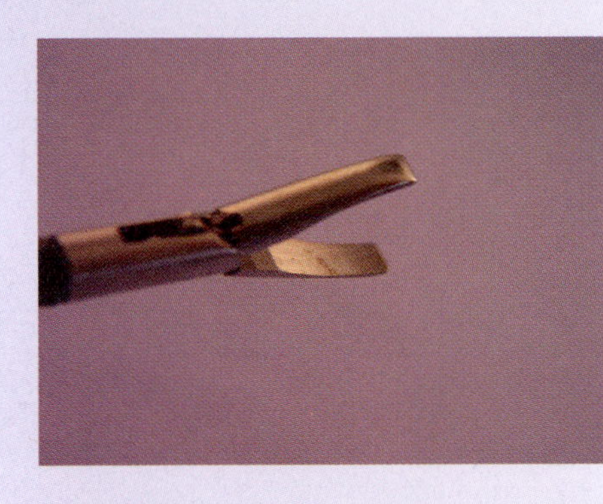

Name: smooth grasper
Alias: none
Category: grasping
Use: grasping tissue or organs
Length: 32 cm
Other: smooth jaws

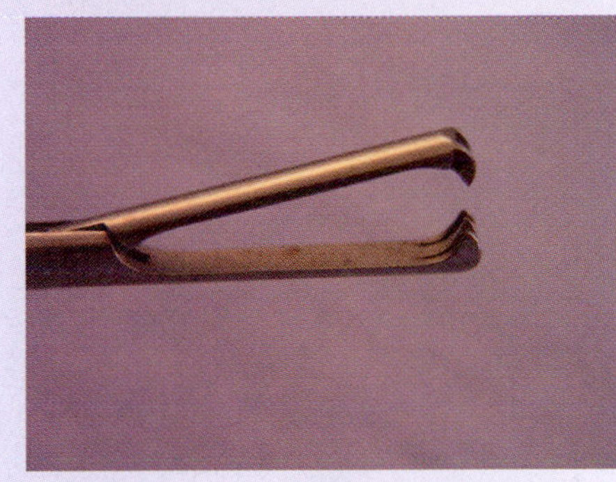

Name: toothed grasper
Alias: claw
Category: grasping
Use: grasping tissue to be removed
Length: 32 cm
Other: 2 × 3 teeth

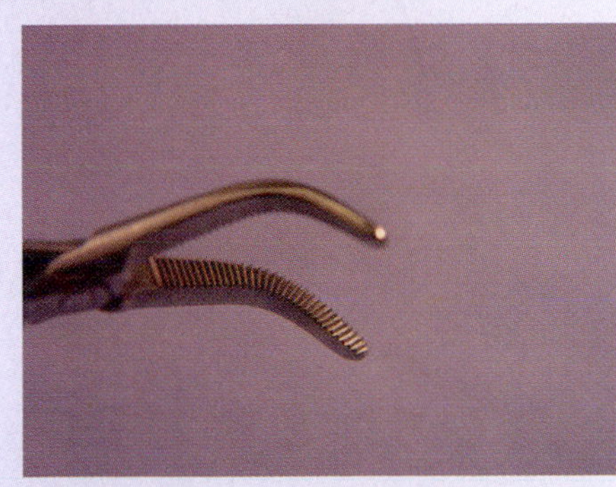

Name: Mixter
Alias: right angle
Category: grasping
Use: grasping tissue around an angle
Length: 32 cm

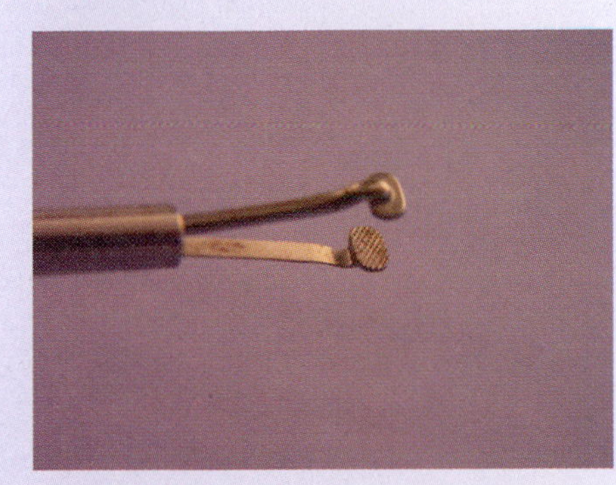

Name: paddle grasper
Alias: none
Category: grasping
Use: grasping tissue
Length: 32 cm

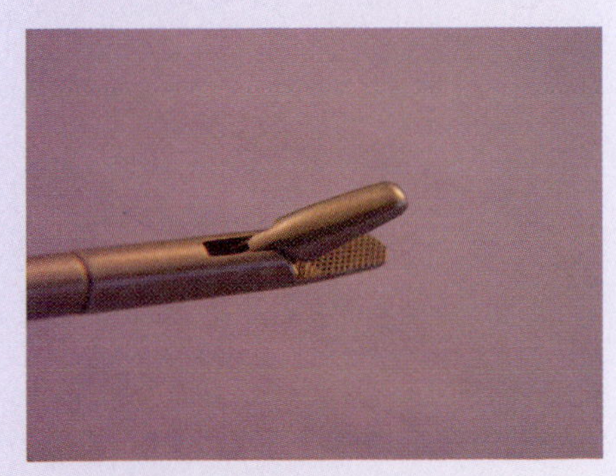

Name: needle holder
Alias: none
Category: suturing
Use: holding suture needles
Length: 32 cm

Name: beaver blade handle
Alias: none
Category: cutting
Use: holding small scalpel blades ("beaver blades")
Length: 32 cm

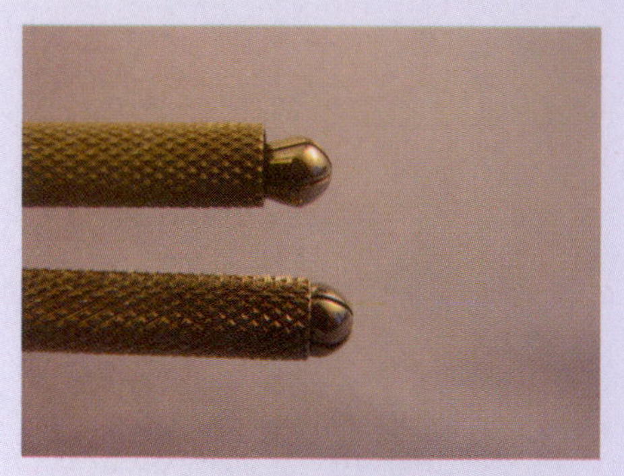

Name: hook scissors
Alias: none
Category: cutting
Use: cutting tissue
Length: 32 cm

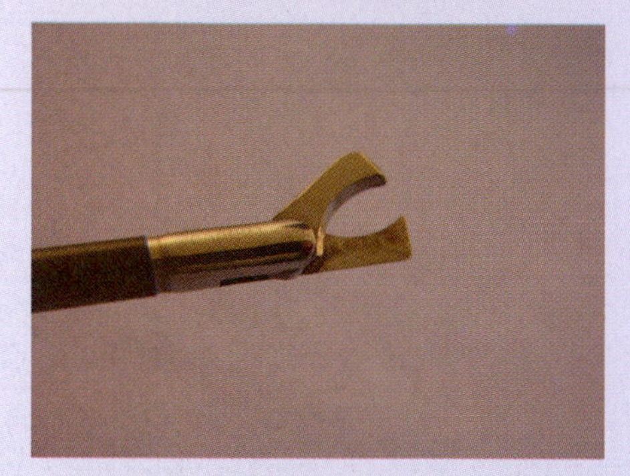

Name: microscissors
Alias: none
Category: cutting
Use: cutting delicate tissue
Length: 32 cm

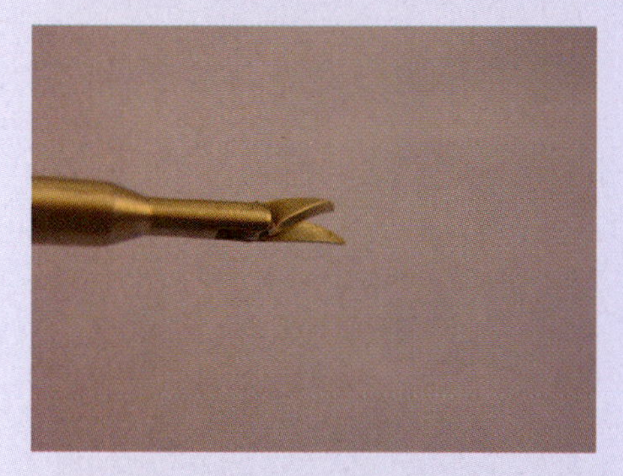

Name: scissors
Alias: none
Category: cutting
Use: cutting tissue or sutures
Length: 32 cm

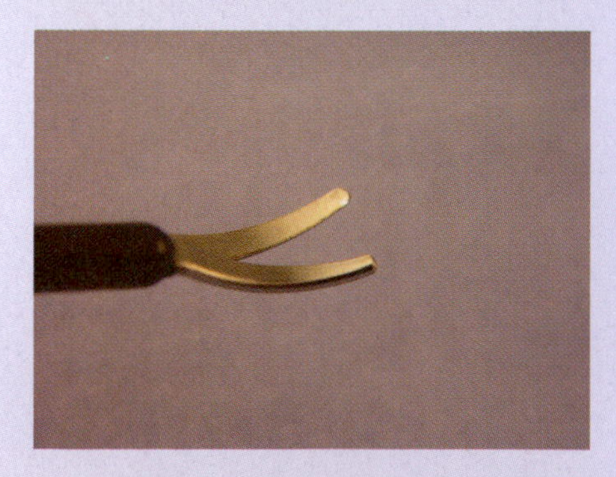

Name: Kleppinger bipolar forceps
Alias: none
Category: accessory
Use: bipolar cauterization of tissue
Length: n/a
Other: used mainly in gynecologic surgery

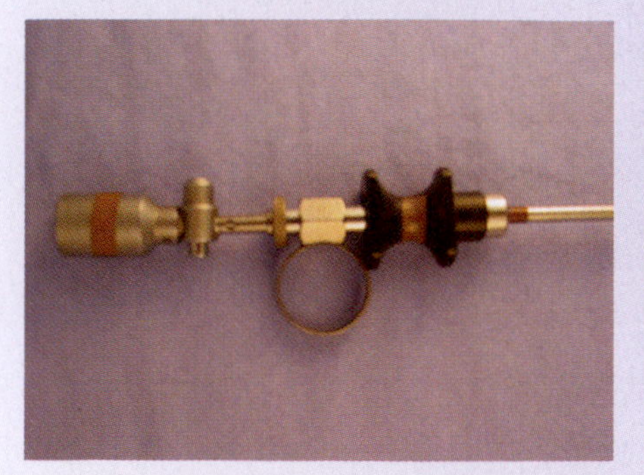

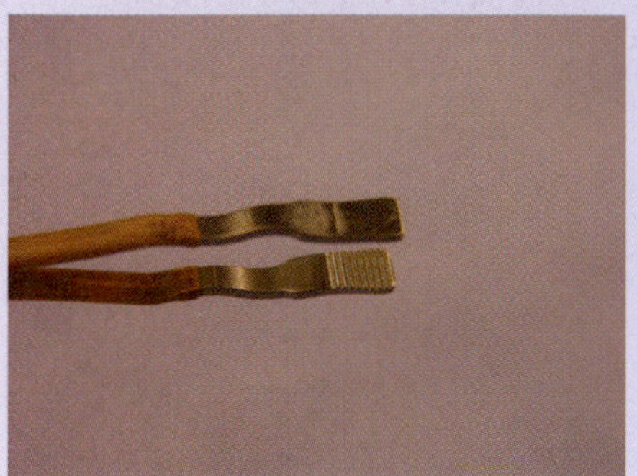

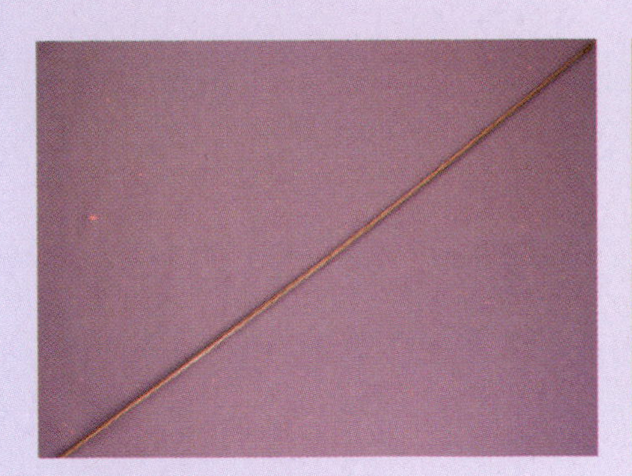
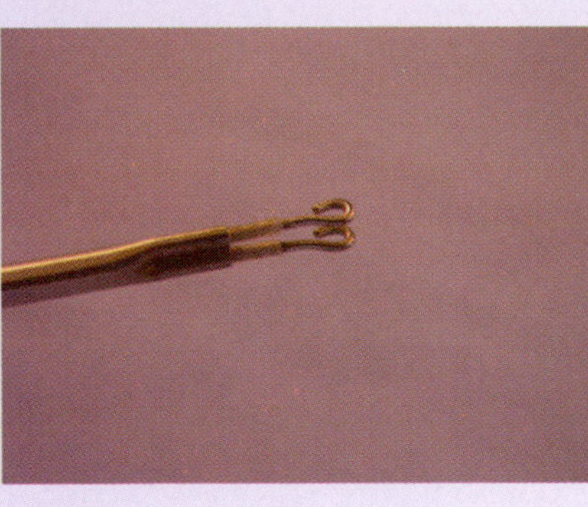

Name: microbipolar
Alias: none
Category: accessory
Use: bipolar cauterization of tissue
Length: 32 cm or 45 cm

STAPLERS

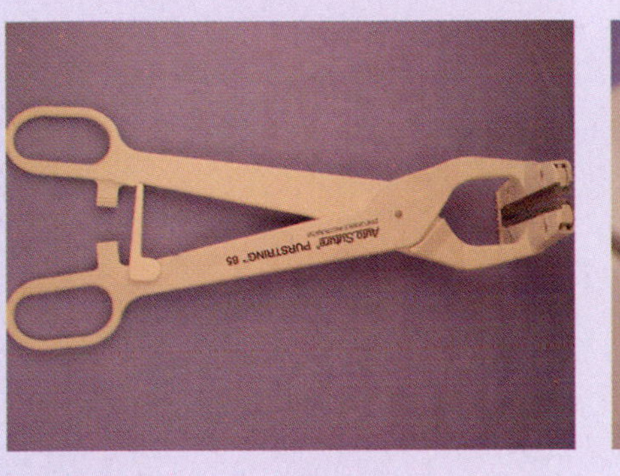
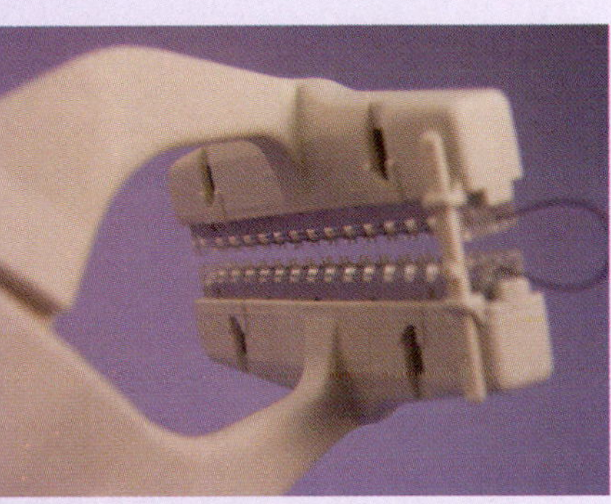

Name: autosuture purse string
Alias: none
Category: suturing
Use: applying a purse-string suture during gastric/colon surgery
Length: n/a
Additional Information: single-patient use

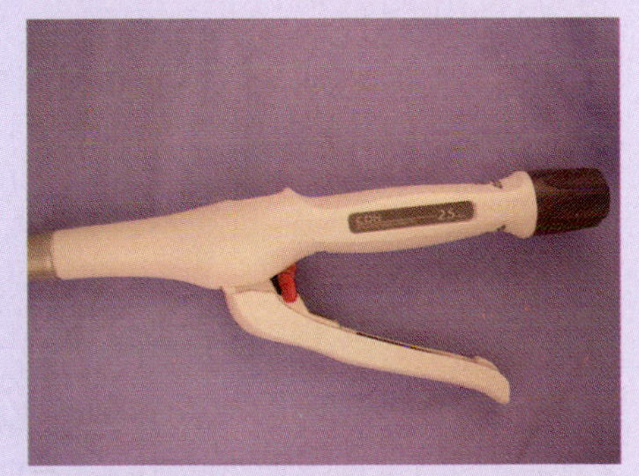
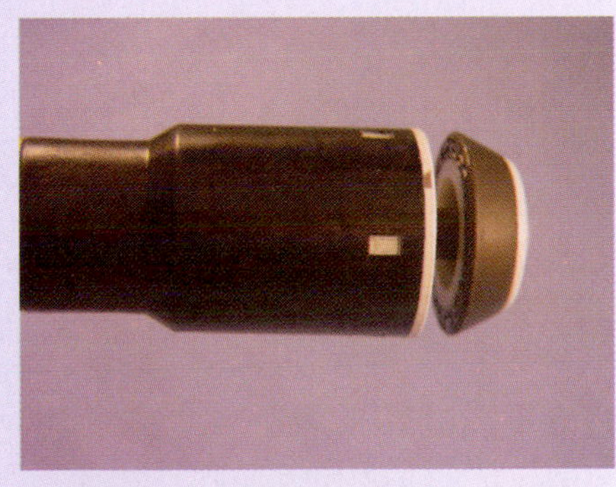

Name: CDH stapler
Alias: eea stapler
Category: stapling
Use: anastomosing bowel to stomach or bowel to bowel
Length: n/a
Additional Information: single-patient use; comes in a variety of diameters (25 mm is pictured)

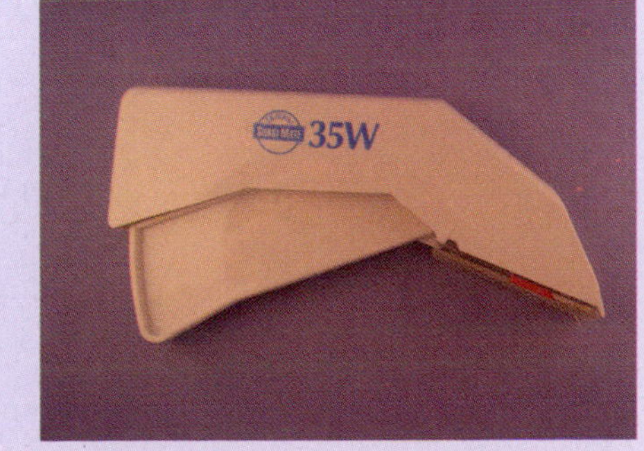

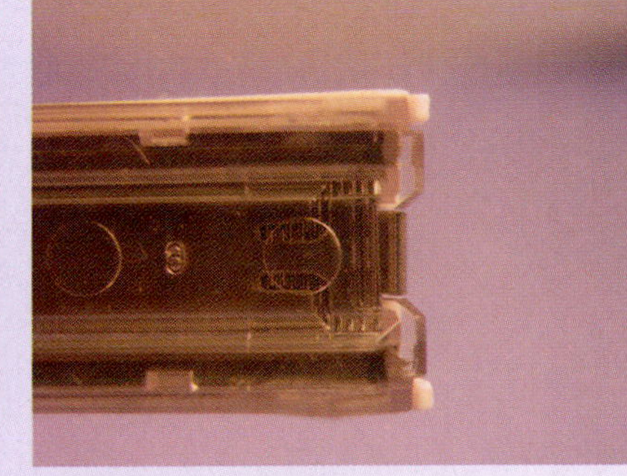

Name: skin stapler
Alias: none
Category: stapling
Use: closing skin incisions
Length: n/a
Additional Information: single-patient use; comes in regular or wide width

Name: Ligaclip stapler

Alias: none

Category: stapling

Use: clipping off vessels or ducts during open procedures

Length: n/a

Additional Information: single-patient use

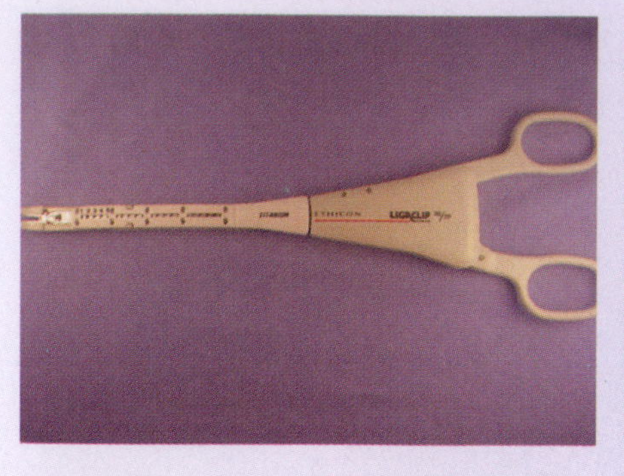

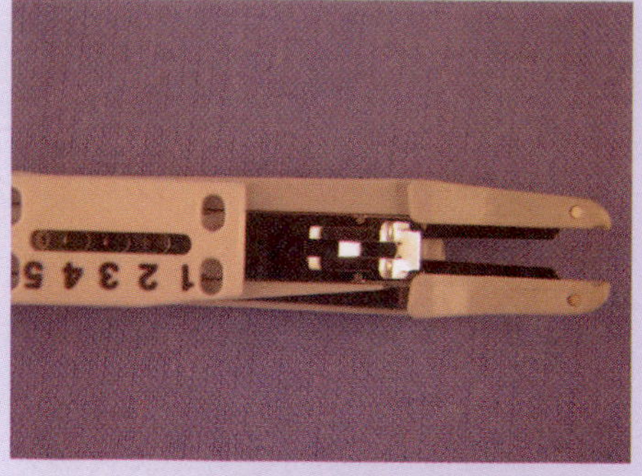

Name: endoscopic ligaclip applier

Alias: none

Category: stapling

Use: clipping off vessels or ducts during endoscopic procedures such as laparoscopic cholecystectomy

Length: n/a

Additional Information: single-patient use; rotary handle allows rotation of the tip of the instrument to the needed position; applies one ligaclip at a time

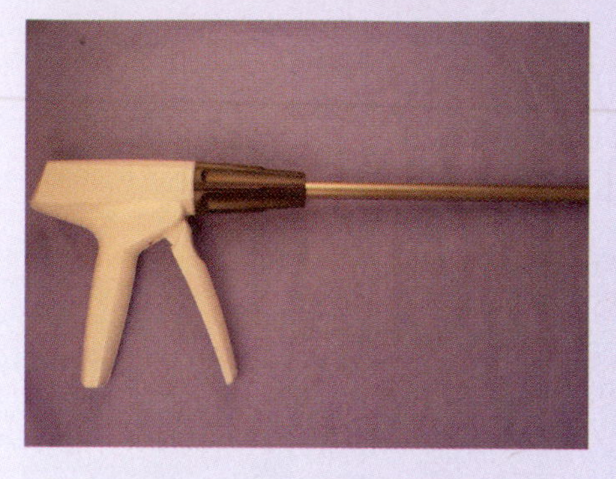

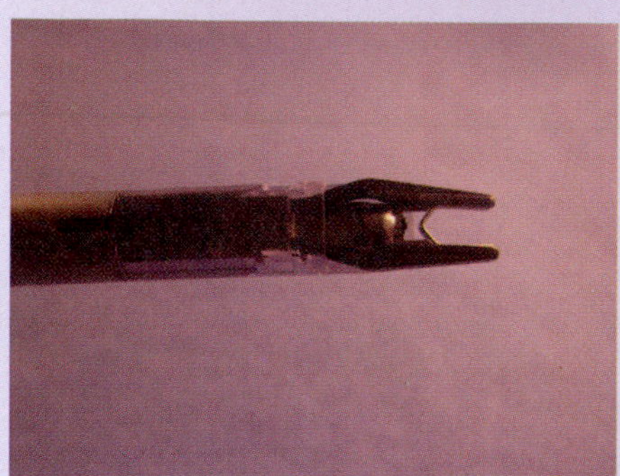

Name: ETS endoscopic stapler

Alias: none

Category: stapling

Use: applying a whole row of staples to tissue during an endoscopic procedure

Length: n/a

Additional Information: single-patient use; reloads available; available in a number of sizes (45 is pictured)

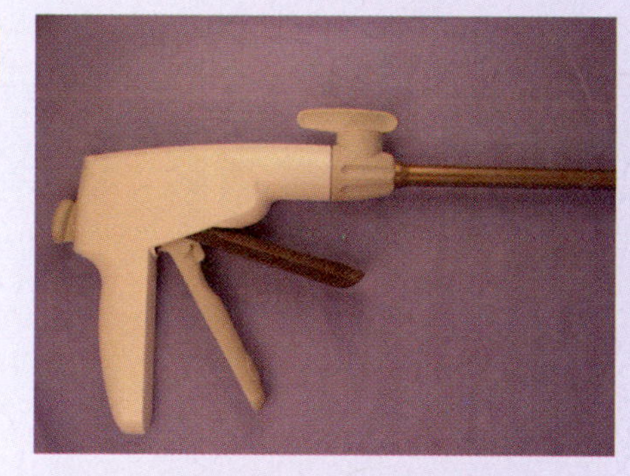

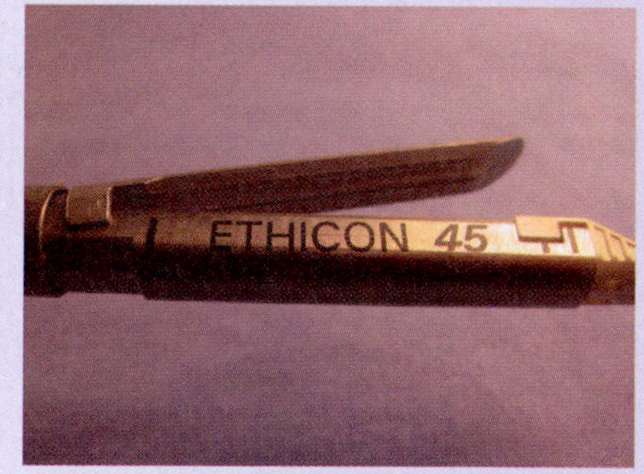

Name: linear stapler

Alias: none

Category: stapling

Use: stapling across a large tissue area such as creating a gastric pouch, anastomosis of bowel or closure of stomach/bowel incisions

Length: n/a

Additional Information: single-patient use; available in a number of sizes

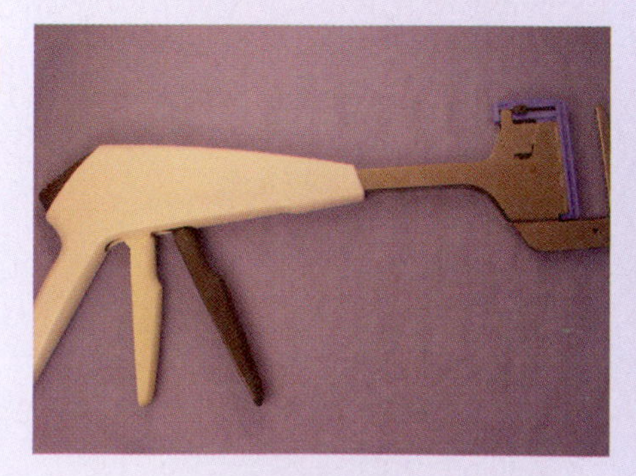

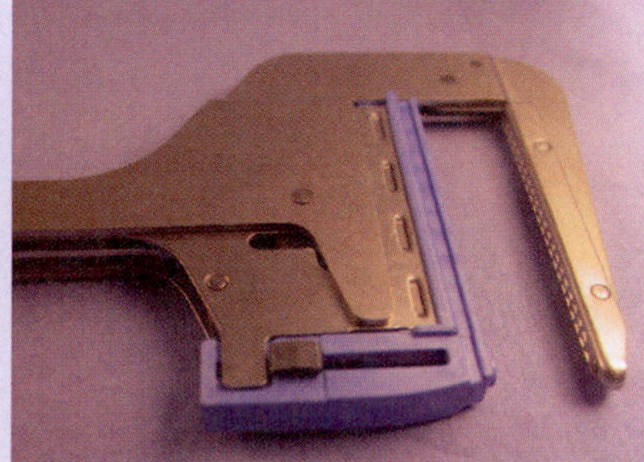

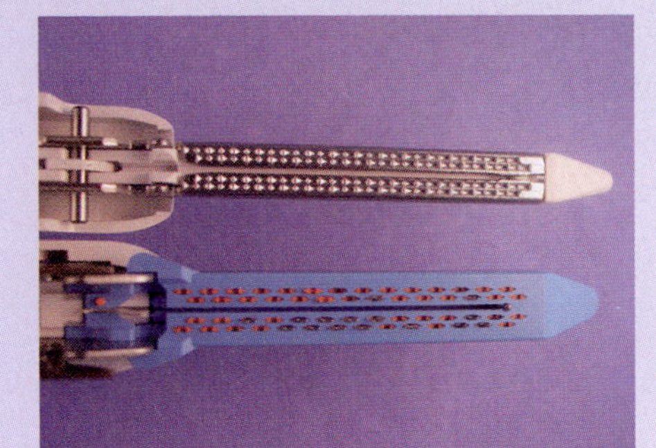

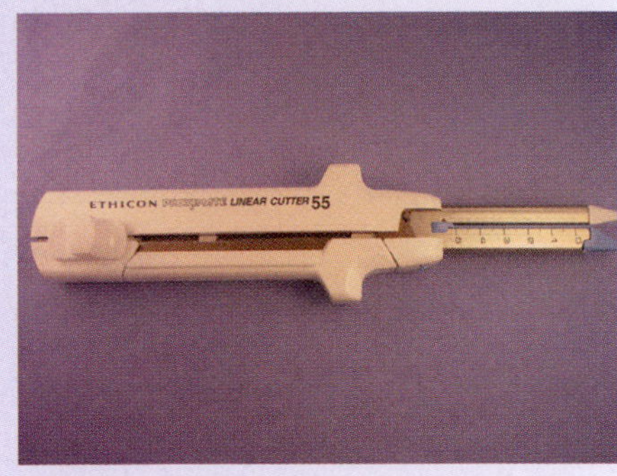

Name: Proximate 2 pieces stapler

Alias: linear cutter
Category: stapling/cutting

Use: stapling anastomoses while creating a linear cut between the two structures

Length: n/a

Additional Information: single-patient use; comes in a variety of sizes; reloads available

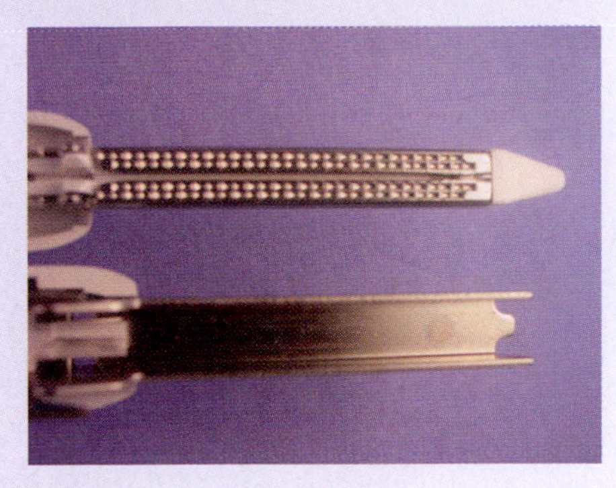

Q&A

Surgical Session—General Instruments

1) You have just handed the surgeon a suture. Which scissors will you have ready to hand to him/her to cut the suture with?
   a. Curved Mayo
   b. Metzenbaum
   c. Potts
   d. Straight Mayo

2) The surgeon is performing a colectomy. He/she has just entered the peritoneal cavity and now requests a large, self-retaining retractor. You would hand him/her a:
   a. Senn
   b. Richardson
   c. Bookwalter
   d. Weitlaner

3) You have a #20 knife blade on your field. What size knife handle do you need to insert the blade onto?
   a. #4
   b. #3
   c. #7
   d. #2

4) The surgeon is getting ready to perform skin closure of an incision. In addition to a stapler, which of the following forceps would generally be used?
   a. Russian
   b. Bonney
   c. Adson
   d. DeBakey

5) The surgeon is about to irrigate the abdomen with large amounts of normal saline. He/she asks for an abdominal suction. What is the other name for this instrument?
   a. Frazier
   b. Poole
   c. Yankauer
   d. Tonsil

6) A mixter is another name for a:
   a. Schnidt
   b. Crile
   c. right angle
   d. Kelly

7) Mosquito is another name for a:
   a. Kelly
   b. Halstead
   c. Pean
   d. Schnidt

8) The surgeon is performing an inguinal herniorrhaphy. He/she has made the skin incision and dissected down a short way into the underlying tissue. The assistant asks for a retractor. Which of the following would *not* be appropriate to hand him/her?
   a. U.S. Army
   b. Volkmann
   c. Bookwalter
   d. Parker

9) Which of the following instruments does *not* have sharp teeth?
   a. Lahey
   b. Kocher
   c. Backhaus
   d. Babcock

10) The nonperforating clip used to hold suction and other cords to the drape is a(n):
   a. Backhaus
   b. Edna
   c. Lahey
   d. Kocher

11) A Foerster is a:
   a. tonsil clamp
   b. tissue forceps
   c. sponge stick
   d. suction tip

12) A Harrington retractor is also known as a:
   a. Richardson
   b. Deaver
   c. Sweetheart
   d. Doyen

13) The surgeon inserts a Blake drain into the incision. Which scissors would you hand him/her to cut the drain?
   a. Metzenbaum
   b. Straight iris
   c. Straight Mayo
   d. Curved iris

14) Which of the following is *not* a type of hand held retractor?
   a. Senn
   b. Volkmann
   c. U.S. Army
   d. Weitlaner

15) The surgeon needs to cut through a heavy muscle. Which scissors would be the most appropriate to hand him/her?
   a. Metzenbaum
   b. Curved Mayo
   c. Curved iris
   d. Straight iris

16) Which of the following would be the most appropriate to hand a surgeon to use to clamp off a very small blood vessel?
   a. Halstead
   b. Kelly
   c. Kocher
   d. Pean

OB-GYN Instruments 2

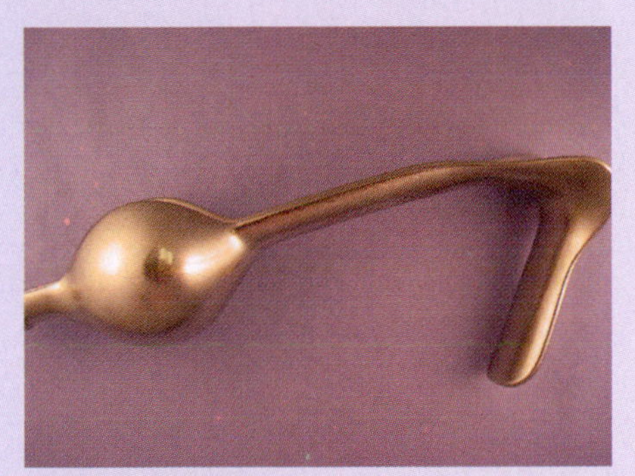
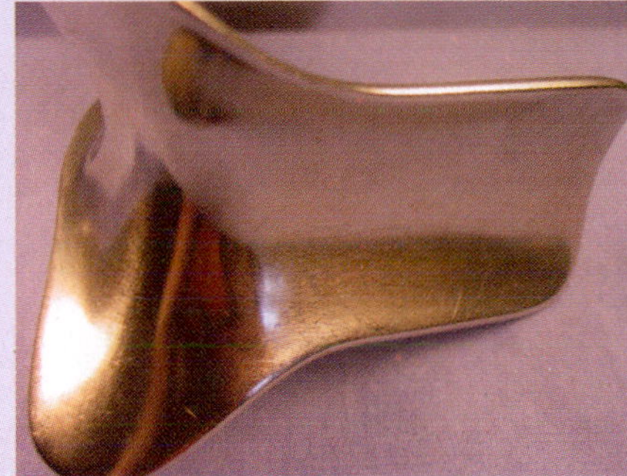

Name: Auvard weighted vaginal speculum

Alias: weighted speculum
Category: retracting

Use: retracting the vaginal floor

Length: n/a

Additional Information: Blades can be 2 $\frac{3}{4}$" × 1.5" or 3" × 1.5"

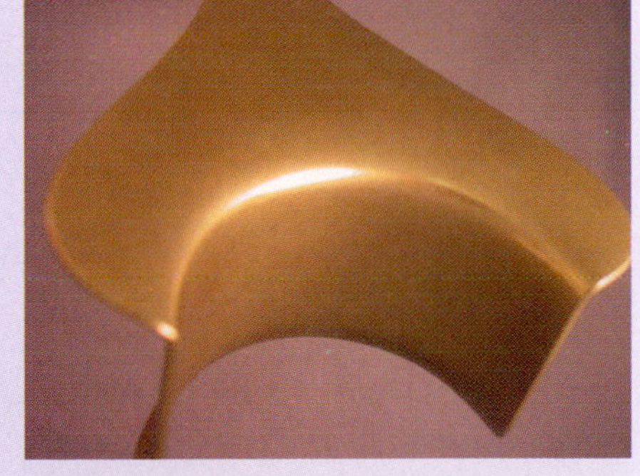

Name: DeLee bladder retractor

Alias: bladder blade
Category: retracting

Use: retracting the bladder during cesarean section

Length: 9.25"

Additional Information: manual retractor; also available with blade offset to left or right

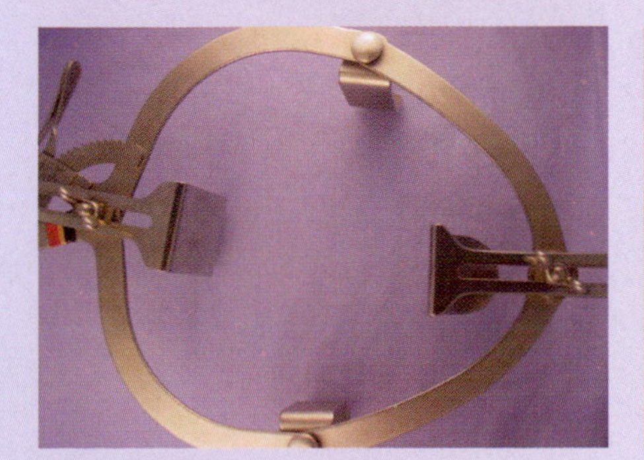
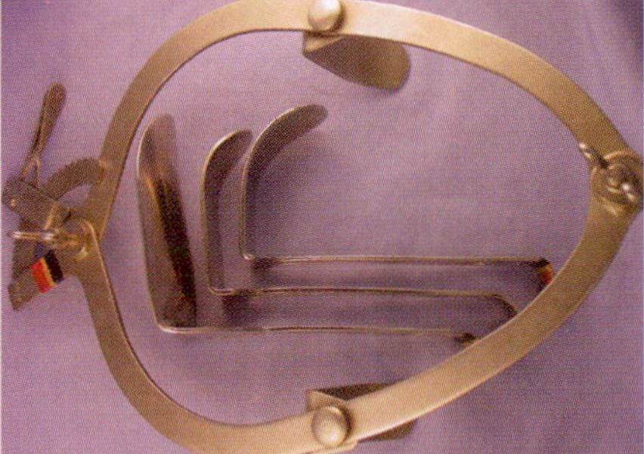

Name: O'Sullivan-O'Connor retractor

Alias: Irish; O'Connor-O'Sullivan
Category: retracting

Length: n/a

Use: retracting abdominal or pelvic wall

Additional Information: self-retaining; interchangeable blades; have moistened lap pads available to hand to the surgeon (to use as padding between the blades and tissue)

Name: Simpson delivery forceps
Alias: none
Category: grasping
Use: delivering baby
Length: 12" or 14"
Additional Information: forceps come in two parts—hand to surgeon as two separate pieces

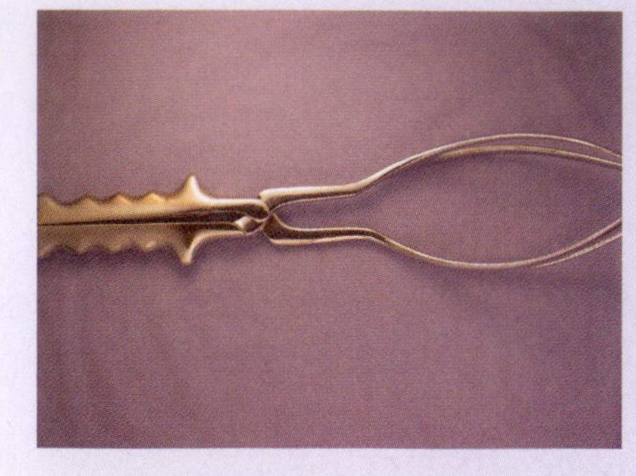
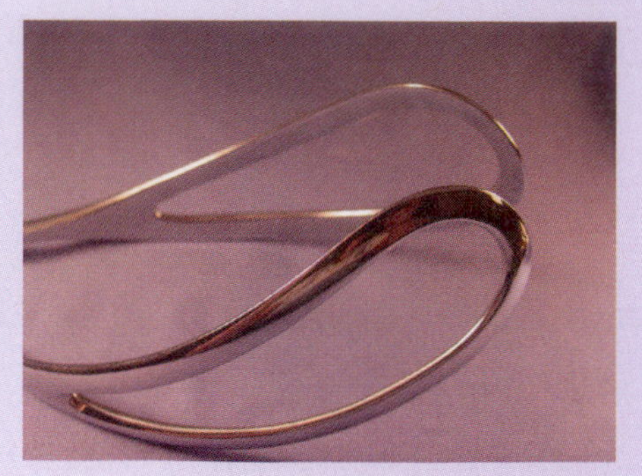

Name: Goodell dilator
Alias: none
Category: dilating
Use: dilating the cervix or uterus
Length: 10" or 13"
Additional Information: self-retaining; corrugated blades

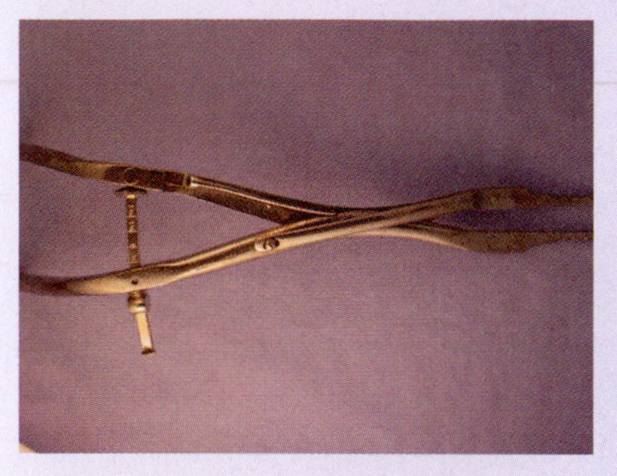
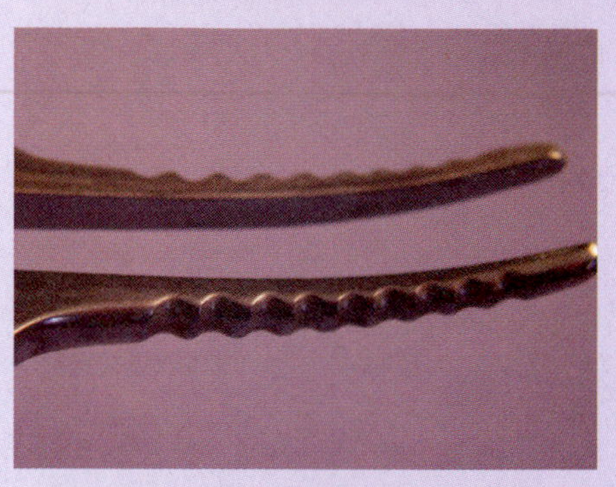

Name: Sims retractor
Alias: none
Category: retracting
Use: retracting vaginal wall
Length:
Additional Information: double ended; blade width and length may vary

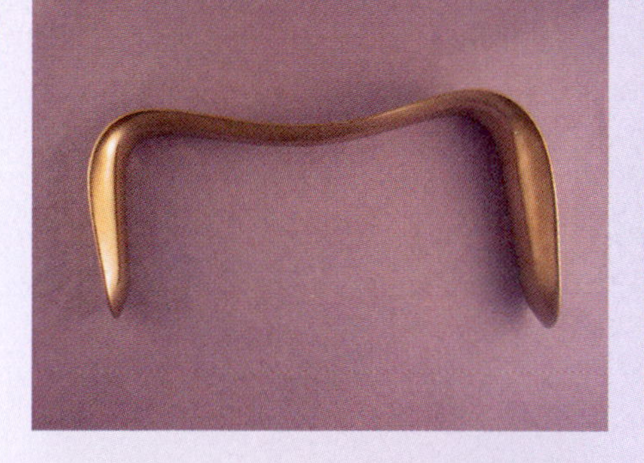
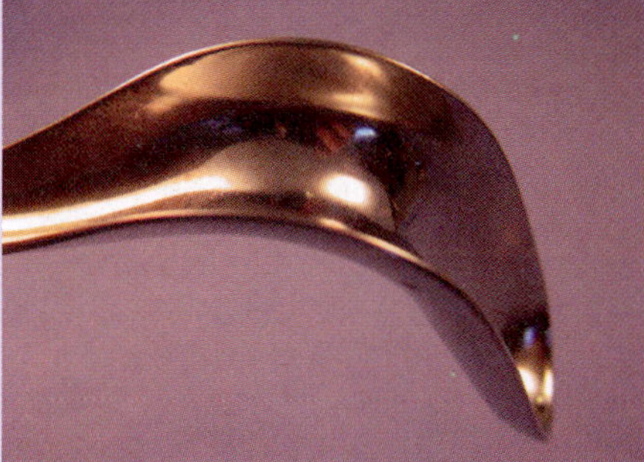

Name: Heaney retractor
Alias: none
Category: retracting
Use: retracting vaginal wall during vaginal hysterectomy
Length: 10"

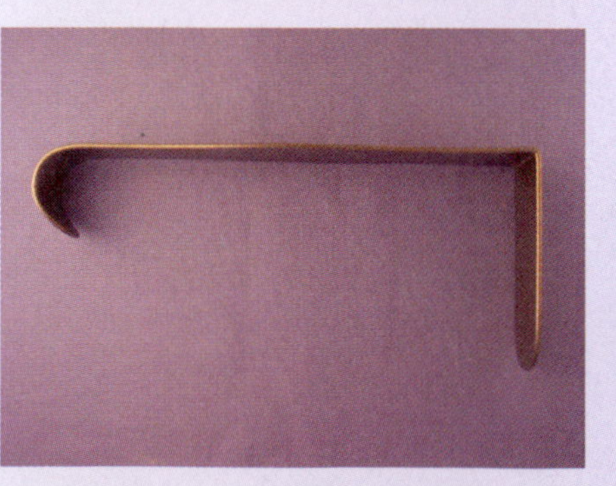
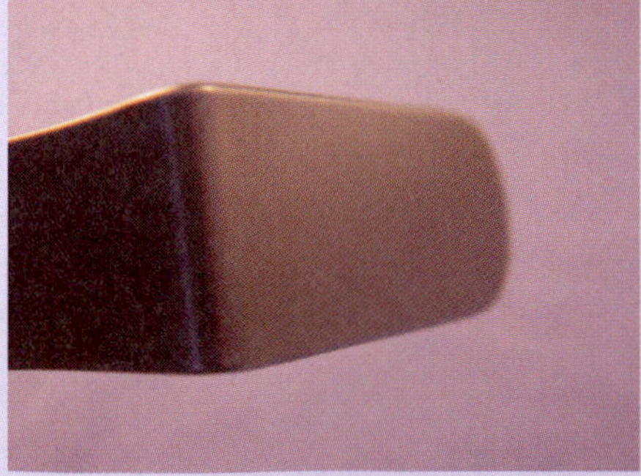

Name: Heaney-Simon retractor
Alias: none
Category: retracting
Use: retracting vaginal wall
Length: 10"
Additional Information: blade 1" wide by 5" long

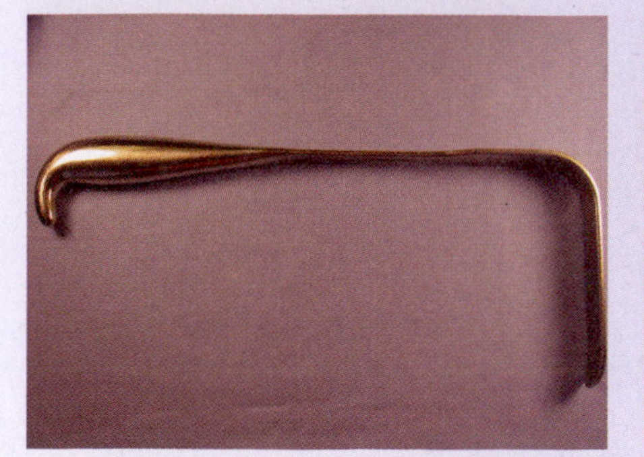
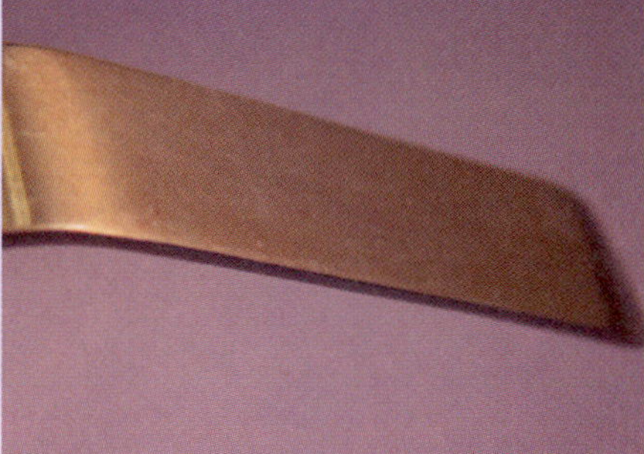

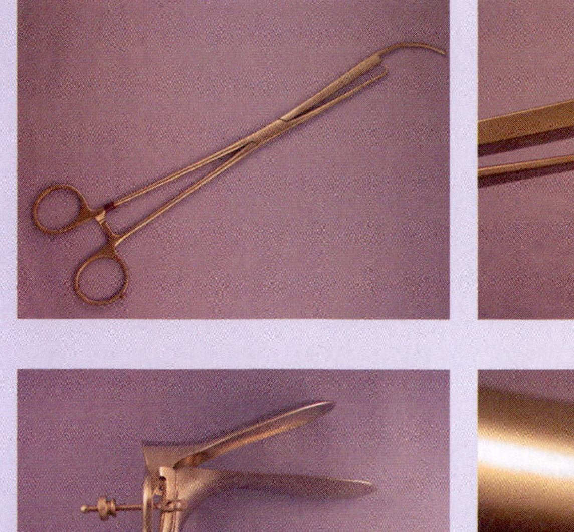

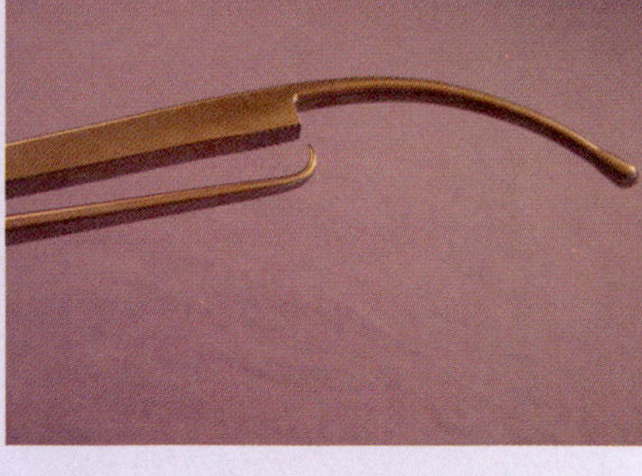

Name: Hulka manipulator

Alias: none
Category: grasping
Use: cervical/uterine measurement (sound); grasping cervix (tenaculum)
Length: 10.75"– 11.5"
Additional Information: combination of uterine sound and single tooth tenaculum

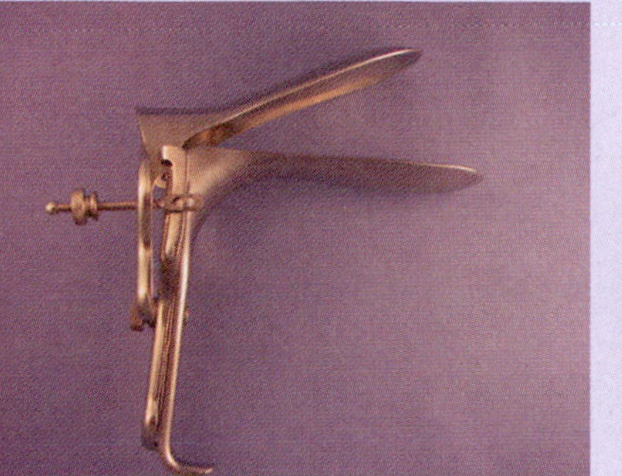

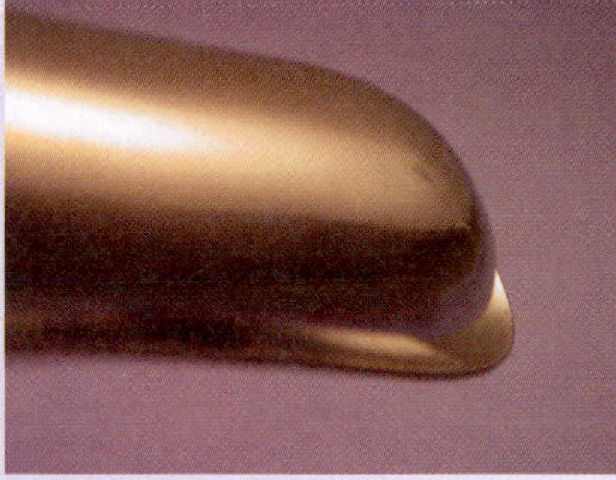

Name: Graves vaginal speculum

Alias: duckbill speculum
Category: retracting
Use: retracting vaginal wall
Length: n/a
Additional width: blade can be $\frac{1}{2}$" to 1.5"in width × and 3" to 4 $\frac{3}{4}$" in length

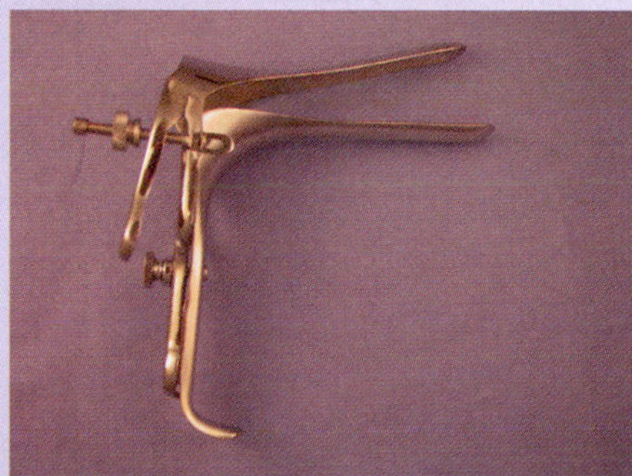

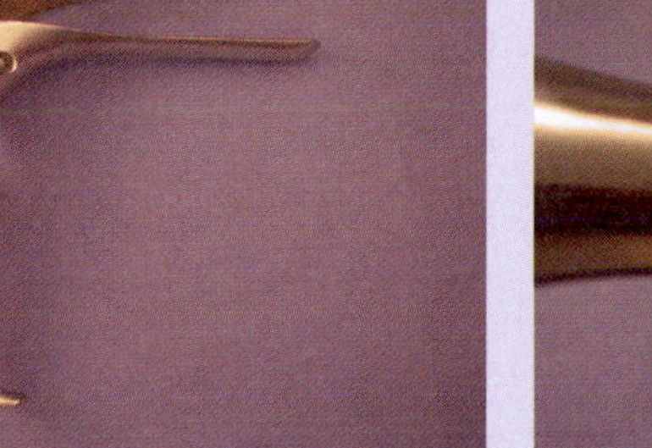

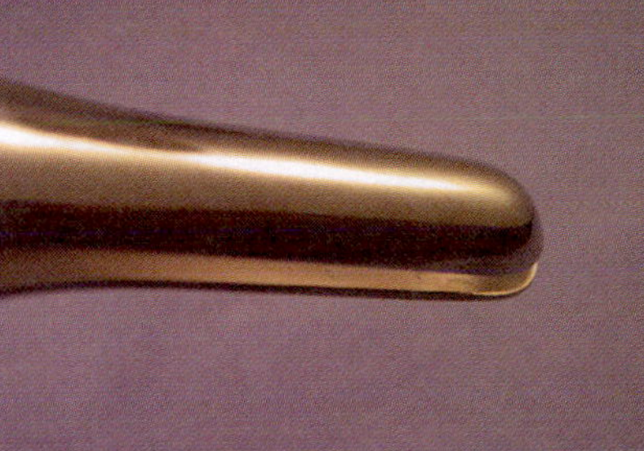

Name: Pederson vaginal speculum

Alias: none
Category: retracting
Use: retracting vaginal wall (narrow); often used for pediatric patients
Length: n/a
Additional Information: narrow; flat, small blades

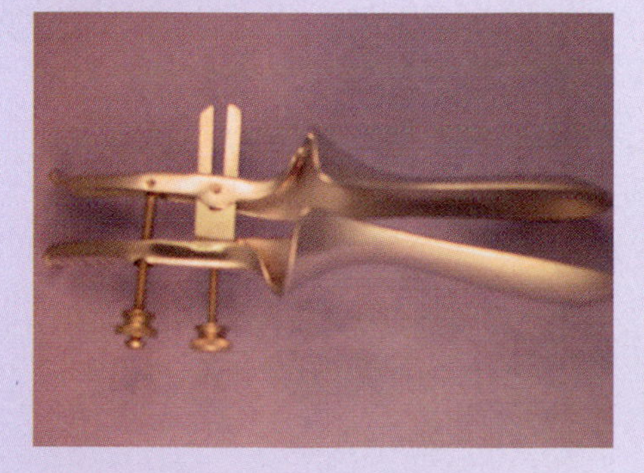

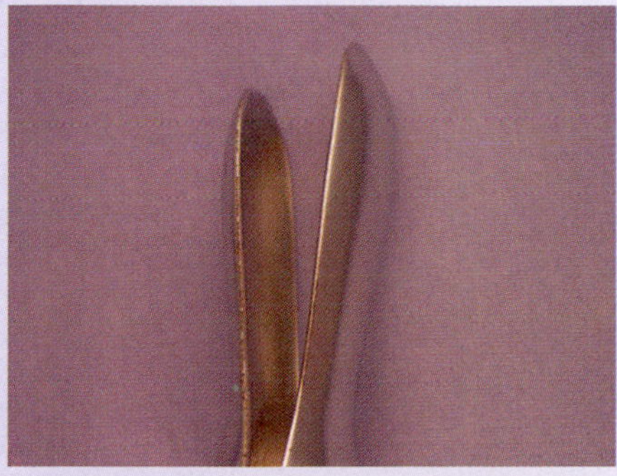

Name: side opening vaginal speculum

Alias: lateral speculum
Category: retracting
Use: retracting vaginal wall
Length: n/a
Additional Information: blades are 1 $\frac{1}{4}$" wide by 4" length

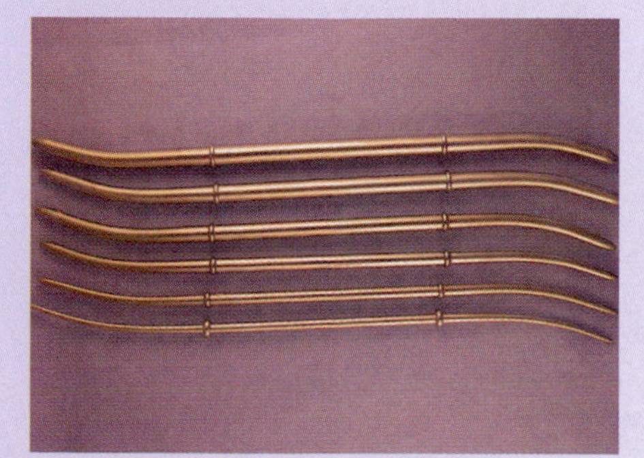

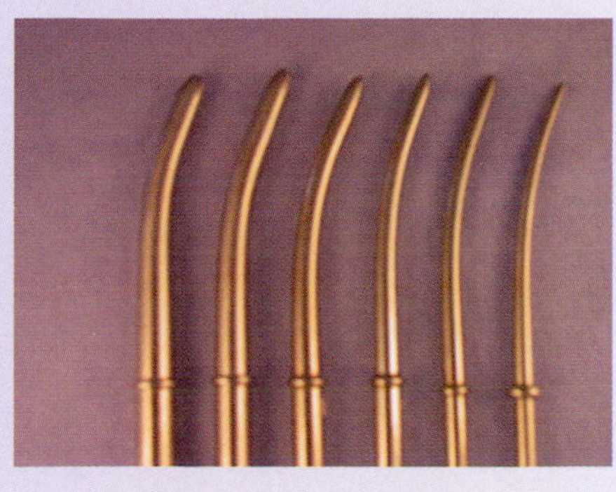

Name: Hank dilators

Alias: none
Category: dilating
Use: dilating cervix
Length: 10"
Additional Information: double ended; solid; have round "stop" on each end; numbered (9/10 Fr to 19/20 Fr); align on your back table by diameter, from smallest to largest

Name: Hegar dilators

Alias: none

Category: dilating

Use: dilating cervix

Length: 7.5"

Additional Information: double ended; hollow; numbered (3/4/Fr to 17/18 Fr); align on your back table by diameter, from smallest to largest

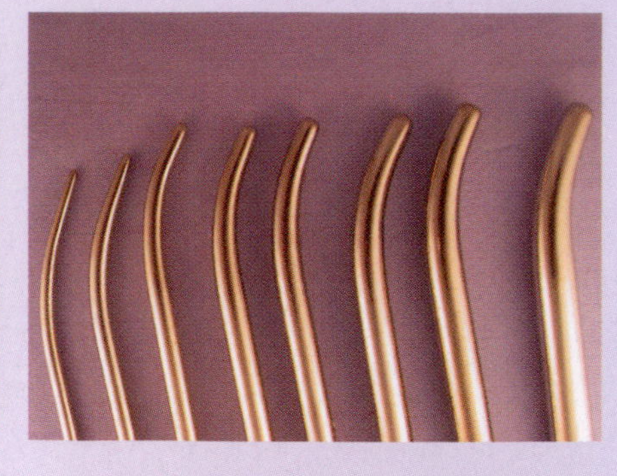

Name: Valtchev uterine mobilizer

Alias: none

Category: accessory

Use: manipulating uterus during surgery

Length: n/a

Additional Information: comes with multiple tips

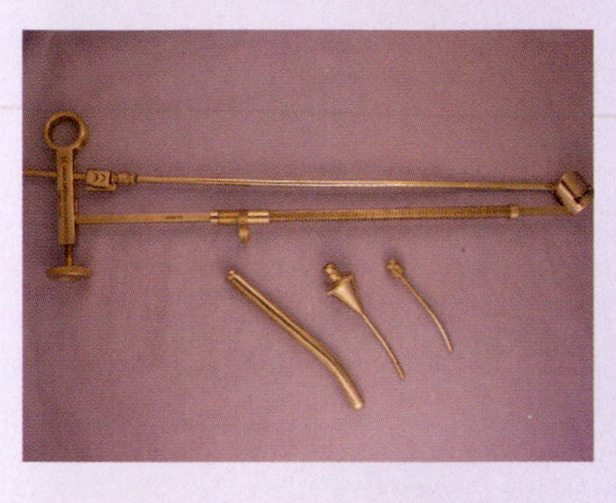

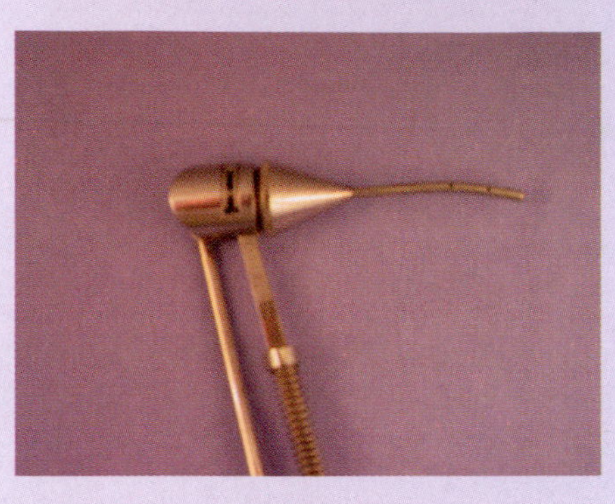

Name: Allis clamp

Alias: none

Category: grasping

Use: grasping organs or tissue that are being removed

Length: 6", 7.5", or 10"

Additional Information 2 X 3, 3 X 4, 4 × 5, 5 × 6 teeth; tips can be straight or angled

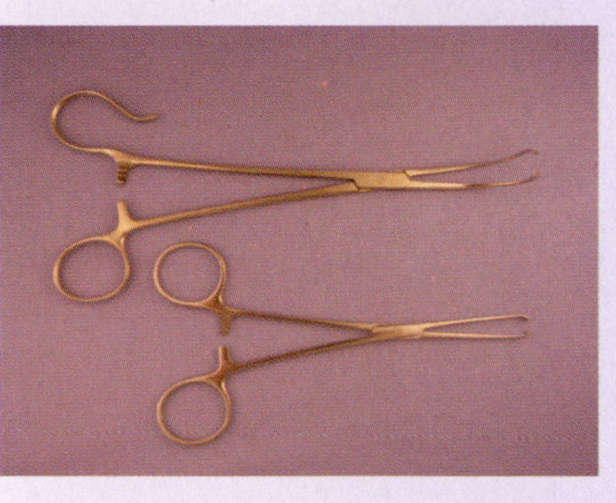

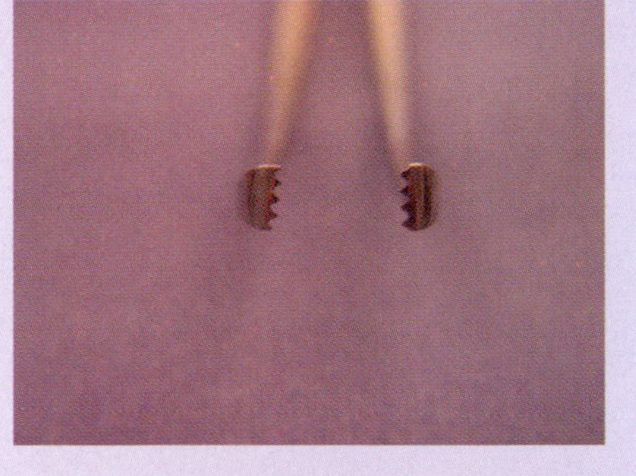

Name: Allis Adair clamp

Alias: T clamp

Category: grasping

Length: 6.5"

Use: grasping tissue

Additional Information: 9 × 10 teeth

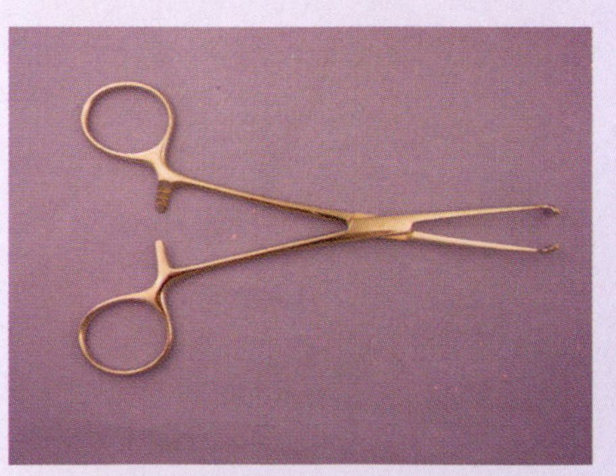

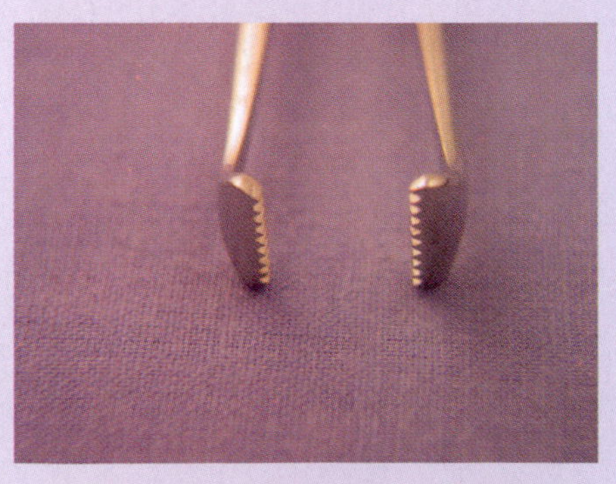

Name: Babcock

Alias: none

Category: grasping

Use: grasping delicate tissue (e.g., fallopian tube, bowel, vas deferens)

Length: 6", 7.5", or 9"

Additional Information: no teeth—atraumatic

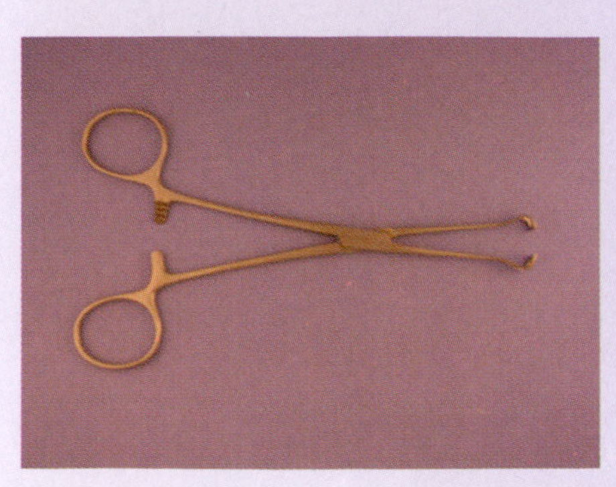

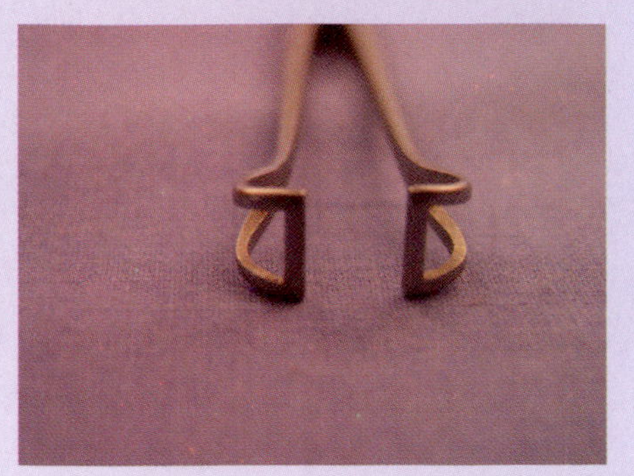

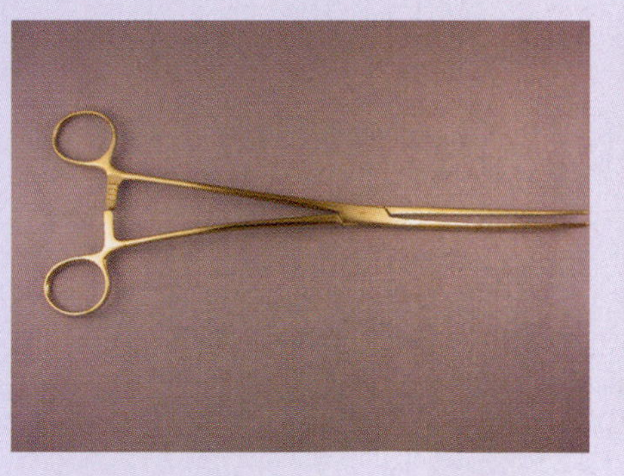
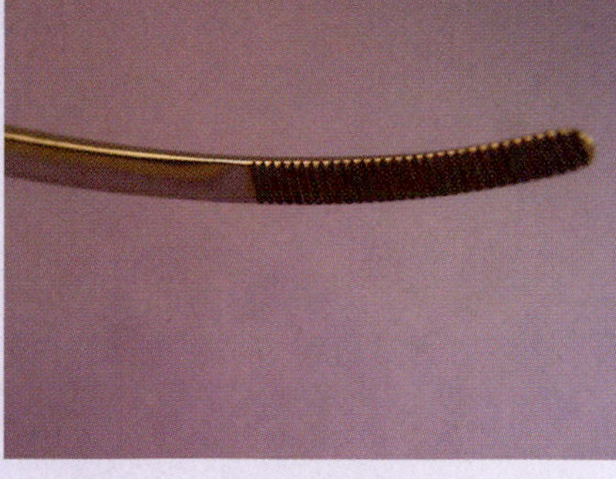

Name: Bozeman dressing forceps
Alias: none
Category: grasping
Use: applying dressing or vaginal packing
Length: 10.5"
Additional Information: double curved

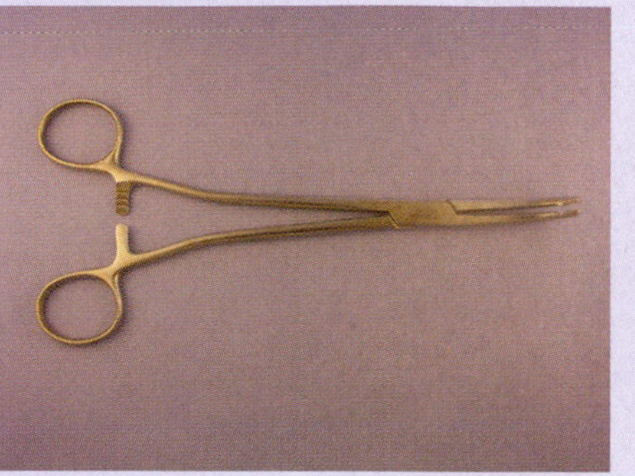

Name: Heaney hysterectomy forceps
Alias: none
Category: clamping
Use: heavy tissue occlusion
Length: 8.25"
Additional Information: longitudinal serrations; single- or double-toothed blade; curved or straight blades

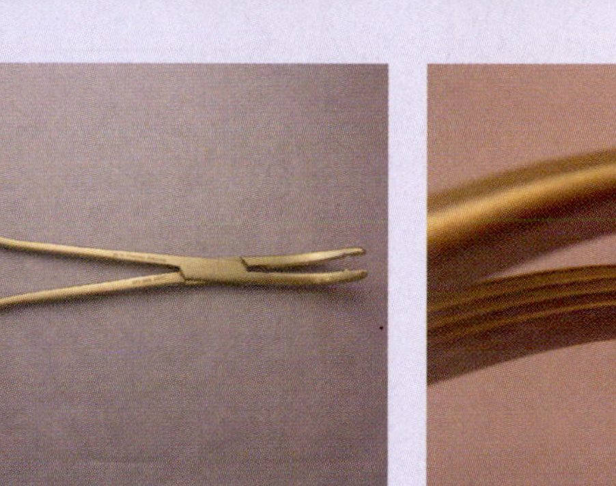
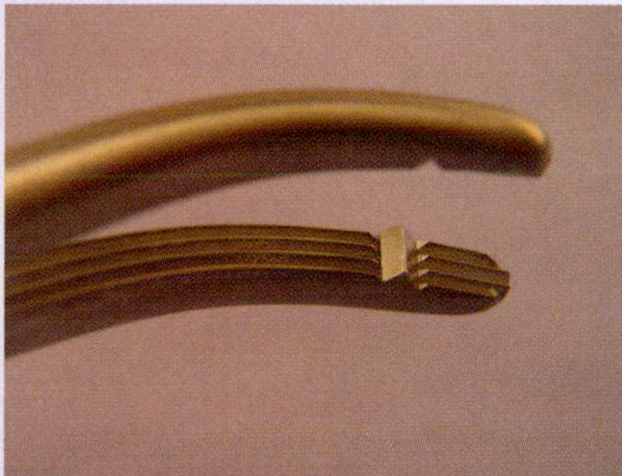

Name: Heaney-Ballentine hysterectomy forceps
Alias: none
Category: clamping
Use: clamping tissue or pedicles during a hysterectomy
Length: 8.5"
Additional Information: curved jaws: 1 X 2 teeth; vertical grooves

Name: Kocher
Alias: Ochsner; Rochester-Ochsner
Category: grasping
Use: grasping heavy tissue (e.g., fascia)
Length: 5.5", 6.25", 7", 8", 9",10"
Additional Information: 1 × 2 teeth

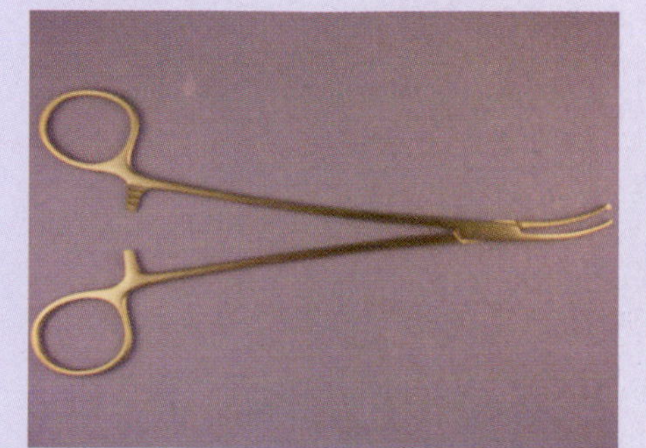
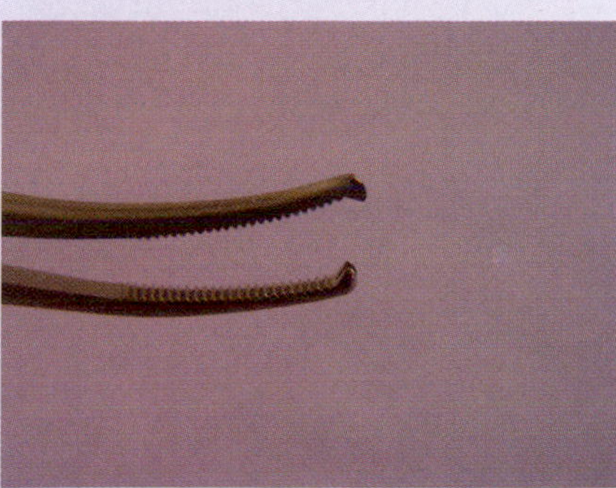

Name: Mikulicz peritoneum forcep
Alias: dandy
Category: grasping
Use: grasping of peritoneum
Length: 7.25"
Additional Information: 1 × 2 teeth

Name: Phaneuf hysterectomy forceps

Alias: none

Category: grasping

Use: grasping heavy tissue during hysterectomy

Length: 8.25" (straight jaw) or 8.5" (angled jaw)

Additional Information: 1 × 2 teeth; jaws can be straight or angled

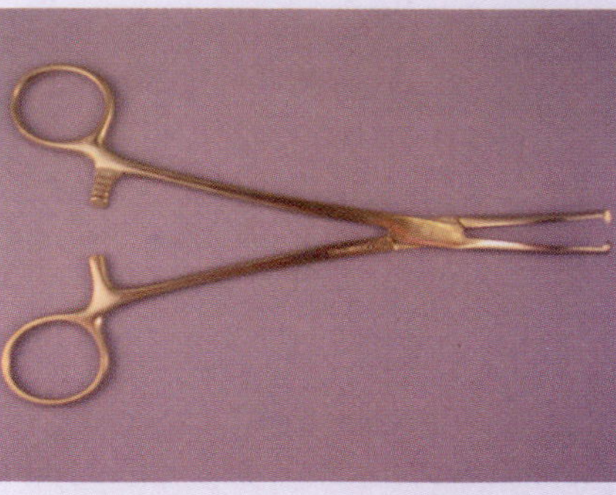

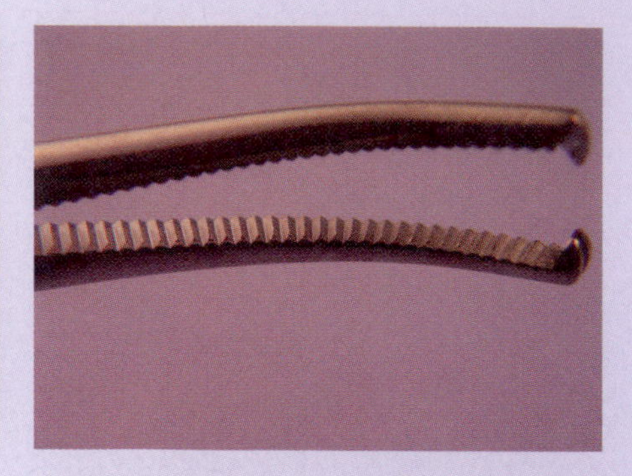

Name: Jacob's uterine vulsellum forcep

Alias: Jacob's heavy tenaculum

Category: grasping

Use: grasping uterus during a hysterectomy

Length: 8.25"

Additional Information: 2 × 2 sharp teeth; can be straight or curved on the side

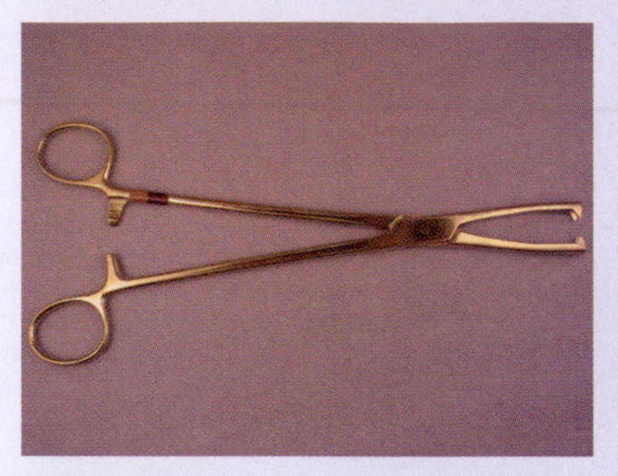

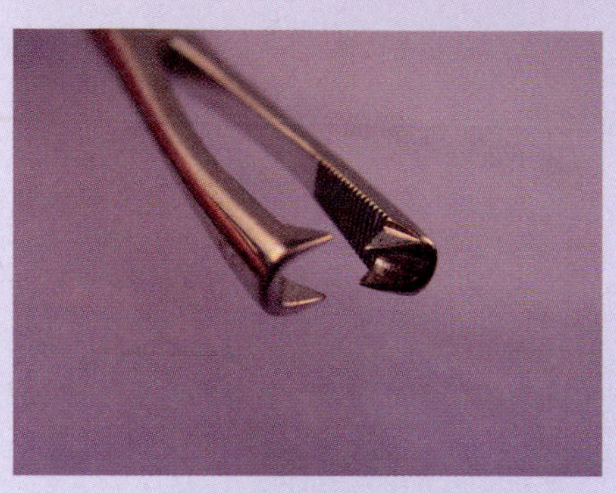

Name: Thoms-Gaylor biopsy punch

Alias: Gaylor biopsy punch

Category: cutting

Length: 9"

Use: obtaining biopsy specimens

Additional Information: angled, sharp jaws

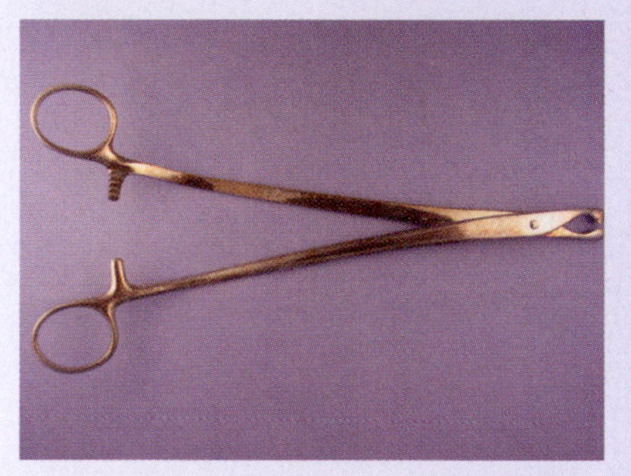

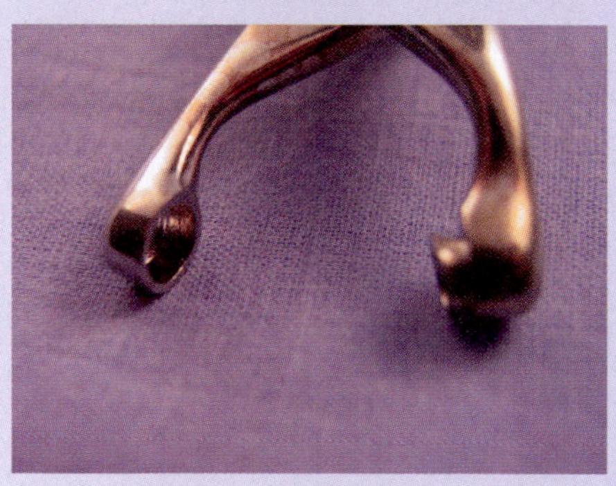

Name: Lahey traction forceps

Alias: tenaculum; Lahey thyroid clamp

Category: grasping

Use: grasping tissue being removed, such as the uterus

Length: 6"

Additional Information: 3 × 3 teeth;

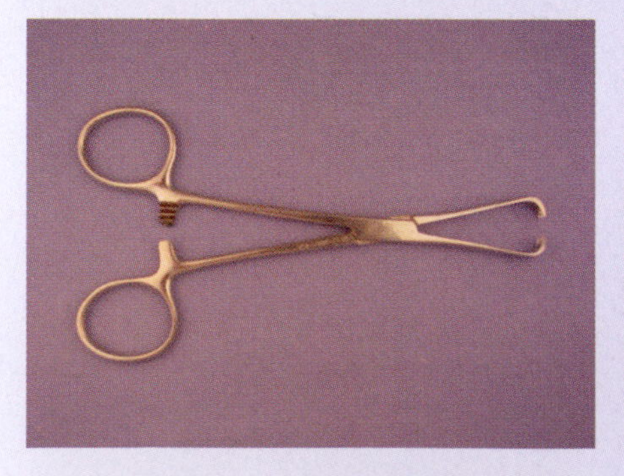

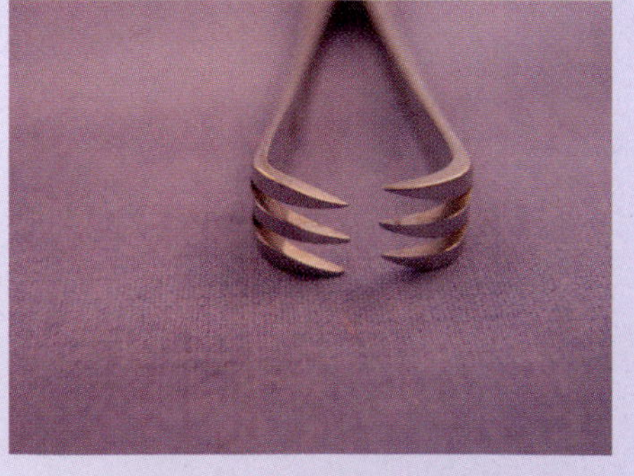

Name: Braun tenaculum

Alias: tenaculum; Schoeder

Category: grasping

Use: grasping cervix; applying traction to the uterus

Length: 9 ½" or 10"

Additional Information: single or double toothed; straight or curved

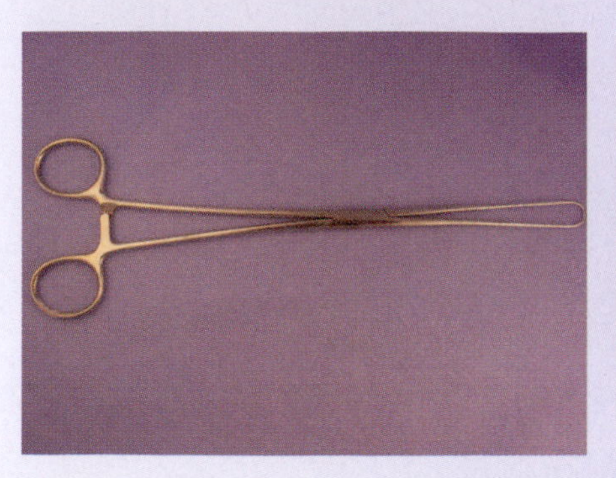

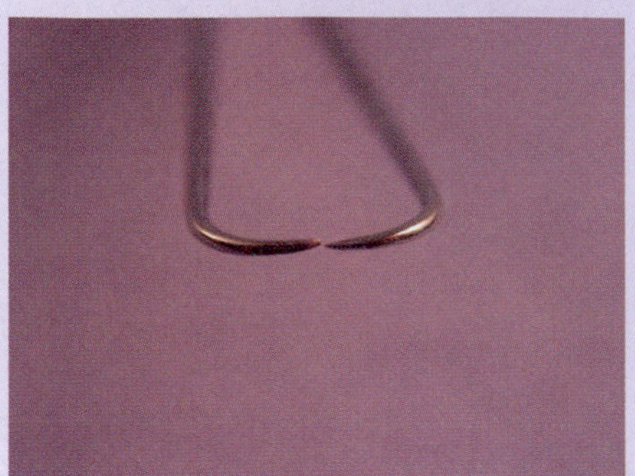

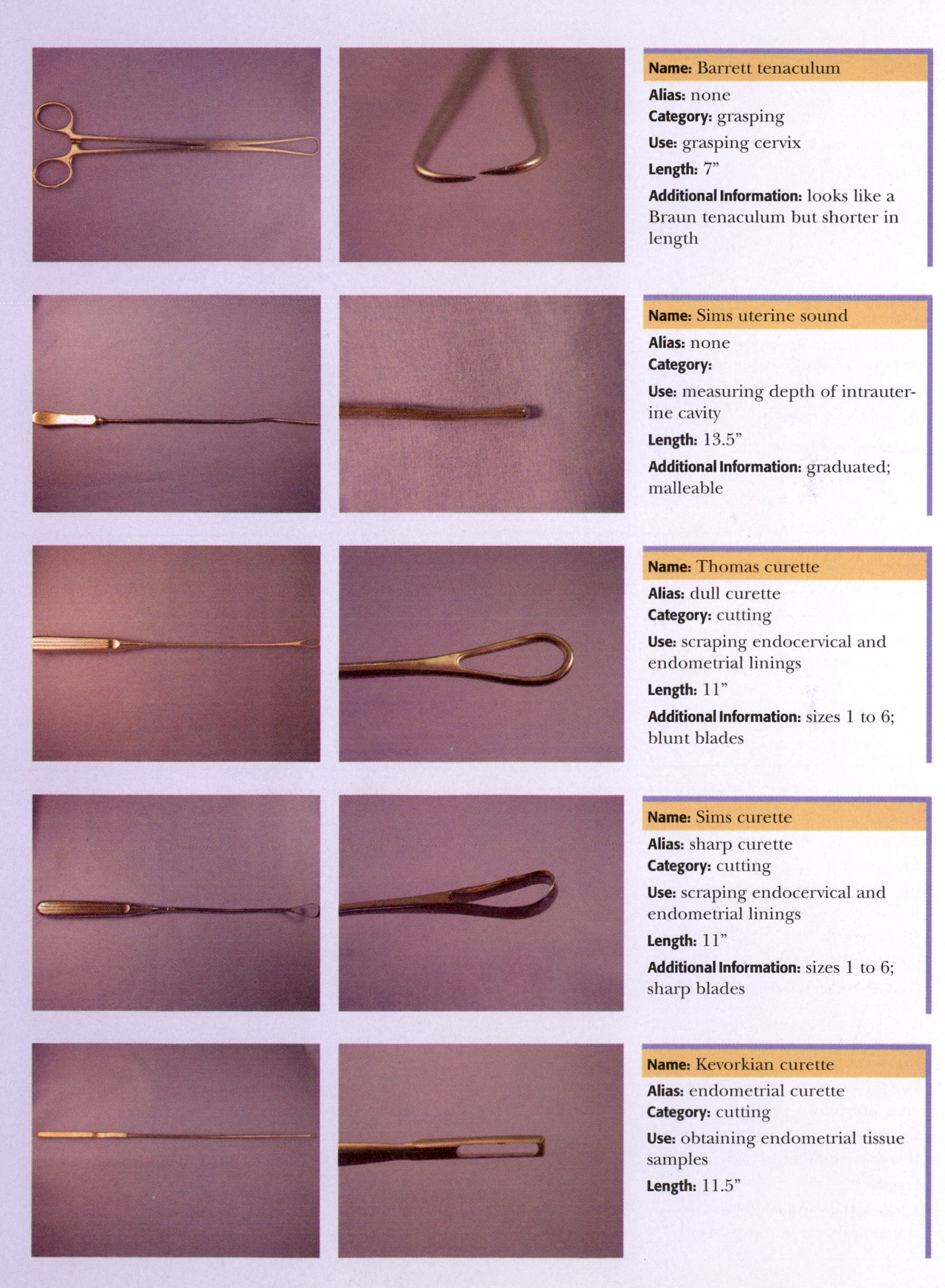

Name: Barrett tenaculum
Alias: none
Category: grasping
Use: grasping cervix
Length: 7"
Additional Information: looks like a Braun tenaculum but shorter in length

Name: Sims uterine sound
Alias: none
Category:
Use: measuring depth of intrauterine cavity
Length: 13.5"
Additional Information: graduated; malleable

Name: Thomas curette
Alias: dull curette
Category: cutting
Use: scraping endocervical and endometrial linings
Length: 11"
Additional Information: sizes 1 to 6; blunt blades

Name: Sims curette
Alias: sharp curette
Category: cutting
Use: scraping endocervical and endometrial linings
Length: 11"
Additional Information: sizes 1 to 6; sharp blades

Name: Kevorkian curette
Alias: endometrial curette
Category: cutting
Use: obtaining endometrial tissue samples
Length: 11.5"

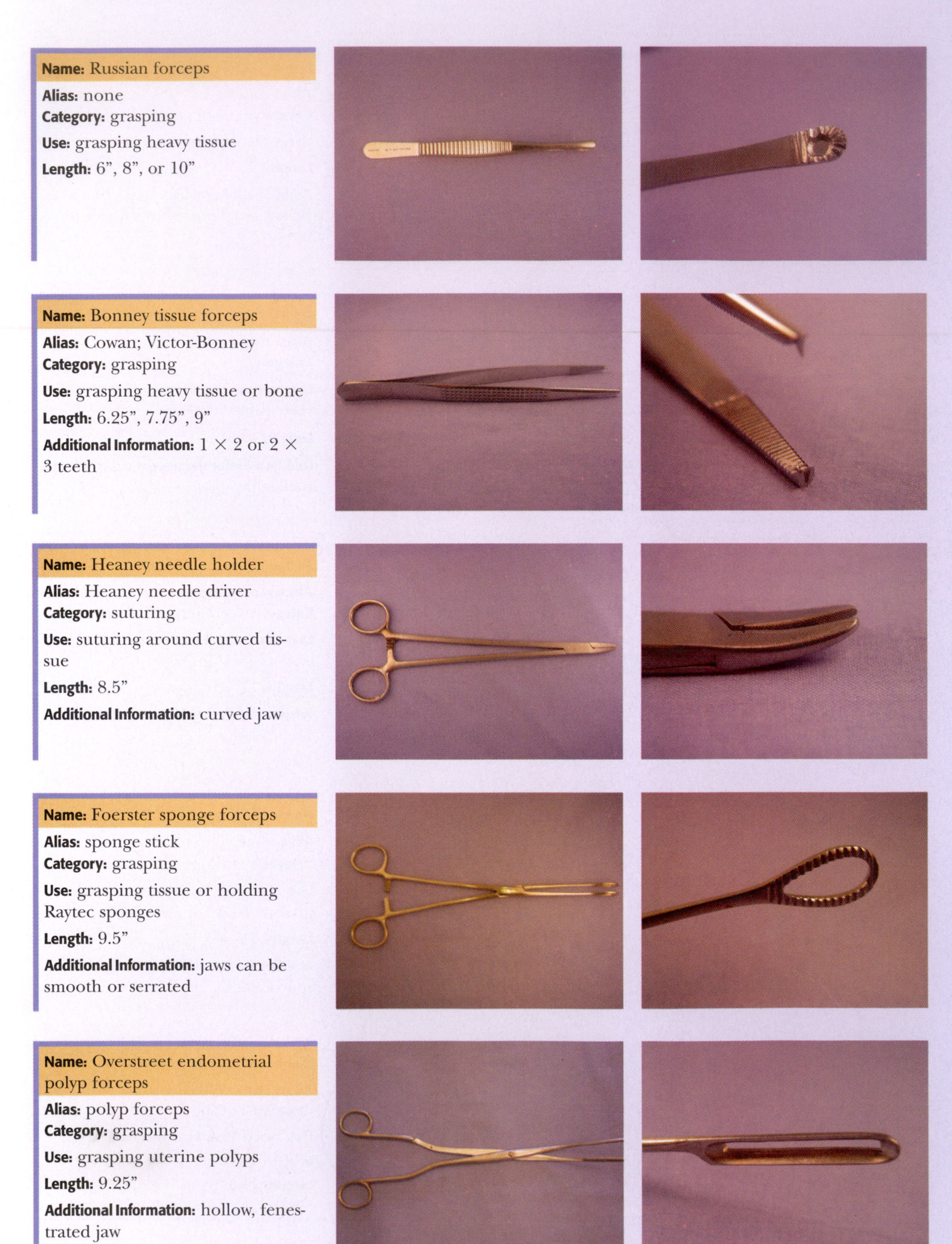

Name: Russian forceps
Alias: none
Category: grasping
Use: grasping heavy tissue
Length: 6", 8", or 10"

Name: Bonney tissue forceps
Alias: Cowan; Victor-Bonney
Category: grasping
Use: grasping heavy tissue or bone
Length: 6.25", 7.75", 9"
Additional Information: 1 × 2 or 2 × 3 teeth

Name: Heaney needle holder
Alias: Heaney needle driver
Category: suturing
Use: suturing around curved tissue
Length: 8.5"
Additional Information: curved jaw

Name: Foerster sponge forceps
Alias: sponge stick
Category: grasping
Use: grasping tissue or holding Raytec sponges
Length: 9.5"
Additional Information: jaws can be smooth or serrated

Name: Overstreet endometrial polyp forceps
Alias: polyp forceps
Category: grasping
Use: grasping uterine polyps
Length: 9.25"
Additional Information: hollow, fenestrated jaw

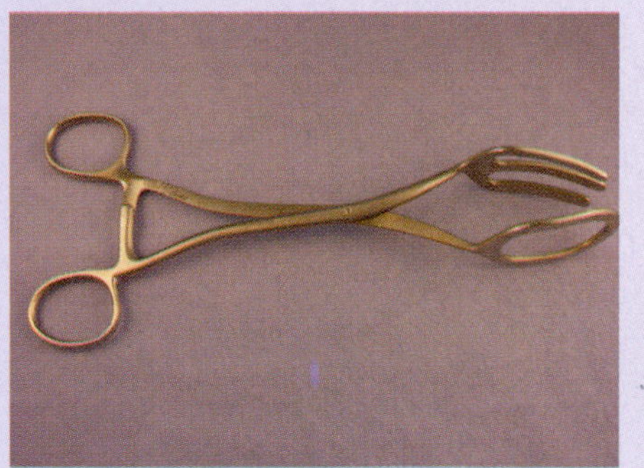
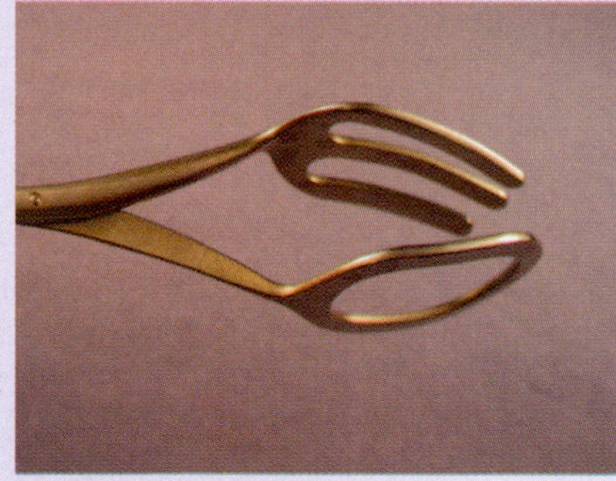

Name: Barrett-Allen uterine elevating forceps
Alias: fork and spoon
Category: grasping
Use: grasping uterus and lifting it out of the way
Length: 8.5”
Additional Information: curved

Name: Lister scissors (large)
Alias: bandage scissors
Category: cutting
Use: opening uterus during cesarean section
Length: 7.5”
Additional Information: guarded blade to protect baby when cutting the uterus

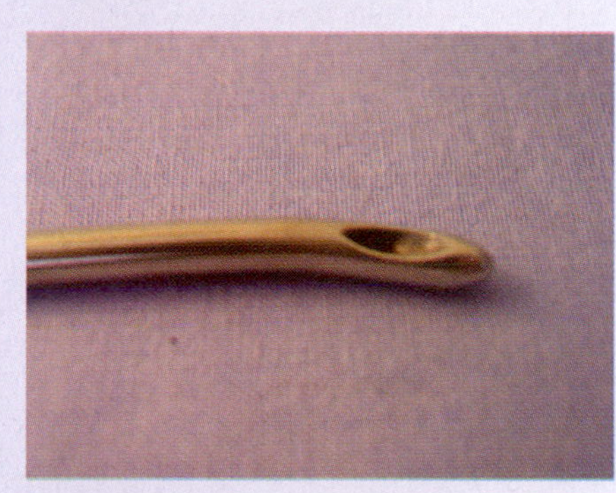

Name: Rubin catheter
Alias: female catheter
Category: accessory
Use: catheterizing female bladder
Length: 6.5”
Additional Information: available in sizes 10 Fr to 18 Fr

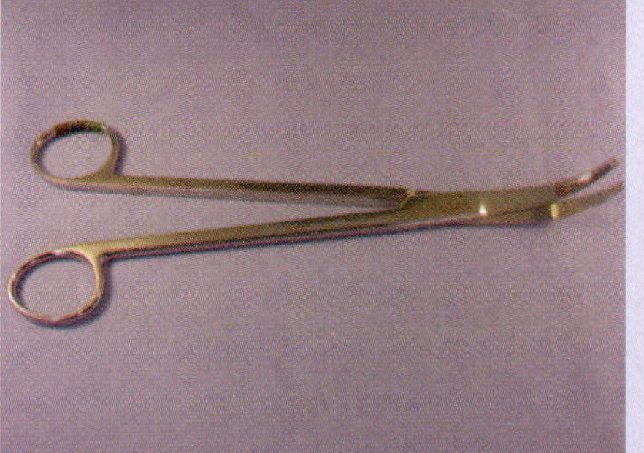
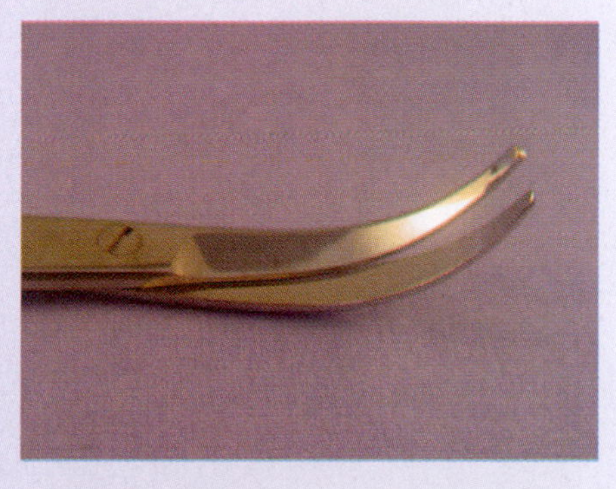

Name: Jorgenson scissors
Alias: none
Category: cutting
Use: cutting heavy tissue
Length: 9”
Additional Information: curved blades

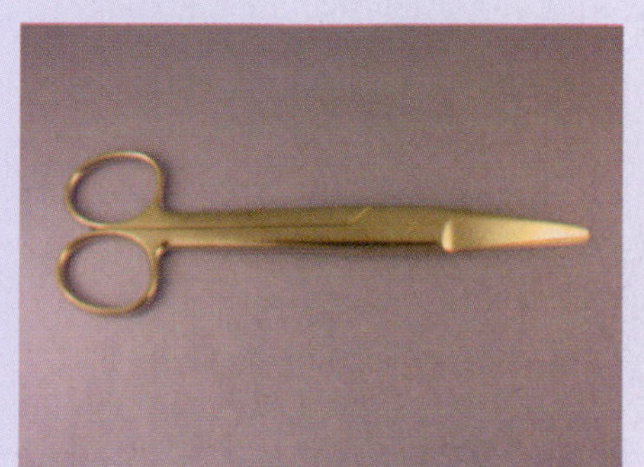
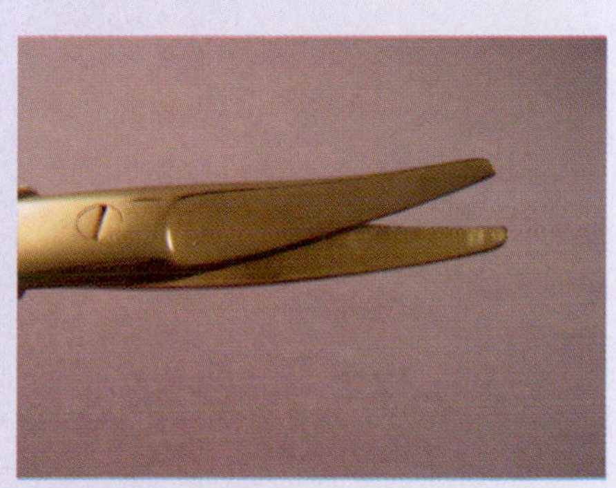

Name: Mayo-Noble scissors
Alias: none
Category: cutting
Use: dissecting heavy tissue
Length: 6.5”
Additional Information: blades can be straight or curved; blunt tips

Q&A

Surgical Session—OB-GYN Instruments

1) You are second scrubbing a cesarean section. The surgeon has reached the bladder and you need to retract it out of the way. Which retractor will you use?
   a. Heaney
   b. DeLee
   c. Sims
   d. U.S. Army
2) The surgeon is performing a D & C. He/she wants to measure the depth of the intrauterine cavity. The instrument you hand him/her is a:
   a. Sims curette
   b. Thomas curette
   c. Sims sound
   d. Goodell
3) During a hysterectomy, the surgeon asks for a "T-clamp." Another name for this instrument is:
   a. Allis
   b. Allis-Adair
   c. Heaney
   d. Heaney-Ballentine
4) You are setting up for an abdominal hysterectomy. You know that once the surgeon enters the peritoneum, he/she will want to have a self-retaining retractor to expose the abdominal/pelvic cavity. Which instrument do you need to make sure you have?
   a. Heaney retractor
   b. Sims retractor
   c. Ribbon retractor
   d. O'Sullivan-O'Connor retractor
5) The surgeon is performing a D & C. He/she asks for the curettes with the *sharp blades*. Which curette do you hand to him/her?
   a. Sims
   b. Thomas
   c. Hegar
   d. Hank
6) A type of endocervical curette is a:
   a. Heaney
   b. Kevorkian
   c. Masterson
   d. Hegar
7) A type of obstetrical forceps used to deliver an infant is a:
   a. Russian
   b. Simpson
   c. Bozeman
   d. Bonney
8) The surgery is completed and you are applying a dressing. The __________ is a type of dressing forceps.
   a. Braun
   b. Schoeder
   c. Bozeman
   d. Simpson
9) Another name for a *weighted* vaginal speculum is a(n):
   a. Graves
   b. Auvard
   c. Pederson
   d. Goodell
10) During a D & C, the surgeon asks for a tenaculum to grasp the cervix. You would hand a(n):
   a. Braun
   b. Bozeman
   c. Allis-Adair
   d. Goodell
11) The surgeon is performing a hysterectomy and needs to suture around a ligament. Which needle holder has an angled tip to facilitate use around structures?
   a. Mayo-Hegar
   b. Heaney
   c. Castroviejo
   d. Crile-Wood
12) During an open tubal ligation, which instrument would be used to grasp or control the fallopian tubes?
   a. Kocher
   b. Kelly
   c. Babcock
   d. Lahey
13) The surgeon is performing a diagnostic laparoscopy. The name of the needle used to insert the carbon dioxide gas into the abdomen is:

a. Verres
b. Steinmann
c. Kirschner
d. Sims

14) A type of cauterizing grasper used during laparoscopic surgery is a:
a. Kevorkian
b. Schubert
c. Kleppinger
d. Wittner

15) During a vaginal hysterectomy, all of the following are hand held retractors that could be used *except:*
a. Sims
b. Heaney
c. Heaney Simon
d. O'Sullivan-O'Connor

16) You are scrubbed on an abdominal hysterectomy. The surgeon requests an instrument to grasp the fallopian tube. The tube is *not* being removed. You would hand the surgeon a:
a. Kocher
b. Babcock
c. Lahey
d. Braun

Urology Instruments 3

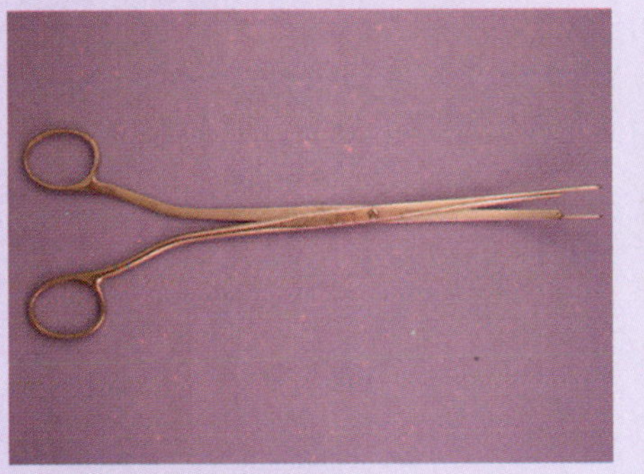

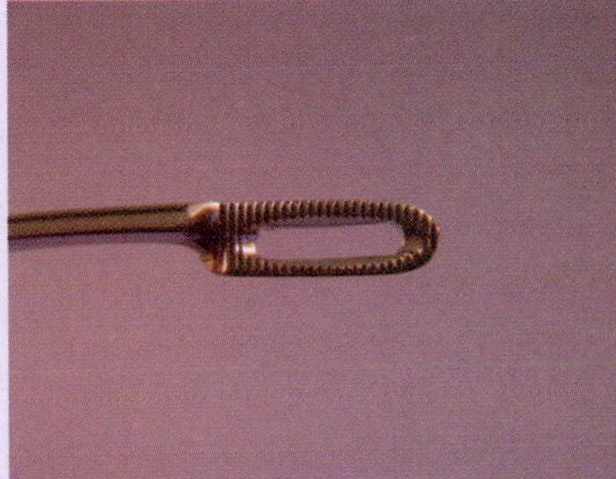

Name: Randall forceps
Alias: kidney stone forceps
Category: grasping
Use: grasping stones or polyps
Length: 9"
Additional Information: curved or straight jaws

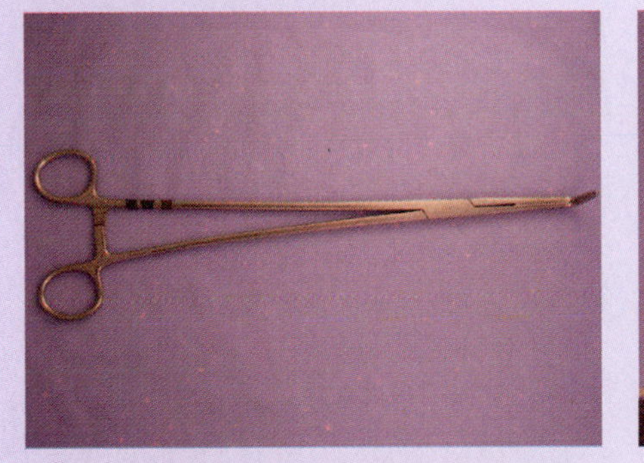

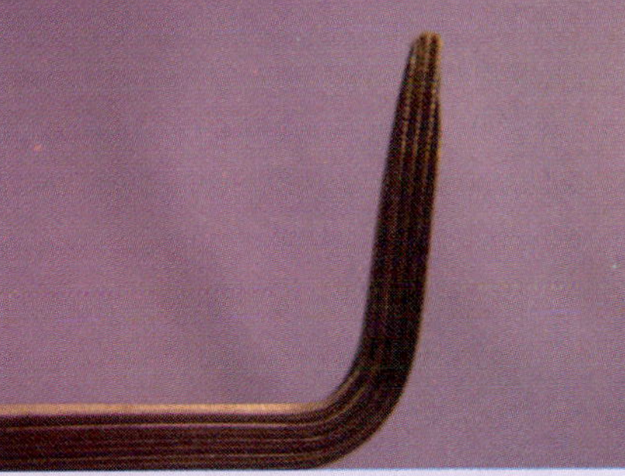

Name: Rochester mixter
Alias: none
Category: clamping
Use: clamping heavy tissue
Length: 10" to 12"
Additional Information: full curve jaws; vertical serrations

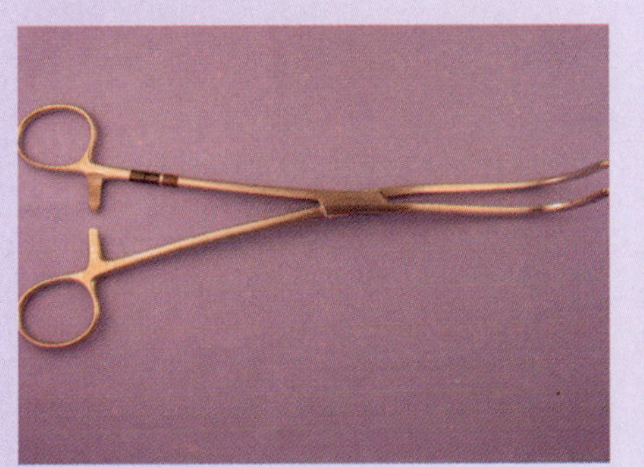

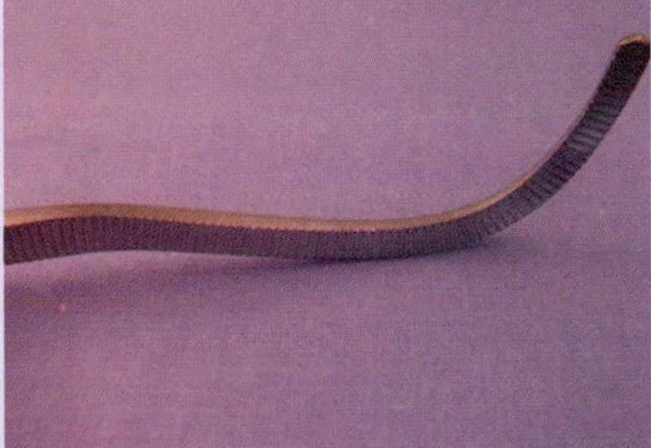

Name: Mayo-Guyon clamp
Alias: kidney clamp
Category: clamping
Use: clamping heavy tissue or organs
Length: 9.25"
Additional Information: heavy jaws; horizontal serrations

Name: McDougal pedicle clamp

Alias: none

Category: clamping

Use: clamping heavy tissue or pedicles

Length: 9.5"

Additional Information: full double curve

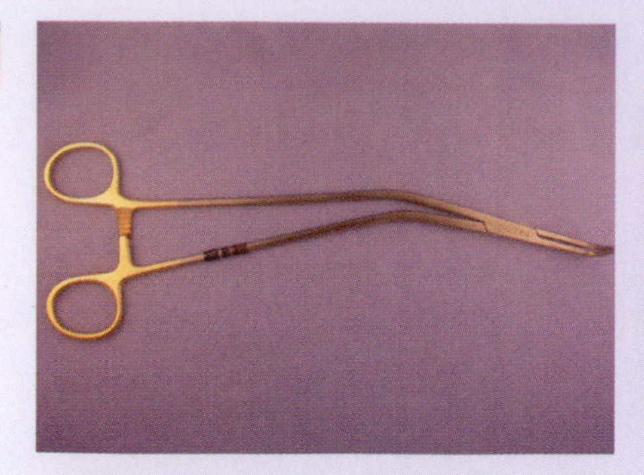

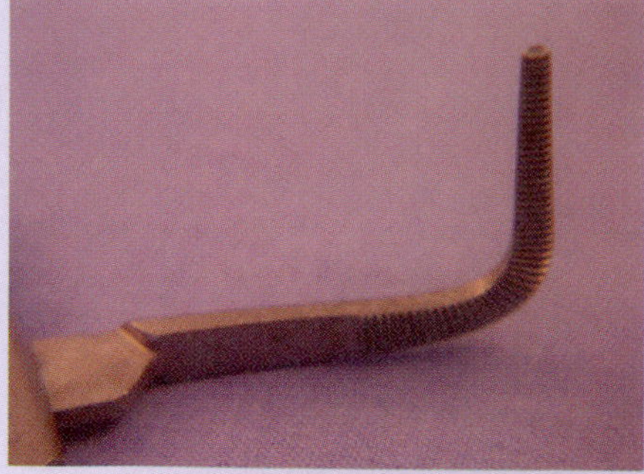

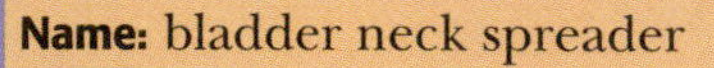

Name: bladder neck spreader

Alias: None

Category: retracting

Use: spreading and retracting bladder neck

Length: n/a

Additional Information: smooth jaws

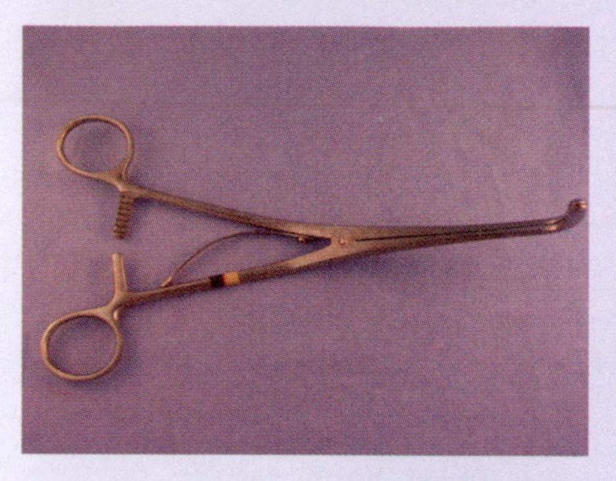

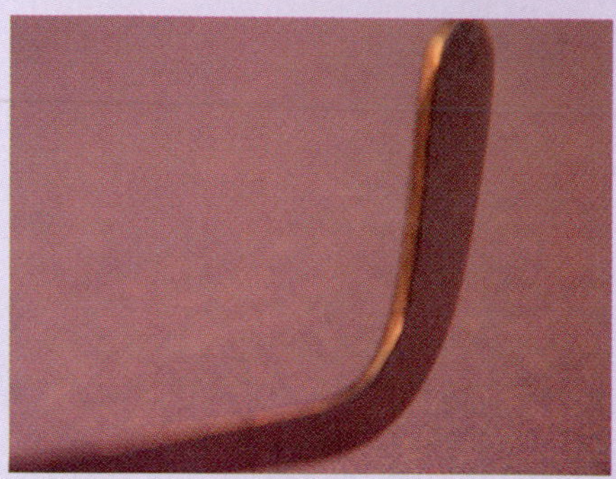

Name: Cushing vein retractor

Alias: none

Category: retracting

Use: retracting blood vessels

Length: 8" or 12"

Additional Information: open handle

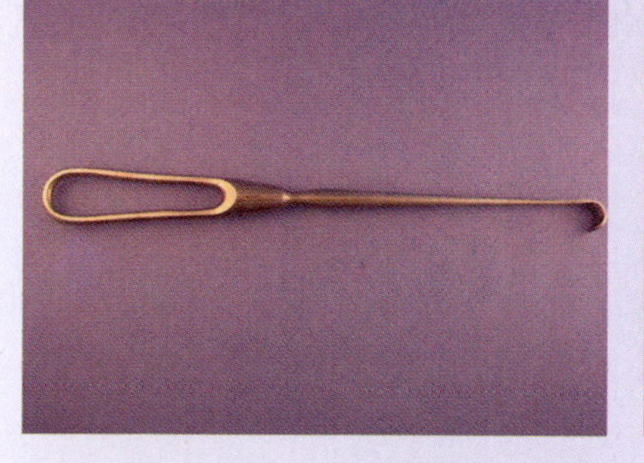

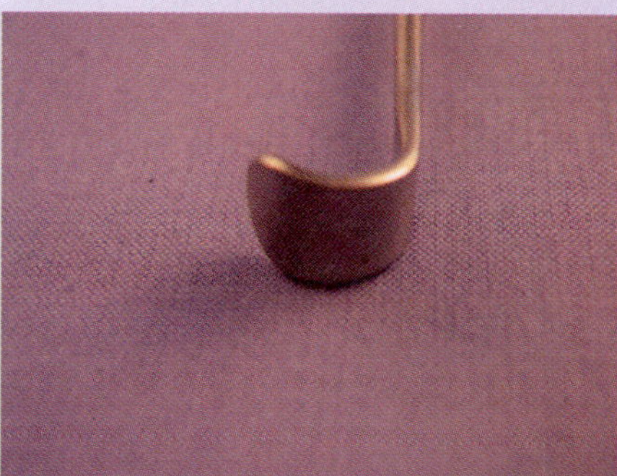

Name: Dandy nerve hook

Alias: none

Category: retracting

Use: retracting nerves

Length: 8.5"

Additional Information: blunt tip; tip can be pointed straight, left, or right

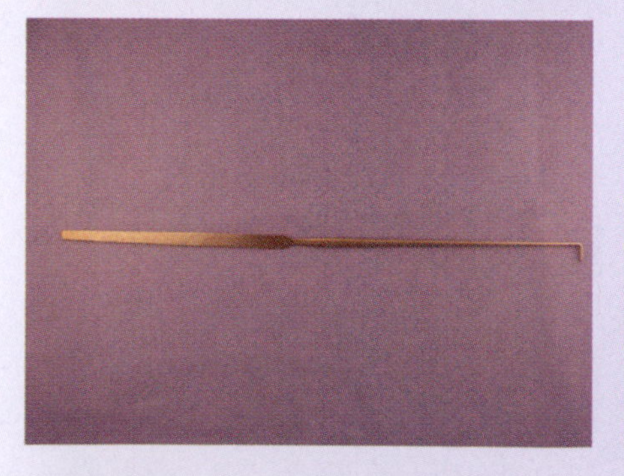

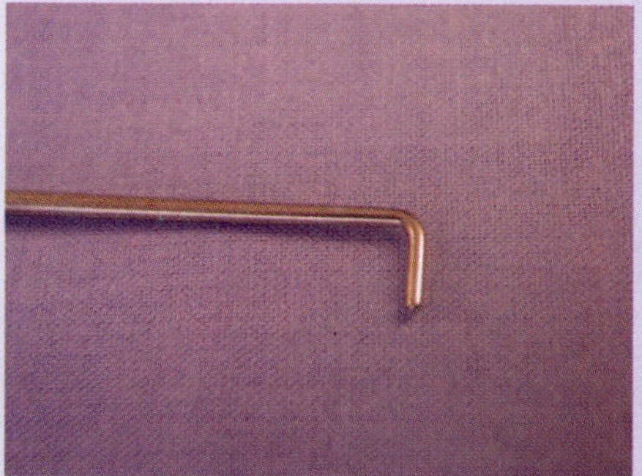

Name: catheter guide

Alias: Mandrin

Category: accessory

Use: inserting catheter

Length: n/a

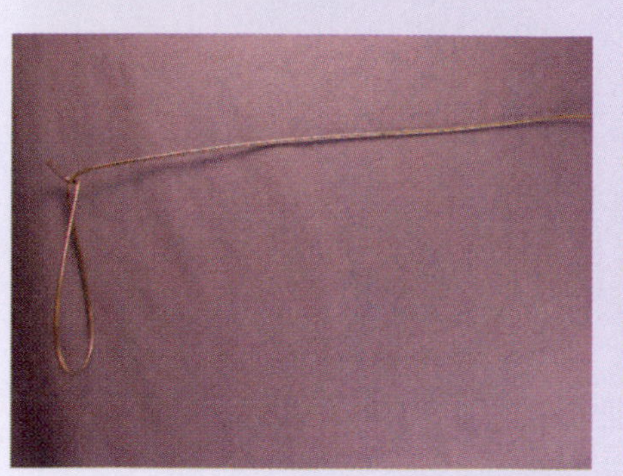

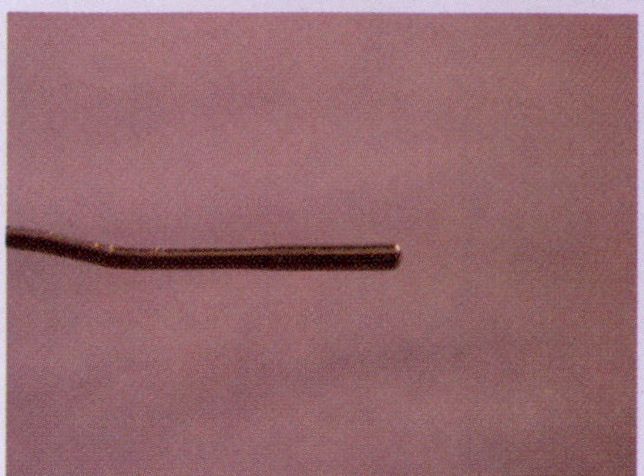

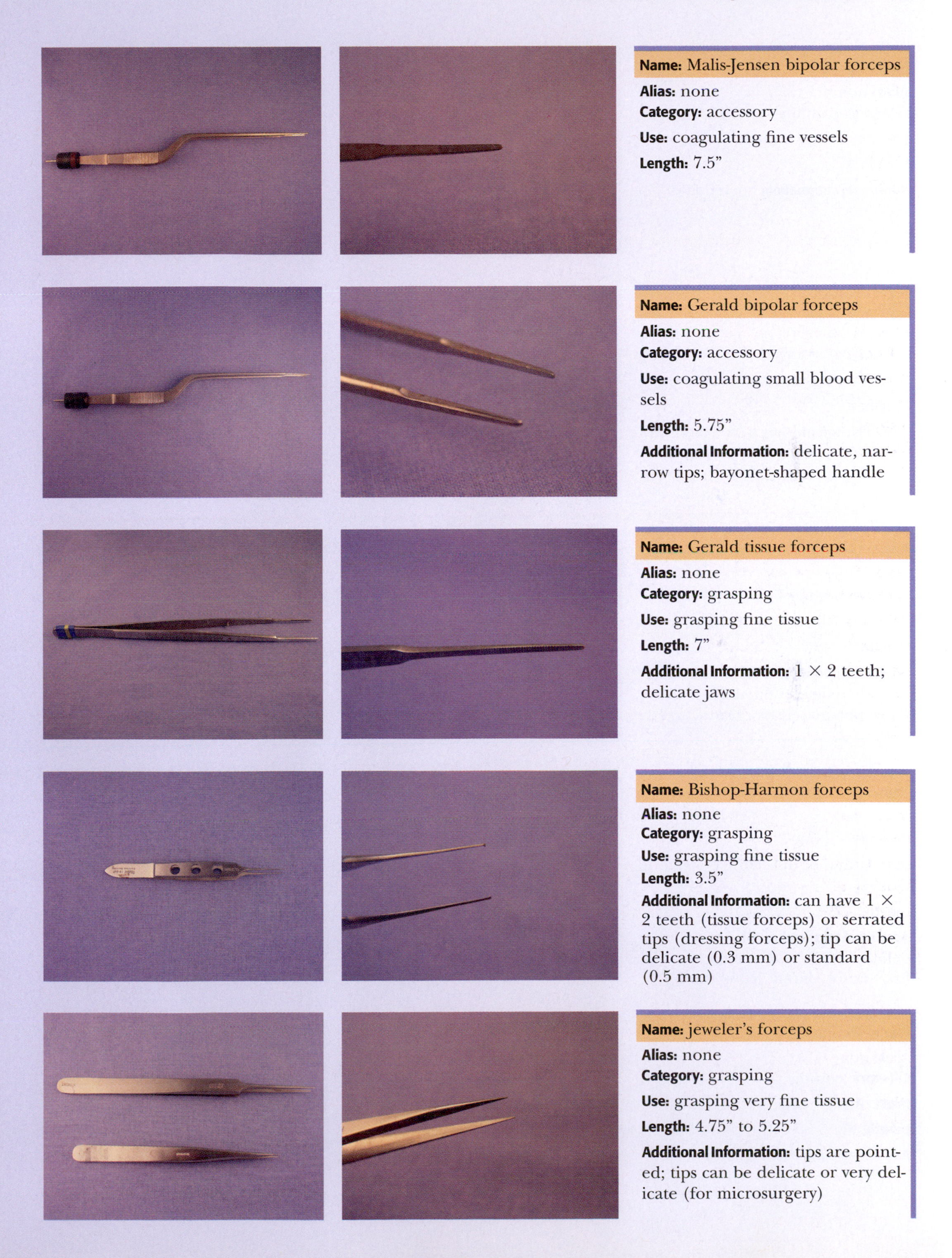

Name: Malis-Jensen bipolar forceps
Alias: none
Category: accessory
Use: coagulating fine vessels
Length: 7.5"

Name: Gerald bipolar forceps
Alias: none
Category: accessory
Use: coagulating small blood vessels
Length: 5.75"
Additional Information: delicate, narrow tips; bayonet-shaped handle

Name: Gerald tissue forceps
Alias: none
Category: grasping
Use: grasping fine tissue
Length: 7"
Additional Information: 1 × 2 teeth; delicate jaws

Name: Bishop-Harmon forceps
Alias: none
Category: grasping
Use: grasping fine tissue
Length: 3.5"
Additional Information: can have 1 × 2 teeth (tissue forceps) or serrated tips (dressing forceps); tip can be delicate (0.3 mm) or standard (0.5 mm)

Name: jeweler's forceps
Alias: none
Category: grasping
Use: grasping very fine tissue
Length: 4.75" to 5.25"
Additional Information: tips are pointed; tips can be delicate or very delicate (for microsurgery)

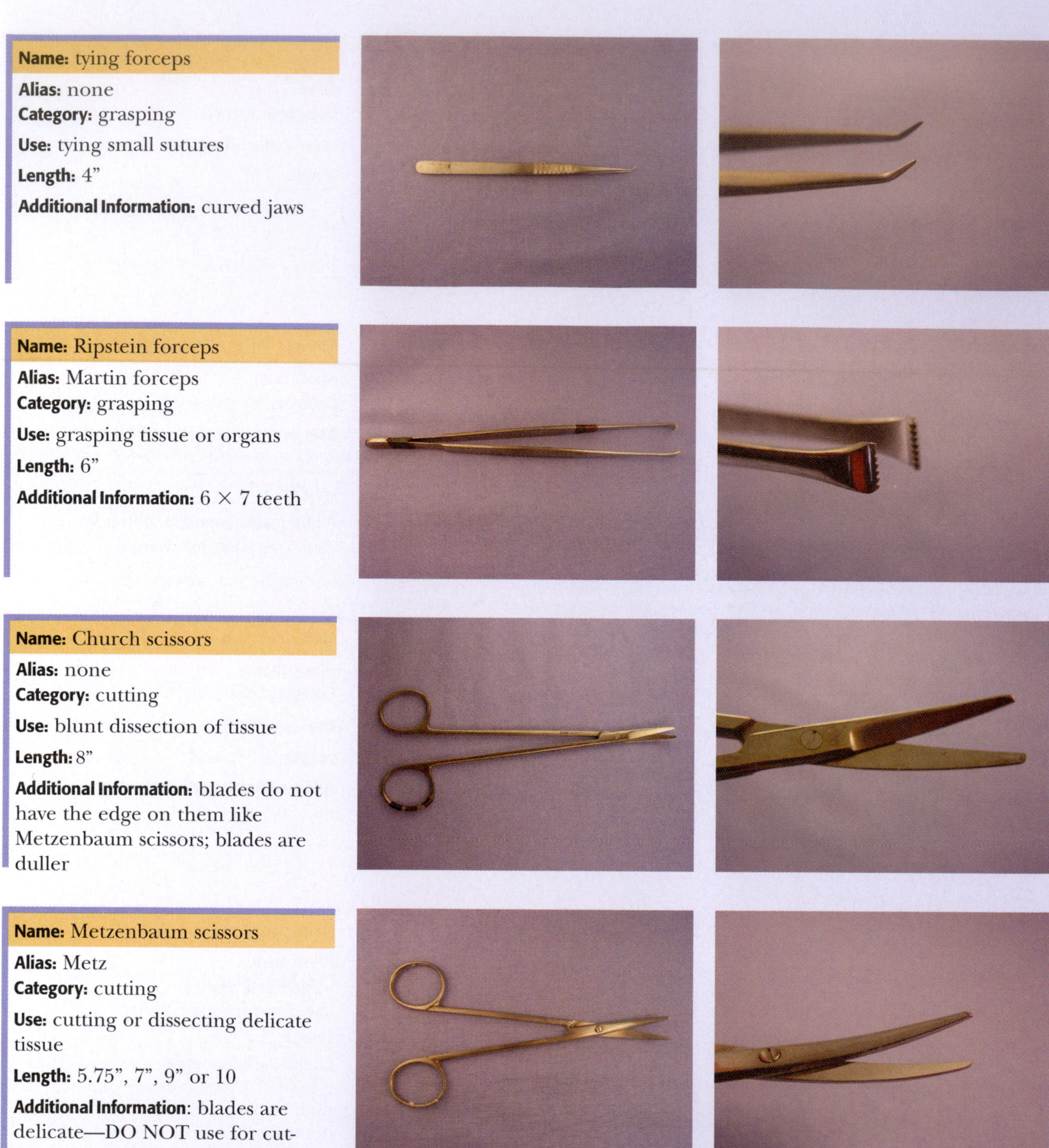

Name: tying forceps

Alias: none

Category: grasping

Use: tying small sutures

Length: 4”

Additional Information: curved jaws

Name: Ripstein forceps

Alias: Martin forceps

Category: grasping

Use: grasping tissue or organs

Length: 6”

Additional Information: 6 × 7 teeth

Name: Church scissors

Alias: none

Category: cutting

Use: blunt dissection of tissue

Length: 8”

Additional Information: blades do not have the edge on them like Metzenbaum scissors; blades are duller

Name: Metzenbaum scissors

Alias: Metz

Category: cutting

Use: cutting or dissecting delicate tissue

Length: 5.75”, 7”, 9” or 10

Additional Information: blades are delicate—DO NOT use for cutting suture, drains, heavy tissue

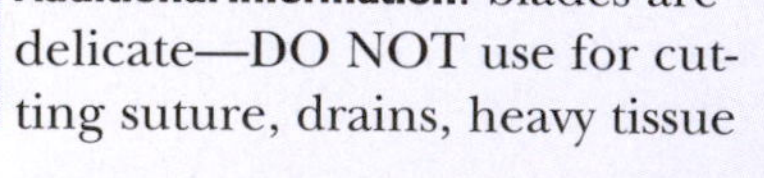

Name: Jorgenson scissors

Alias: none

Category: cutting

Use: cutting heavy tissue

Length: 9”

Additional Information: curved blades

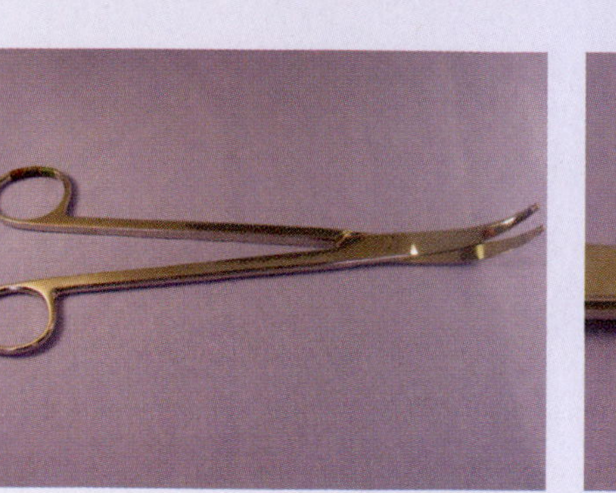

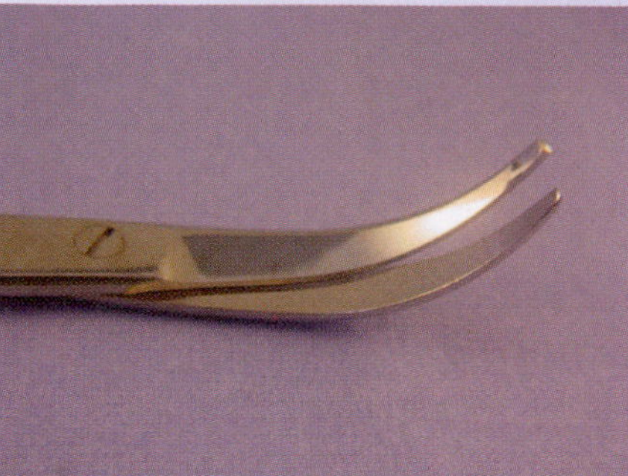

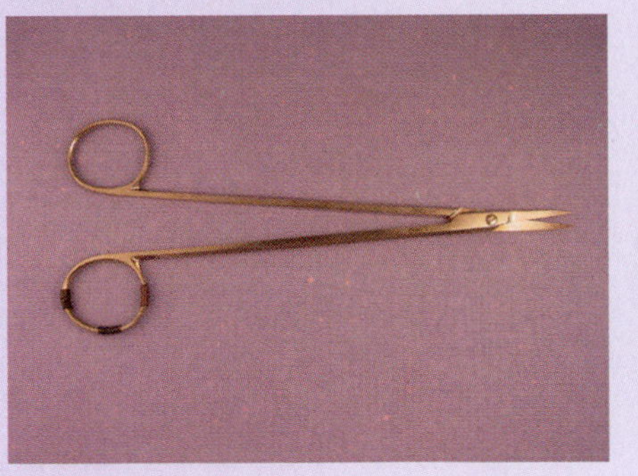
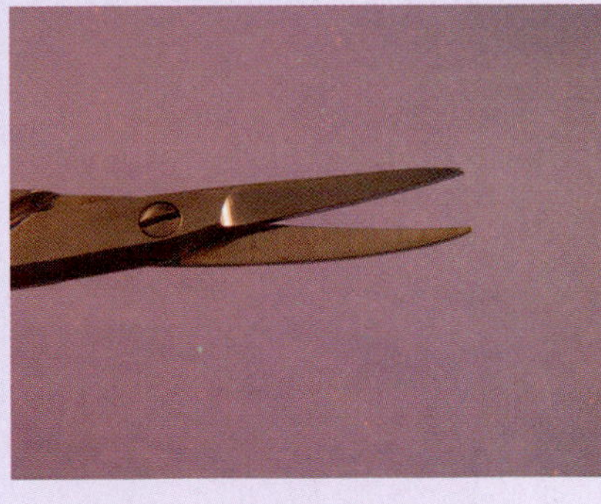

Name: Joseph scissors
Alias: none
Category: cutting
Use: cutting tissue
Length: 5.75"
Additional Information: can have straight or curved blades; sharp tips

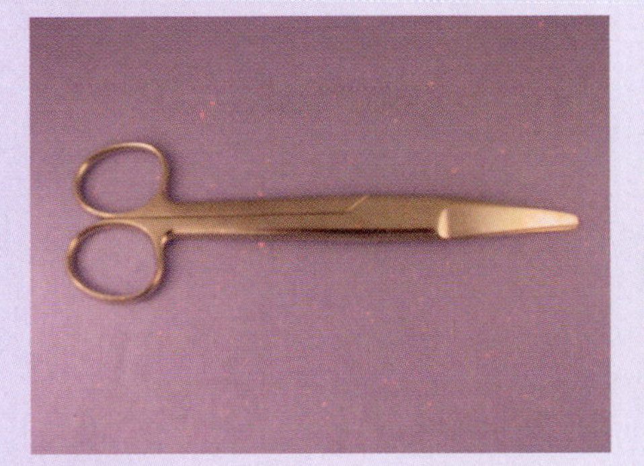
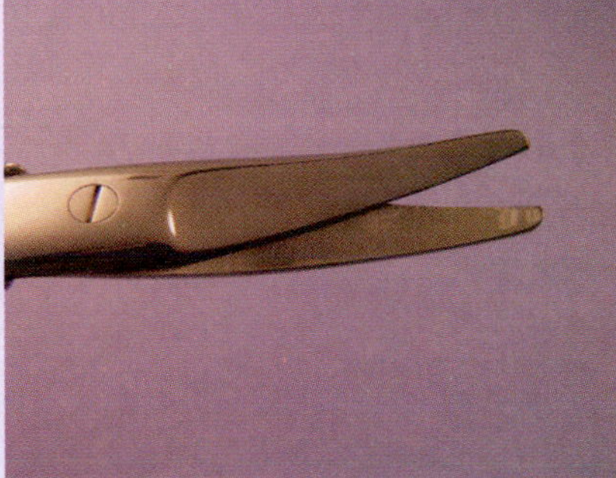

Name: Mayo-Noble scissors
Alias: none
Category: cutting
Use: dissecting heavy tissue
Length: 6.5"
Additional Information: blades can be straight or curved; blunt tips

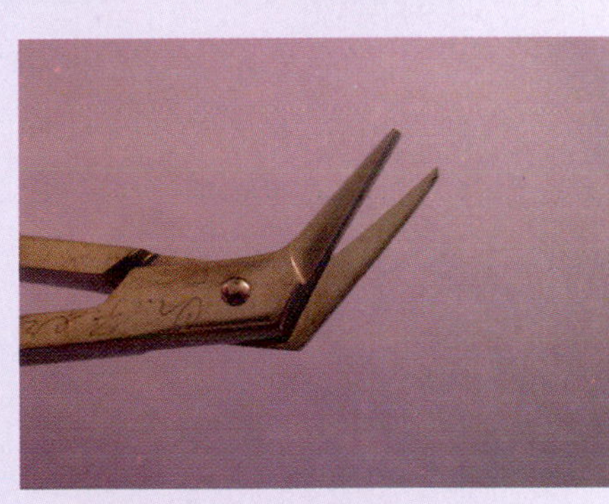

Name: Potts-Smith scissors
Alias: none
Category: cutting
Use: cutting fine blood vessels
Length: 5.25" to 7"
Additional Information: blades can have 25, 40, or 60 degree angle; blades can be delicate or standard

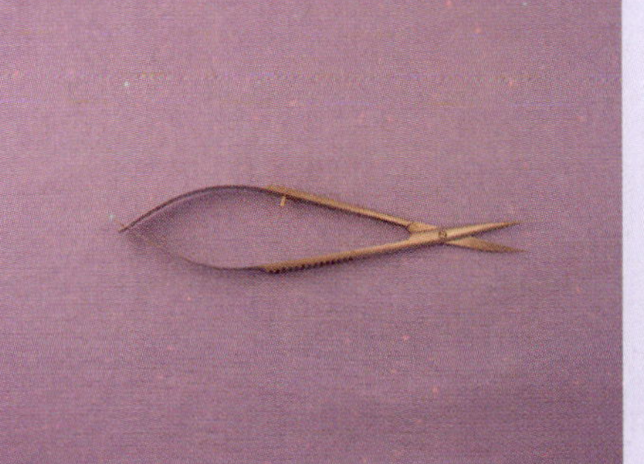
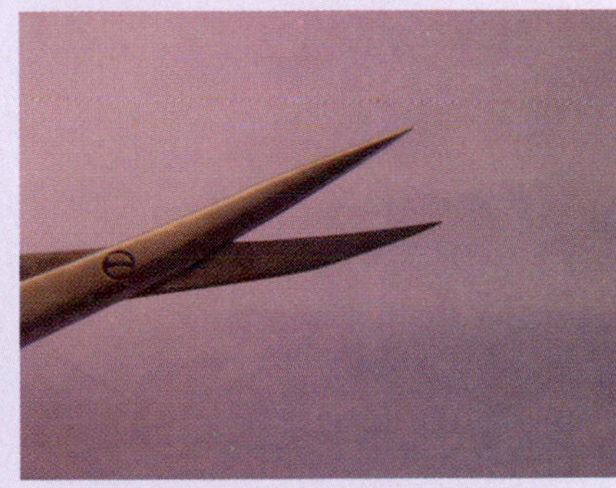

Name: Wescott utility scissors
Alias: none
Category: cutting
Use: cutting and dissecting fine tissue; cutting fine suture
Length: 5"
Additional Information: 25 mm from mid-screw to tip

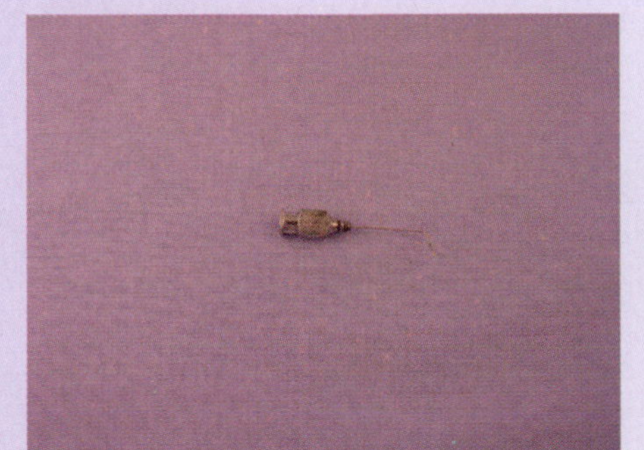
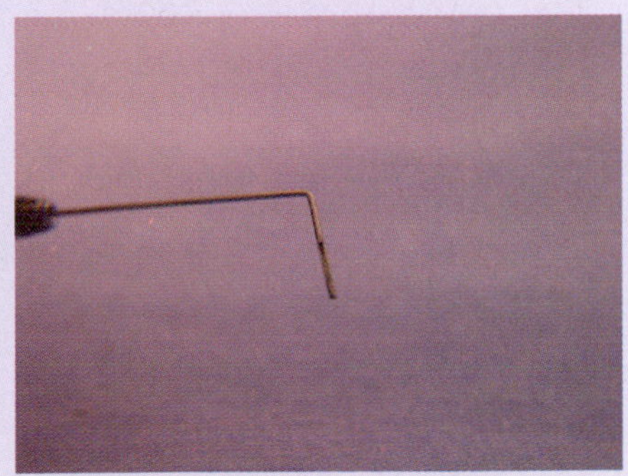

Name: micro needles
Alias: none
Category: accessory
Use: injecting or irrigating fluids into small vessels
Length: n/a
Additional Information: angle tip

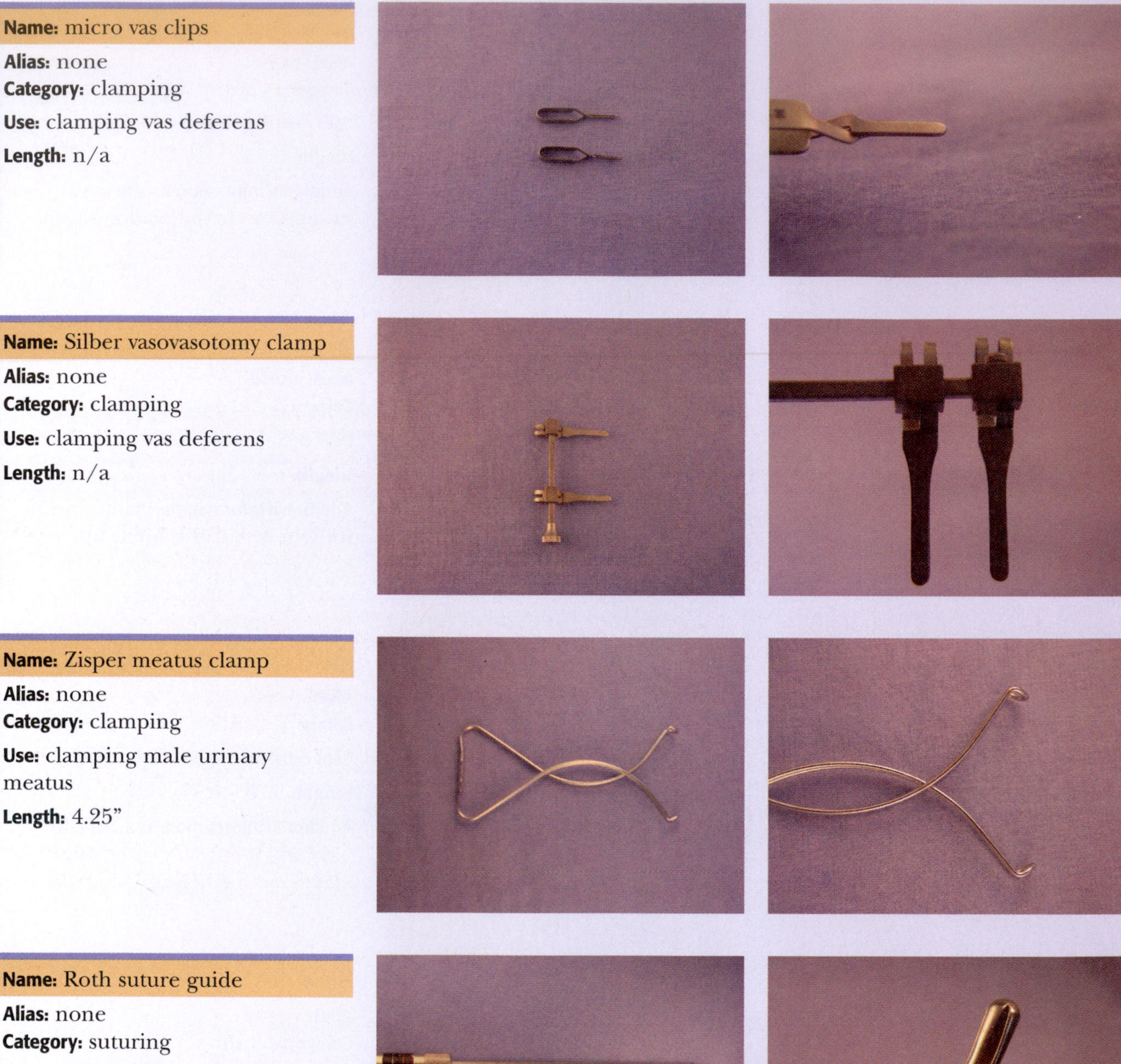

Name: micro vas clips
Alias: none
Category: clamping
Use: clamping vas deferens
Length: n/a

Name: Silber vasovasotomy clamp
Alias: none
Category: clamping
Use: clamping vas deferens
Length: n/a

Name: Zisper meatus clamp
Alias: none
Category: clamping
Use: clamping male urinary meatus
Length: 4.25"

Name: Roth suture guide
Alias: none
Category: suturing
Use: guiding sutures during prostate surgery
Length: 11.25"

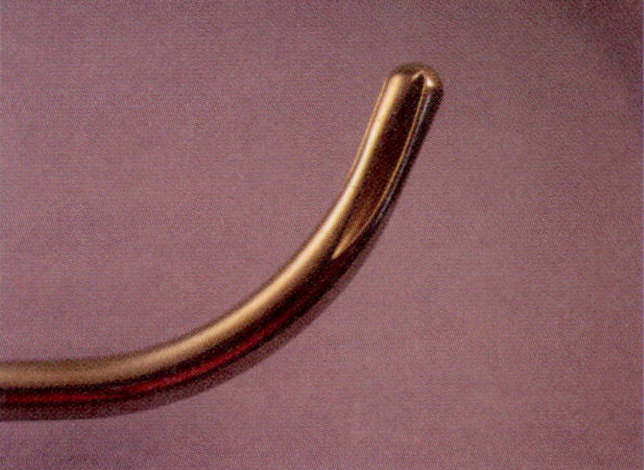

Name: Van Buren urethral sounds
Alias: Van Buren dilators
Category: dilating
Use: dilating urethra
Length: 10.5"
Additional Information: come in diameters of 8 to 40 Fr; arrange on your back table by sizes, starting with the smallest

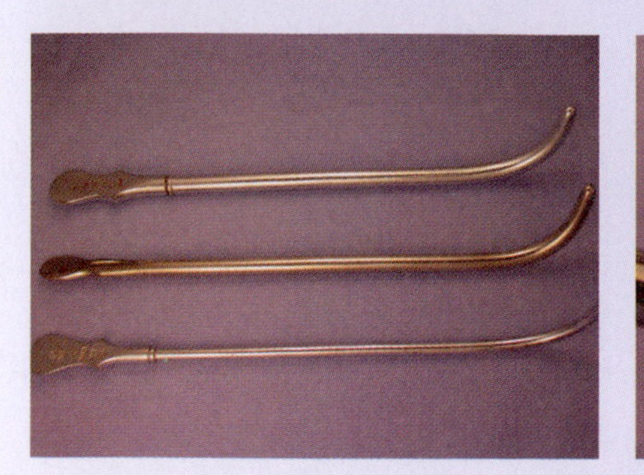

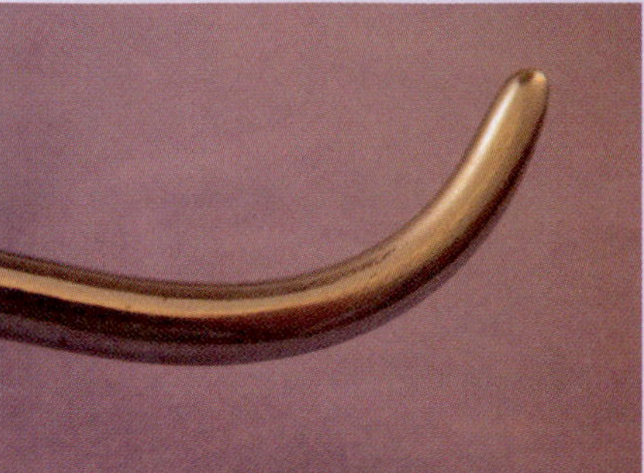

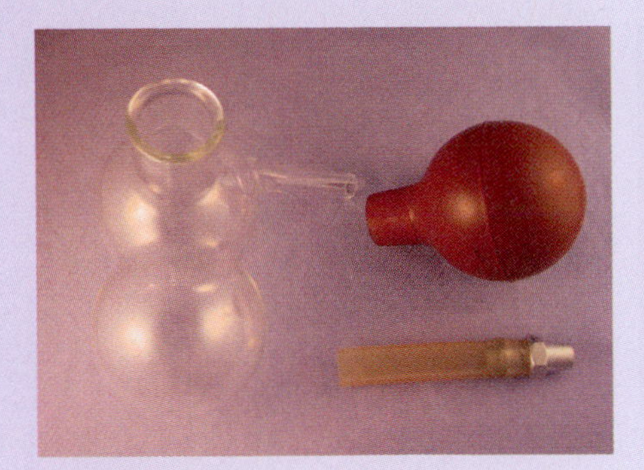

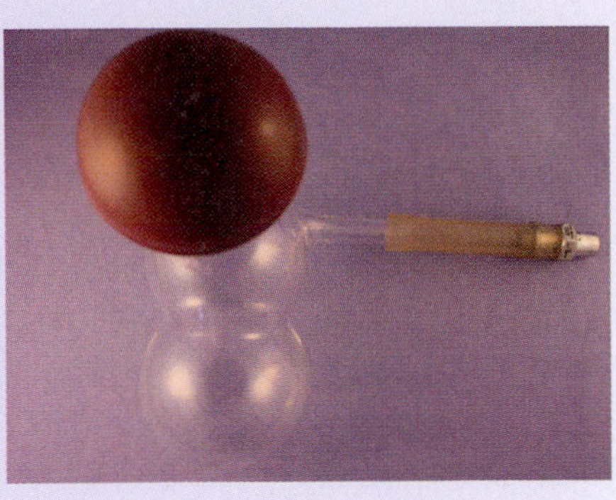

Name: Ellik evacuator

Alias: none

Category: accessory

Use: collecting fluid and resected prostate tissue during TURP

Length: n/a

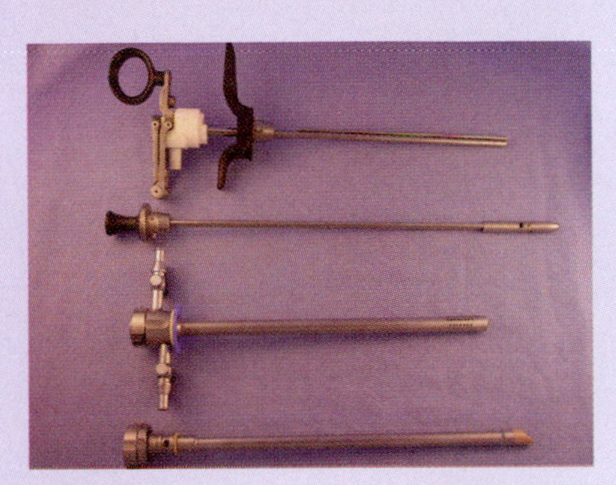

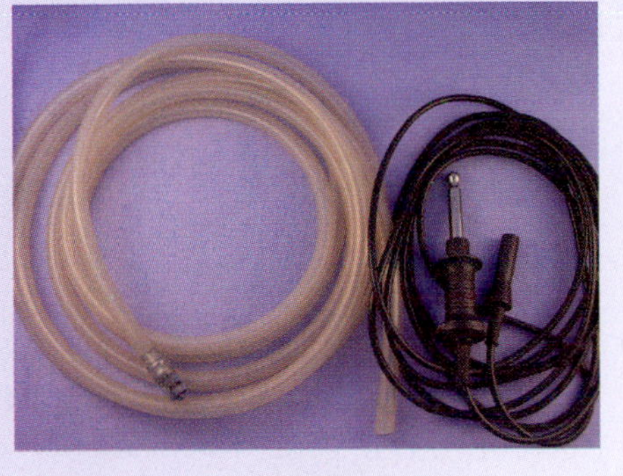

Name: resectoscope

Alias: none

Category: cutting

Use: cutting and coagulating tissue during TURP or TURB

Length: n/a

Additional Information: used with various styles cutting loops, depending on procedure

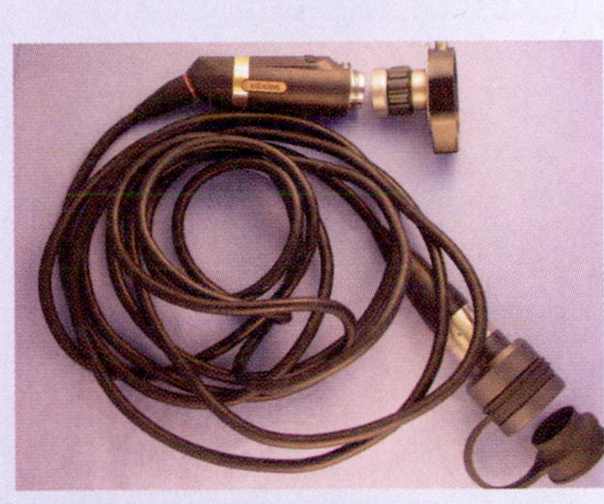

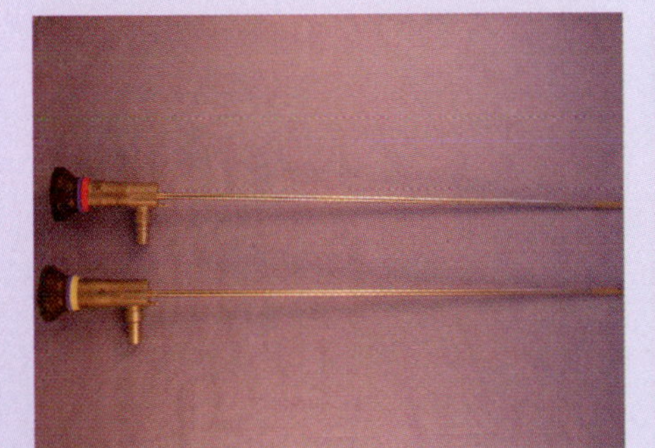

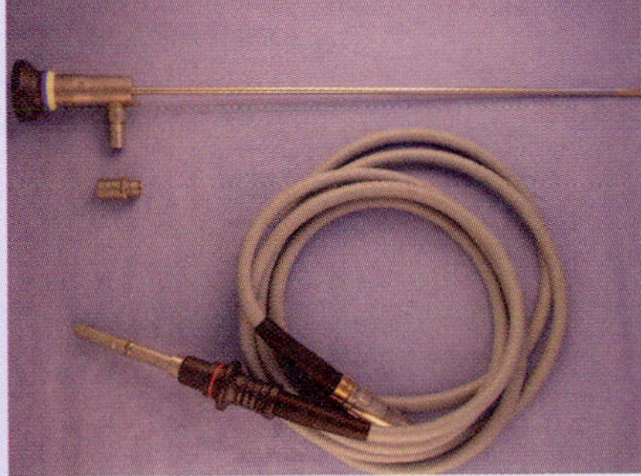

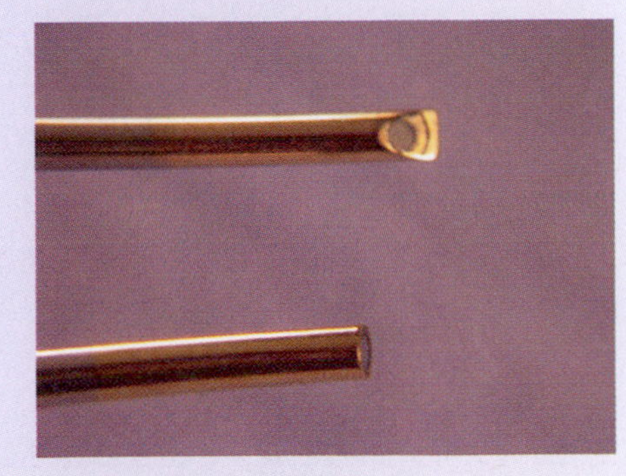

Name: cystoscopy system

Alias: none

Category: accessory

Use: viewing into bladder during transurethral procedures

Length: n/a

Additional Information: used with various degree scopes, depending on procedure

Name: collagen injection system

Alias: none

Category: accessory

Use: injecting collagen for treatment of incontinence

Length: n/a

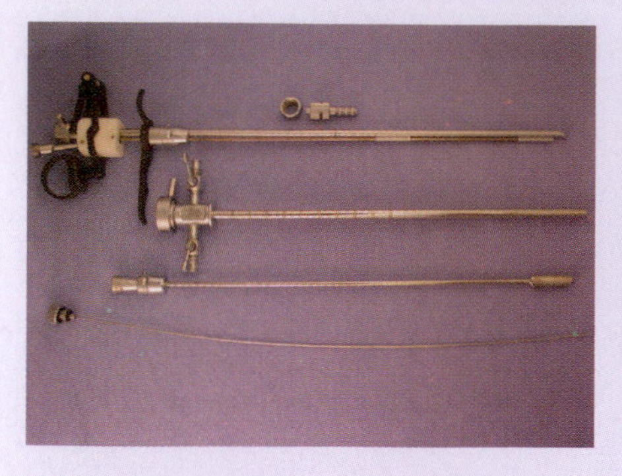

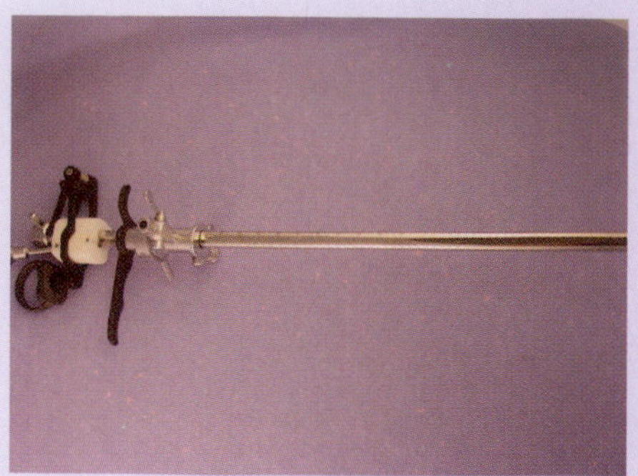

Name: semi-rigid ureteroscope

Alias: none

Category: accessory

Use: viewing into ureter during transurethral procedures

Length: n/a

Additional Information: long, thin shaft

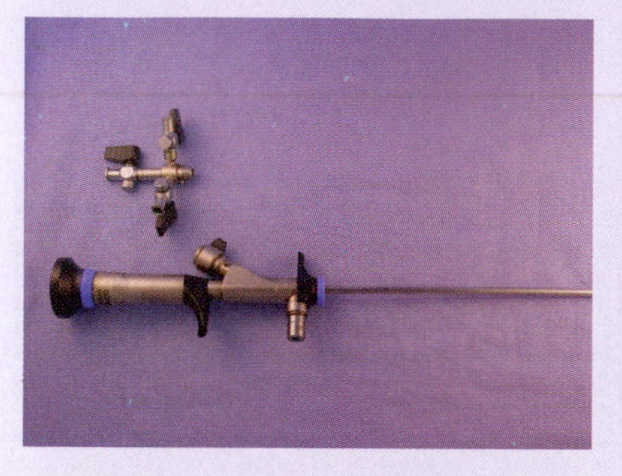

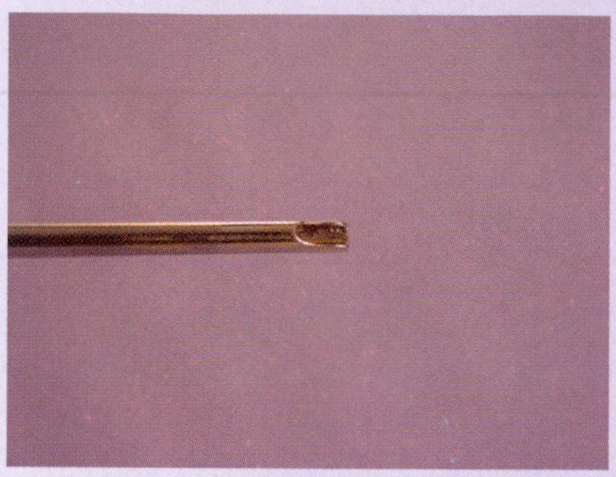

Name: Lowsley prostatic tractors

Alias: none

Category: retracting

Use: inserting through bladder to push prostate down toward perineum

Length: 13"

Additional Information: can be curved or straight

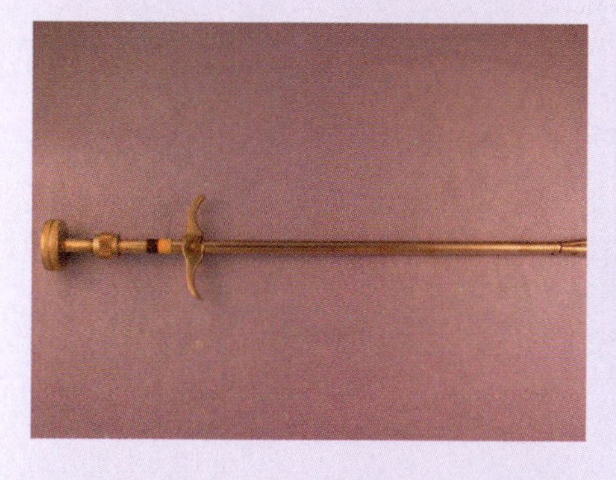

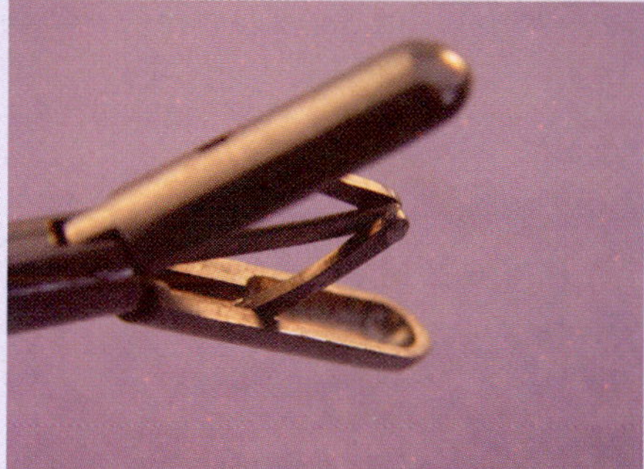

Name: Miller-Bacon retropubic prostatectomy retractor

Alias: none

Category: retracting

Use: retracting prostate during retropubic surgery

Length: n/a

Additional Information: side blades come in 2" and 2.5" lengths; self-retaining

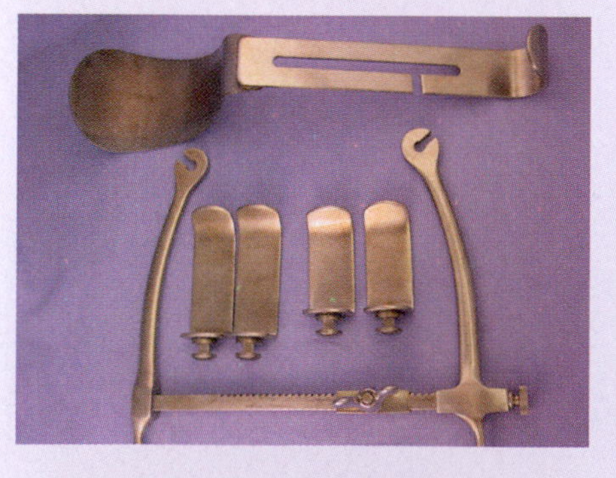

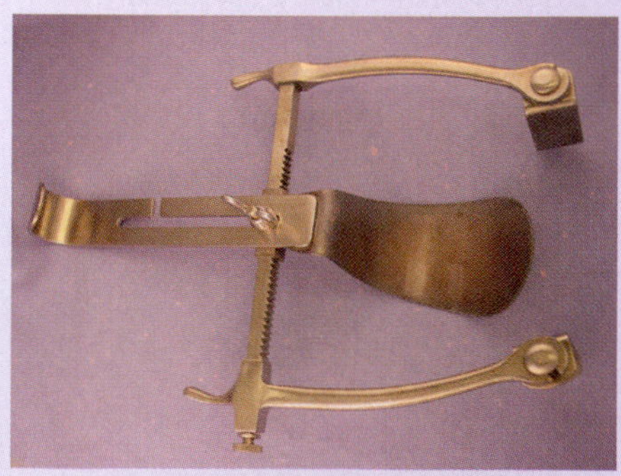

Name: Young anterior retractor

Alias: none

Category: retracting

Use: retracting prostate

Length: 7.5"

Additional Information: blade 2.5" or 3" wide; blade acutely angled

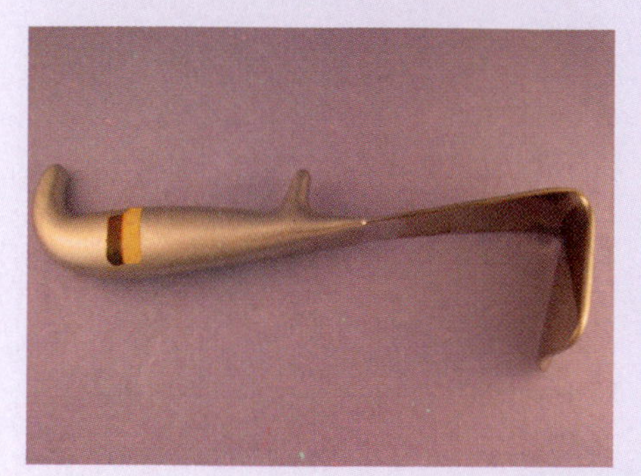

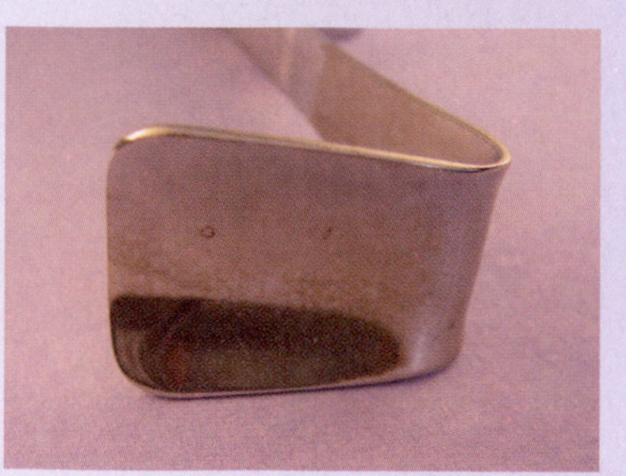

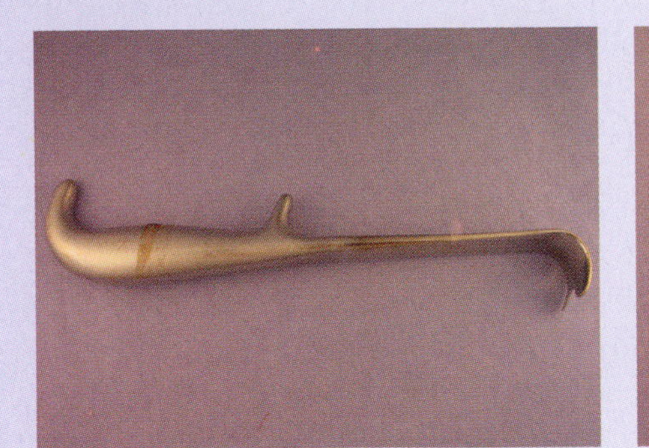

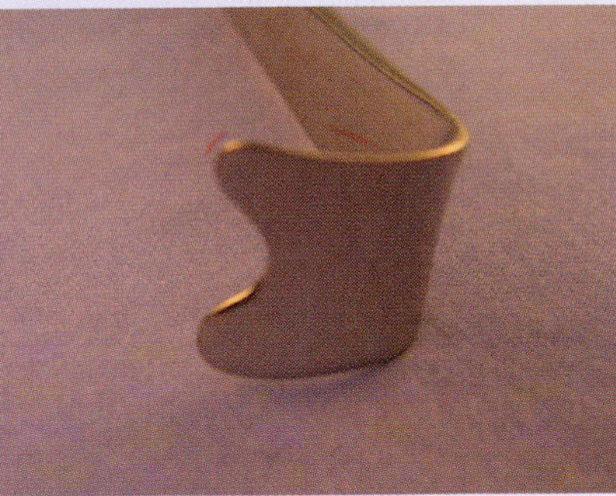

Name: Young bulb retractor

Alias: none

Category: retracting

Use: retracting prostate

Length: 8.5"

Additional Information: notched to go around the urethra

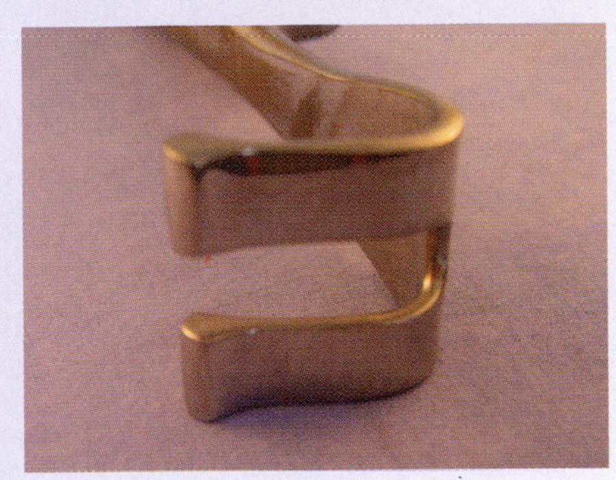

Name: Young bifed retractor

Alias: None

Category: retracting

Use: prostate retraction

Length: 8"

Additional Information: notched to go around the urethra

Q&A

Surgical Session—Urology Instruments

1) The surgeon needs to dilate the patient's urethra. You would hand him/her a:
   a. Van Dyne
   b. Van Buren
   c. Randall
   d. Cushing
2) All of the following are scissors *except:*
   a. Potts-Smith
   b. Jorgenson
   c. Wescott
   d. Dandy
3) A __________ is used to cut and coagulate prostate tissue during a TURP.
   a. cystoscope
   b. resectoscope
   c. ureteroscope
   d. malis-jensen bipolar
4) Which instrument is used to collect fluid and resected tissue during a TURP?
   a. Ellik evacuator
   b. Roth
   c. Jorgenson
   d. Randall
5) A __________ is a type of stone forceps.
   a. Roth
   b. Randall
   c. Ripstein
   d. Rochester
6) __________ scissors would be used on heavy tissue.
   a. Wescott utility
   b. Metzenbaum
   c. Potts
   d. Mayo-Noble
7) The surgeon requests a meatus clamp. You would hand him/her a:
   a. Silber
   b. Roth
   c. Zisper
   d. McDougal
8) You are assisting on a vasovasotomy. Which of the following would be used to clamp/hold the vas deferens?

a. Roth
b. Van Buren
c. Cushing
d. Silber

9) The surgeon requests a right angle clamp. You would hand a:
a. Mayo-Guyon
b. McDougal
c. Rochester mixter
d. Ripstein

10) All of the following are forceps *except:*
a. Bishop Harmon
b. Ripstein
c. Church
d. Gerald

11) __________ is a type of bipolar forceps.
a. Ripstein
b. Malis-Jensen
c. Mayo-Guyon
d. Van Buren

12) Which of the following is a prostate tractor?
a. Roth
b. Van Buren
c. Lowsley
d. Randall

13) All of the following could be used in a transurethral procedure *except*:
a. cystoscope
b. resectoscope
c. Ellik evacuator
d. Jorgenson scissors

14) During a radical nephrectomy, the surgeon requests a vein retractor. You hand him/her a:
a. Dandy
b. Young
c. Cushing
d. Ripstein

15) You are setting up for open prostate surgery. You need a self-retaining prostate retractor. Which of the following would you set out?
a. Young bifed
b. Young bulb
c. Miller-Bacon
d. Young anterior

16) A suture guide used in prostate surgery is a:
a. Roth
b. Van Buren
c. Van Dyne
d. McDougal

Orthopedic Instruments 4

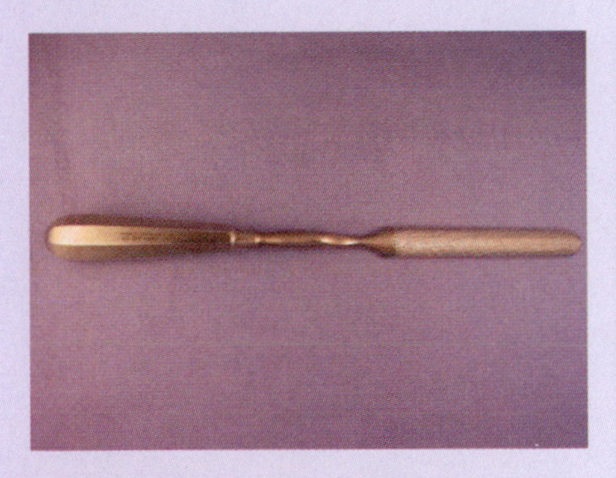

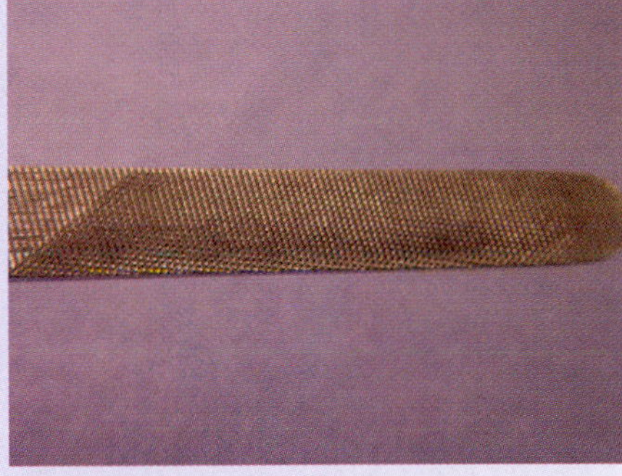

Name: bone file

Alias: none

Category: cutting

Use: smoothing bone

Length: 9.5”

Additional Information: half round blade; fine teeth

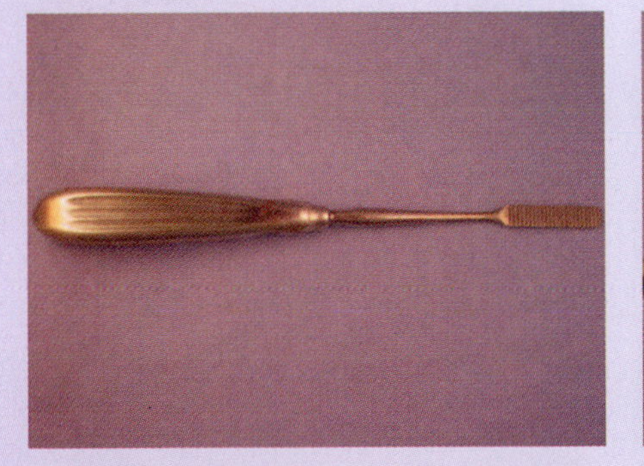

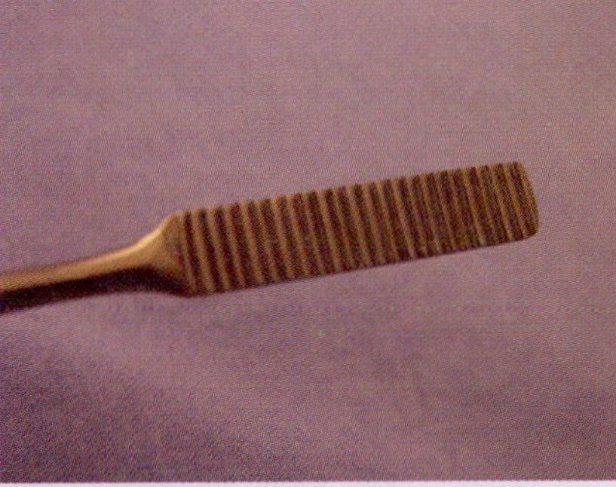

Name: Parkes rasp

Alias: none

Category: cutting

Use: cutting bone

Length: 8.5”

Additional Information: cuts on the downstroke

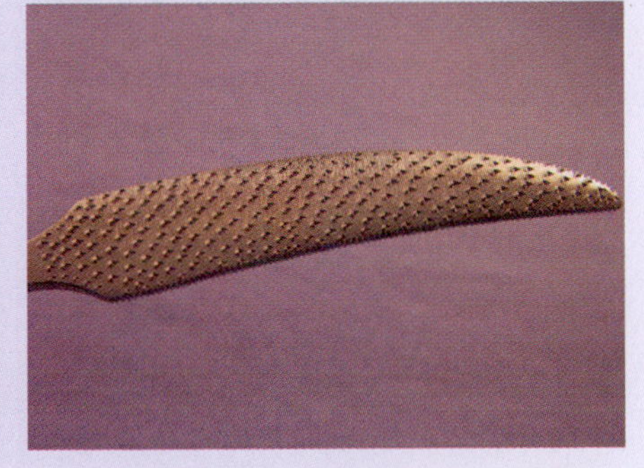

Name: Putti rasp

Alias: rat tail

Category: cutting

Use: smoothing the surface of bone

Length: 10.5” or 12”

Additional Information: double ended; flat blades

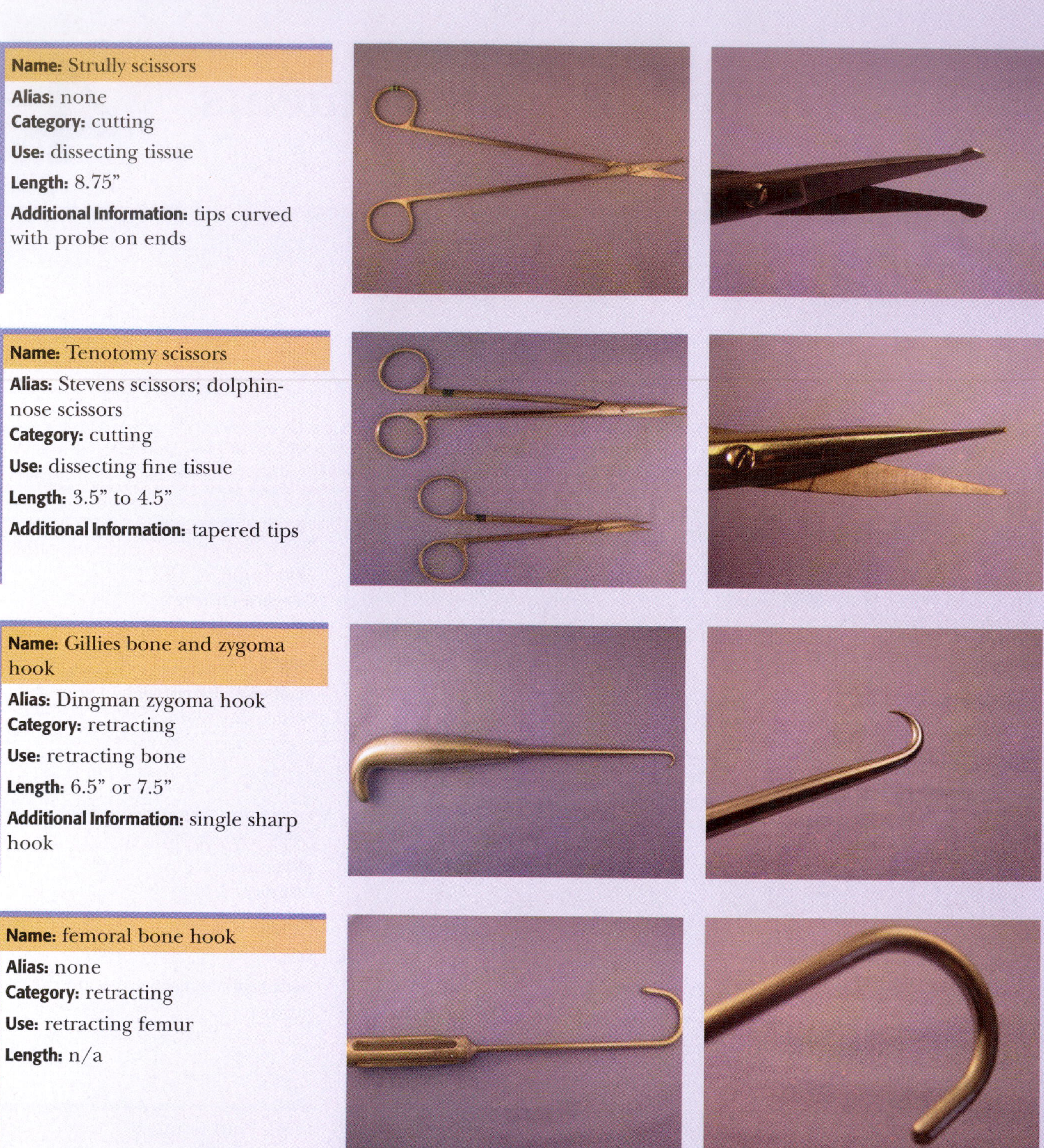

Name: Strully scissors

Alias: none

Category: cutting

Use: dissecting tissue

Length: 8.75"

Additional Information: tips curved with probe on ends

Name: Tenotomy scissors

Alias: Stevens scissors; dolphin-nose scissors

Category: cutting

Use: dissecting fine tissue

Length: 3.5" to 4.5"

Additional Information: tapered tips

Name: Gillies bone and zygoma hook

Alias: Dingman zygoma hook

Category: retracting

Use: retracting bone

Length: 6.5" or 7.5"

Additional Information: single sharp hook

Name: femoral bone hook

Alias: none

Category: retracting

Use: retracting femur

Length: n/a

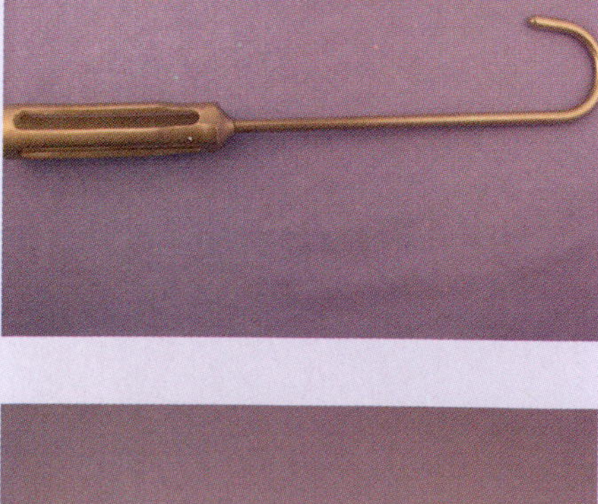

Name: Cushing little joker periosteal elevator

Alias: little joker

Category: cutting

Use: removing periosteum from bone

Length: 6" or 7.5"

Additional Information: can have solid or hollow handle

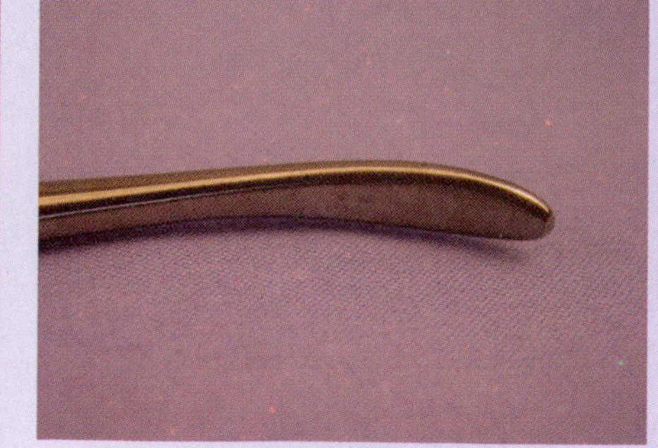

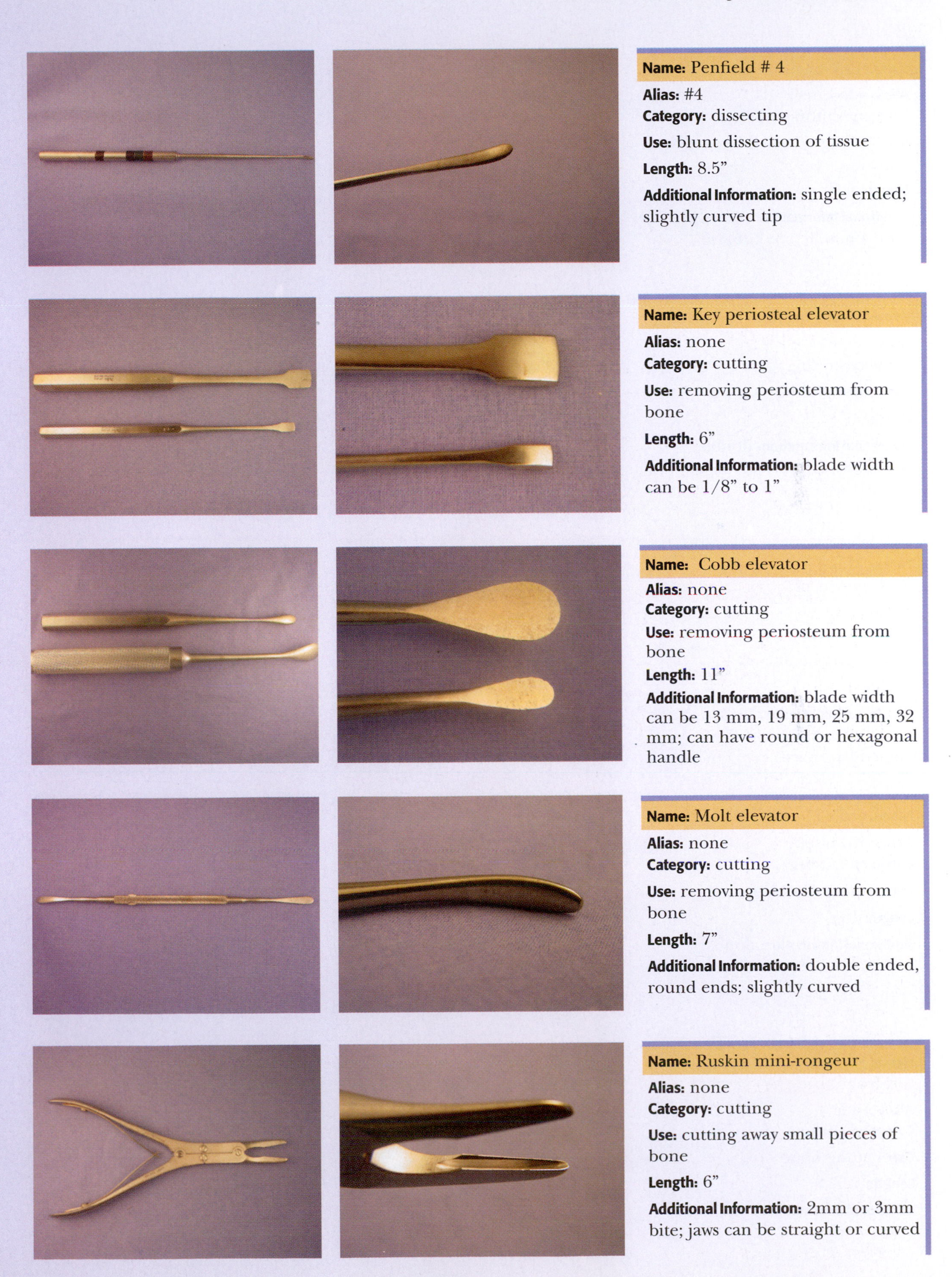

Name: Penfield # 4
Alias: #4
Category: dissecting
Use: blunt dissection of tissue
Length: 8.5”
Additional Information: single ended; slightly curved tip

Name: Key periosteal elevator
Alias: none
Category: cutting
Use: removing periosteum from bone
Length: 6”
Additional Information: blade width can be 1/8” to 1”

Name: Cobb elevator
Alias: none
Category: cutting
Use: removing periosteum from bone
Length: 11”
Additional Information: blade width can be 13 mm, 19 mm, 25 mm, 32 mm; can have round or hexagonal handle

Name: Molt elevator
Alias: none
Category: cutting
Use: removing periosteum from bone
Length: 7”
Additional Information: double ended, round ends; slightly curved

Name: Ruskin mini-rongeur
Alias: none
Category: cutting
Use: cutting away small pieces of bone
Length: 6”
Additional Information: 2mm or 3mm bite; jaws can be straight or curved

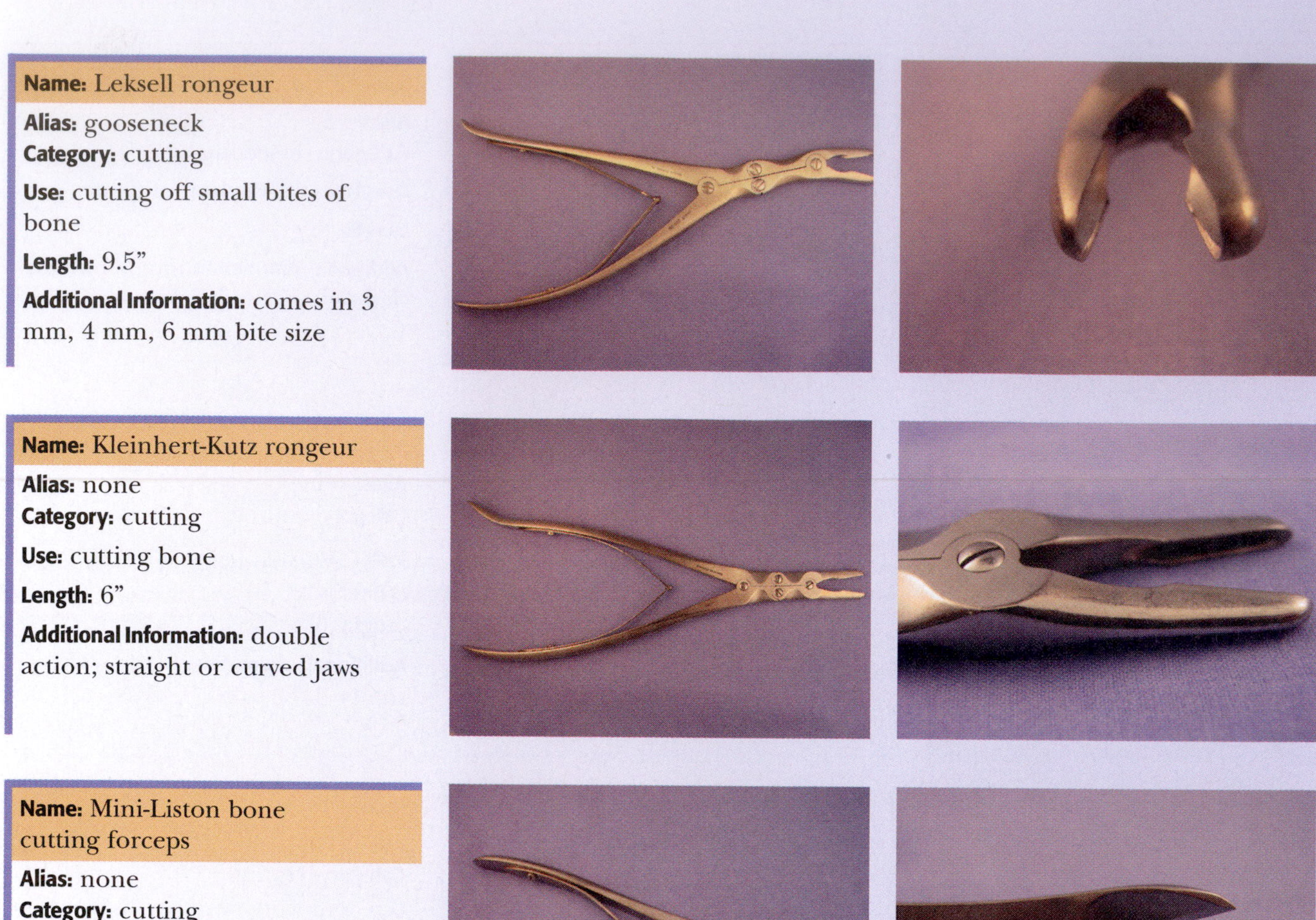

Name: Leksell rongeur
Alias: gooseneck
Category: cutting
Use: cutting off small bites of bone
Length: 9.5”
Additional Information: comes in 3 mm, 4 mm, 6 mm bite size

Name: Kleinhert-Kutz rongeur
Alias: none
Category: cutting
Use: cutting bone
Length: 6”
Additional Information: double action; straight or curved jaws

Name: Mini-Liston bone cutting forceps
Alias: none
Category: cutting
Use: cutting bone
Length: 6”
Additional Information: blades can be straight, angled forward or angled backward

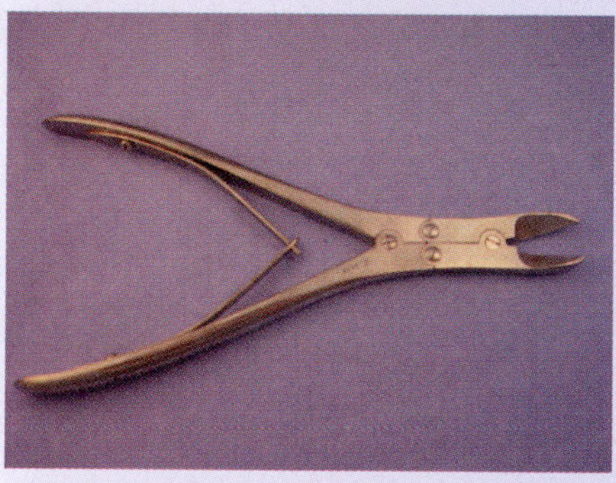

Name: Stille-Horsley rongeur
Alias: rib cutter
Category: cutting
Use: cutting ribs or bone
Length: 10”
Additional Information: double action; double curved

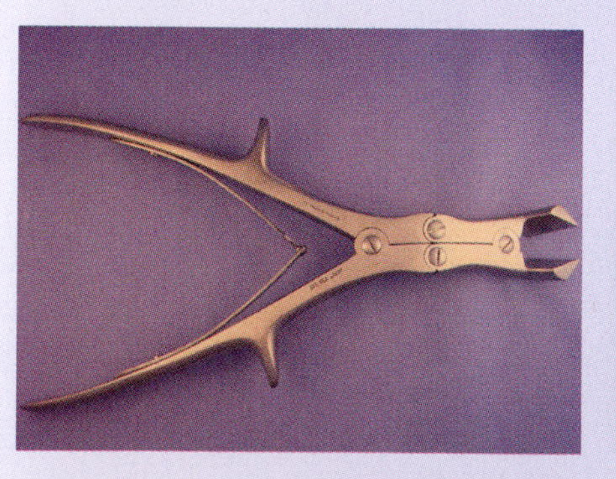

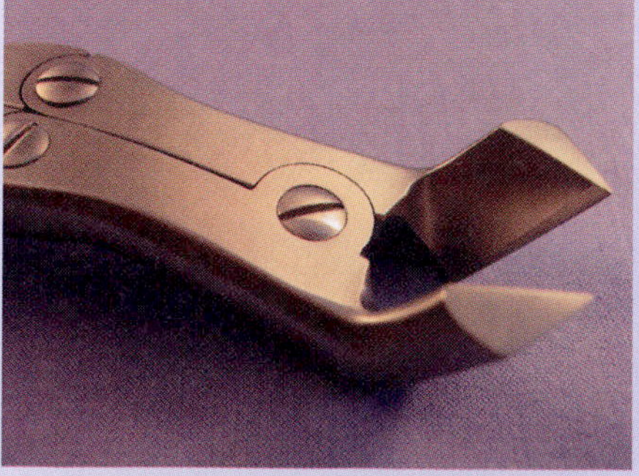

Name: Horsley bone cutting forceps
Alias: none
Category: cutting
Use: cutting bone
Length: 7.5”
Additional Information: straight tips

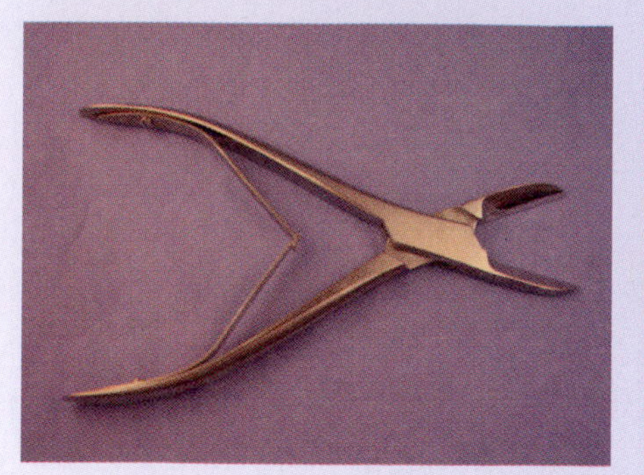

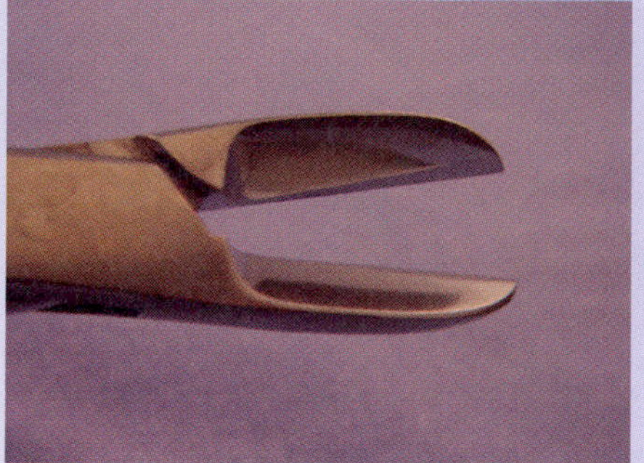

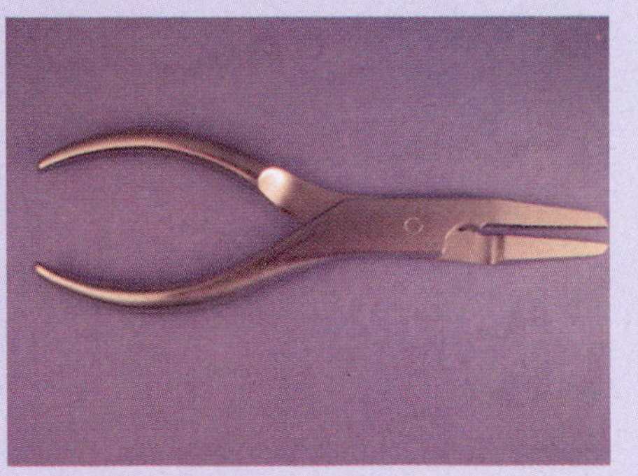

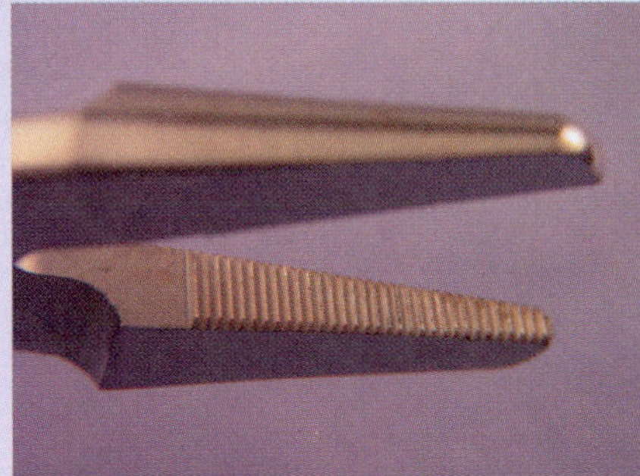

Name: needle-nose pliers/ wire cutter

Alias: none

Category: cutting

Use: cutting or twisting wires

Length: 6.5"

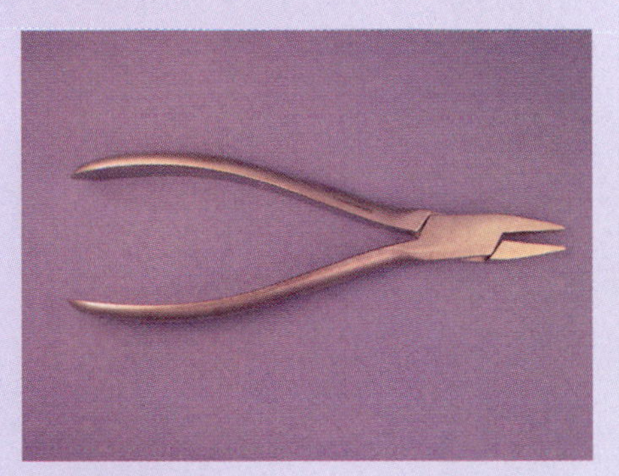

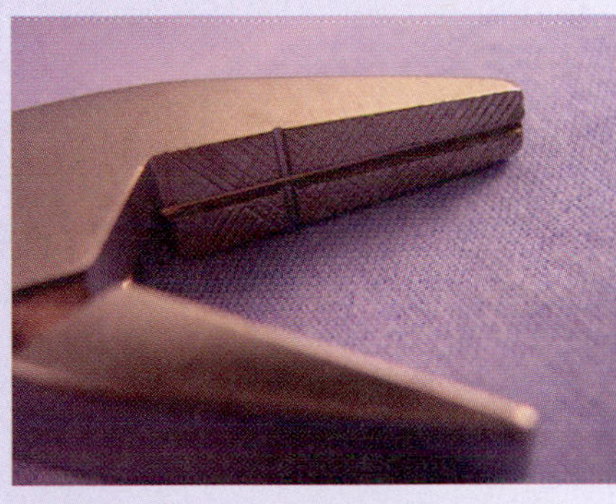

Name: flat-nose K wire pliers

Alias: none

Category: grasping

Use: pulling or bending Kirschner wires

Length: 6.75"

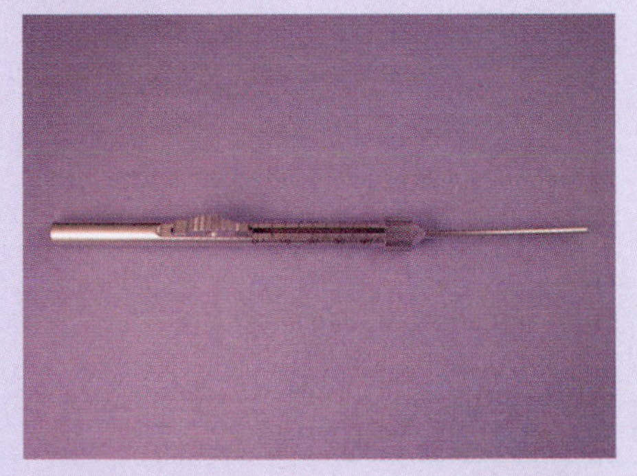

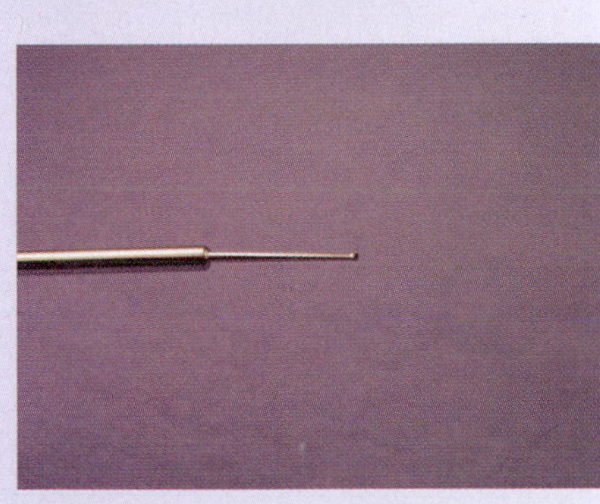

Name: depth gauge

Alias: none

Category: accessory

Use: measuring depth of drill holes

Length: 6.5"

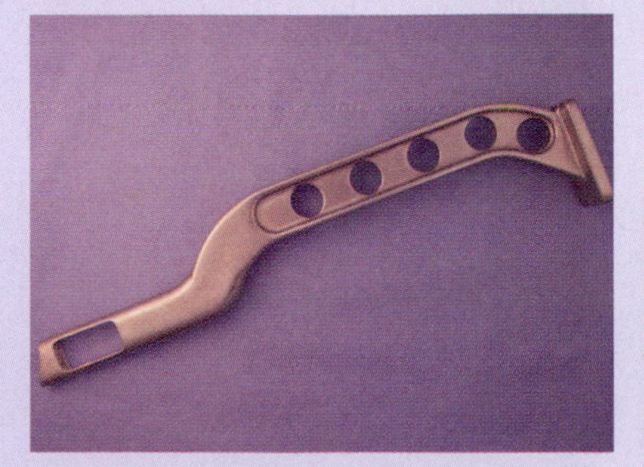

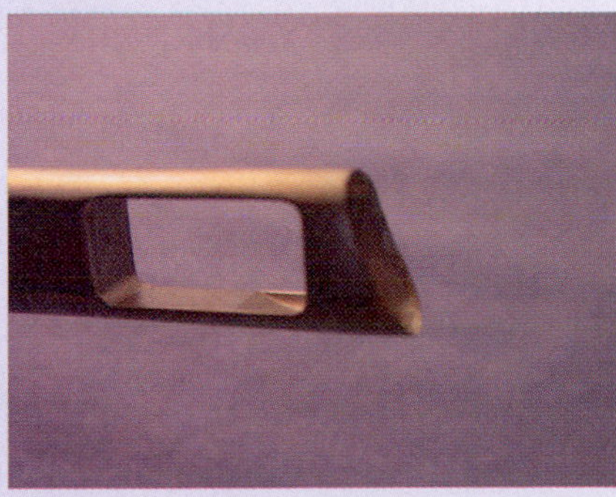

Name: box osteotome

Alias: none

Category: cutting

Use: inserted into femoral canal to create a pilot hole for femoral reaming

Length: n/a

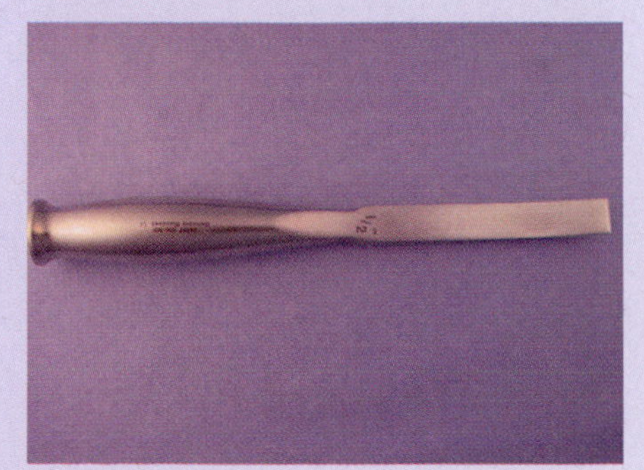

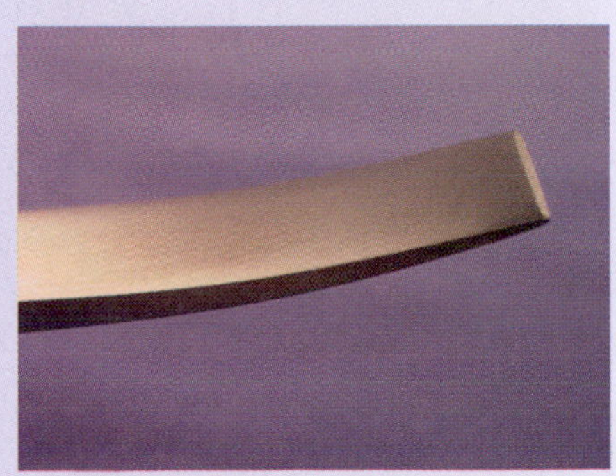

Name: Hibbs osteotome

Alias: none

Category: cutting

Use: cutting bone

Length: 9.5"

Additional Information: can be straight or curved; blade width 0.25" to 1.5"

Name: Lambotte osteotomes

Alias: none

Category: cutting

Use: scoring or cutting bone

Length: straight—5" (mini) or 9"; curved—9"

Additional Information: mini osteotomes come in blade width 4 mm to 20 mm; 9" Lambotte tips can be straight or curved—come in blade widths of 1/4" to 1.5"

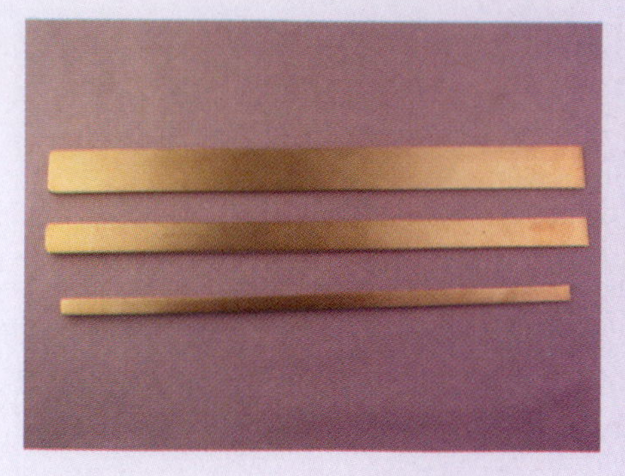

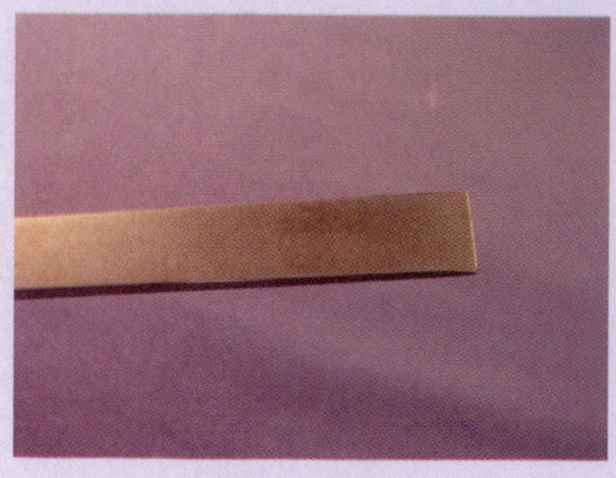

Name: Lexer gouge

Alias: none

Category: cutting

Use: cutting bone

Length: 7", 8.5", or 11.75"

Additional Information: blade width can be 5 mm to 30 mm

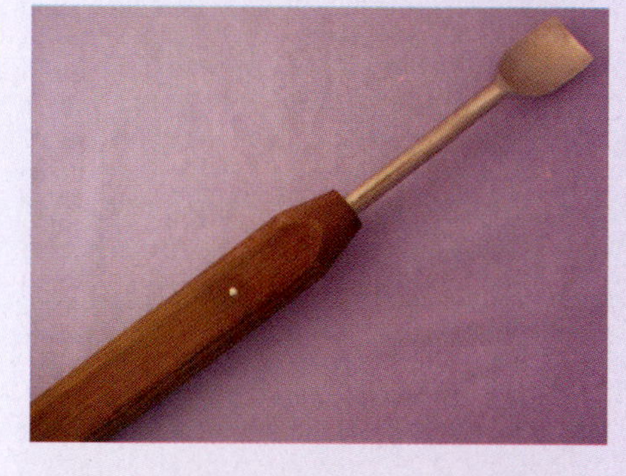

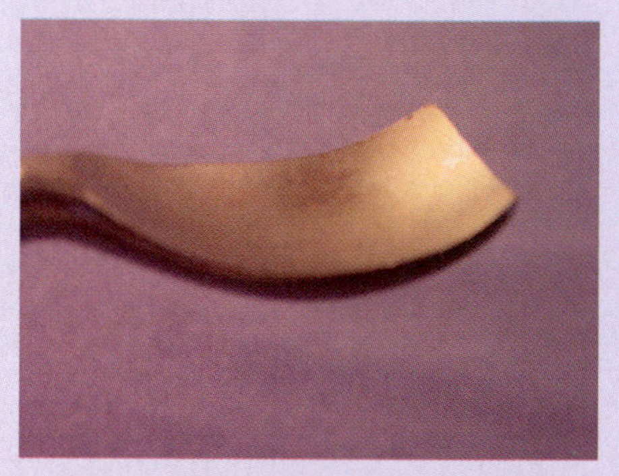

Name: Cushing pituitary rongeur

Alias: upbiter (jaws angled up); downbiter (jaws angled down)

Category: cutting

Length: shaft can be 6", 7", or 8"

Use: removing pieces of intervertebral disc or bone

Additional Information: jaws can be straight or angled up or down; jaw bite can be 1.5 mm or 2 mm

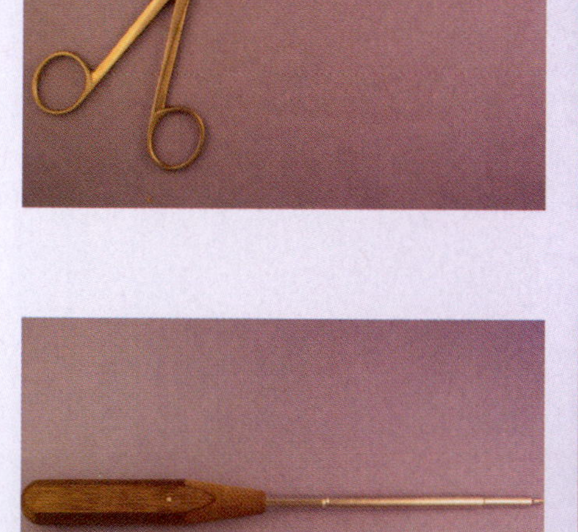

Name: hand-held screwdriver

Alias: none

Category: accessory

Length: n/a

Use: advancing screws into bone

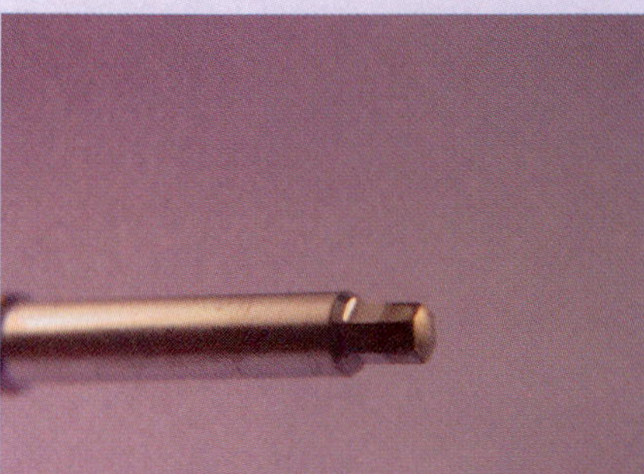

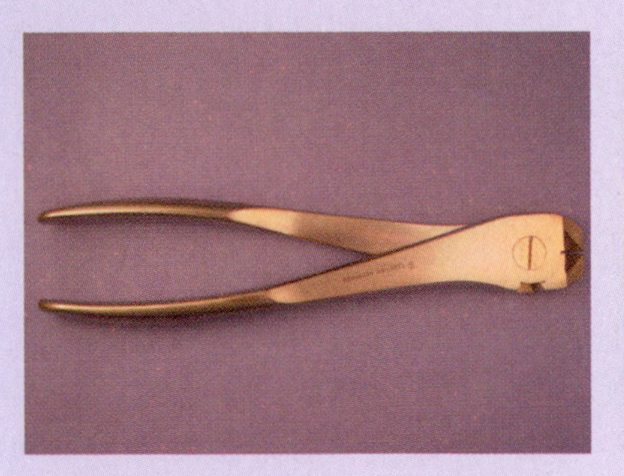

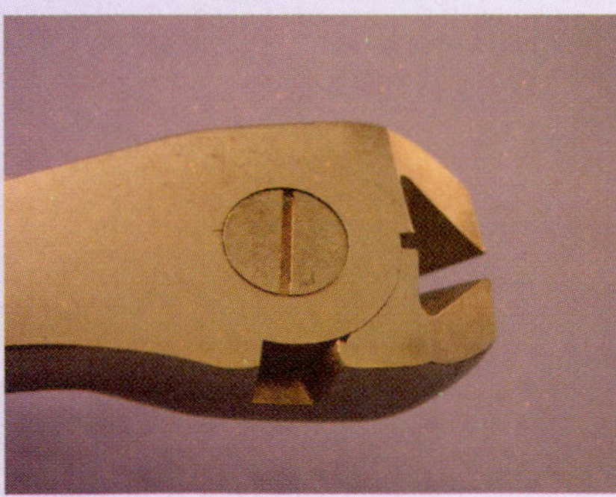

Name: cannulated pin cutter

Alias: none

Category: cutting

Use: cutting wires, pins

Length: 7.25"

Additional Information: 1.6 mm capacity; end cutting; designed to slide over inserted wire, cut piece remains inside the channel

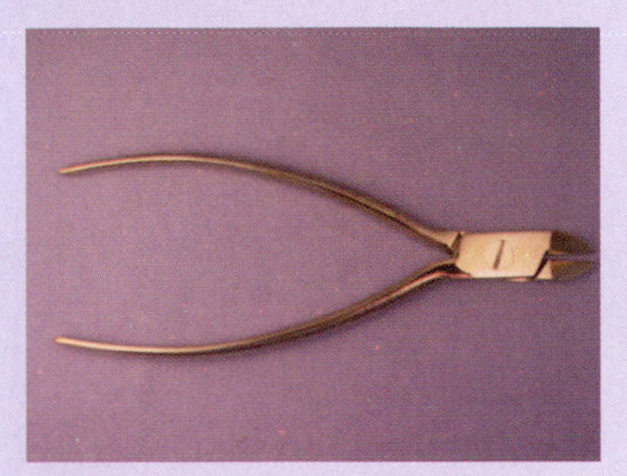

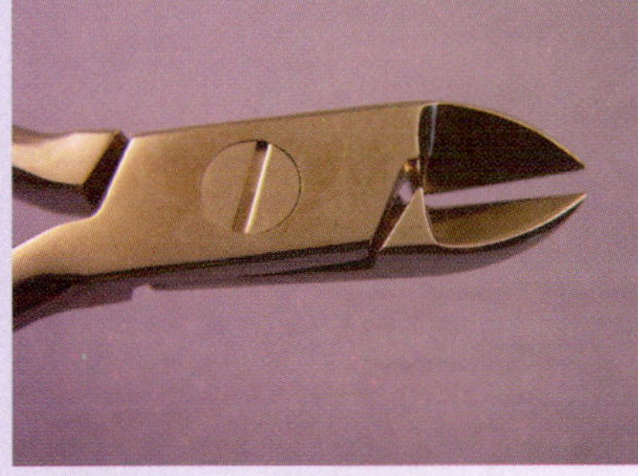

Name: delicate wire cutter

Alias: none

Category: cutting

Use: cutting small wires

Length: n/a

Additional Information: end or side cut

Name: Martin diamond wire cutter

Alias: diamond pin cutter

Category: cutting

Use: cutting wires

Length: 6.5"

Additional Information: maximum capacity 1.25 mm

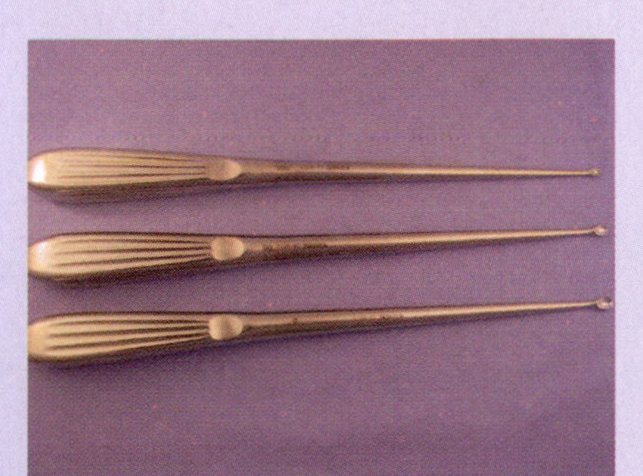

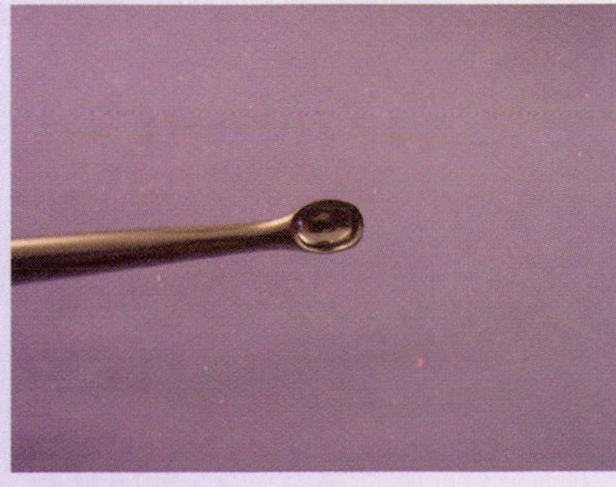

Name: Bruns bone curette

Alias: none

Category: cutting

Use: scraping away pieces of bone

Length: 9"

Additional Information: comes in sizes 0000 to 6; tip can be straight or angled

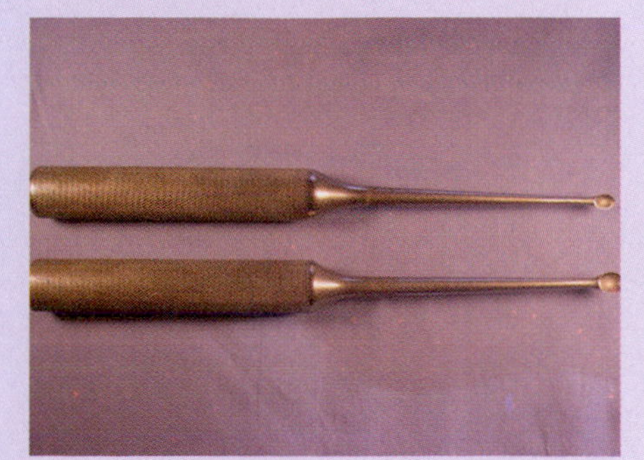

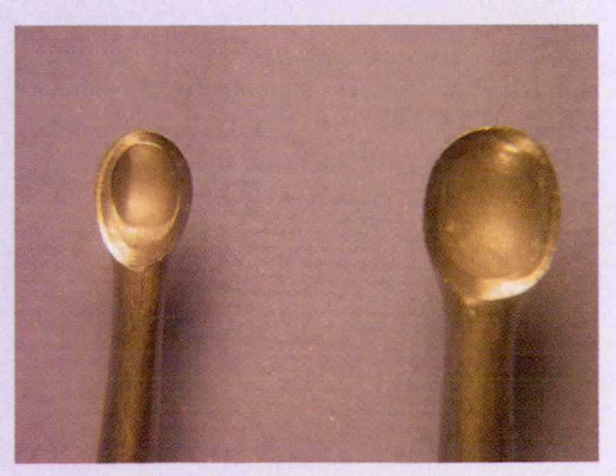

Name: Cobb bone curettes

Alias: Dawson-Yuhl curettes

Category: cutting

Use: scraping away pieces of bone

Length: 11"

Additional Information: cup sizes 2 mm to 8mm

Name: bone tamp

Alias: none

Category: accessory

Use: tamping bone

Length: 6”

Additional Information: comes in 2 mm to 10 mm sizes

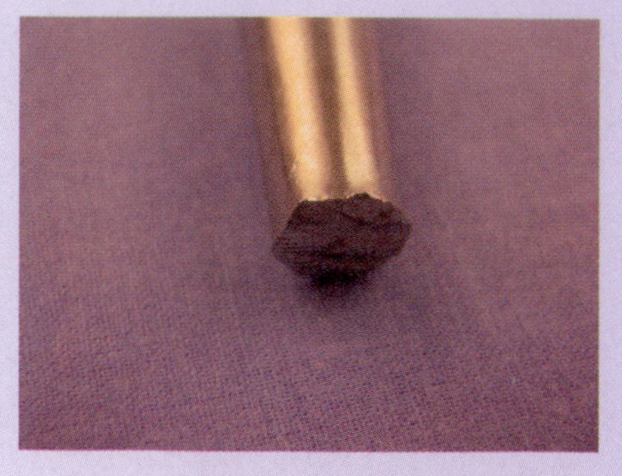

Name: orthopedic mallet

Alias: none

Category: accessory

Use: tapping on osteotomes or chisels, or inserting pins

Length: 7.25” or 7.5”

Other: head diameter 1.5”; weight 1 pound or 2 pounds

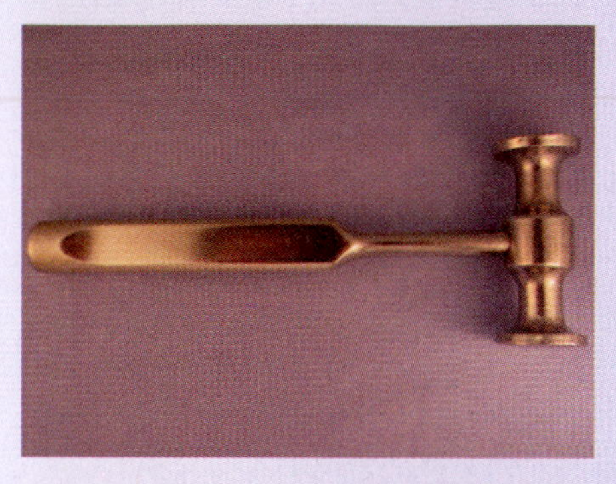

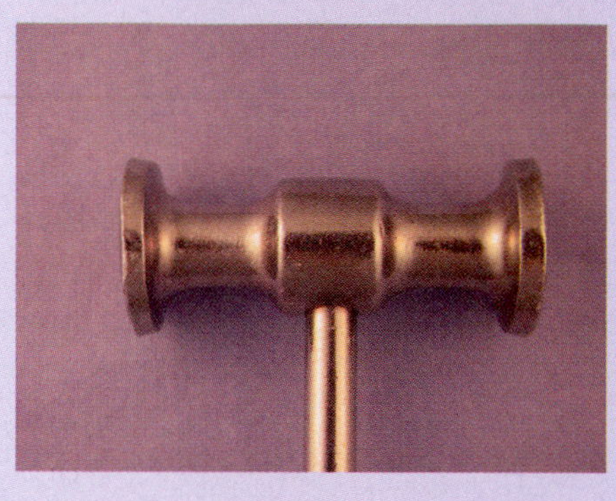

Name: bone mallet

Alias: none

Category: accessory

Use: tapping on osteotomes or chisels, or inserting pins

Length: 7.5”

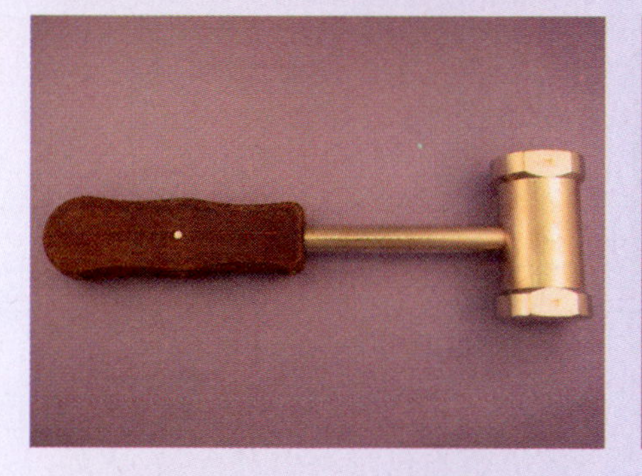

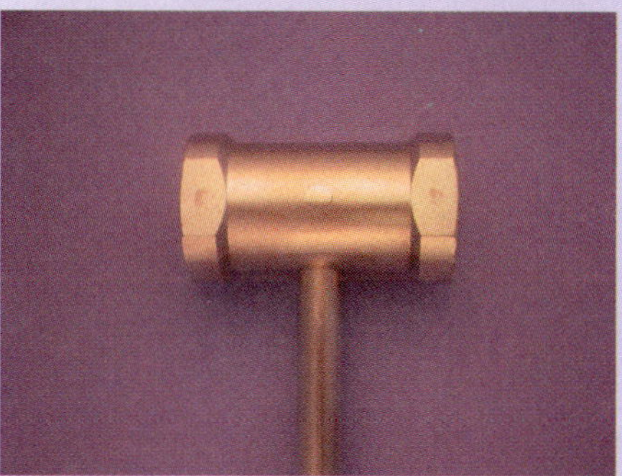

Name: Townley caliper

Alias: caliper

Category: accessory

Use: measuring

Length: 4”

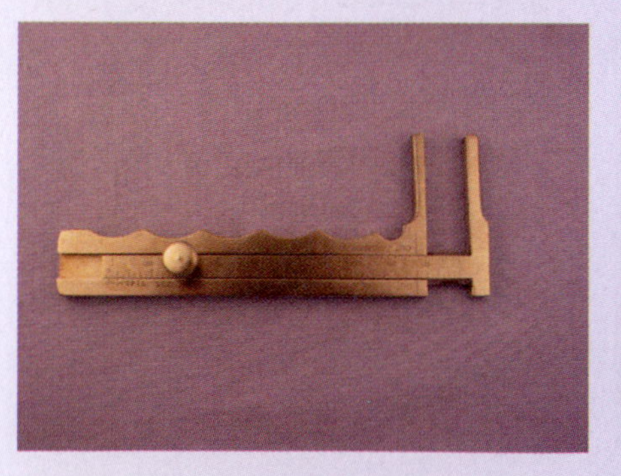

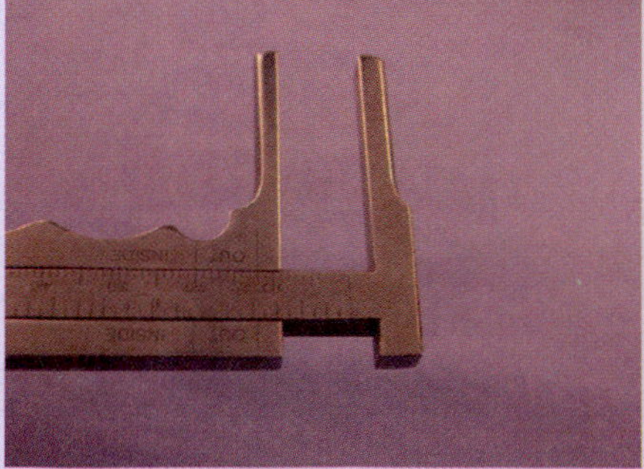

Name: Lewin bone clamp

Alias: Lewin spinal perforating forceps

Category: clamping

Use: temporary clamping of bone fragments

Length: 7”

Additional Information: jaws extend in a curve

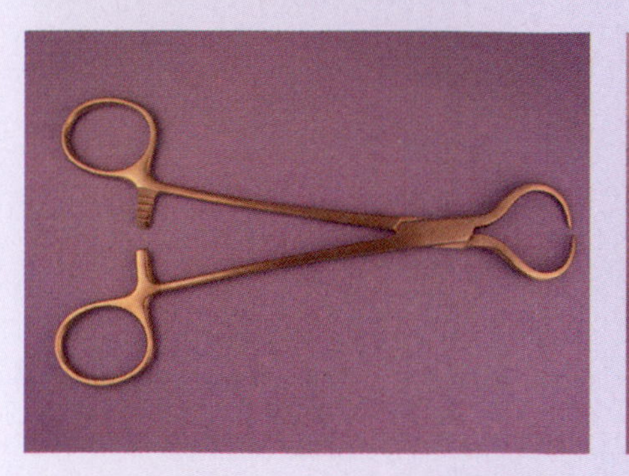

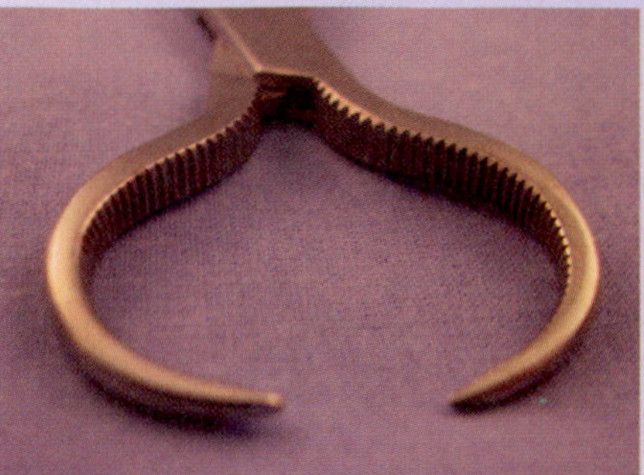

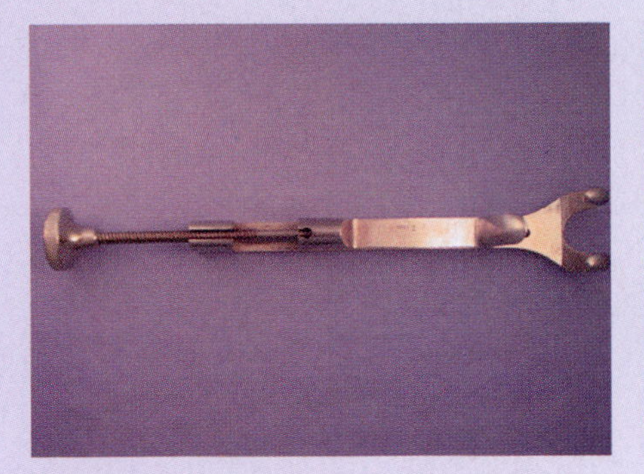

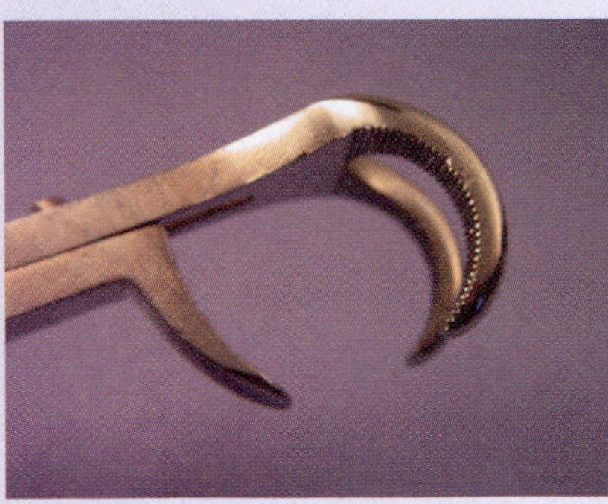

Name: Lowman bone-holding clamp

Alias: none

Category: clamping

Use: holding bone in place

Length: 4.75", 7.25", or 8"

Additional Information: 1 × 2 jaws

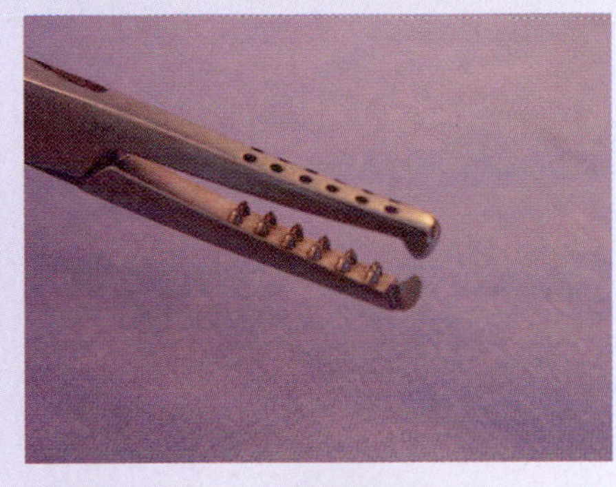

Name: Walton meniscus clamp

Alias: none

Category: clamping

Use: clamping meniscus tissue

Length: 7"

Additional Information: 1 × 2 teeth at tips of the jaw

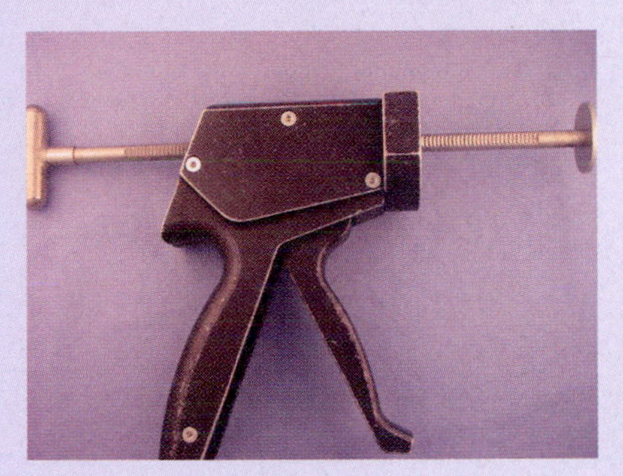

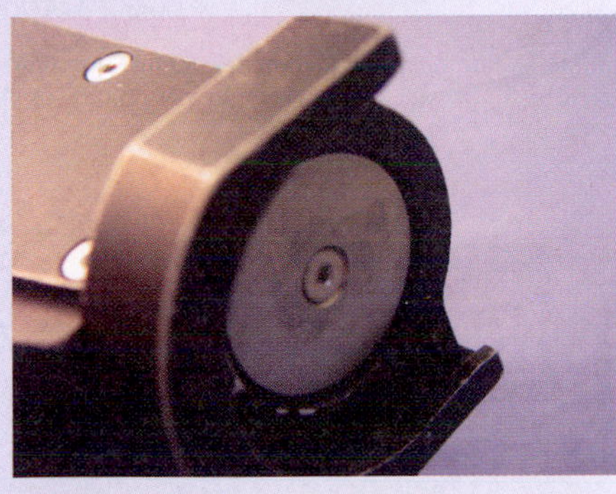

Name: cement gun

Alias: none

Category: accessory

Use: holding bone cement applicator; applying bone cement

Length: n/a

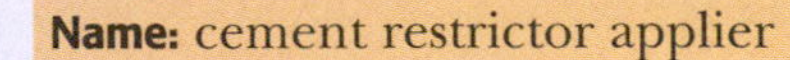

Name: cement restrictor applier

Alias: none

Category: accessory

Use: applying cement restrictor into femoral canal

Length: n/a

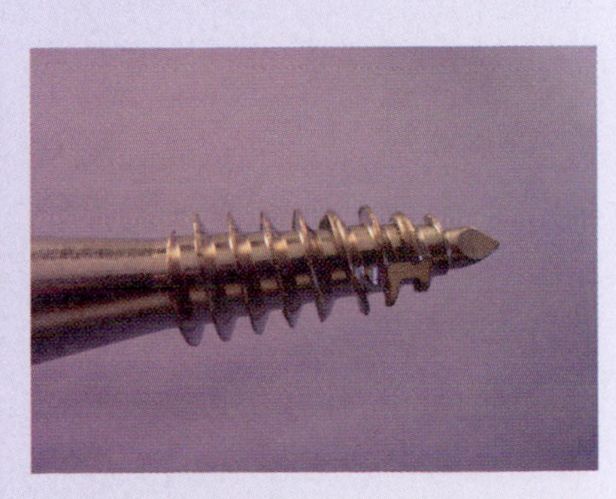

Name: femoral head remover

Alias: none

Category: accessory

Use: removing femoral head during hip surgery

Length: n/a

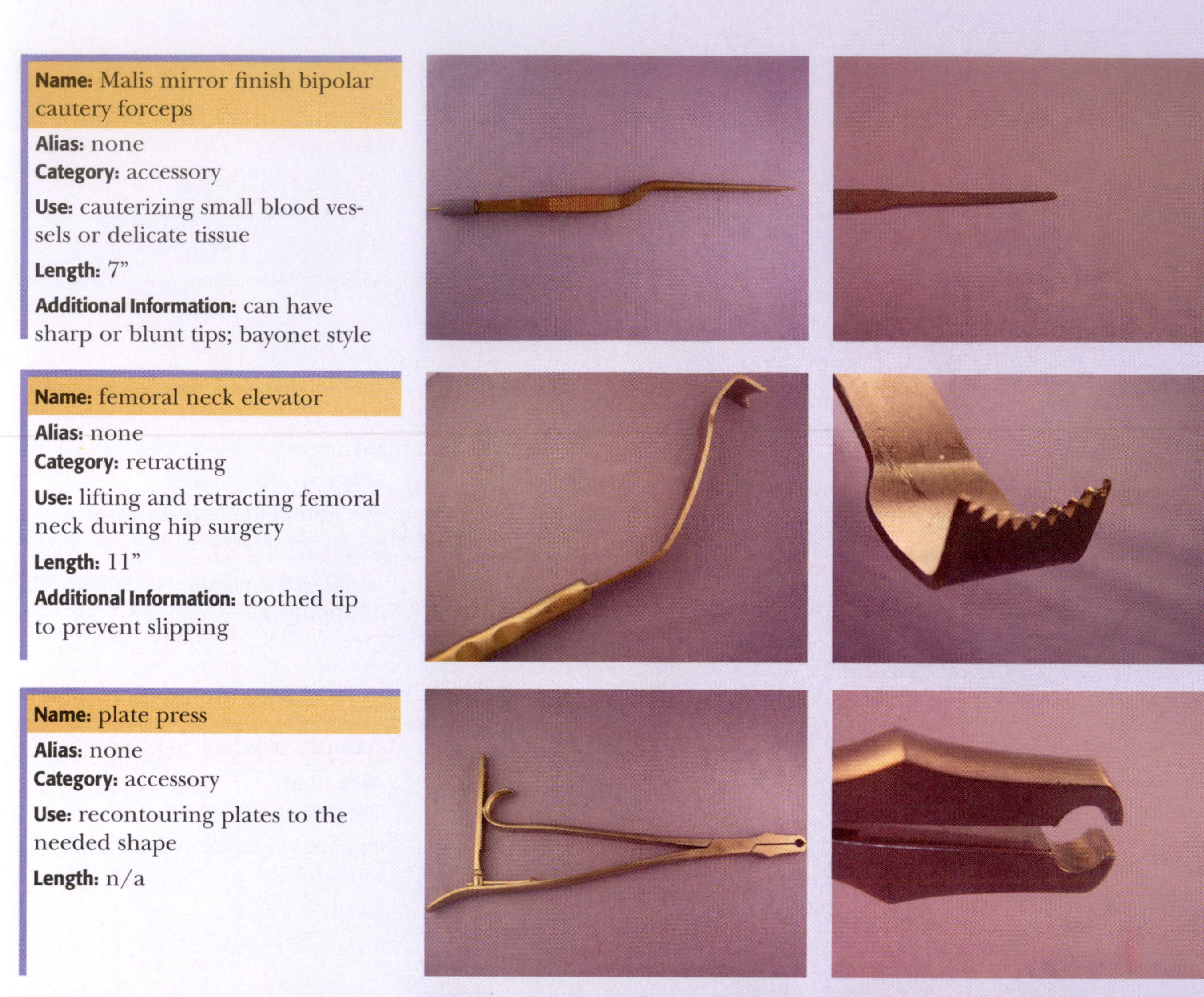

Name: Malis mirror finish bipolar cautery forceps
Alias: none
Category: accessory
Use: cauterizing small blood vessels or delicate tissue
Length: 7"
Additional Information: can have sharp or blunt tips; bayonet style

Name: femoral neck elevator
Alias: none
Category: retracting
Use: lifting and retracting femoral neck during hip surgery
Length: 11"
Additional Information: toothed tip to prevent slipping

Name: plate press
Alias: none
Category: accessory
Use: recontouring plates to the needed shape
Length: n/a

Name: Stryker drill
Alias: Stryker power system
Category: accessory
Use: provide power for drilling, sawing, or reaming during surgery
Length: n/a
Additional Information: has adapters so it can be used as a drill, saggital saw, or with reamers; battery operated

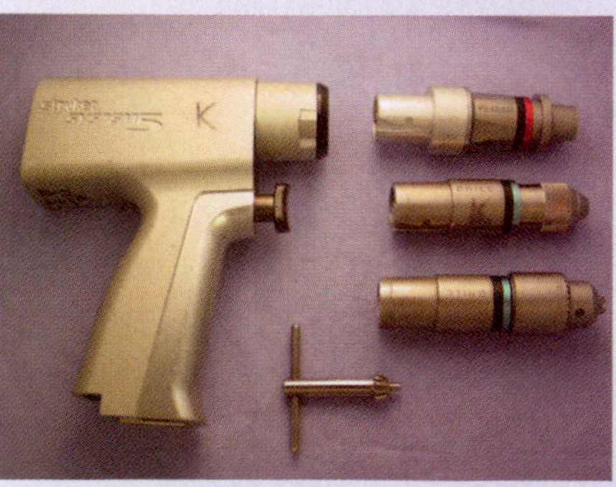

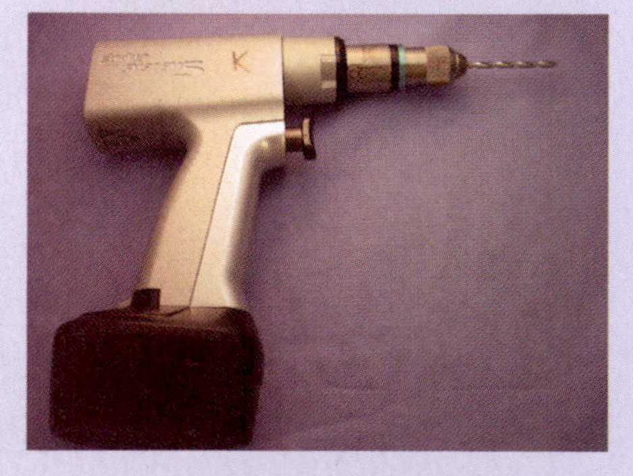

ORTHOPEDIC RETRACTORS

Name: Beckmann retractor
Alias: none
Category: retracting
Use: retracting soft tissue
Length: 5.5" or 6.5"
Additional Information: 3 × 4 prongs; prongs can be sharp or blunt; hinged arms

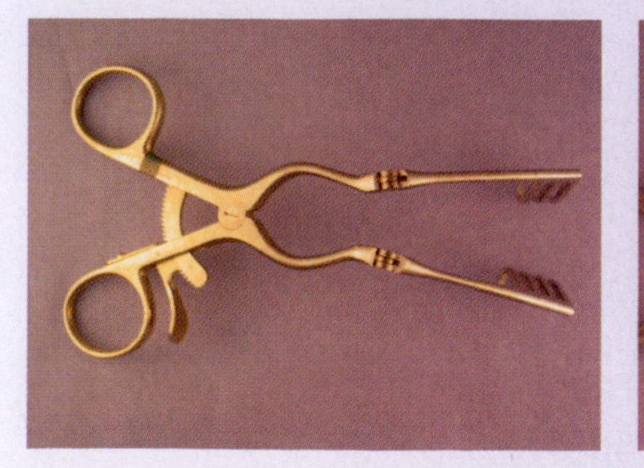

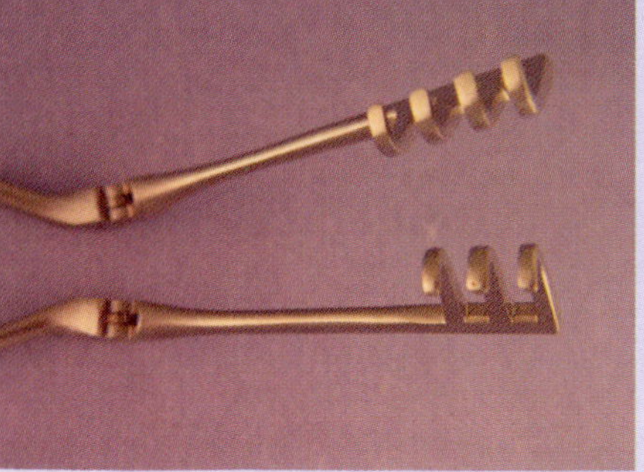

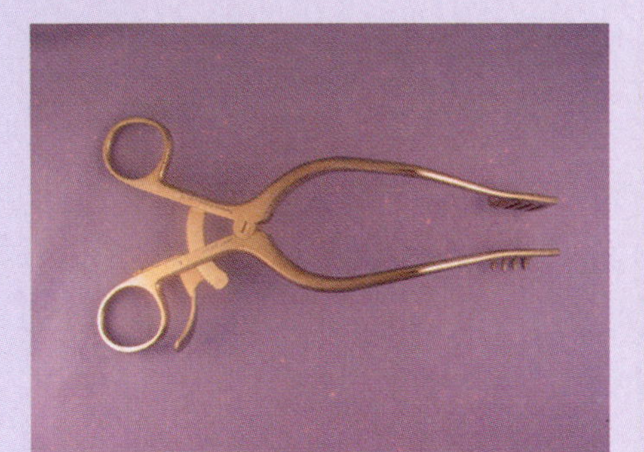
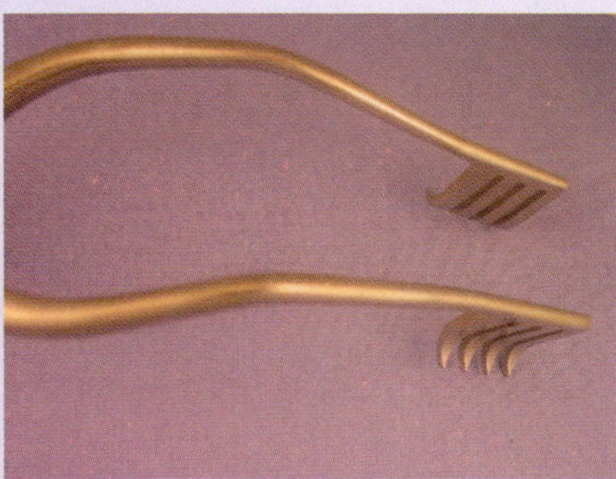

Name: Cerebellar retractor
Alias: Adson retractor
Category: retracting
Use: exposing wound
Length: 8”
Additional Information: 4 × 4 prongs; shanks are angled

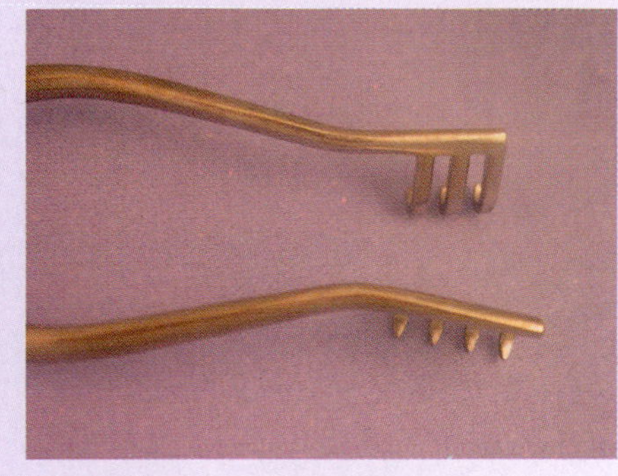

Name: Weitlaner retractor
Alias: none
Category: retracting
Use: superficial wound exposure
Length: 4”, 5.5”, 6.5”, 8”, or 9.5”
Additional Information: self-retaining; prongs can be sharp or dull; 2 × 3 prongs (4”), 3 × 4 prongs (all other sizes)

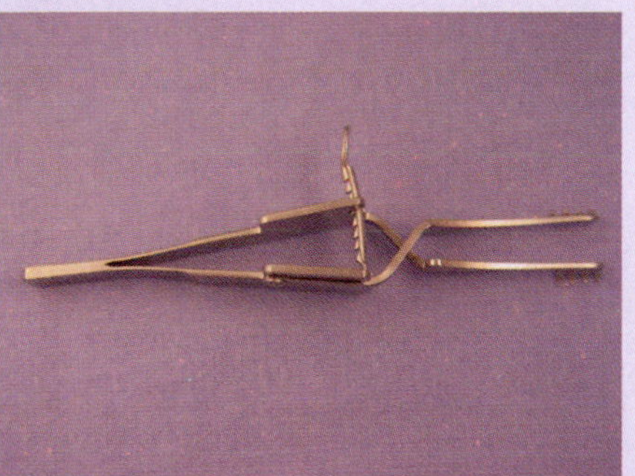
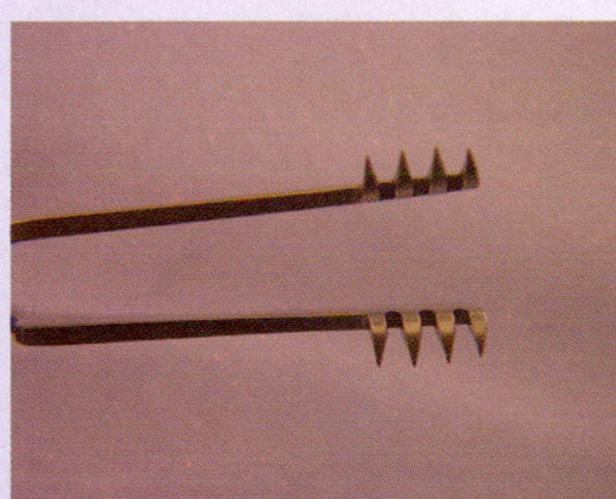

Name: Heiss skin retractor
Alias: none
Category: retracting
Use: retracting skin during hand surgery
Length: 4”
Additional Information: 4 × 4 prongs

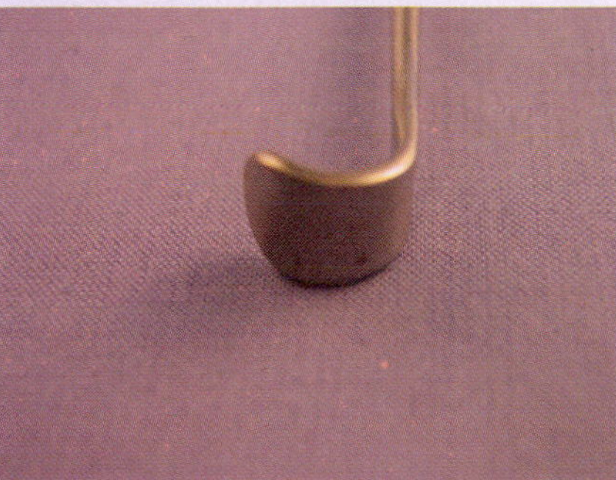

Name: Cushing vein retractor
Alias: none
Category: retracting
Use: retracting blood vessels
Length: 8” or 12”
Additional Information: open handle

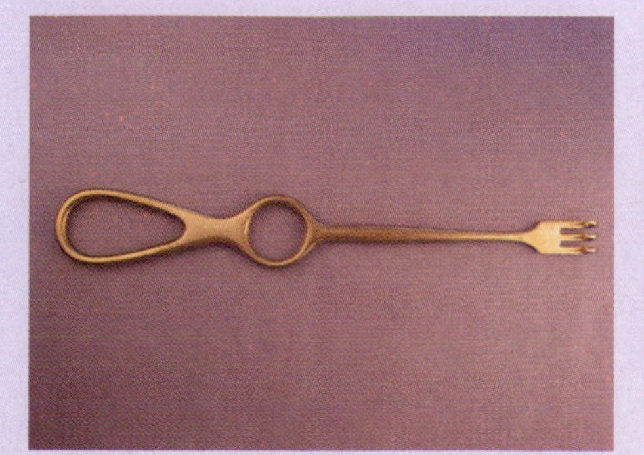
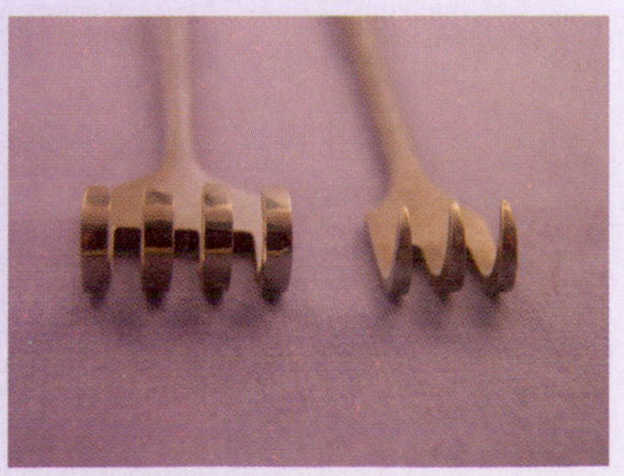

Name: Volkmann retractor
Alias: rake
Category: retracting
Use: superficial wound exposure
Length: 8.5”
Other: sharp or blunt tips; can have 2 to 6 teeth

Name: Senn Retractor
Alias: none
Category: retracting
Use: superficial wound exposure (hand or foot surgery)
Length: 6”
Additional Information: hand held; double ended; prongs can be sharp or dull; usually used in pairs

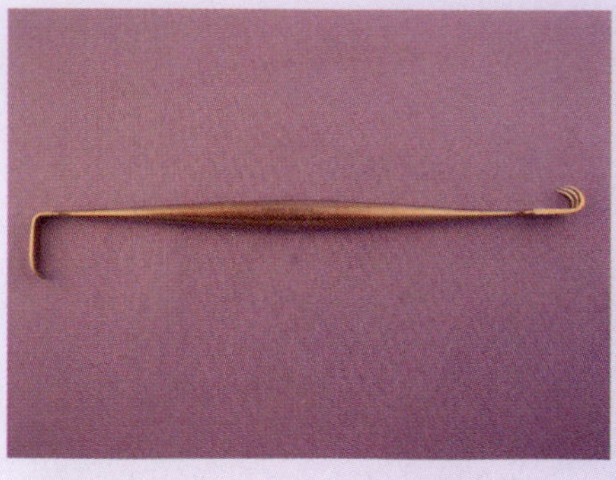
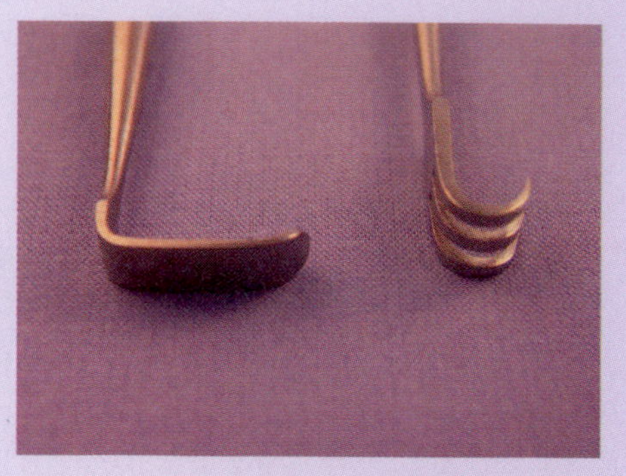

Name: Ragnell retractor
Alias: none
Category: retracting
Use: superficial wound exposure
Length: 6”
Additional Information: double ended; blunt on both ends

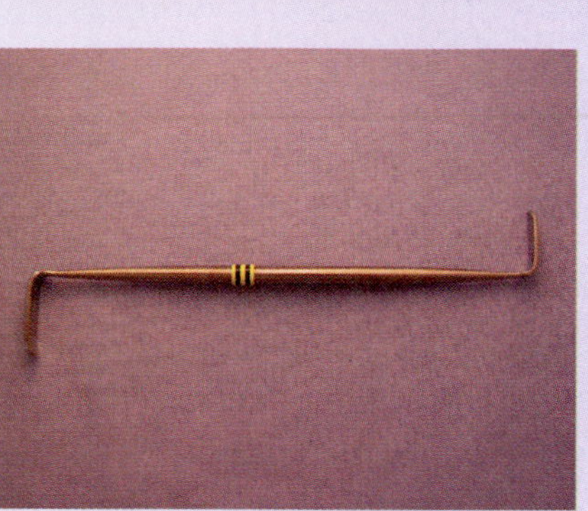
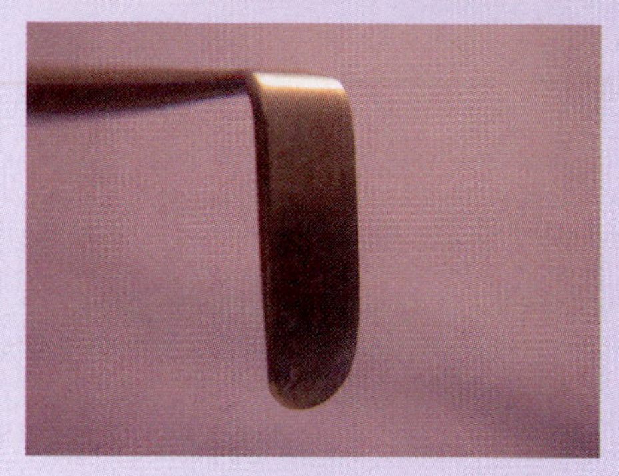

Name: Dandy nerve hook
Alias: none
Category: retracting
Use: retracting nerves
Length: 8.5”
Additional Information: blunt tip; tip can be pointed straight, left, or right

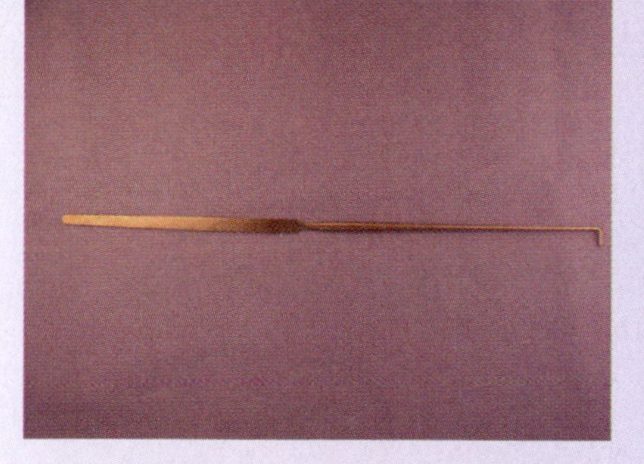
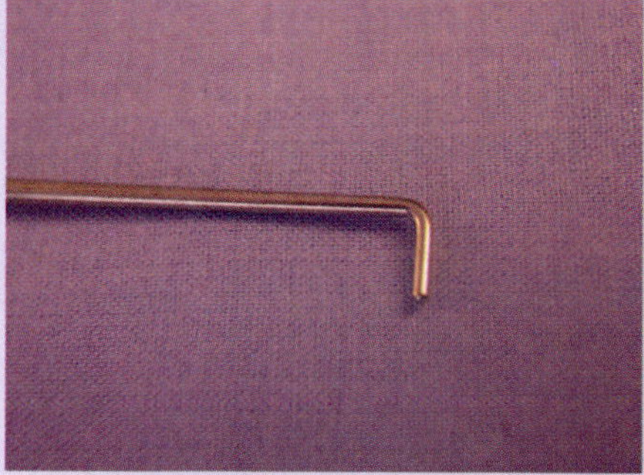

Name: Hohmann retractor
Alias: none
Category: retracting
Use: wound exposure during hip or knee surgery
Length: 9.5” to 11”
Additional Information: pointed blade; blade width varies

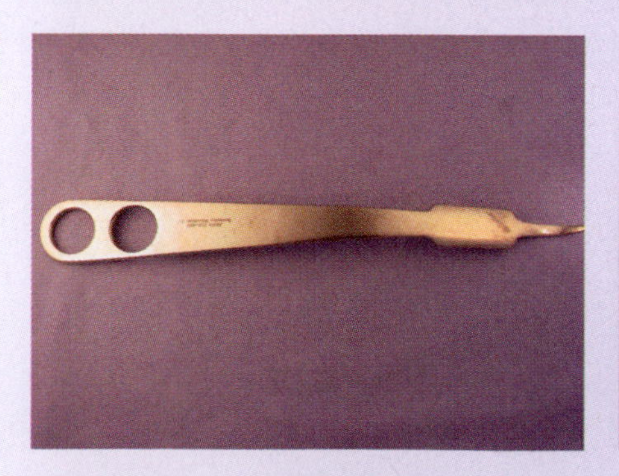
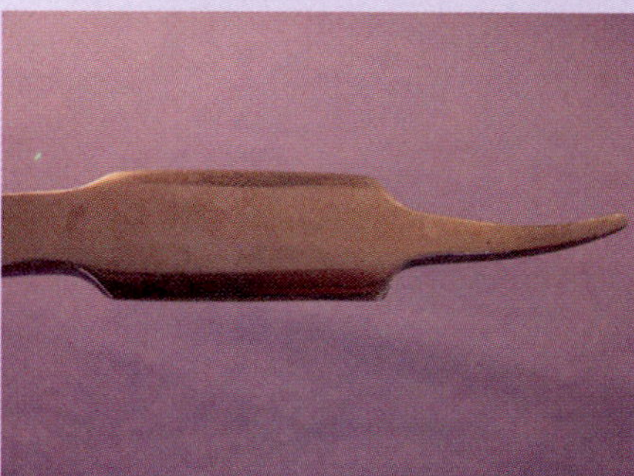

Name: Hohmann retractor
Alias: none
Category: retracting
Use: wound exposure during hip or knee surgery
Length: 9.5” to 11”
Additional Information: blunt blade; blade width varies

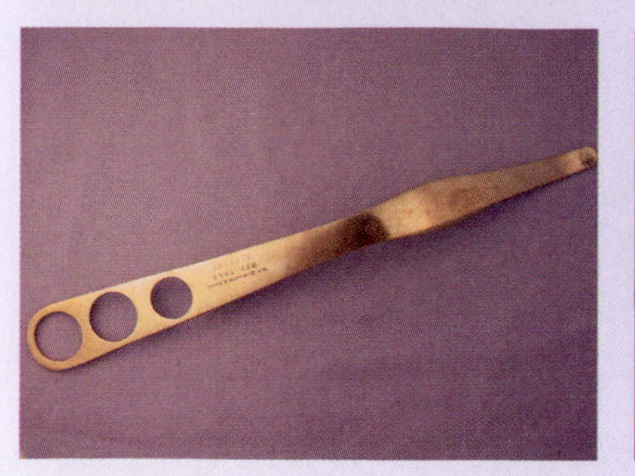
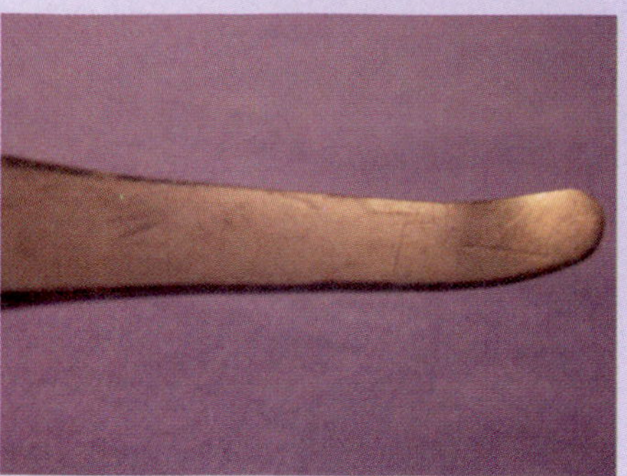

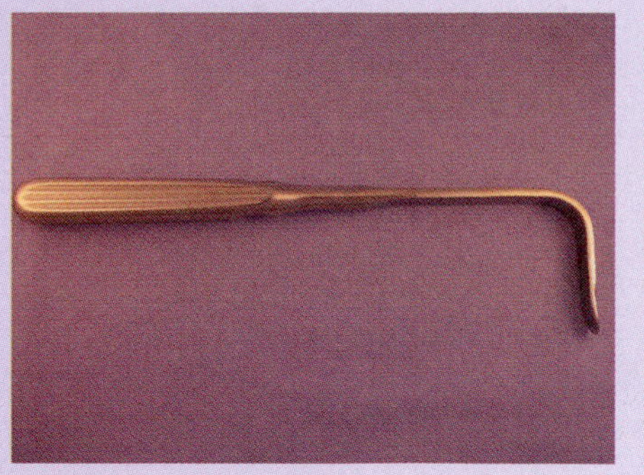

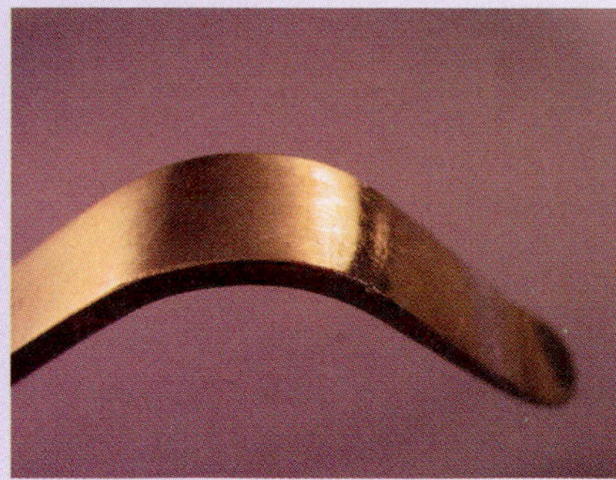

Name: Sauerbruch retractor
Alias: none
Category: retracting
Use: retracting soft tissue
Length: 9.5"
Additional Information: blade is slightly curved on the end; blade can be 1.75" to 3" wide

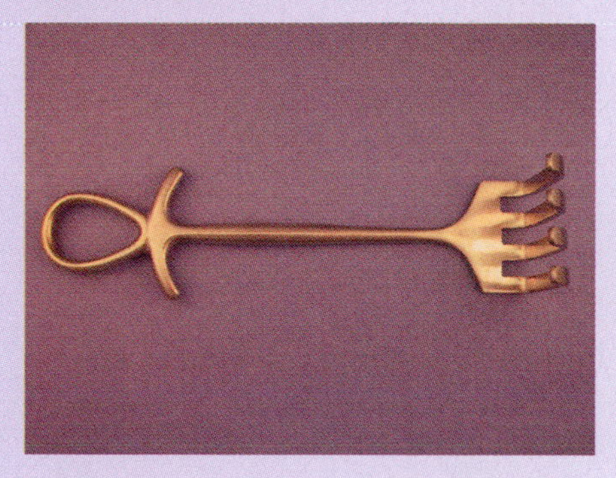

Name: Israel retractor
Alias: none
Category: retracting
Use: retracting heavy tissue
Length: 8"
Additional Information: rake can have 4 or 5 prongs; blades are 1.75" × 1.75"

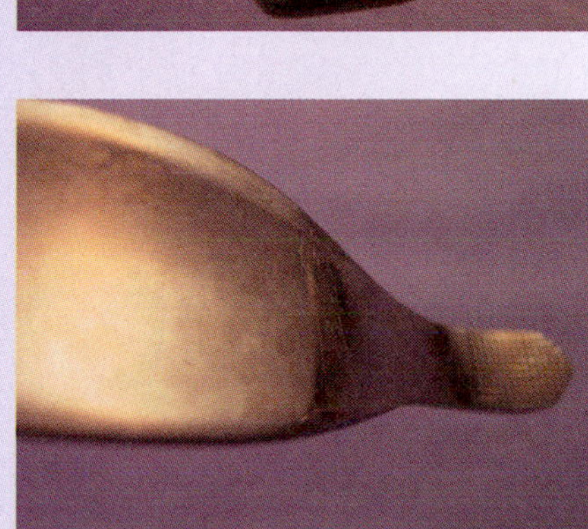

Name: Aufranc retractor
Alias: Cobra
Category: retracting
Use: wound exposure during knee or hip surgery
Length: 8.5"
Additional Information: hollow handle; three tip styles

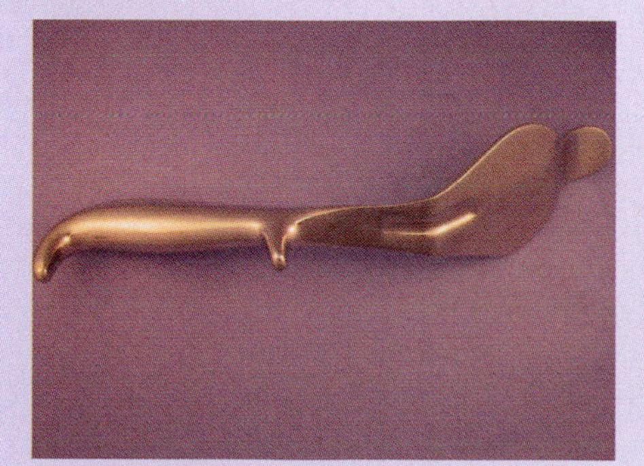

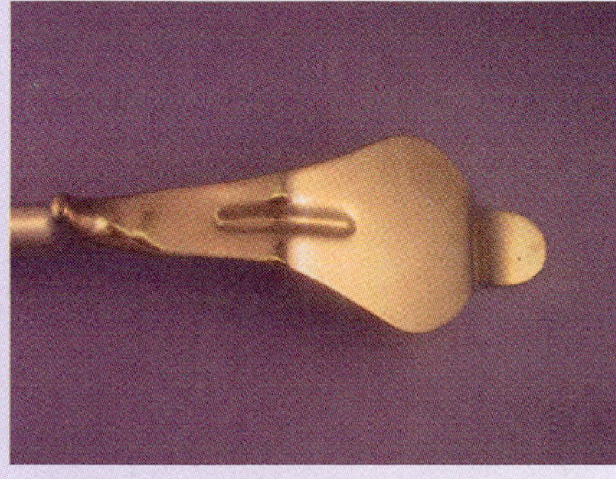

Name: Bennett retractor
Alias: none
Category: retracting
Use: tibial retraction
Length: 10"
Additional Information: blade width 1.75" or 2.5"

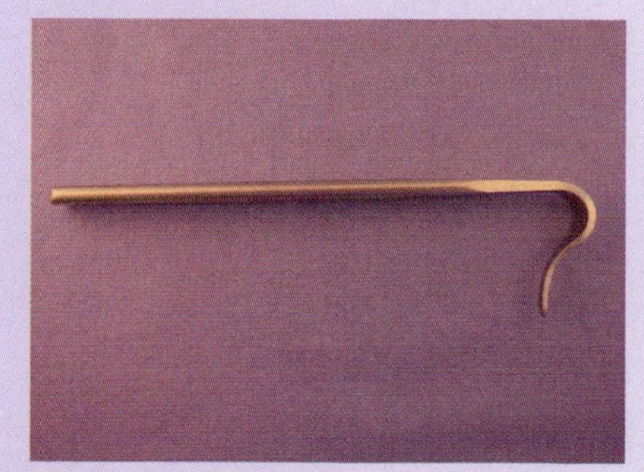

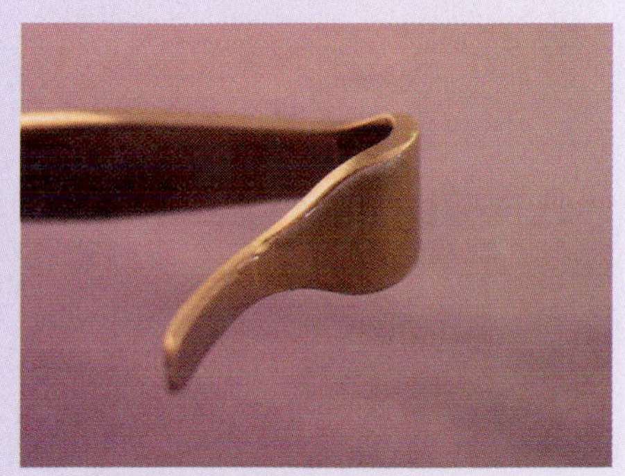

Name: Blount knee retractor
Alias: none
Category: retracting
Use: wound exposure during knee surgery
Length: 8.75"
Additional Information: notched blade

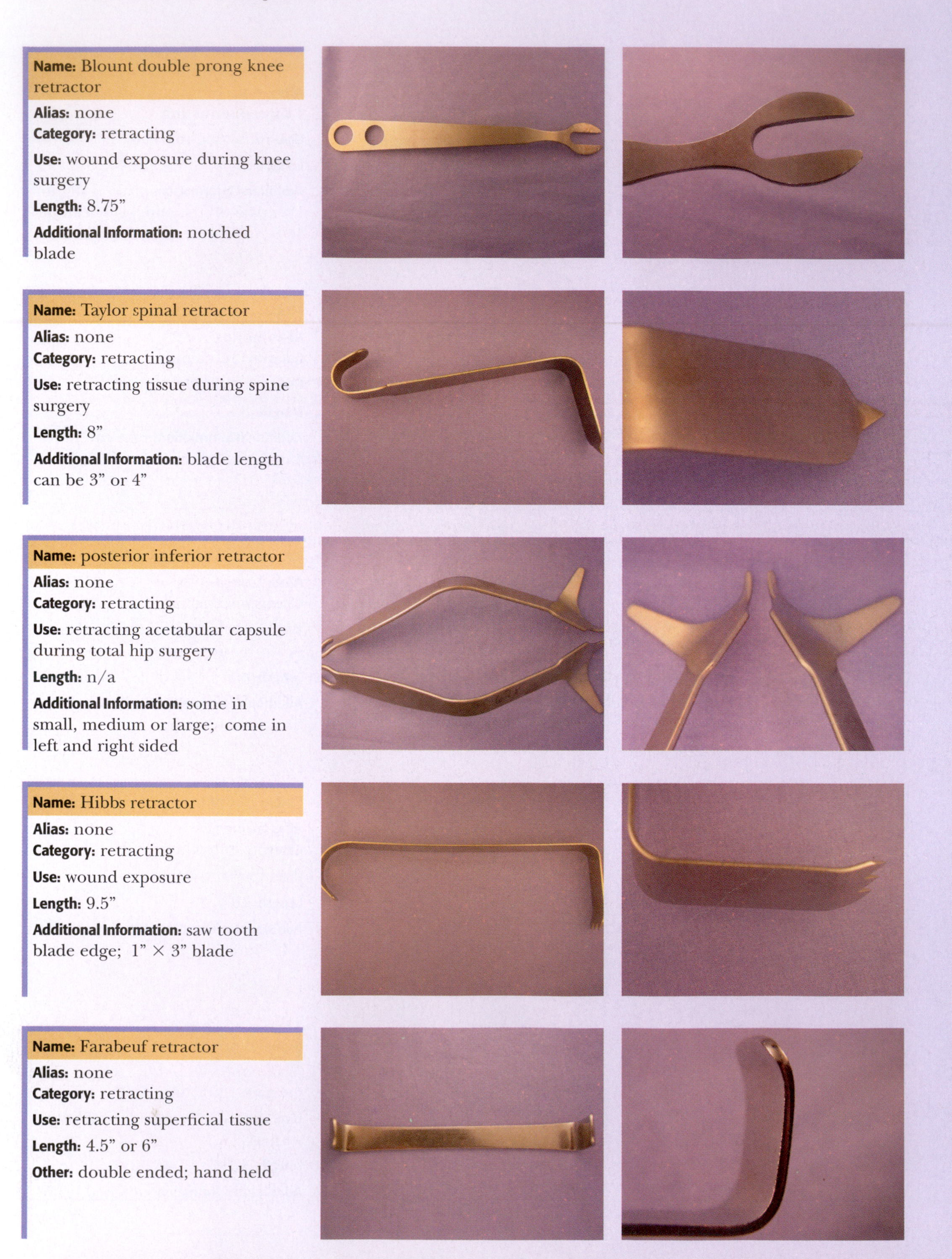

Name: Blount double prong knee retractor
Alias: none
Category: retracting
Use: wound exposure during knee surgery
Length: 8.75"
Additional Information: notched blade

Name: Taylor spinal retractor
Alias: none
Category: retracting
Use: retracting tissue during spine surgery
Length: 8"
Additional Information: blade length can be 3" or 4"

Name: posterior inferior retractor
Alias: none
Category: retracting
Use: retracting acetabular capsule during total hip surgery
Length: n/a
Additional Information: some in small, medium or large; come in left and right sided

Name: Hibbs retractor
Alias: none
Category: retracting
Use: wound exposure
Length: 9.5"
Additional Information: saw tooth blade edge; 1" × 3" blade

Name: Farabeuf retractor
Alias: none
Category: retracting
Use: retracting superficial tissue
Length: 4.5" or 6"
Other: double ended; hand held

Q&A

Surgical Session—Orthopedic Instruments

1) You are scrubbed on shoulder surgery. The surgeon asks for a rasp to smooth the bone. You would hand him/her a:
   a. Putti
   b. Penfield
   c. Molt
   d. Bennett

2) All of the following are hand-held (manual) retractors *except*:
   a. Hohmann
   b. Blout
   c. Beckmann
   d. Israel

3) Which of the following would you NOT expect to find on a set-up for hip surgery?
   a. femoral head extractor
   b. femoral neck elevator
   c. posterior inferior retractor
   d. Taylor retractor

4) A small self-retaining skin retractor used in hand surgery is a:
   a. Heiss
   b. Beckmann
   c. Senn
   d. Ragnell

5) The surgeon asks for a "cobra" retractor. Another name for this is a:
   a. Bennett
   b. Aufranc
   c. Hibbs
   d. Israel

6) A ____________ is a type of meniscus clamp.
   a. Waller
   b. Walton
   c. Waldron
   d. Wallstein

7) You hand the surgeon a Hibbs osteotome. The next instrument you need to have ready to hand him/her is a:
   a. pin cutter
   b. mallet
   c. curette
   d. pliers

8) Dawson-Yuhl curettes are more commonly known as:
   a. Cobb
   b. Brun
   c. Hibbs
   d. Lambotte

9) All of the following are rongeurs *except*:
   a. Ruskin
   b. Stille-Horsley
   c. Molt
   d. Luksell

10) A Stevens scissors is also known as a _________ scissors.
    a. Mayo
    b. Metzenbaum
    c. Tenotomy
    d. Strully

11) The surgeon wishes to measure the femoral head. You hand him/her a:
    a. Hibbs
    b. Townley
    c. Molt
    d. Key

12) The instrument used to create a pilot hole for femoral reaming is a:
    a. Senn
    b. Lambotte
    c. Box osteotome
    d. Brun

13) A ____________ is a type of gouge.
    a. Lexer
    b. Luxor
    c. Lambotte
    d. Little

14) A type of self-retaining retractor with hinged arms is a:
    a. Weitlaner
    b. Cerebellar

c. Beckmann

d. Farabeuf

15) You are scrubbed on a total knee replacement. The surgeon asks for a tibial retractor. You would hand him/her a:

a. Senn

b. Bennett

c. Farabeuf

d. Taylor

16) All of the following are periosteal elevators *except*:

a. Molt

b. Key

c. Cushing "little joker"

d. Putti

Neurosurgical Instruments 5

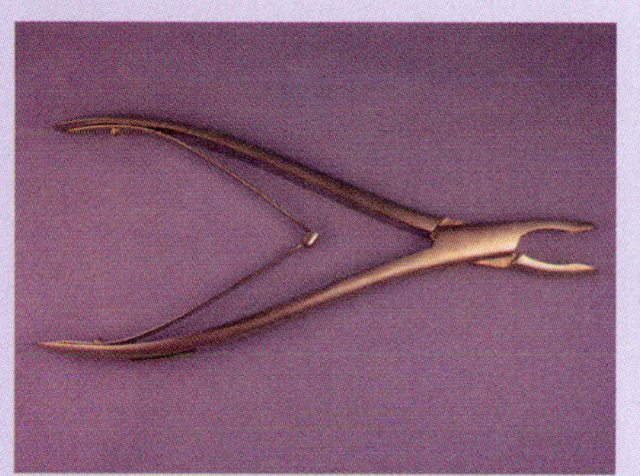

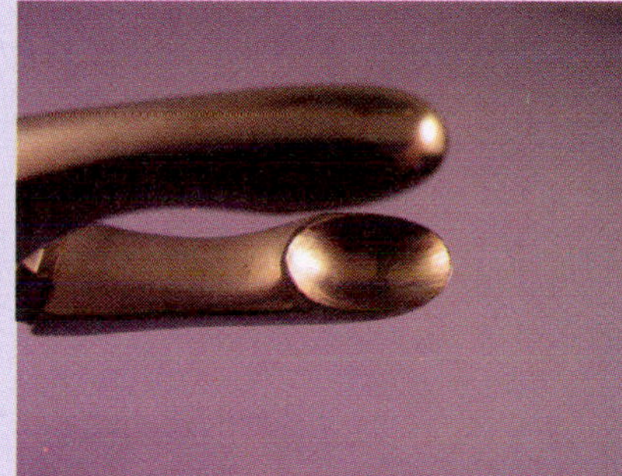

Name: Adson cranial rongeur
Alias: none
Category: cutting
Use: removing pieces of cranial bone
Length: 8"
Additional Information: straight jaw; 8 mm bite

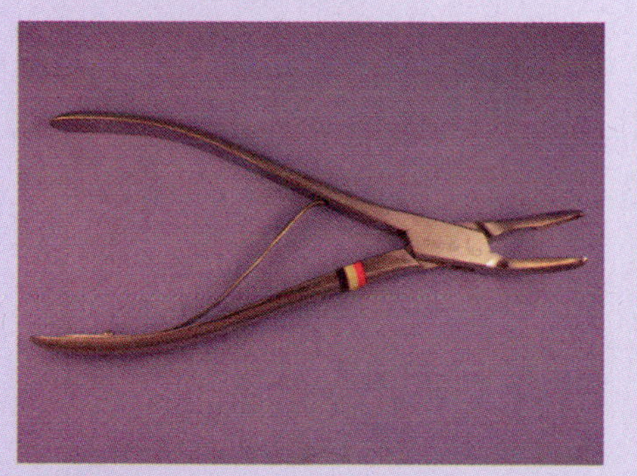

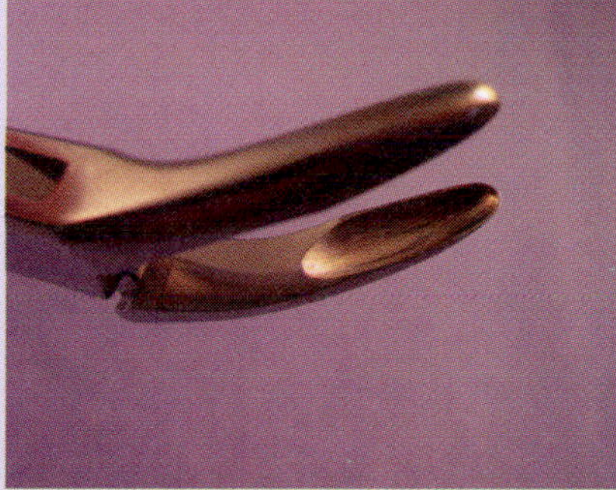

Name: Bacon cranial rongeur
Alias: none
Category: cutting
Use: removing pieces of cranial bone
Length: 7.75"
Additional Information: angled jaw; 5 mm bite

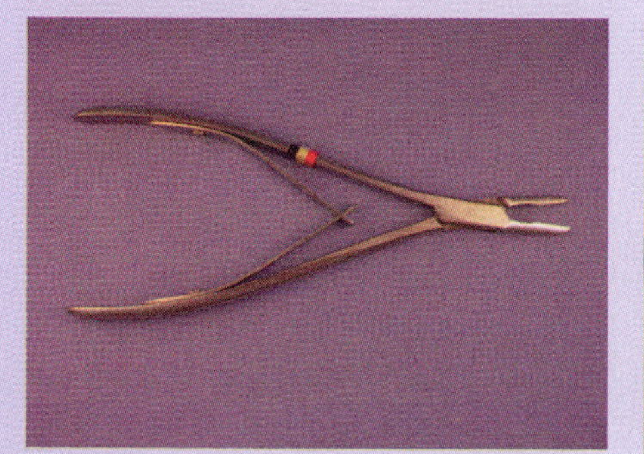

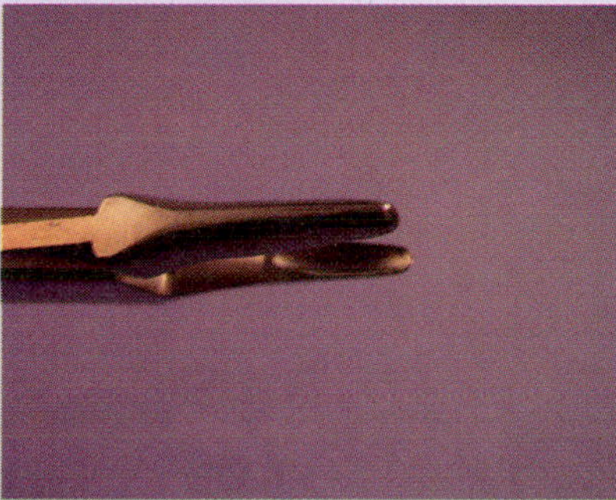

Name: Beyer rongeur
Alias: Lamprey rongeur
Category: cutting
Use: removing small pieces of bone
Length: 6"
Additional Information: 2 mm bite

Name: Stookey cranial rongeur
Alias: none
Category: cutting
Use: removing pieces of cranial bone
Length: 7.5"
Additional Information: angled jaw; 3 mm bite

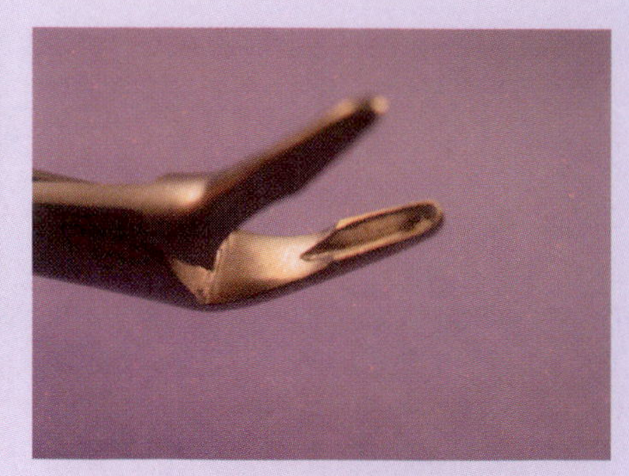

Name: Leksell rongeur
Alias: Gooseneck
Category: cutting
Use: cutting off small bites of bone
Length: 9.5"
Additional Information: comes in 3 mm, 4 mm, 6 mm bite size

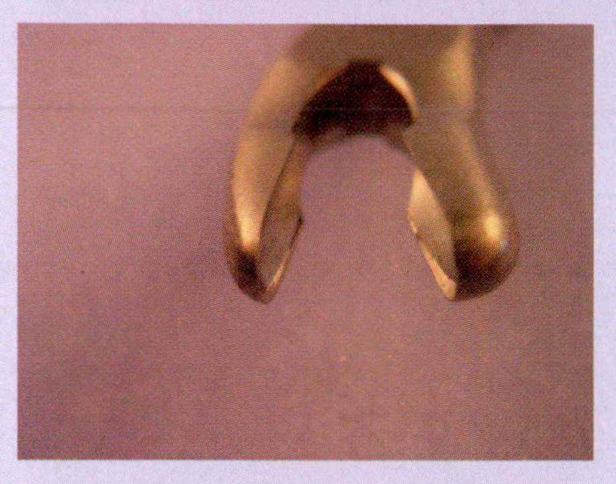

Name: Kerrison rongeur
Alias: none
Category: cutting
Use: removing pieces of bone
Length: 6", 7", or 8"
Additional Information: bite size can be 2 mm to 5 mm; plate can be 40 degrees up or 90 degrees up or down

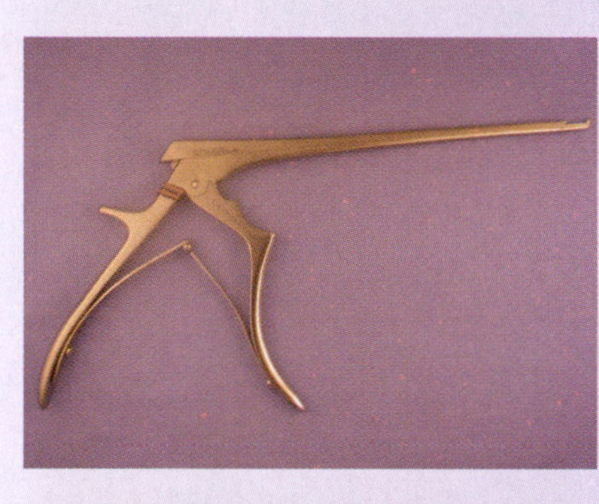

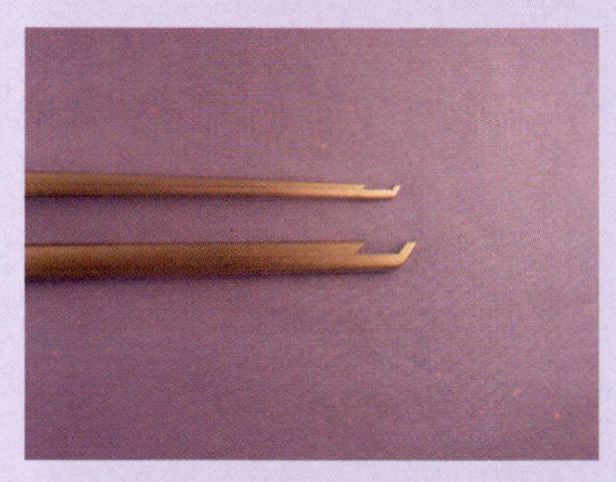

Name: Cushing pituitary rongeur
Alias: upbiter (jaws angled up); downbiter (jaws angled down)
Category: cutting
Use: removing pieces of intervertebral disc or bone
Length: shaft can be 6", 7", or 8"
Additional Information: jaws can be straight or angled up or down; jaw bite can be 1.5 mm or 2 mm

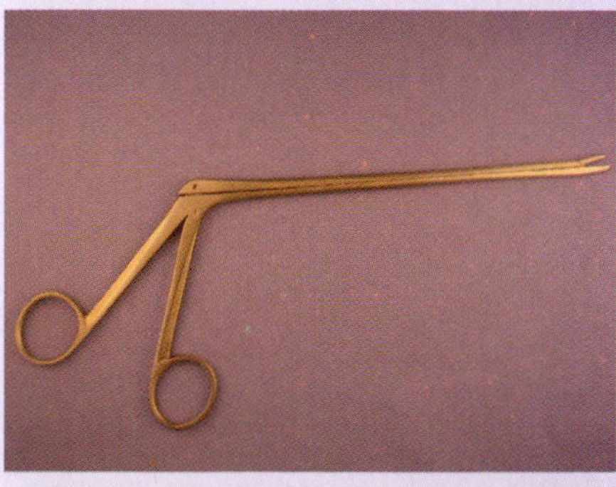

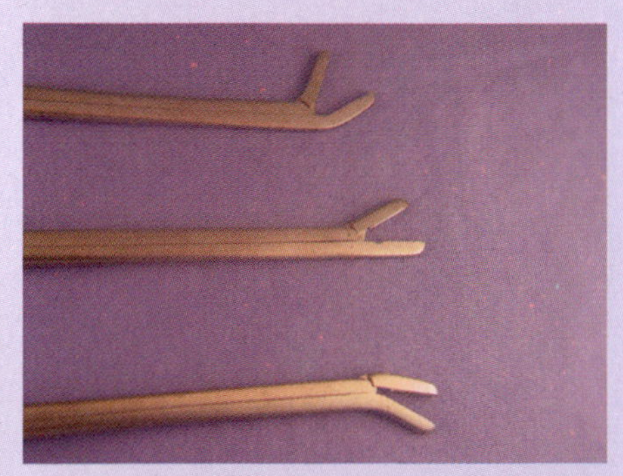

Name: Spurling rongeur
Alias: Spurling intervertebral disc rongeur
Category: cutting
Use: removing bits of intervertebral disc
Length: shaft is 6" or 7"
Additional Information: jaws can be straight, up, or down; jaw bite 4 mm × 10 mm

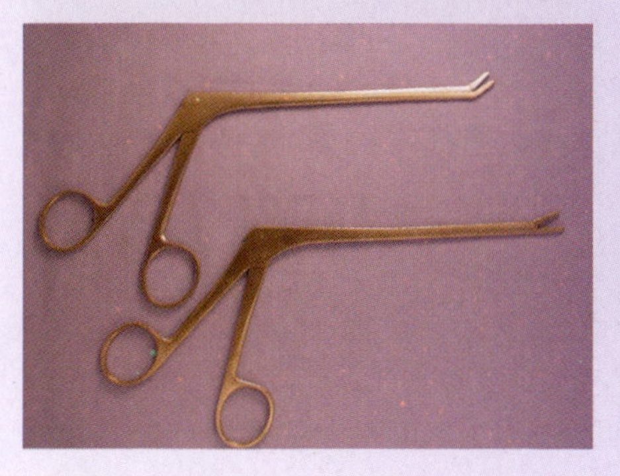

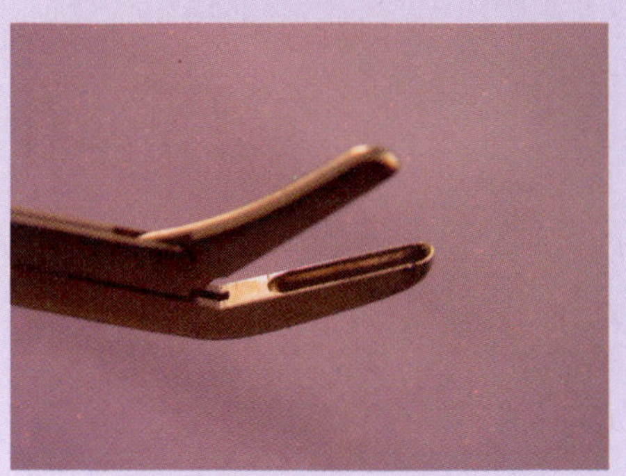

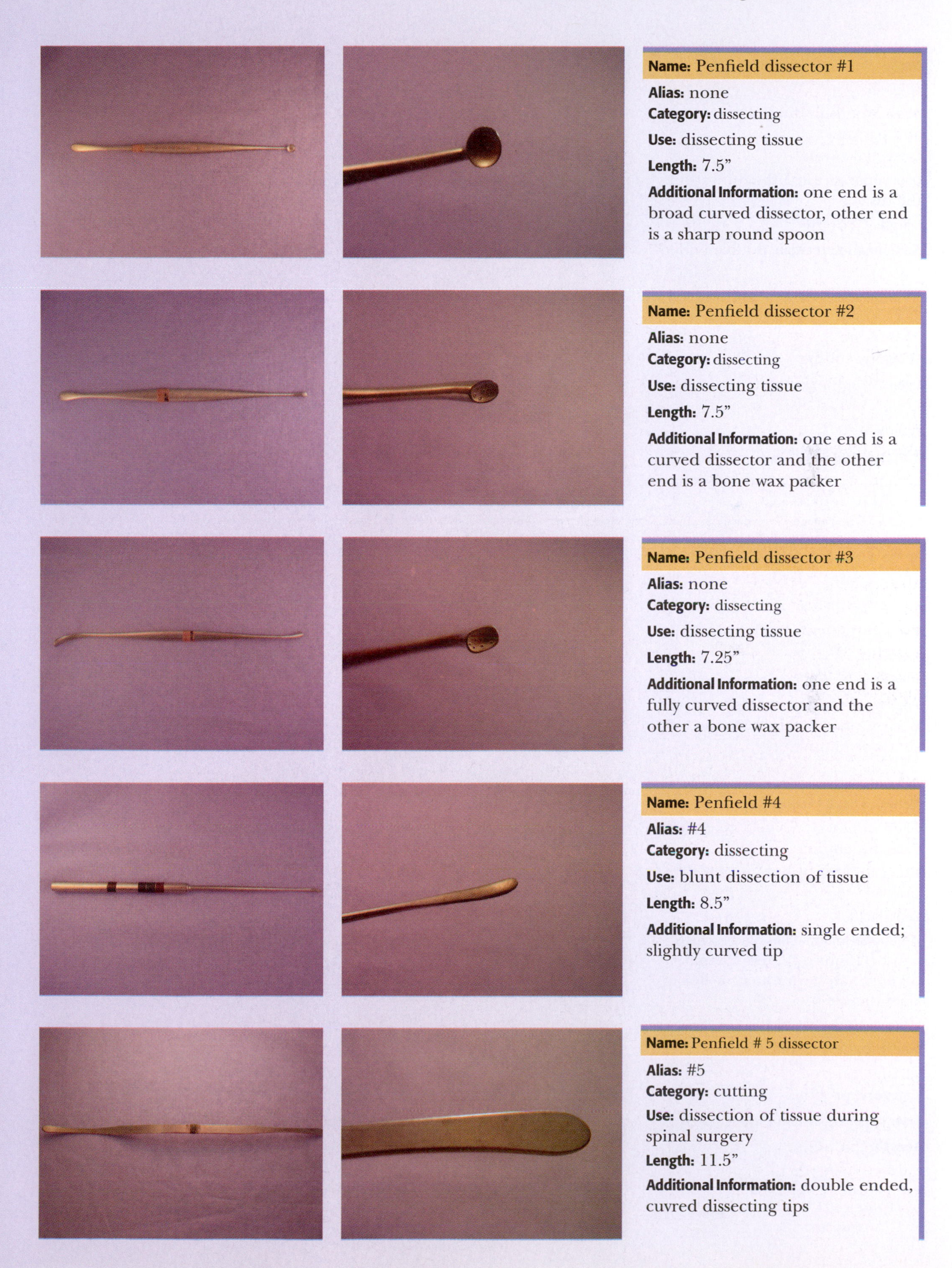

Name: Penfield dissector #1

Alias: none

Category: dissecting

Use: dissecting tissue

Length: 7.5"

Additional Information: one end is a broad curved dissector, other end is a sharp round spoon

Name: Penfield dissector #2

Alias: none

Category: dissecting

Use: dissecting tissue

Length: 7.5"

Additional Information: one end is a curved dissector and the other end is a bone wax packer

Name: Penfield dissector #3

Alias: none

Category: dissecting

Use: dissecting tissue

Length: 7.25"

Additional Information: one end is a fully curved dissector and the other a bone wax packer

Name: Penfield #4

Alias: #4

Category: dissecting

Use: blunt dissection of tissue

Length: 8.5"

Additional Information: single ended; slightly curved tip

Name: Penfield # 5 dissector

Alias: #5

Category: cutting

Use: dissection of tissue during spinal surgery

Length: 11.5"

Additional Information: double ended, cuvred dissecting tips

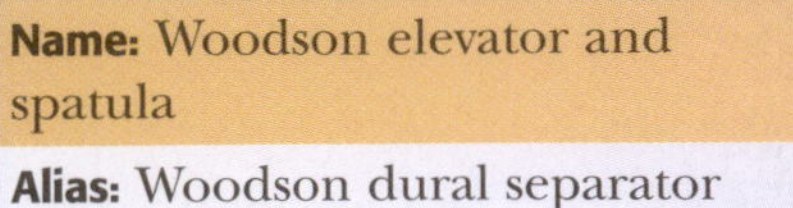
Name: Woodson elevator and spatula

Alias: Woodson dural separator and packer
Category: cutting
Use: separate (lift) the dura from the disk
Length: 7" or 10"
Additional Information: double ended

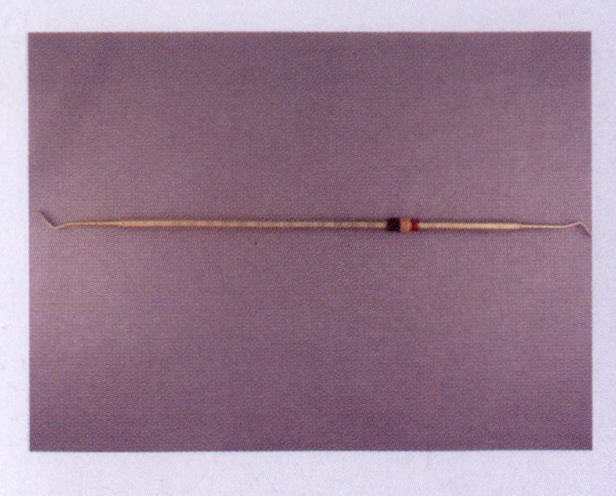

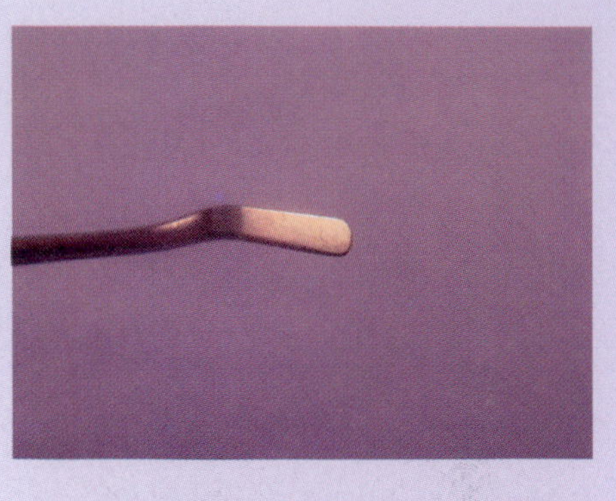

Name: Adson periosteal elevator

Alias: none
Category: cutting
Use: lifting periosteum from the bone
Length: 6.5"
Additional Information: blade can be straight or curved; end can be round or square

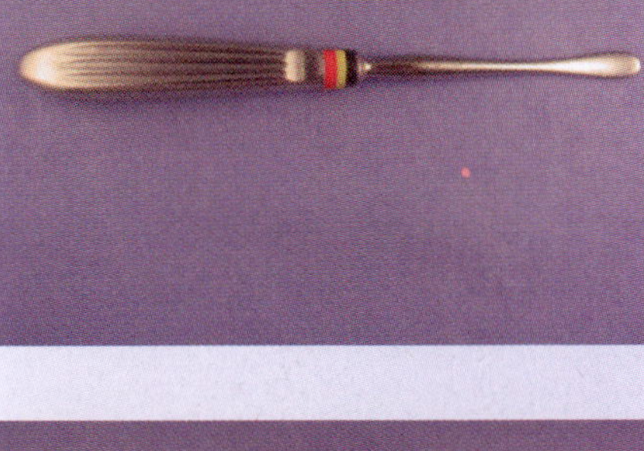

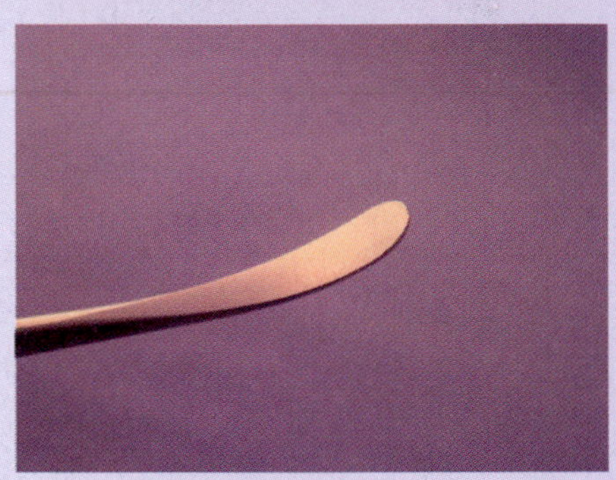

Name: Cushing periosteal elevator

Alias: none
Category: cutting
Use: lifting periosteum from the bone
Length: 7.5"
Additional Information: blade can be narrow or wide; blade can be sharp or blunt

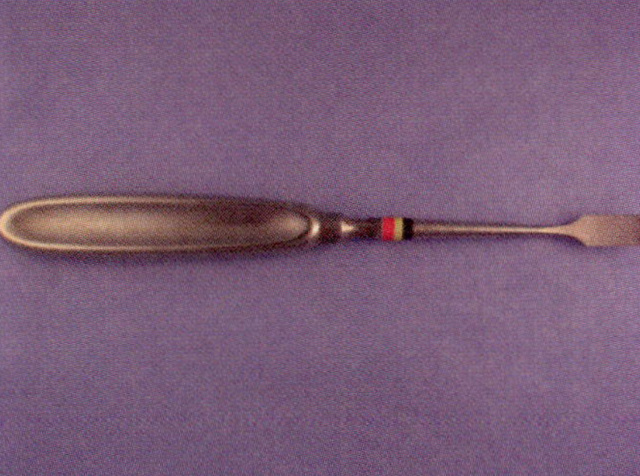

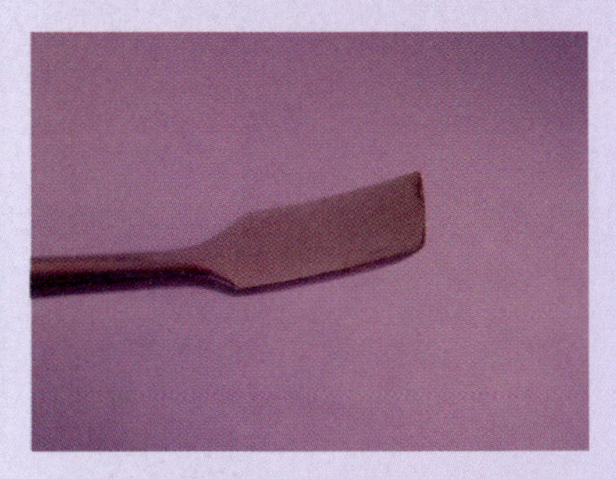

Name: Cobb elevator

Alias: none
Category: cutting
Use: Elevating and removing soft tissue
Length: 11"
Additional Information: blade width can be 13 mm, 19 mm, 25 mm, 32 mm; can have round or hexagonal handle

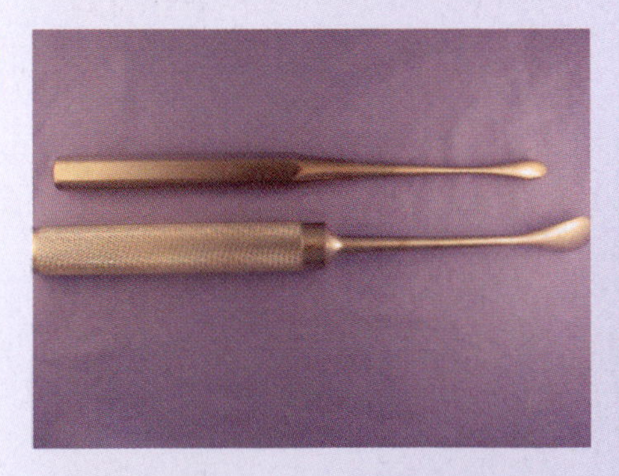

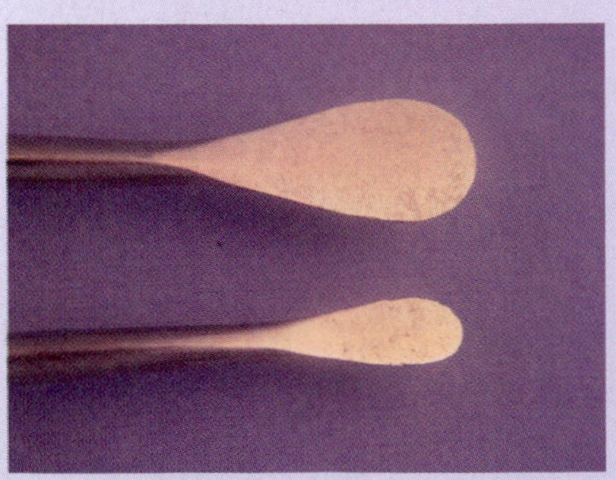

Name: ball tip probe

Alias: none
Category: probing
Use: probing during back surgery
Length: 9.5"

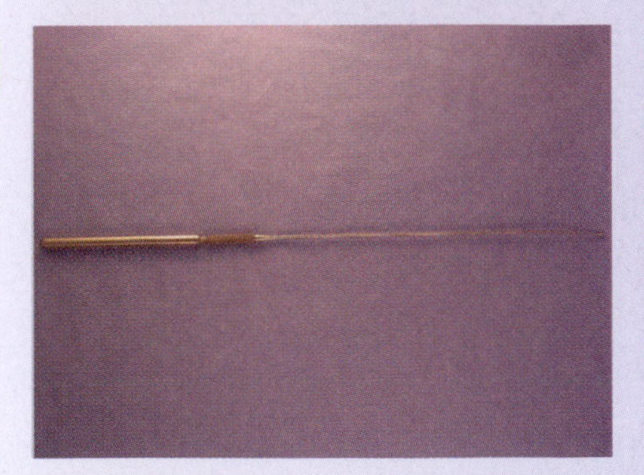

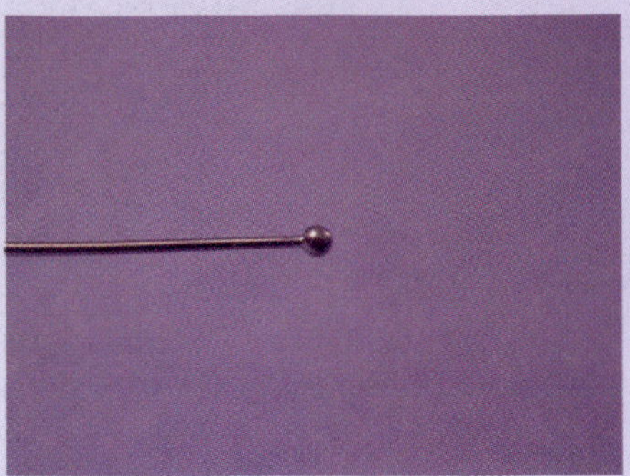

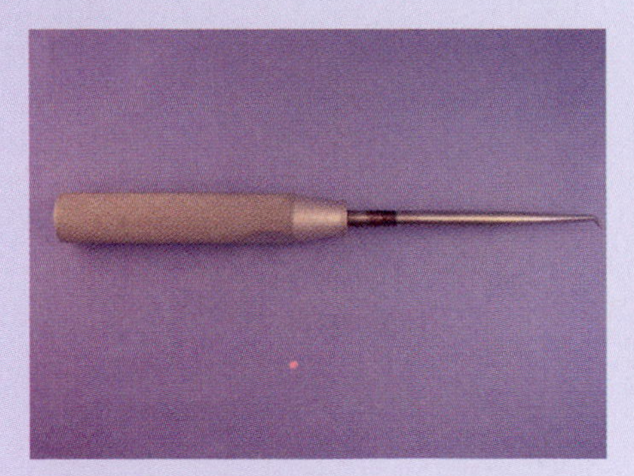
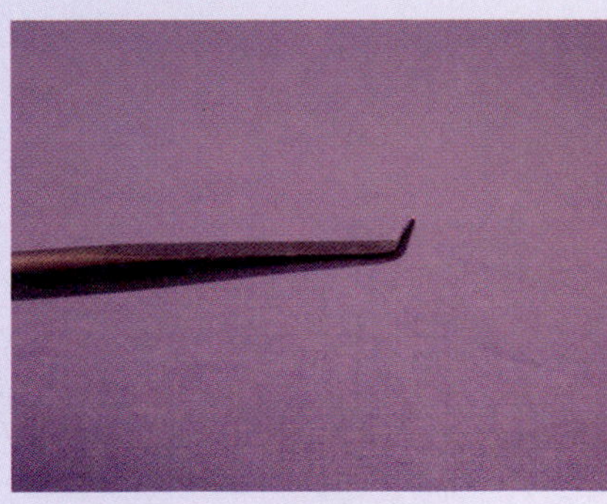

Name: Annular dissector perforator

Alias: none

Category: cutting

Use: reducing annular bulge following discectomy; dissecting scar tissue from dural sac

Length: 8.75"

Additional Information: tapered tip

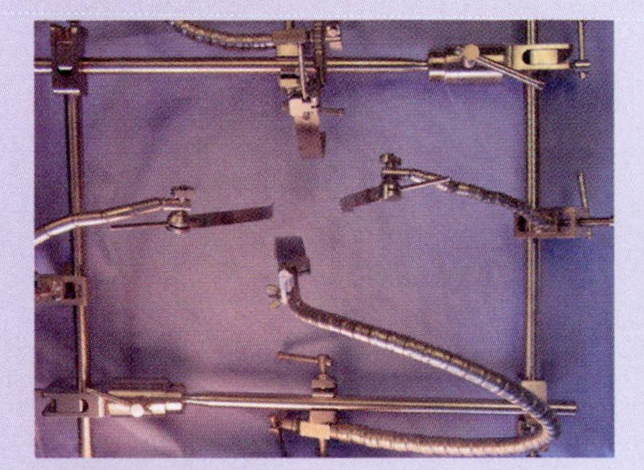
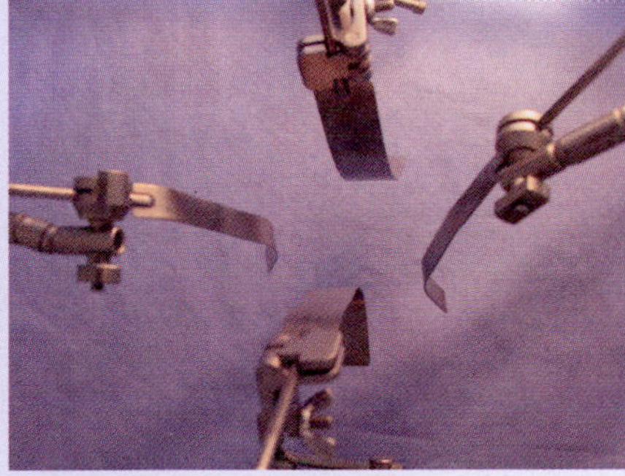

Name: Greenberg retractor

Alias: none

Category: retracting

Use: retraction of cranium during neurosurgery

Length: n/a

Additional Information: self retaining; has additional pieces (not pictured) to mount on bed/frame

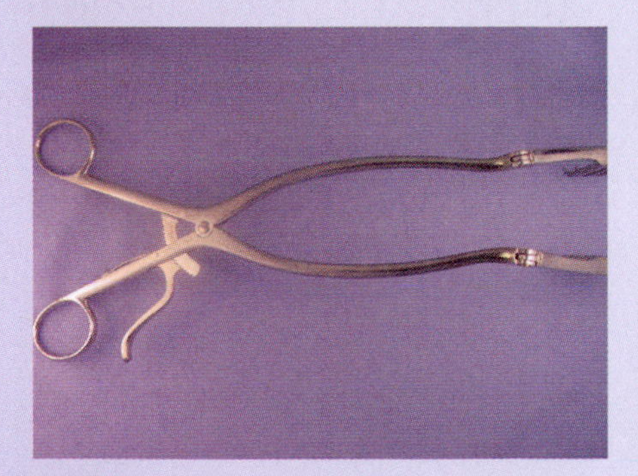
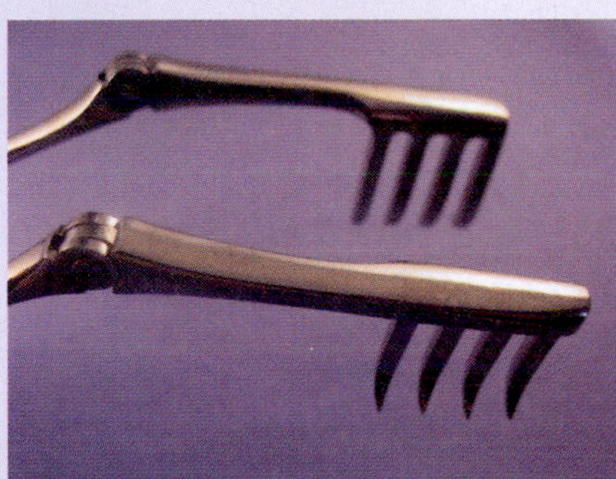

Name: Beckmann-Adson laminectomy retractor

Alias: Beckmann goiter retractor

Category: retracting

Use: wound exposure

Length: 12"

Additional Information: hinged shanks; 4 × 4 sharp prongs

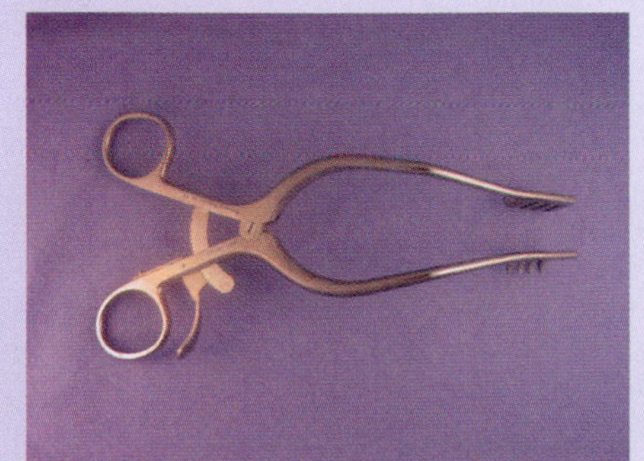

Name: Cerebellar retractor

Alias: Adson retractor

Category: retracting

Use: wound exposure

Length: 8"

Additional Information: 4 × 4 prongs; shanks are angled

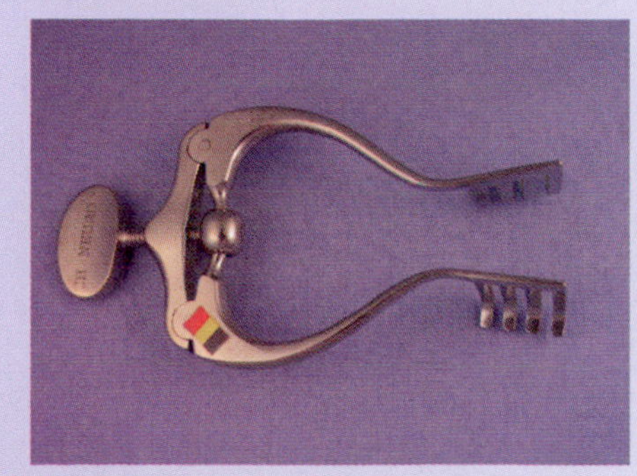
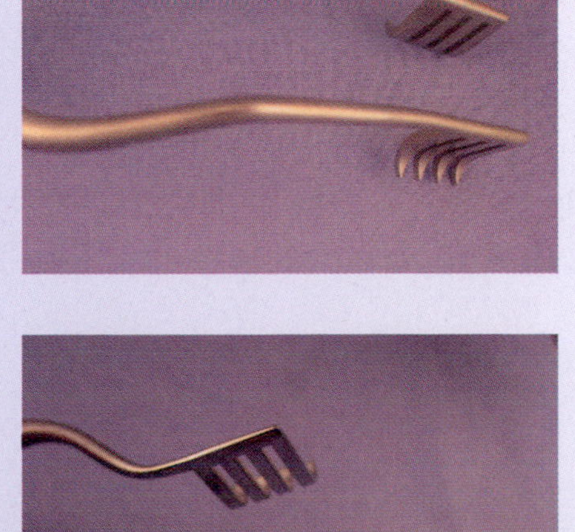

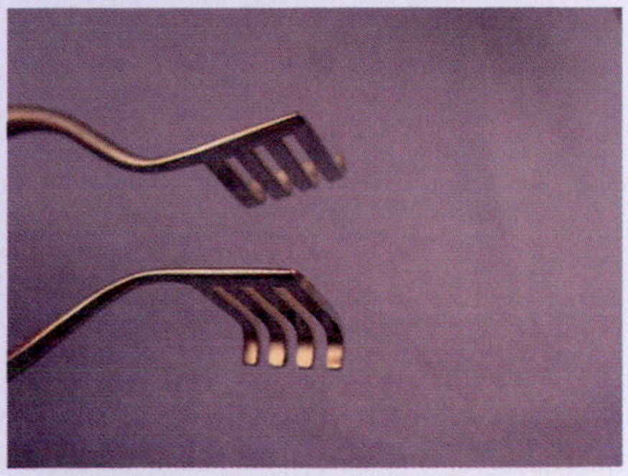

Name: Jansen retractor

Alias: Gifford; Allport; mastoid

Category: retracting

Use: retracting mastoid or scalp

Length: 4" or 4.5"

Additional Information: blunt; 3 × 3 or 4 × 4 prongs; self-retaining

Name: Taylor spinal retractor
Alias: none
Category: retracting
Use: retracting tissue during spine surgery
Length: 8"
Additional Information: blade length can be 3" or 4"

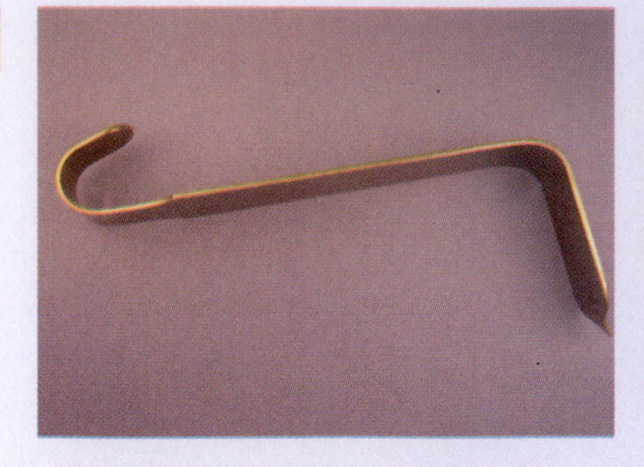
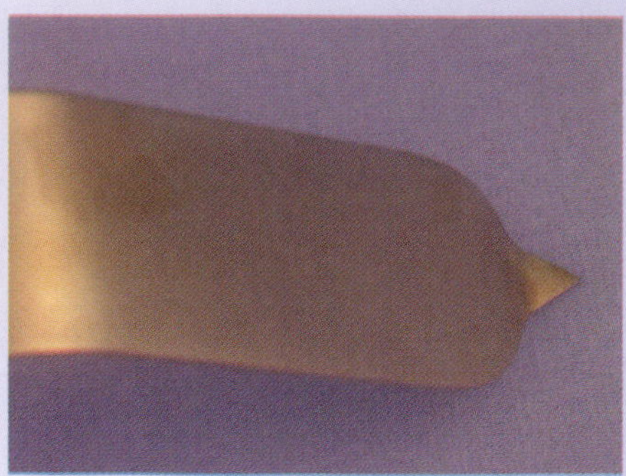

Name: Williams retractor
Alias: none
Category: retracting
Use: deep wound exposure during disk surgery
Length: 7"
Additional Information: blade width 1 cm or 2 cm; blade length 5 cm or 7 cm

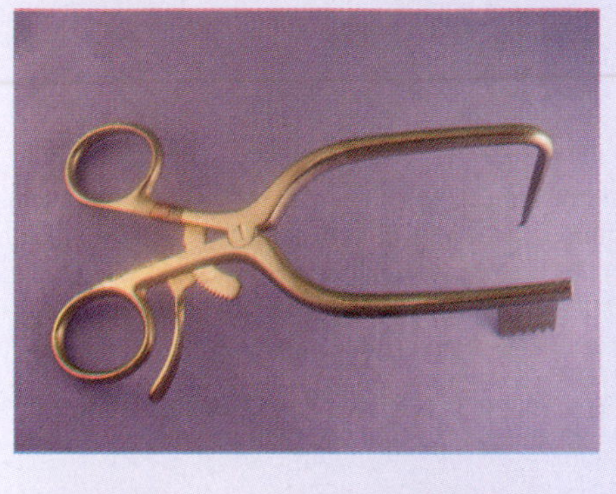
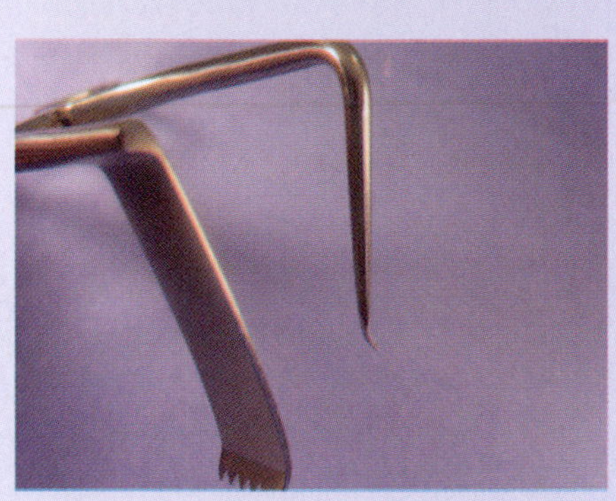

Name: Scoville hemi-laminectomy retractor
Alias: Scoville-Haverfield
Category: retracting
Use: deep retraction of tissue during laminectomy
Length: arms 8" long
Additional Information: comes with flat or 4 prong blades

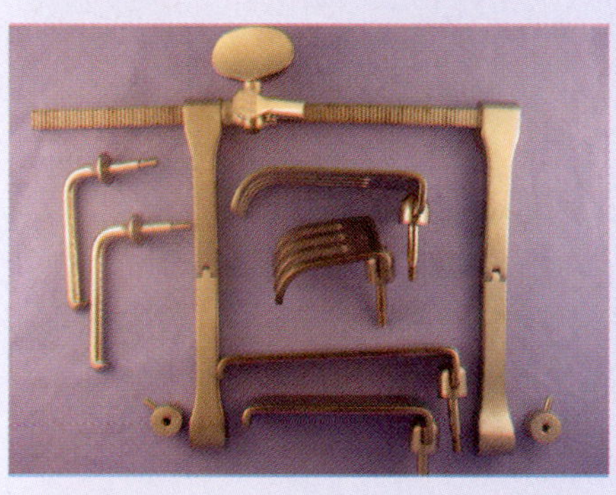
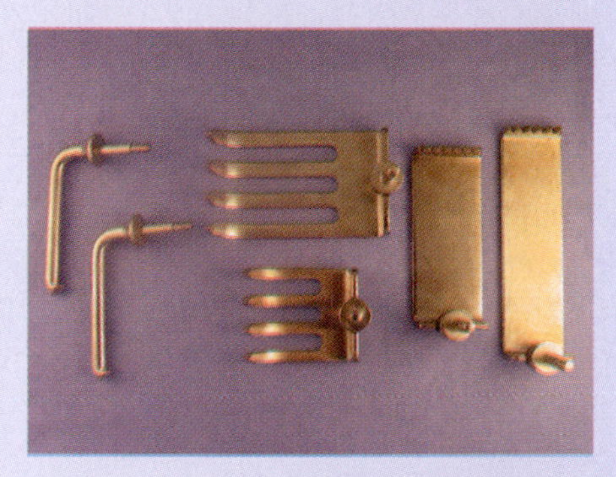

Name: Meyerding retractor
Alias: none
Category: retracting
Use: wound exposure
Length: 9" or 10"
Additional Information: blade width varies from $^3/_4$" to 2"; saw-toothed edge

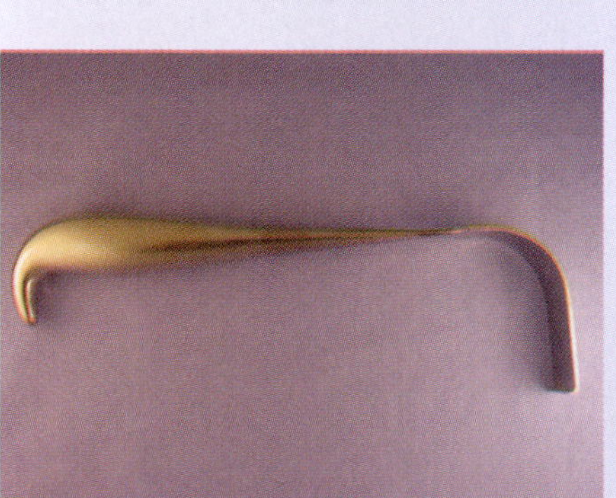
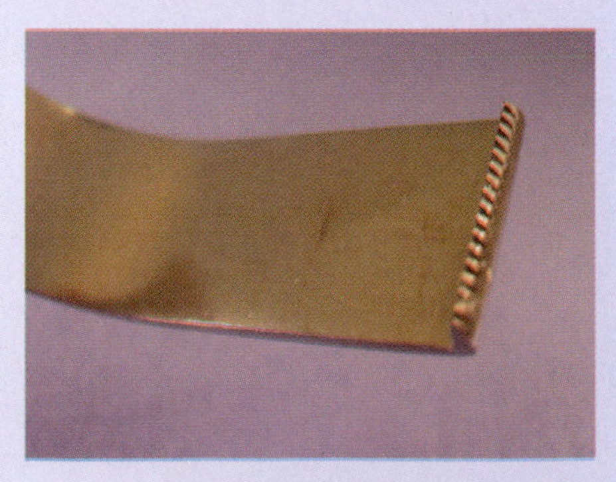

Name: Scoville brain spatula
Alias: none
Category: retracting
Use: retracting brain tissue
Length: 8"
Additional Information: double ended; blade widths 10/13 mm or 16/19 mm; malleable; should be moistened with saline before handing to the surgeon

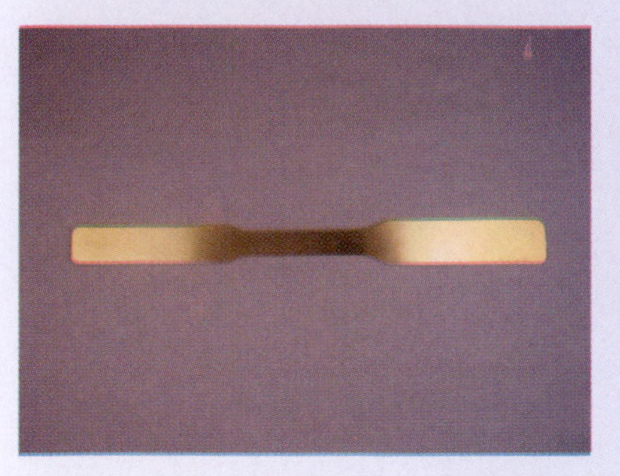
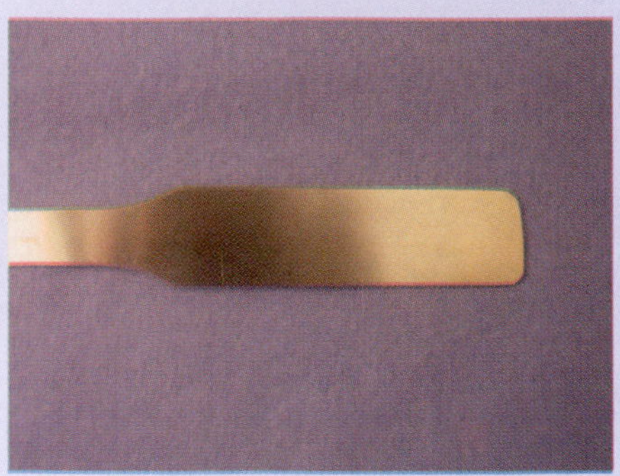

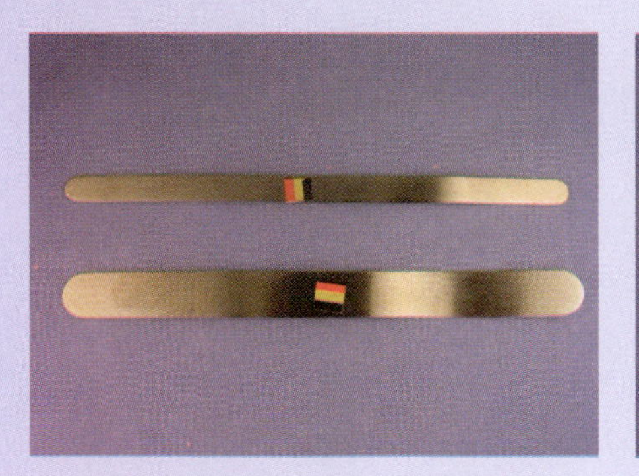
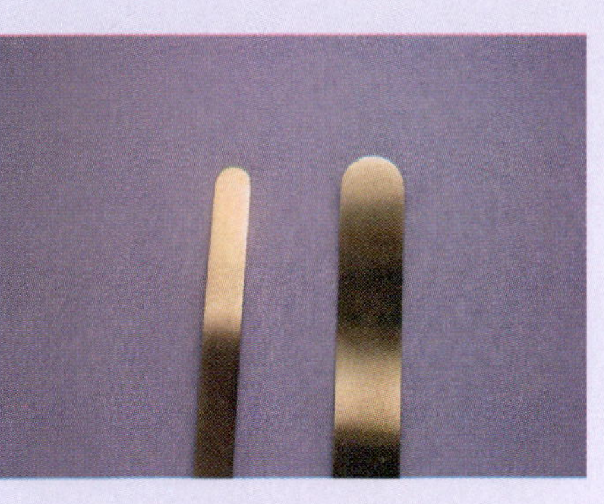

Name: Davis brain spatula
Alias: none
Category: retracting
Use: retracting brain tissue
Length: 7"
Additional Information: double ended; comes in blade widths of 0.25" to 1.5"; malleable; should be moistened with saline before handing to the surgeon

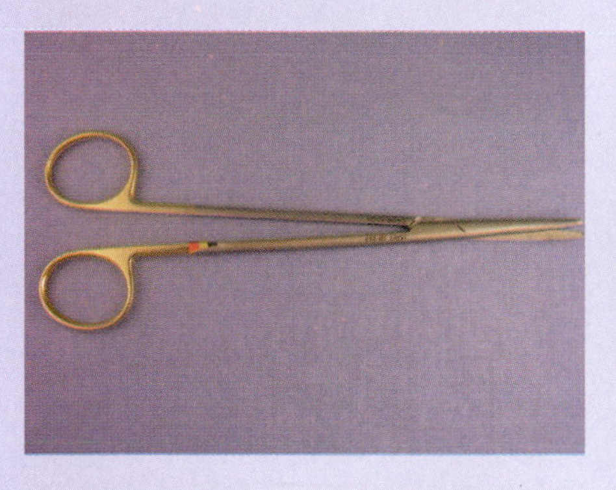
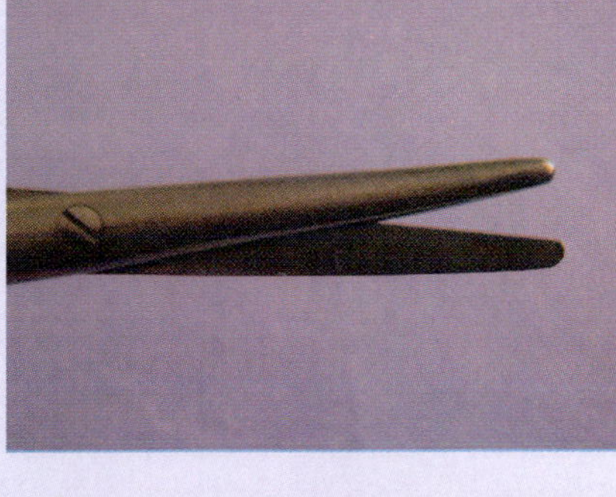

Name: Adson dural scissors
Alias: none
Category: cutting
Use: cutting or dissecting dura
Length: 7"
Additional Information: curved, blunt blades

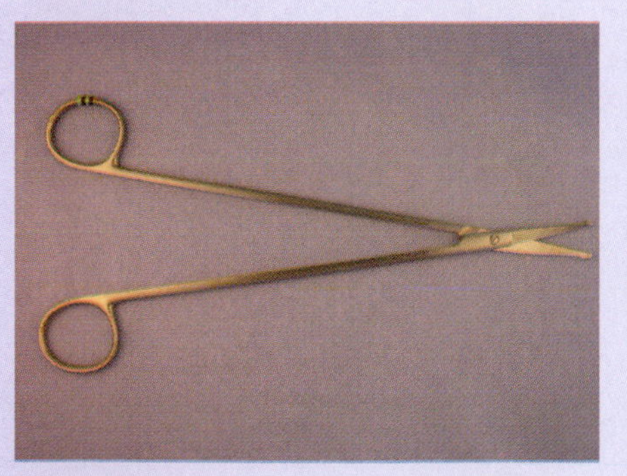
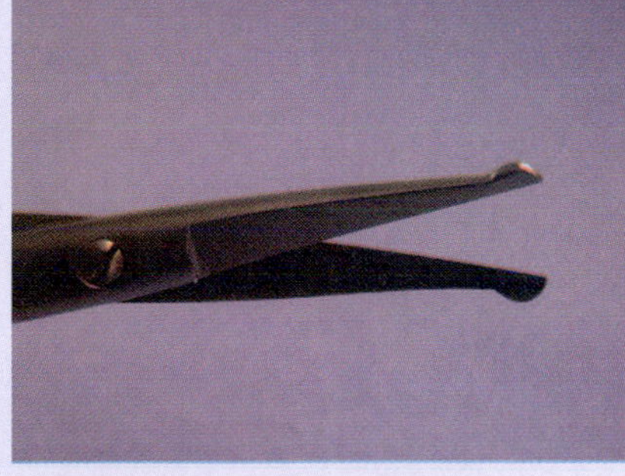

Name: Strully scissors
Alias: none
Category: cutting
Use: dissecting tissue
Length: 8.75"
Additional Information: ball tip (probe) on points; curved blades

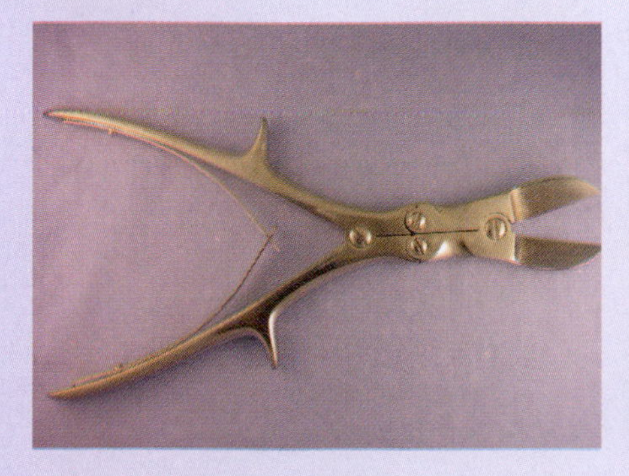
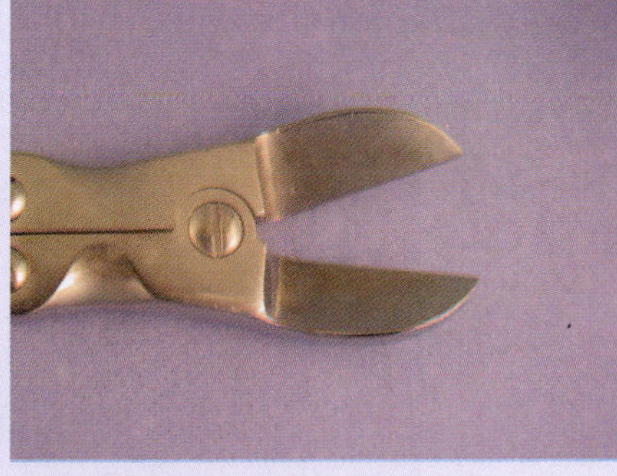

Name: Liston-Stille bone cutter
Alias: none
Category: cutting
Use: cut bone
Length: 10.5"
Additional Information: can have straight or angled blades

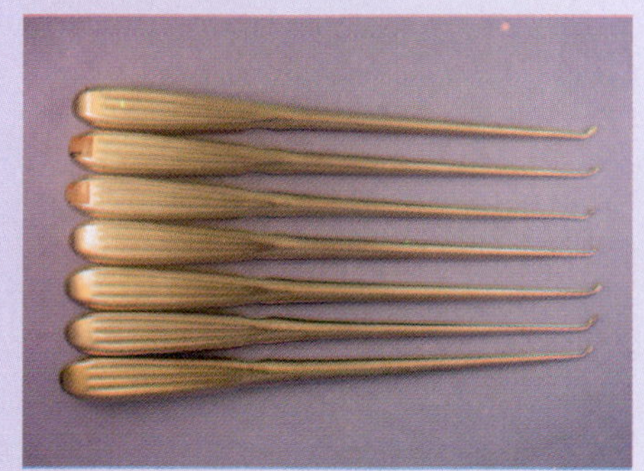
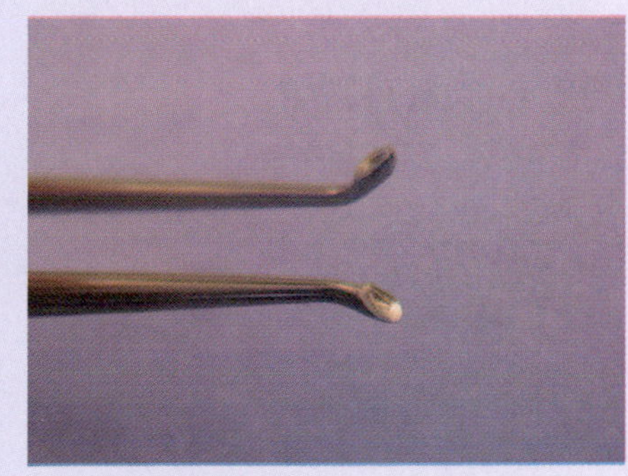

Name: Bruns bone curette
Alias: none
Category: cutting
Use: scraping bone
Length: 9"
Additional Information: comes in sizes 0000 to 6; tip can be straight or angled

Name: spinal curettes

Alias: none

Category: cutting

Use: removing pieces of bone during spinal surgery

Length: 6.5"

Additional Information: come with various diameter cups

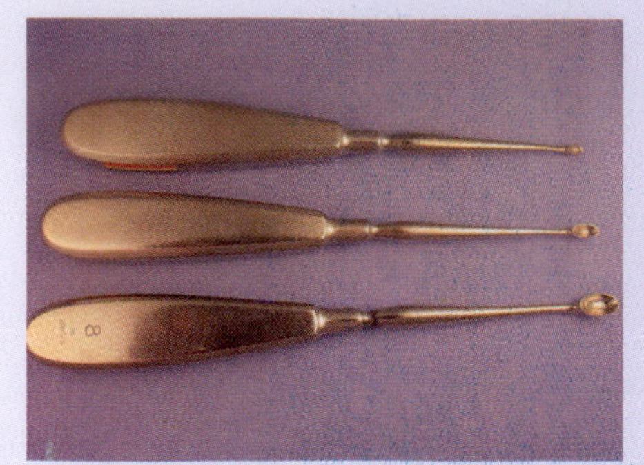

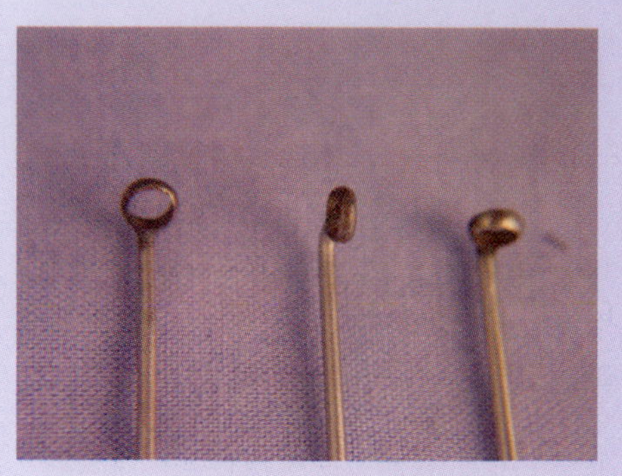

Name: corkscrew dural hook

Alias: none

Category: accessory

Use: hooking and lifting dural layer

Length: 6.5"

Additional Information: comes as 2 separate pieces—hook can be stored inside handle

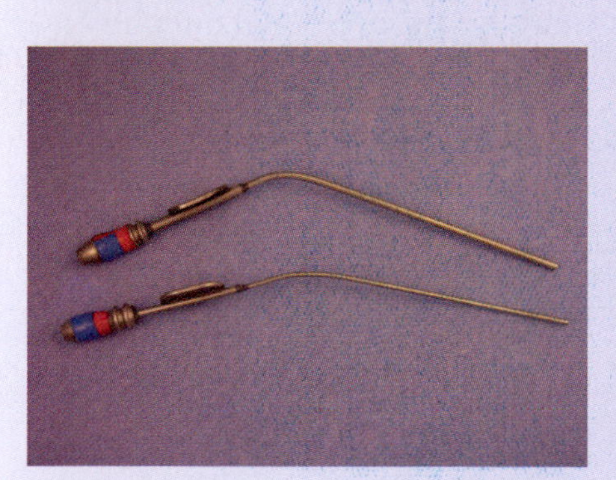

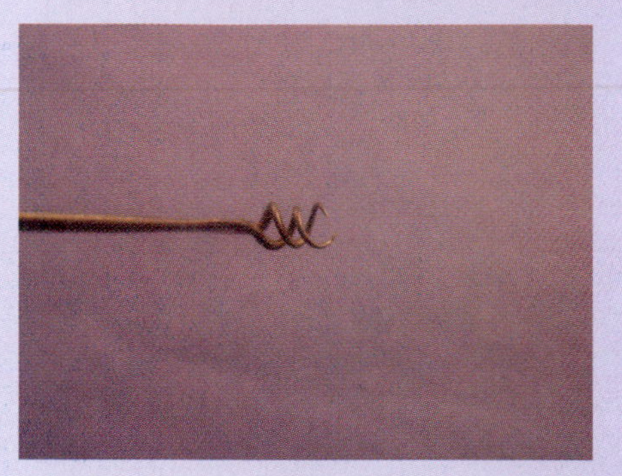

Name: Adson suction

Alias: none

Category: suctioning

Use: fine suctioning during neuro or spine surgery

Length: 6"

Additional Information: comes in 7, 9, 11, or 15 Fr sizes; blade can be straight or curved

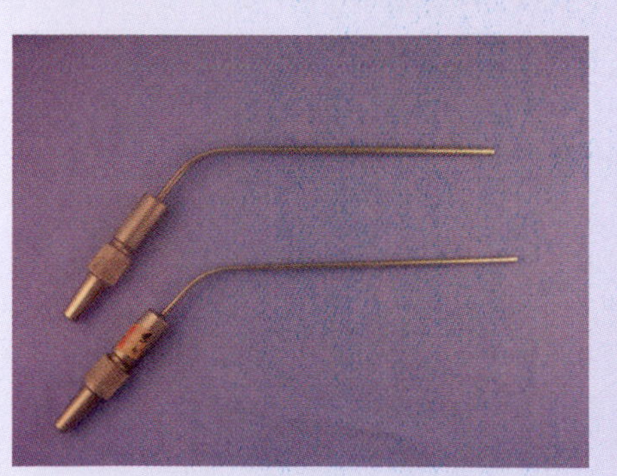

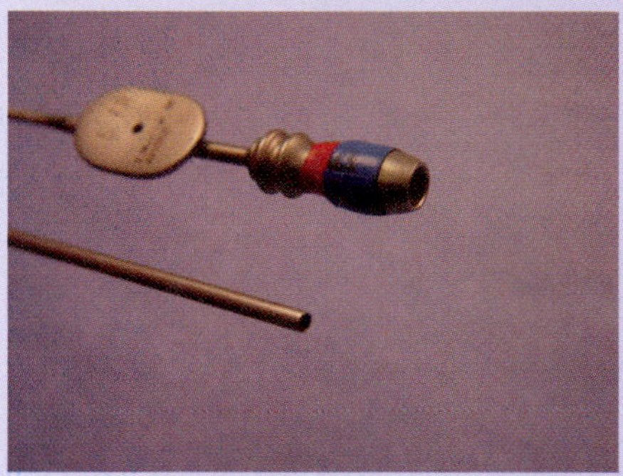

Name: Frazier suction

Alias: nasal suction; neuro suction

Category: suctioning

Use: suctioning small quantities of fluid from nose or ears; suctioning in small areas

Length: 6.5"

Additional Information: short or long tips; 6 Fr to 16 Fr diameter; can be metal or disposable; angled

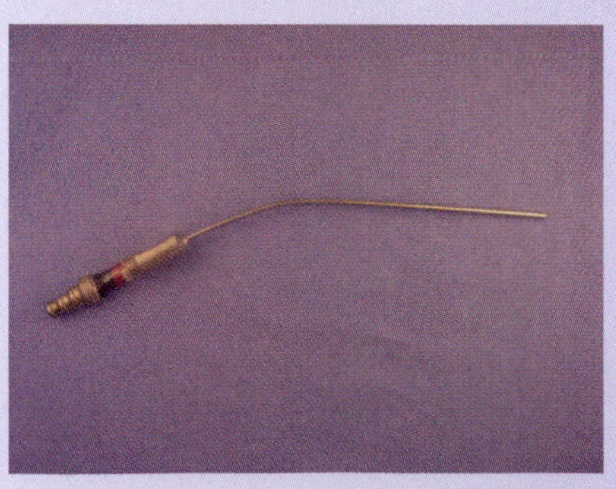

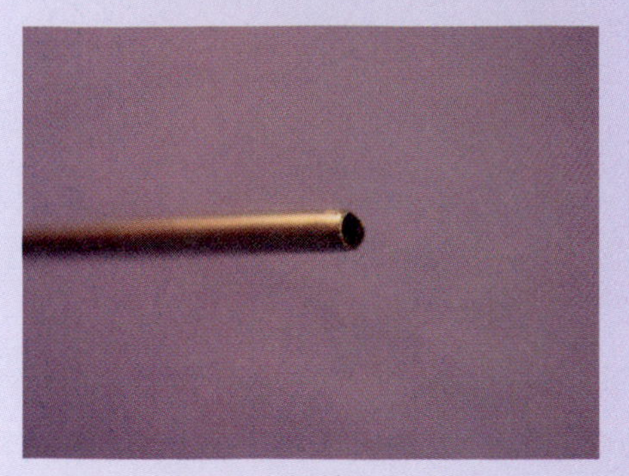

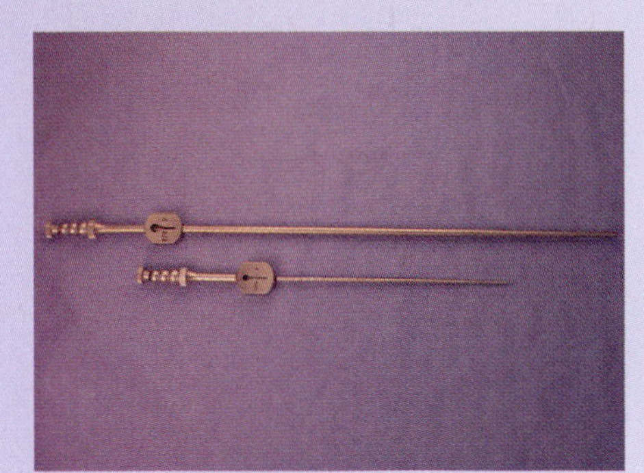
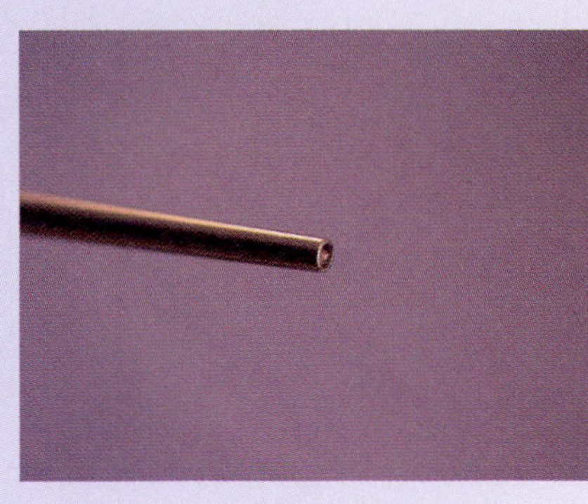

Name: Fukushima suction
Alias: teardrop suction
Category: suctioning
Use: suctioning of blood/fluid during neurosurgery
Length: 5" or 9"
Additional Information: has stylet for insertion

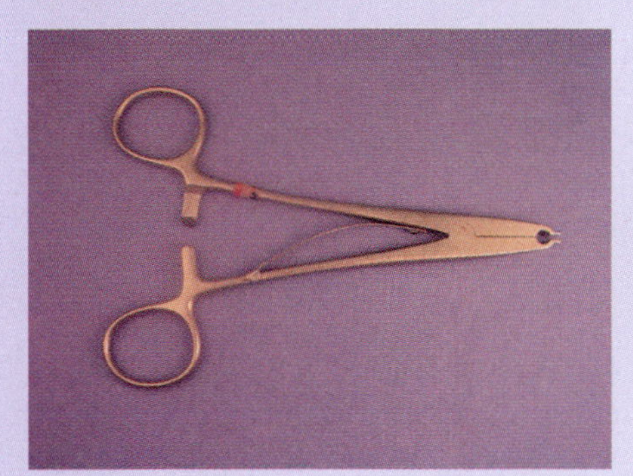
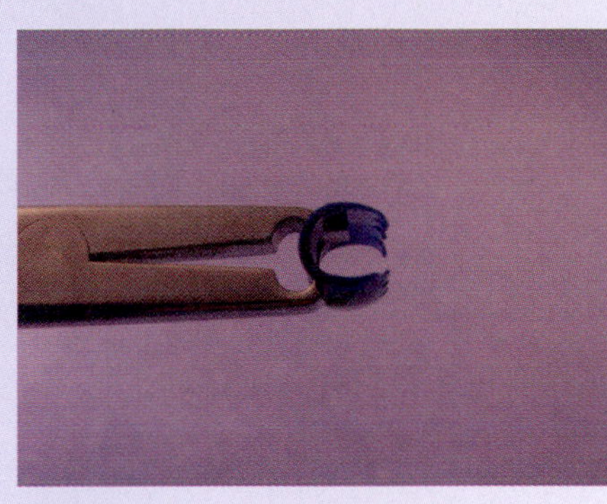

Name: Raney scalp clip applying forceps
Alias: Raney clip appliers
Category: accessory
Use: applying Raney retracting clips
Length: 6.25"
Additional Information: clips can be stainless or plastic

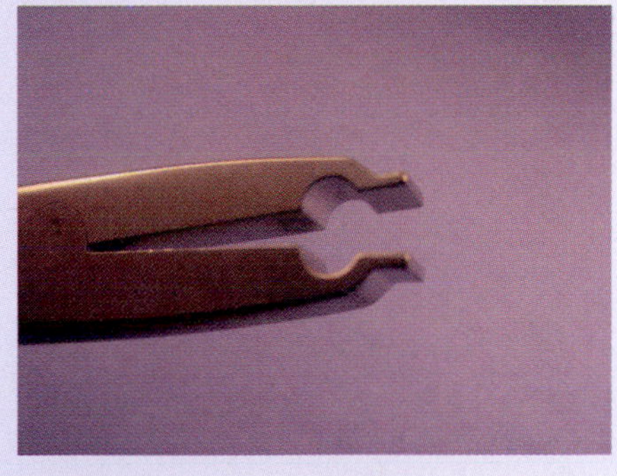

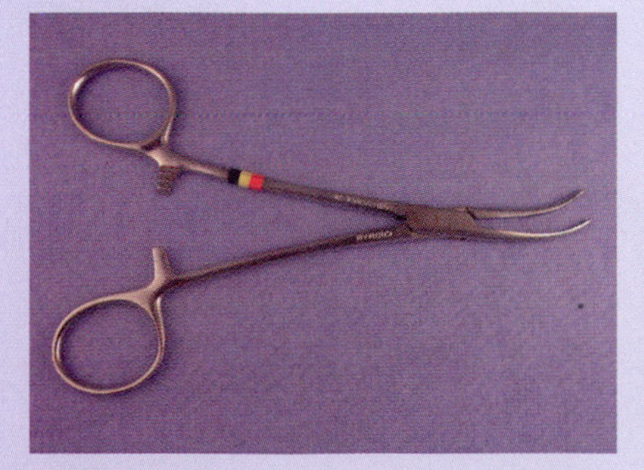
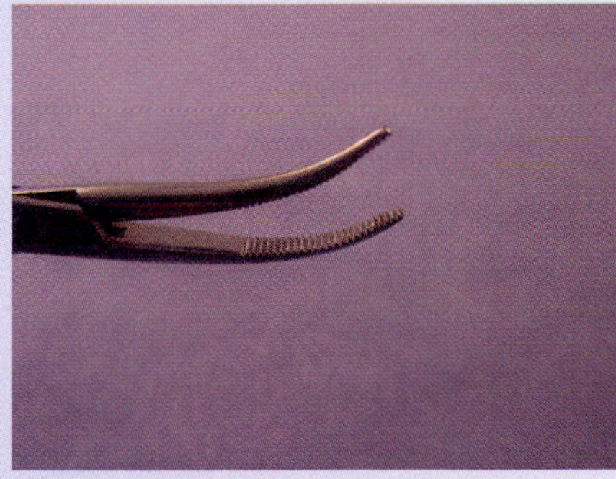

Name: Dandy clamp
Alias: Cairn clamp
Category: clamping
Use: retracting dura out of the way; scalp hemostasis
Length: 5.5"
Additional Information: jaw curved on the side; can have serrated tips or 1 × 2 teeth

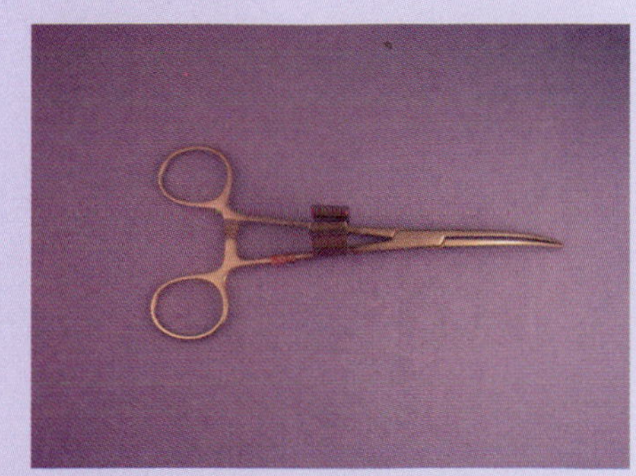
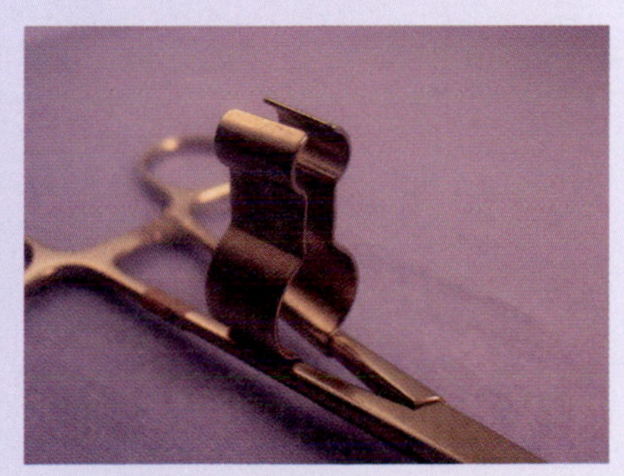

Name: Greene tubing holding clamp
Alias: none
Category: clamping
Use: attaching tubing to drapes
Length: 6.5"

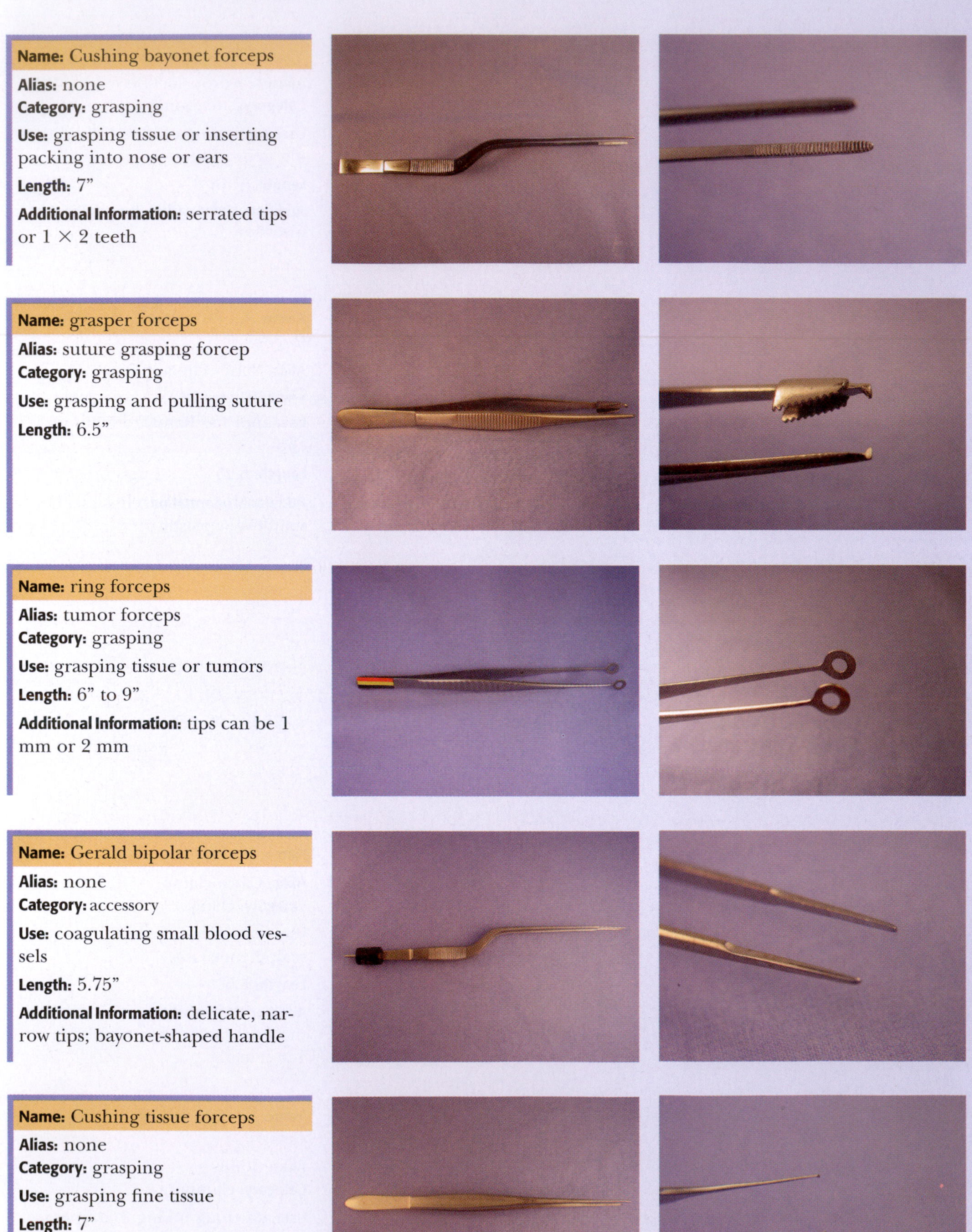

Name: Cushing bayonet forceps

Alias: none

Category: grasping

Use: grasping tissue or inserting packing into nose or ears

Length: 7"

Additional Information: serrated tips or 1 × 2 teeth

Name: grasper forceps

Alias: suture grasping forcep

Category: grasping

Use: grasping and pulling suture

Length: 6.5"

Name: ring forceps

Alias: tumor forceps

Category: grasping

Use: grasping tissue or tumors

Length: 6" to 9"

Additional Information: tips can be 1 mm or 2 mm

Name: Gerald bipolar forceps

Alias: none

Category: accessory

Use: coagulating small blood vessels

Length: 5.75"

Additional Information: delicate, narrow tips; bayonet-shaped handle

Name: Cushing tissue forceps

Alias: none

Category: grasping

Use: grasping fine tissue

Length: 7"

Additional Information: can be smooth or have 1 × 2 teeth

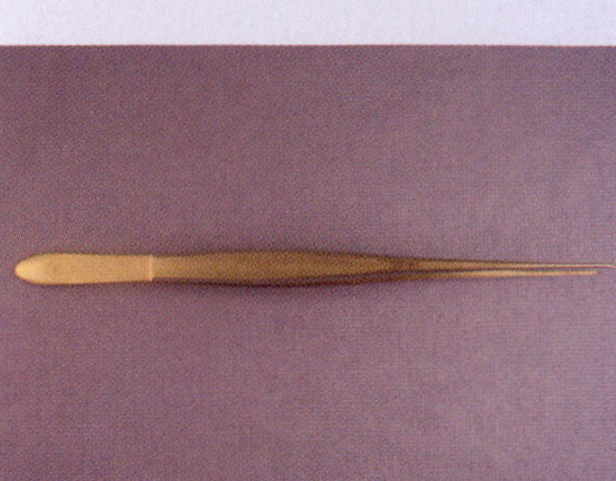

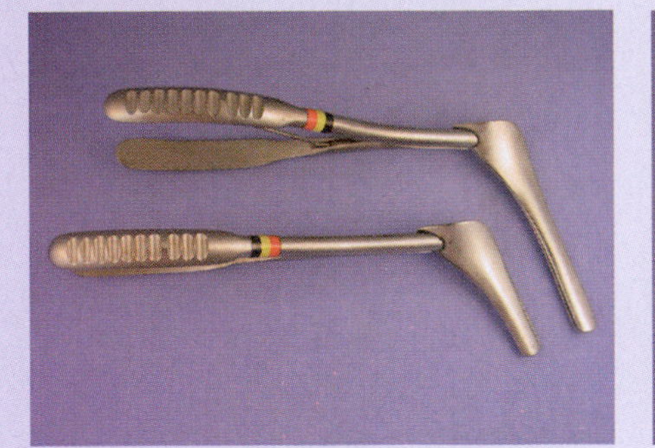
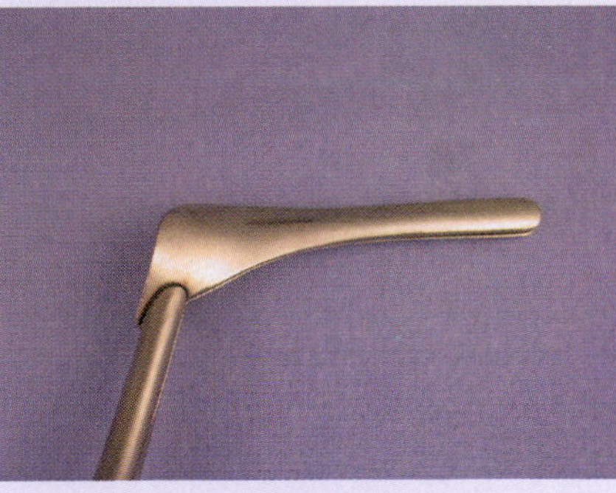

Name: Vienna nasal speculum

Alias: none

Category: retracting

Use: retracting nasal walls

Length: 5.5"

Additional Information: blades can be small (9.5 mm × 27 mm), medium (11 mm × 30 mm), or large (13 mm × 32 mm)

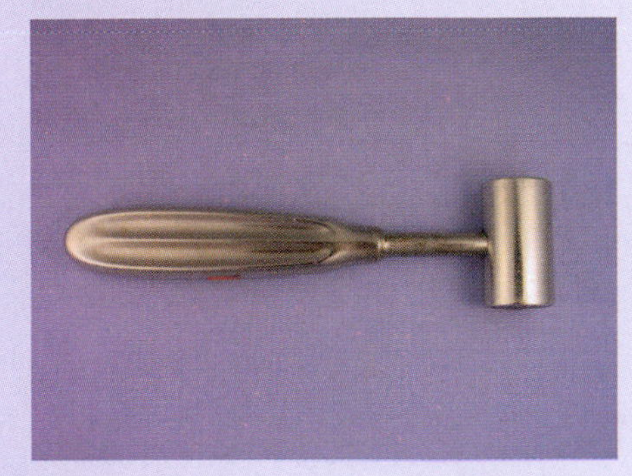
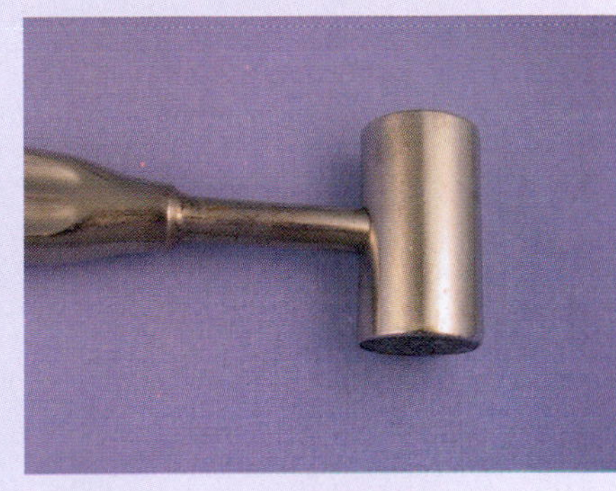

Name: Gerzog mallet

Alias: none

Category: accessory

Use: pounding other instruments (like osteotomes) or driving in pins

Length: 6.75"

Additional Information: head diameter 1"; head is lead filled

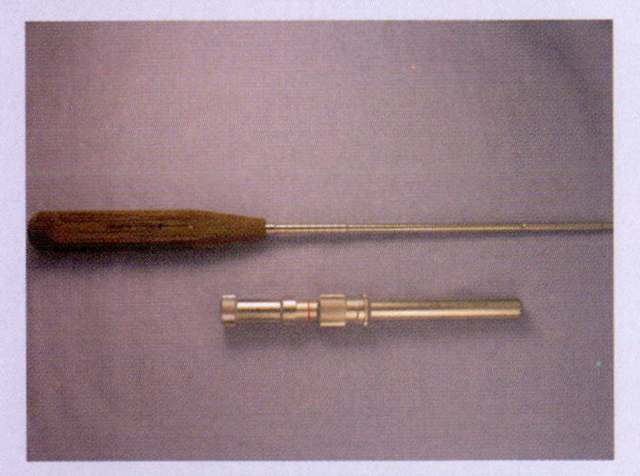
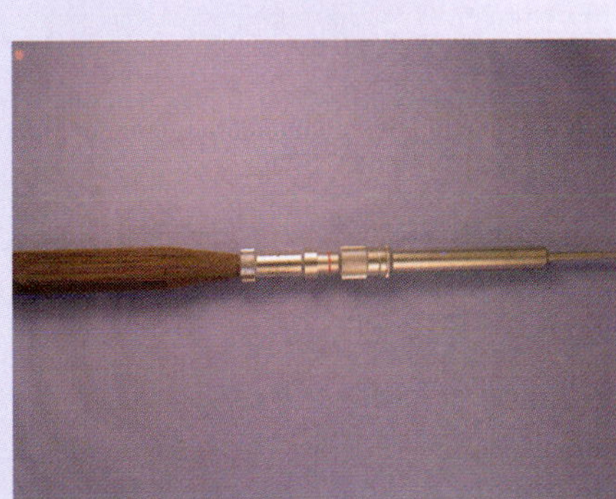

Name: screwdriver with sleeve

Alias: none

Category: grasping

Use: holding and inserting screws during instrumentation

Length: n/a

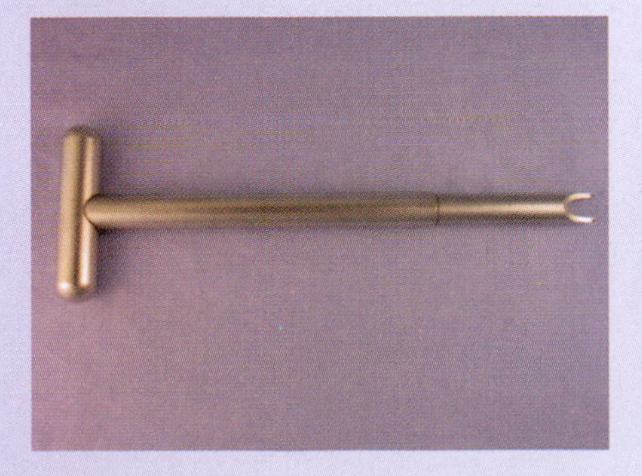
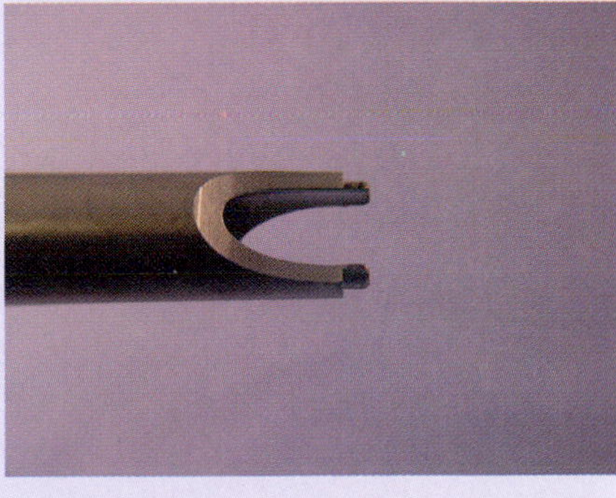

Name: locking cap screwdriver

Alias: none

Category: accessory

Use: tightening locking caps

Length: n/a

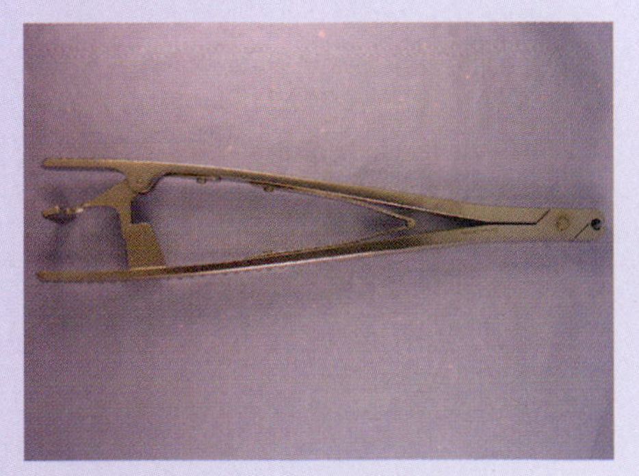
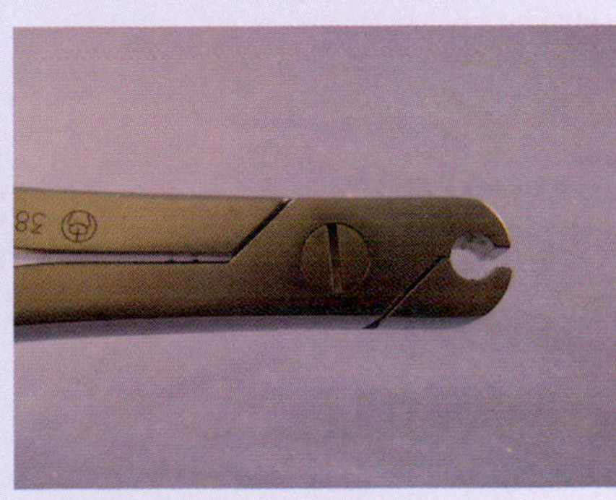

Name: bar-holding forcep

Alias: none

Category: grasping

Use: holding rods

Length: n/a

Name: bending iron
Alias: none
Category: accessory
Use: contouring rods during spinal procedures
Length: n/a
Additional Information: come in left- and right-sided

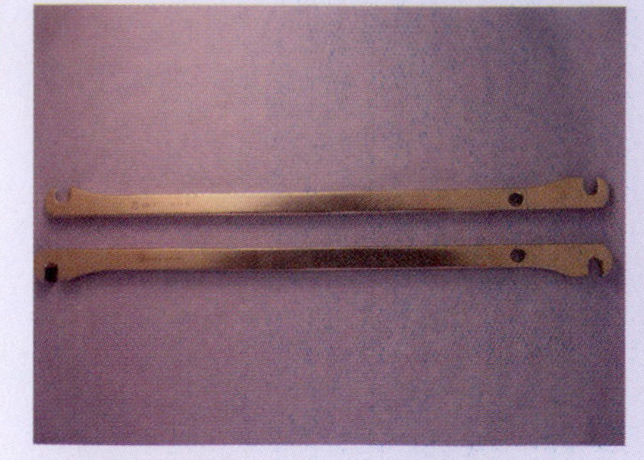
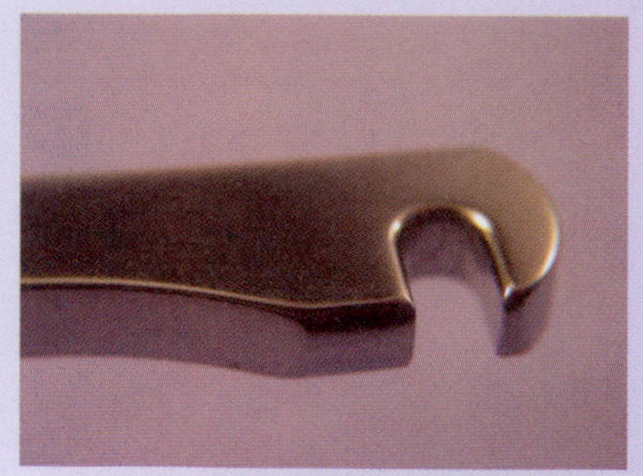

Name: rod bender
Alias: none
Category: accessory
Use: contouring rods during spinal procedures
Length: n/a

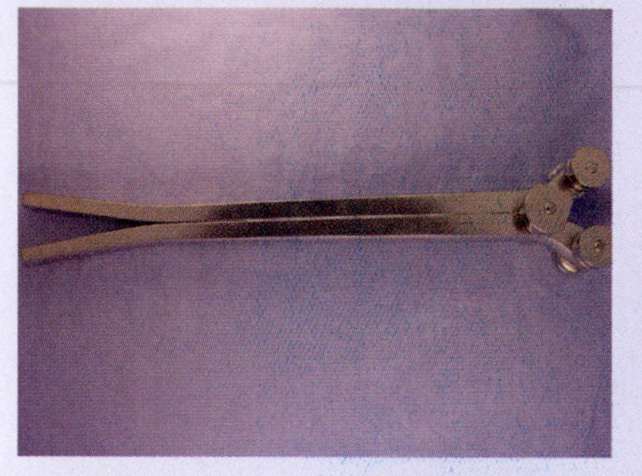
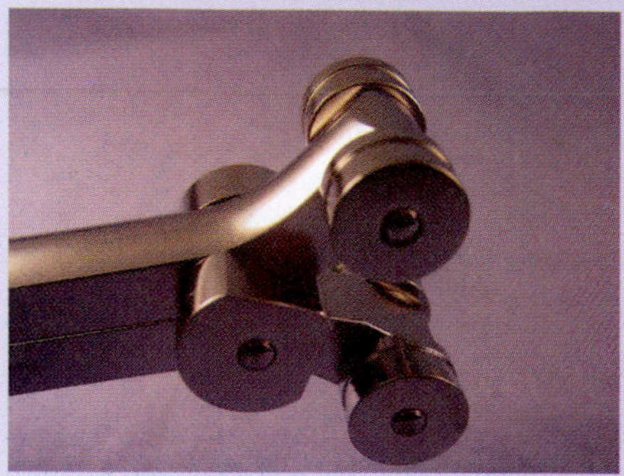

Name: extraction pliers
Alias: none
Category: grasping
Use: removing screws
Length: n/a

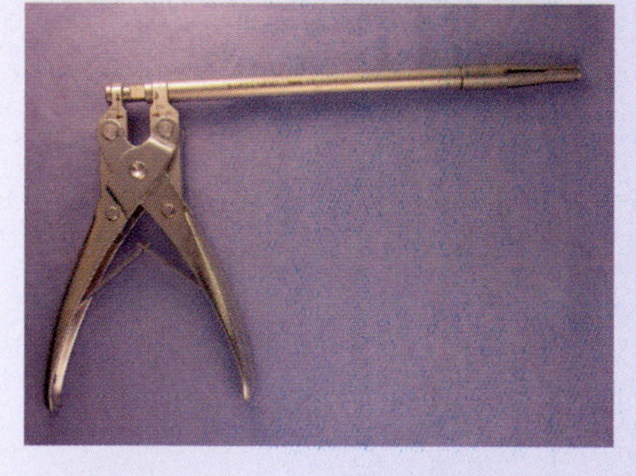
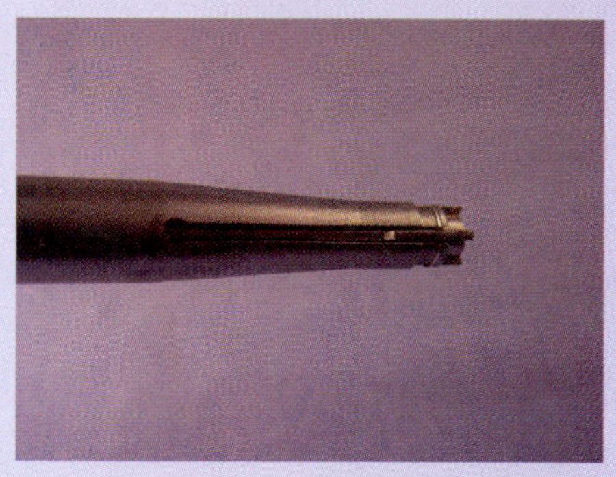

Name: cannulated tap and handle
Alias: tap
Category: accessory
Use: tapping the hole for insertion of cannulated screws
Length: n/a

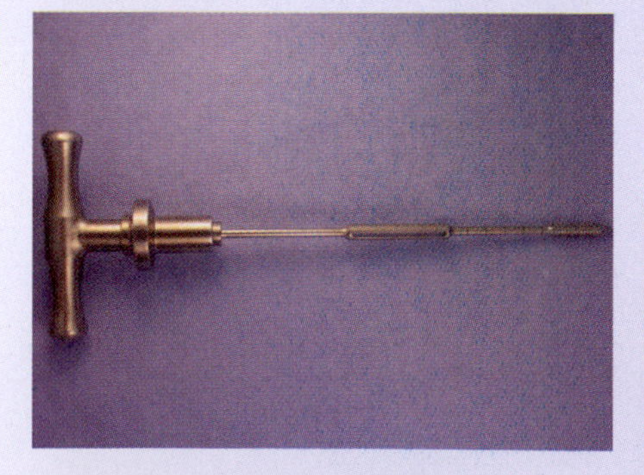
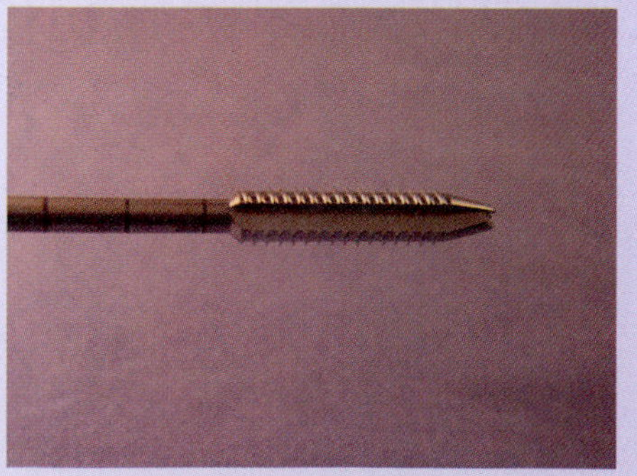

Name: hexagonal screwdriver
Alias: none
Category: accessory
Use: inserting/removing screws with hexagonal heads
Length: n/a

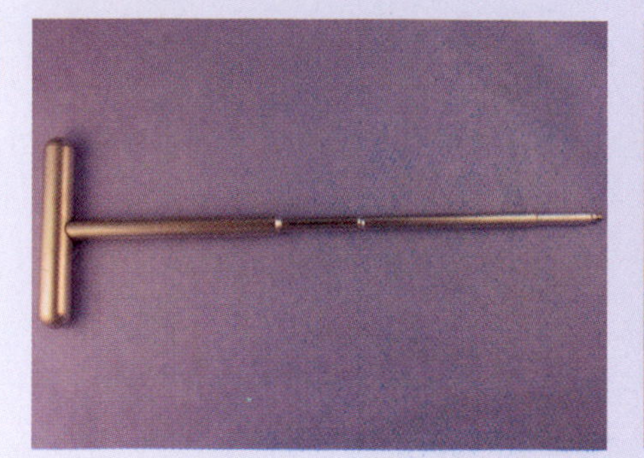
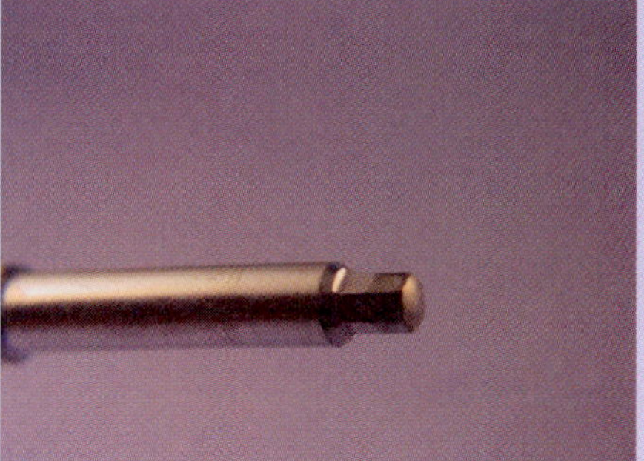

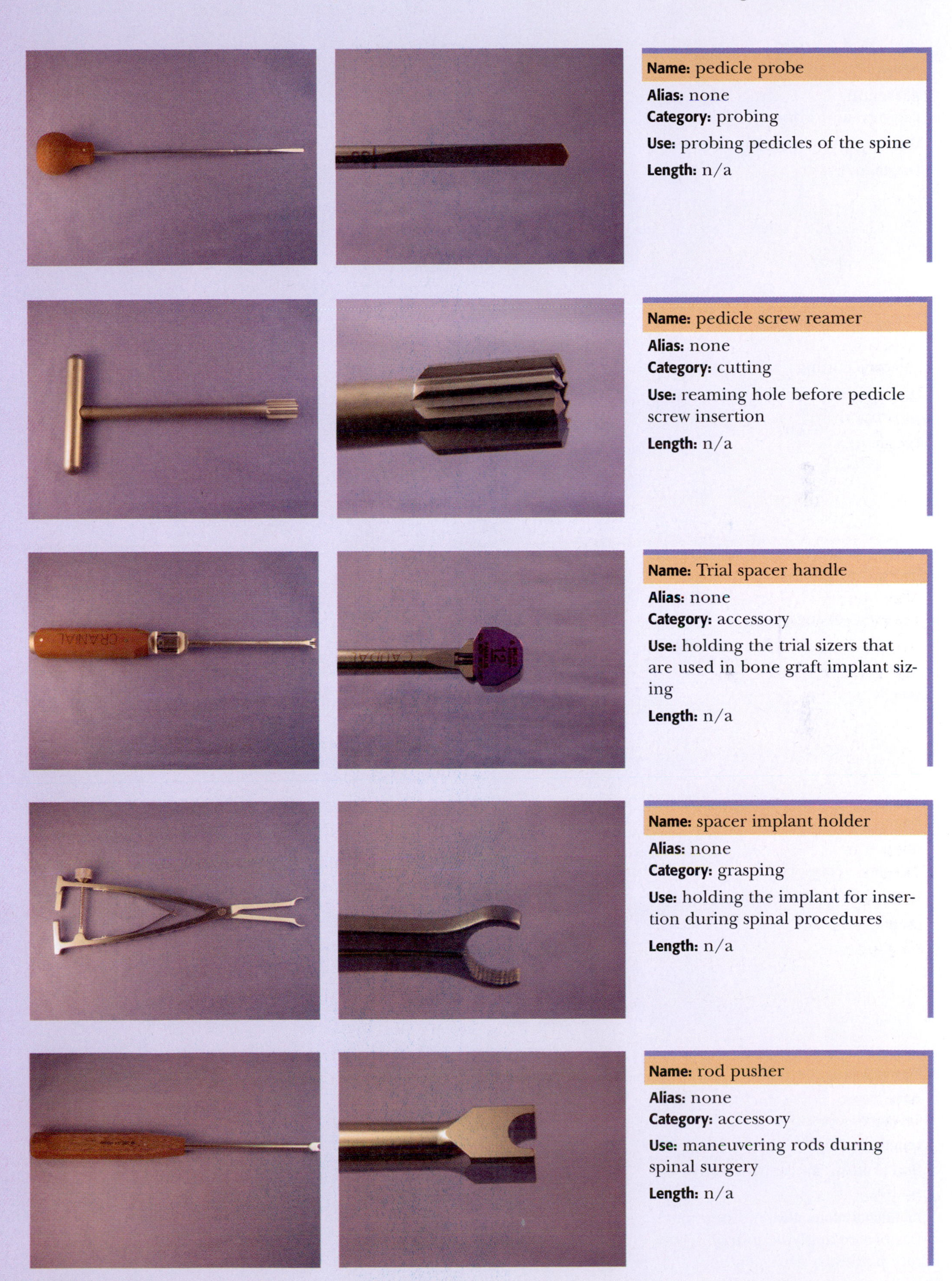

Name: pedicle probe
Alias: none
Category: probing
Use: probing pedicles of the spine
Length: n/a

Name: pedicle screw reamer
Alias: none
Category: cutting
Use: reaming hole before pedicle screw insertion
Length: n/a

Name: Trial spacer handle
Alias: none
Category: accessory
Use: holding the trial sizers that are used in bone graft implant sizing
Length: n/a

Name: spacer implant holder
Alias: none
Category: grasping
Use: holding the implant for insertion during spinal procedures
Length: n/a

Name: rod pusher
Alias: none
Category: accessory
Use: maneuvering rods during spinal surgery
Length: n/a

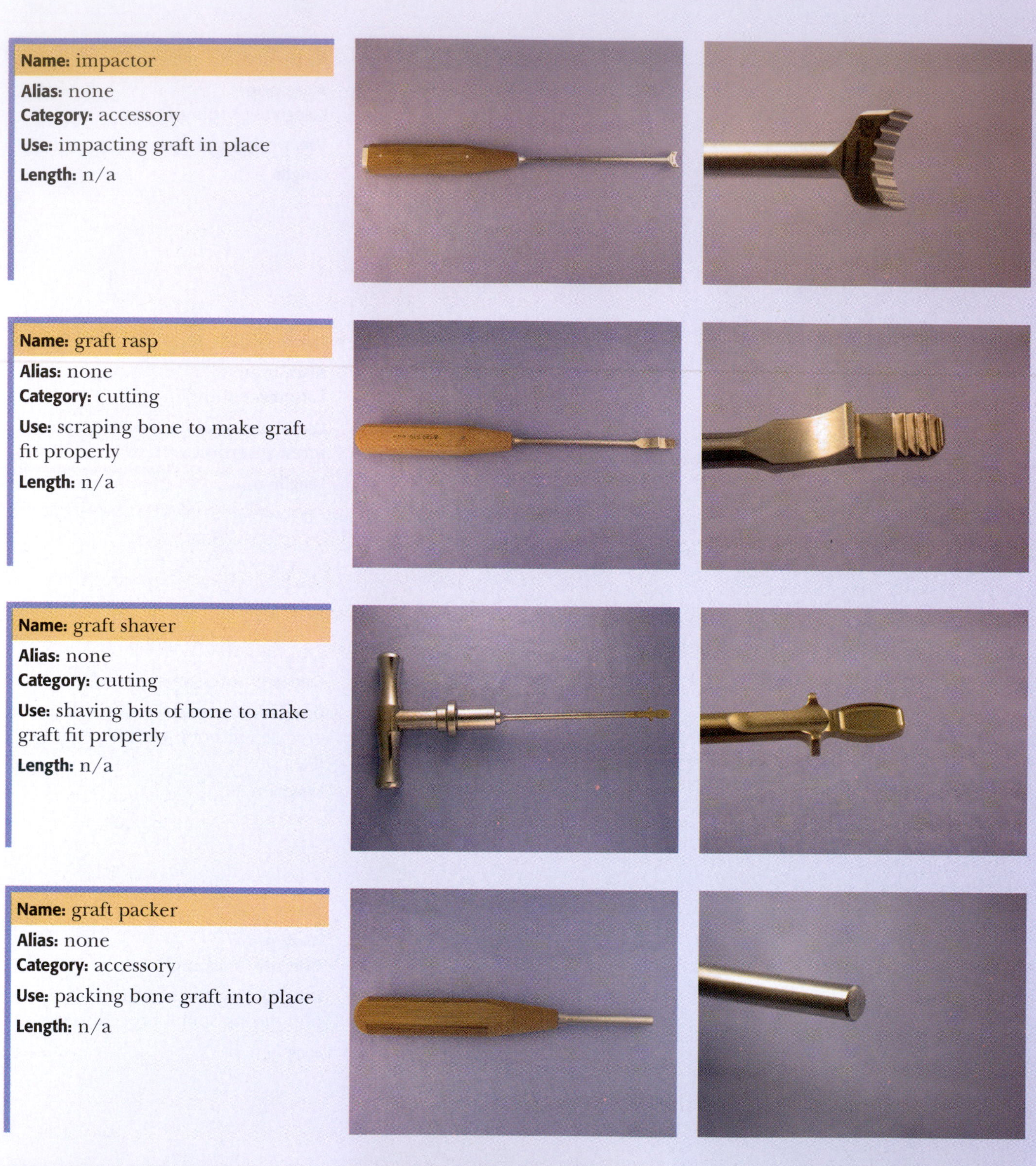

Name: impactor
Alias: none
Category: accessory
Use: impacting graft in place
Length: n/a

Name: graft rasp
Alias: none
Category: cutting
Use: scraping bone to make graft fit properly
Length: n/a

Name: graft shaver
Alias: none
Category: cutting
Use: shaving bits of bone to make graft fit properly
Length: n/a

Name: graft packer
Alias: none
Category: accessory
Use: packing bone graft into place
Length: n/a

Name: neuro pattie tray
Alias: none
Category: accessory
Length: n/a
Use: holding moistened neuro patties
Additional Information: moisten patties before applying to tray; separate patties by size

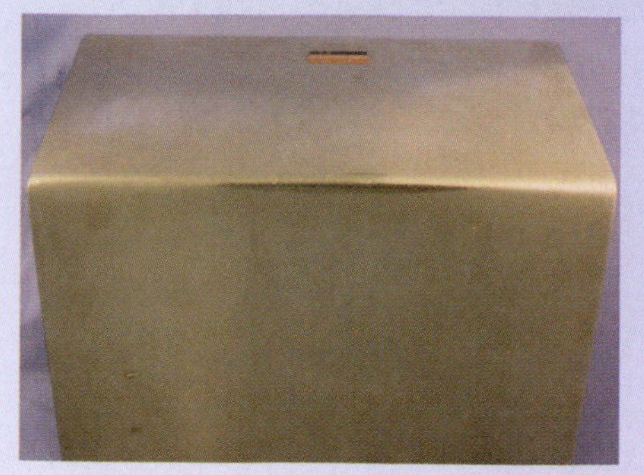

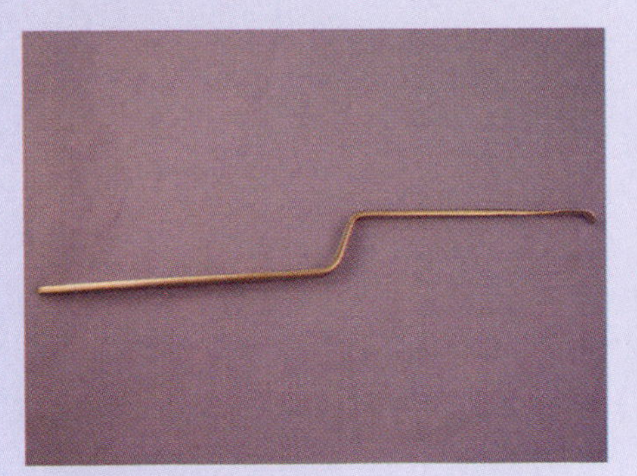

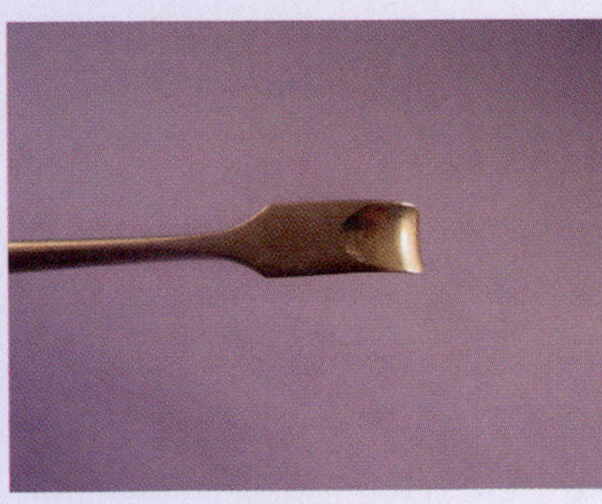

Name: Love nerve root retractor

Alias: none

Category: retracting

Use: retracting nerve root

Length: 8”

Additional Information: can be straight, 45 degrees, or 90 degrees

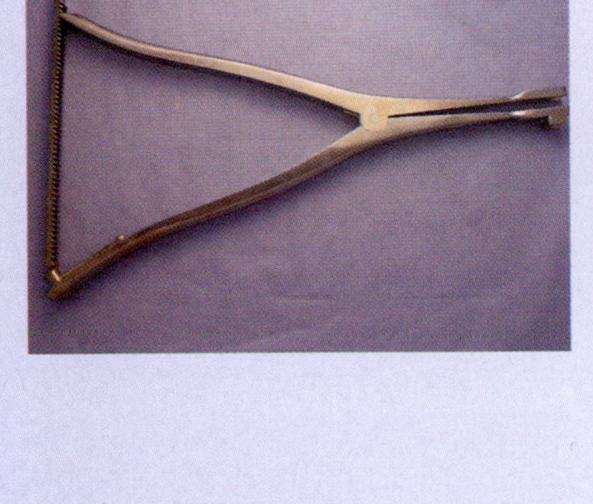

Name: lamina spreader

Alias: none

Category: accessory

Use: disk exposure during spinal surgery

Length: 11”

Additional Information: The one pictured is used during instrumentation; Jaws may have be flat instead of ringed to be used without instrumentation

Transsphenoidal Instruments

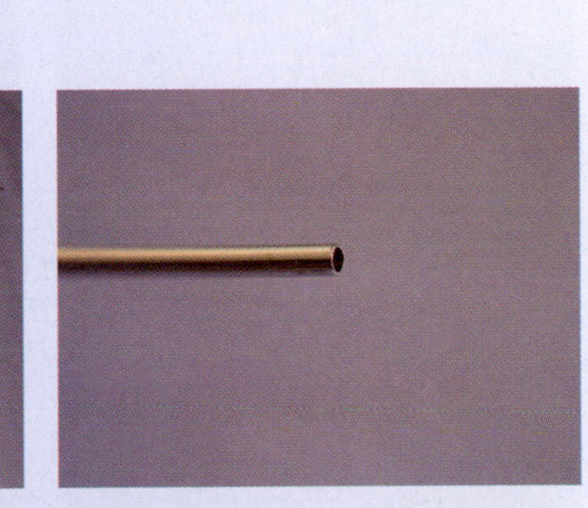

Name: Frazier suction and obturator

Alias: none

Category: suctioning

Use: removing fluids and tissue from the wound

Length: 7.5”

Additional Information: come in a variety of Fr diameters

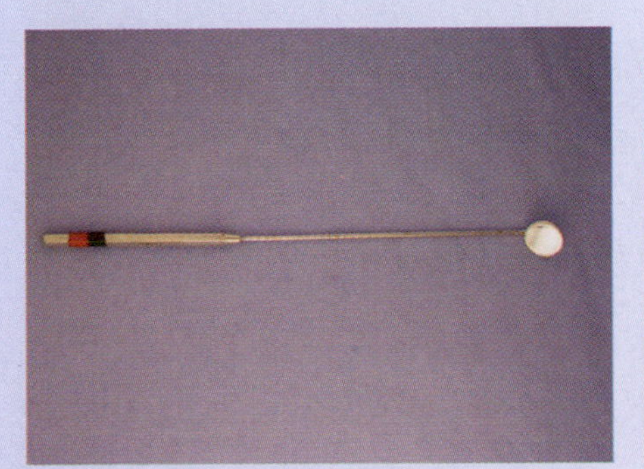

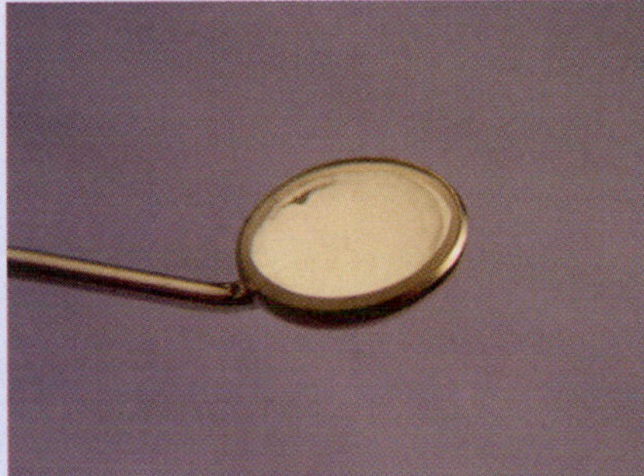

Name: Mirror

Alias: none

Category: accessory

Use: visualizing inside a wound

Length: 9.5”

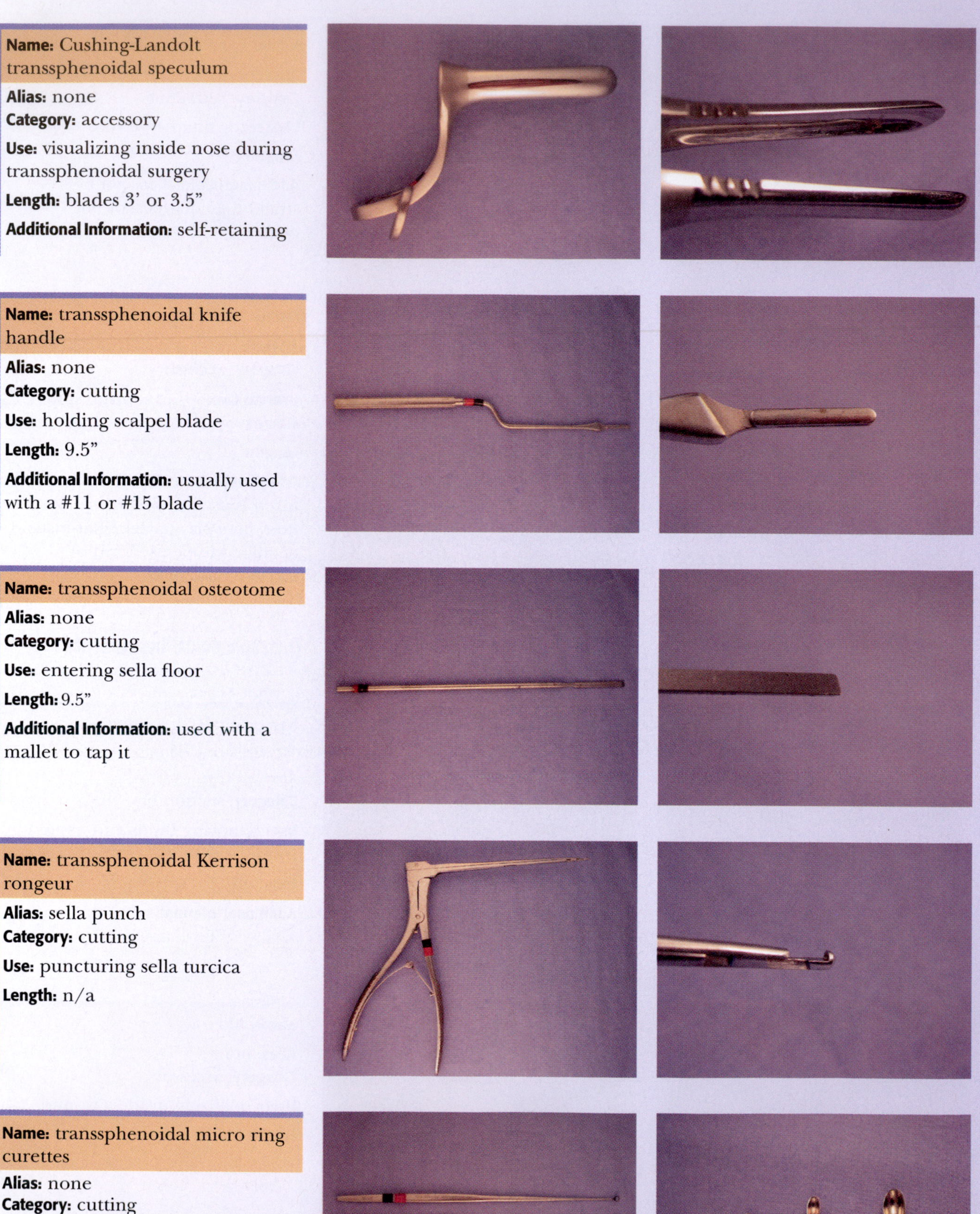

Name: Cushing-Landolt transsphenoidal speculum

Alias: none

Category: accessory

Use: visualizing inside nose during transsphenoidal surgery

Length: blades 3' or 3.5"

Additional Information: self-retaining

Name: transsphenoidal knife handle

Alias: none

Category: cutting

Use: holding scalpel blade

Length: 9.5"

Additional Information: usually used with a #11 or #15 blade

Name: transsphenoidal osteotome

Alias: none

Category: cutting

Use: entering sella floor

Length: 9.5"

Additional Information: used with a mallet to tap it

Name: transsphenoidal Kerrison rongeur

Alias: sella punch

Category: cutting

Use: puncturing sella turcica

Length: n/a

Name: transsphenoidal micro ring curettes

Alias: none

Category: cutting

Use: removing small pieces of tumor

Length: 9.5"

Additional Information: straight handles; tips can be curved up or down or angled up, down, or to the right; rings 3 mm diameter

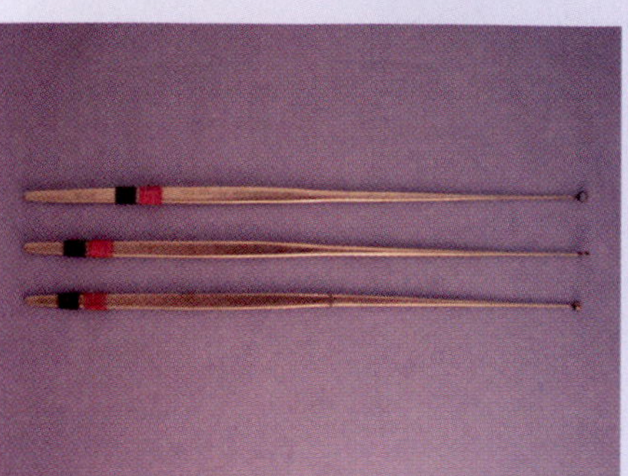

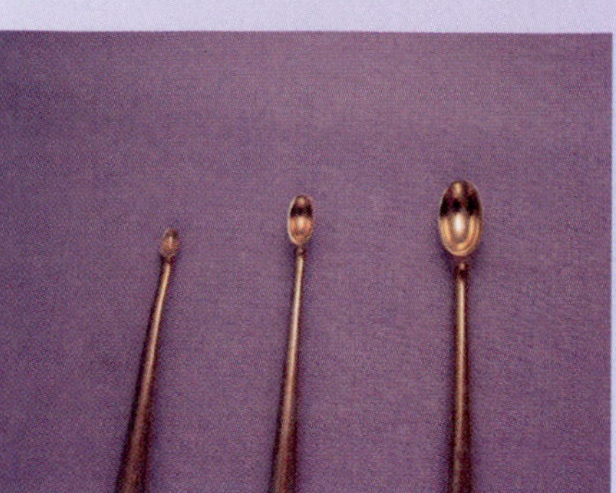

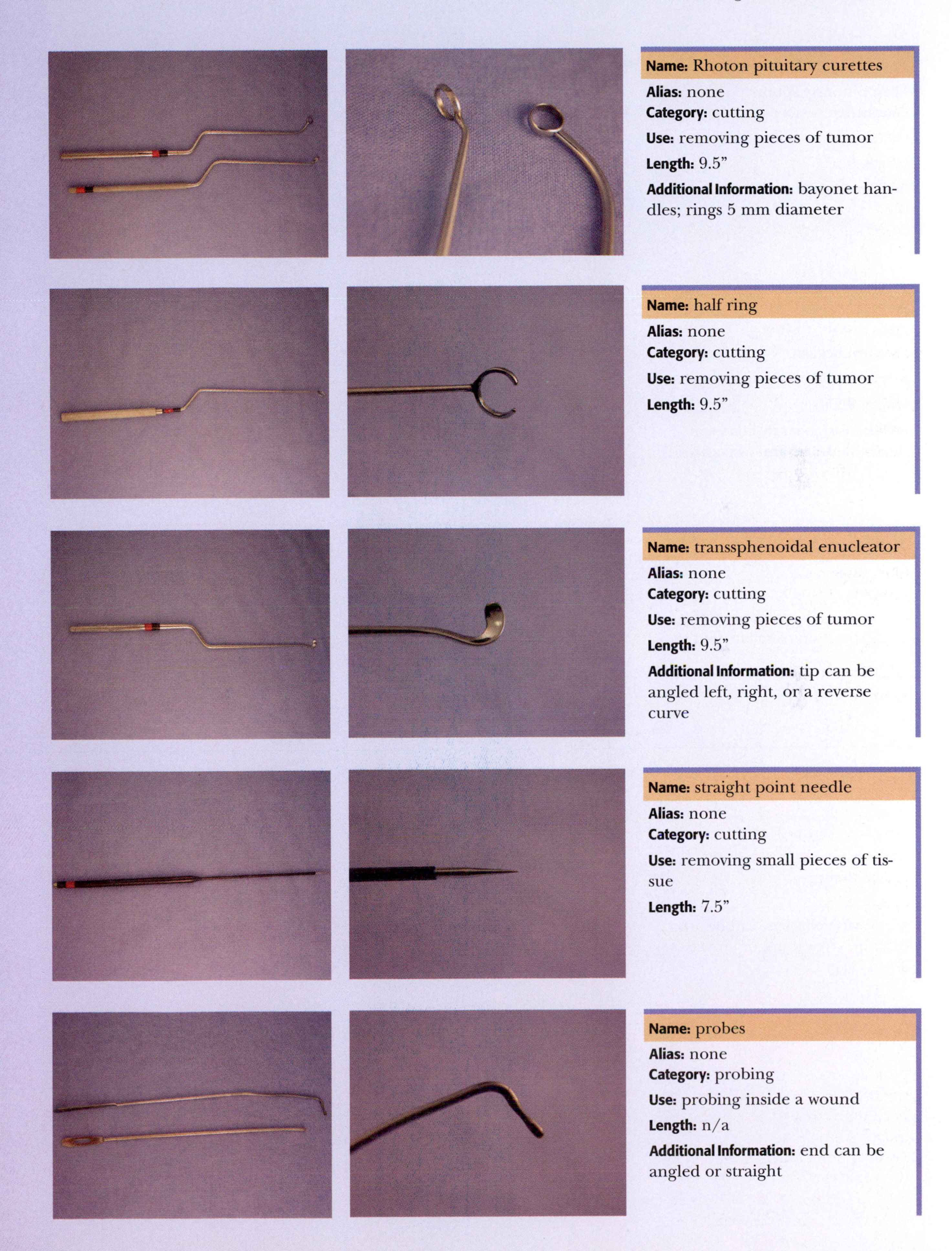

Name: Rhoton pituitary curettes
Alias: none
Category: cutting
Use: removing pieces of tumor
Length: 9.5"
Additional Information: bayonet handles; rings 5 mm diameter

Name: half ring
Alias: none
Category: cutting
Use: removing pieces of tumor
Length: 9.5"

Name: transsphenoidal enucleator
Alias: none
Category: cutting
Use: removing pieces of tumor
Length: 9.5"
Additional Information: tip can be angled left, right, or a reverse curve

Name: straight point needle
Alias: none
Category: cutting
Use: removing small pieces of tissue
Length: 7.5"

Name: probes
Alias: none
Category: probing
Use: probing inside a wound
Length: n/a
Additional Information: end can be angled or straight

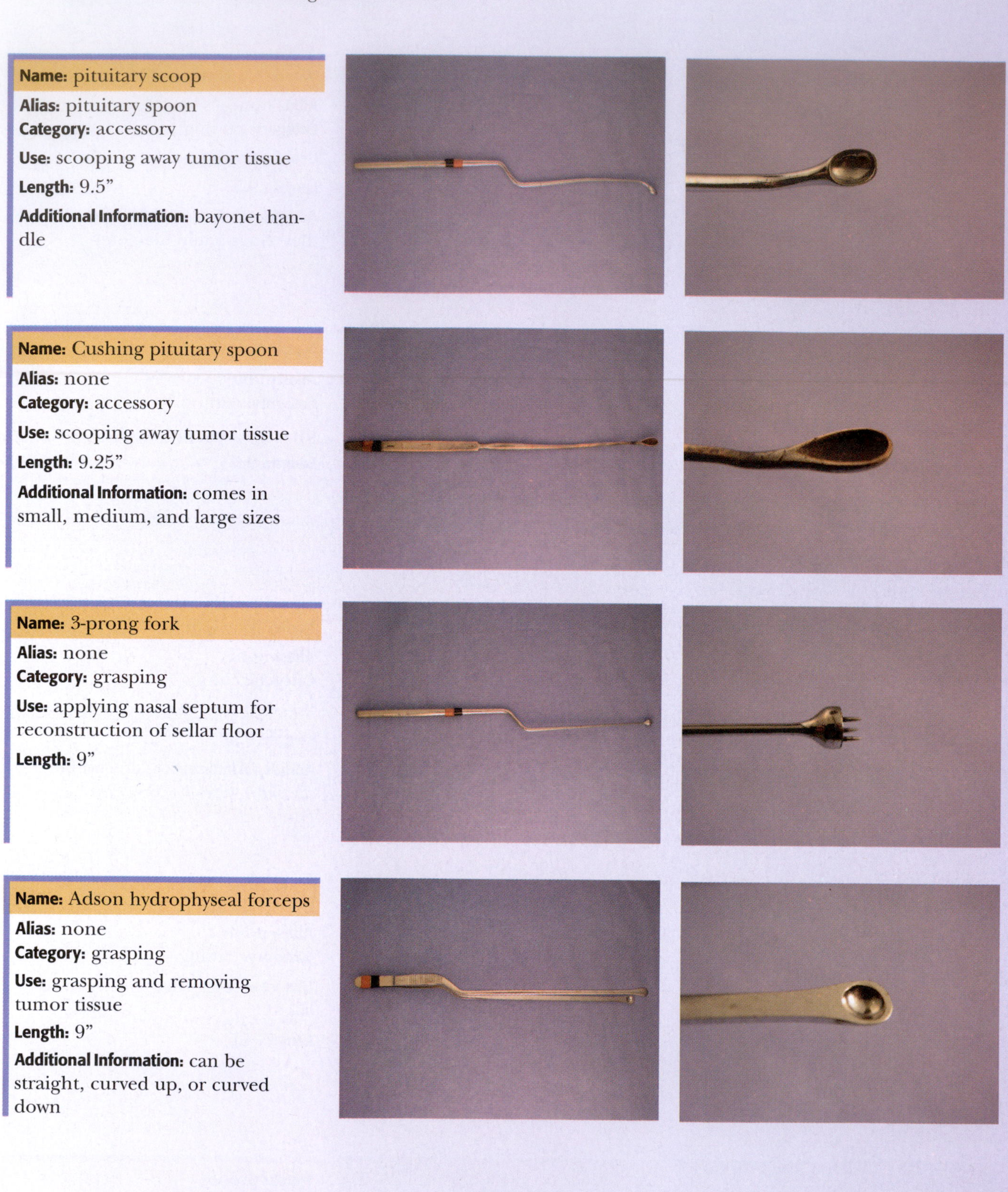

Name: pituitary scoop
Alias: pituitary spoon
Category: accessory
Use: scooping away tumor tissue
Length: 9.5"
Additional Information: bayonet handle

Name: Cushing pituitary spoon
Alias: none
Category: accessory
Use: scooping away tumor tissue
Length: 9.25"
Additional Information: comes in small, medium, and large sizes

Name: 3-prong fork
Alias: none
Category: grasping
Use: applying nasal septum for reconstruction of sellar floor
Length: 9"

Name: Adson hydrophyseal forceps
Alias: none
Category: grasping
Use: grasping and removing tumor tissue
Length: 9"
Additional Information: can be straight, curved up, or curved down

Q&A

Surgical Session—Neurosurgical/ Spinal Instruments

1) The neurosurgeon is performing a craniotomy. He/she asks for the clamps used to retract the dura and hold it out of the way. You would hand him/her:
   a. Kelley clamps
   b. Cairn (dandy) clamps
   c. Peans
   d. Laheys
2) While performing a craniotomy, the neurosurgeon asks for a "brain spatula." You would hand him/her a:
   a. ribbon
   b. Scoville
   c. Green
   d. Beckman
3) Before handing the neurosurgeon the brain spatula, you need to first:
   a. moisten it with sterile water
   b. moisten it with alcohol
   c. moisten it with normal saline
   d. moisten it with betadine
4) While performing a lumbar discectomy, the surgeon asks for a Leksell. You hand him/her a:
   a. retractor
   b. rongeur
   c. clamp
   d. periosteal elevator
5) Which of the following instruments is NOT a cranial rongeur?
   a. Bacon
   b. Adson
   c. Beyer
   d. Gerzog
6) All of the following are self-retaining retractors *except*:
   a. Williams
   b. Beckman-Adson
   c. cerebellar
   d. Taylor
7) You hand the surgeon the scissors with a "ball tip" on them. You just handed him/her the ___________ scissors.
   a. Potts
   b. Adson
   c. Strully
   d. Mayo
8) The surgeon needs to shave a little bit of bone from the graft. You would hand him/her a graft________.
   a. packer
   b. rasp
   c. sizer
   d. impactor
9) You are first scrubbing a lumbar laminectomy. The surgeon needs a large hinged self-retaining retractor. What would you hand to him/her?
   a. Jansen
   b. cerebellar
   c. Taylor
   d. Beckman-Adson
10) During neurosurgery the surgeon requests the "ring forceps." The other name for this forceps is:
    a. tumor forceps
    b. Cushing forceps
    c. Gerald forceps
    d. grasper forceps
11) The name for the tubing holding forceps is:
    a. Cushing
    b. Greene
    c. ring
    d. grasper
12) Which cranial rongeur has the largest bite size?
    a. Adson
    b. Bacon
    c. Beyer
    d. Stookey

13) The cranial rongeur with a 2-mm bite size is a(n):
   a. Adson
   b. Bacon
   c. Beyer
   d. Stookey

14) Which Penfield dissector is single ended?
   a. #1
   b. #2
   c. #3
   d. #4

15) The surgeon is placing a pin. You hand him/her the pin and the next instrument you have ready is the:
   a. Gerzog
   b. Taylor
   c. Cushing
   d. Jansen

16) All of the following are jaw types for the Cushing pituitary *except*:
   a. straight
   b. left
   c. upbiting
   d. downbiting

Ear, Nose, and Throat Instruments

6

EAR INSTRUMENTS

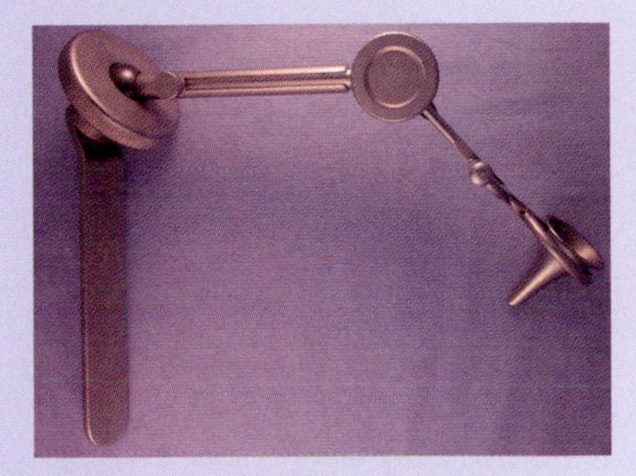
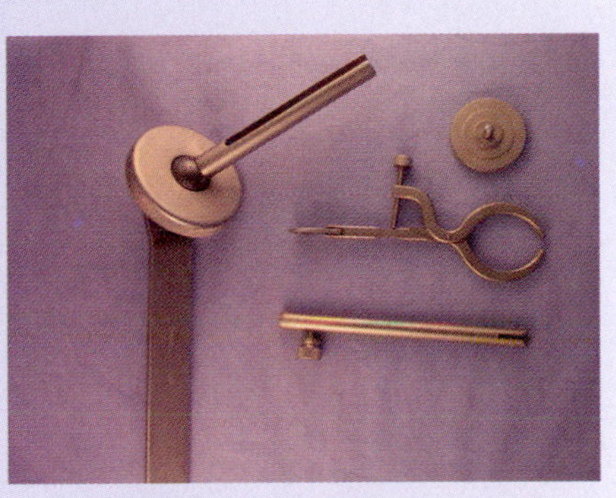

Name: Shea speculum holder

Alias: none

Category: accessory

Use: holding ear speculum in place, leaving surgeon's hands free

Length: n/a

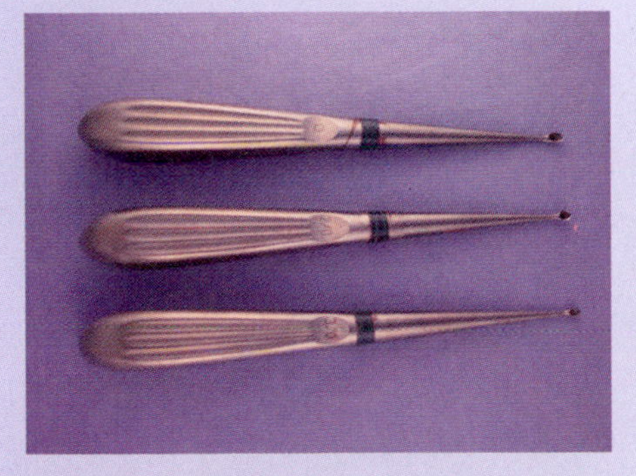
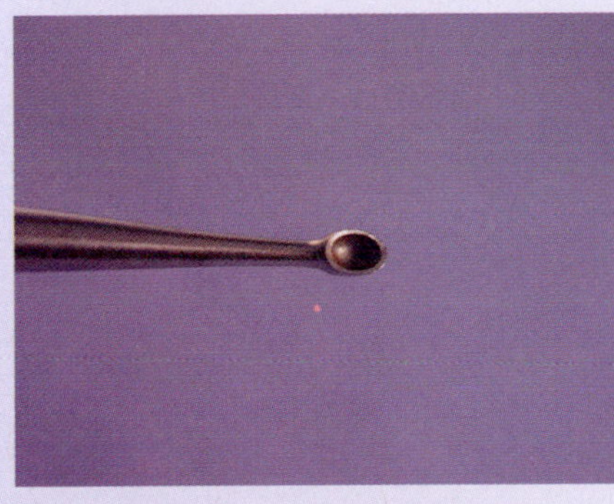

Name: Spratt mastoid curette

Alias: none

Category: cutting

Use: removing pieces of mastoid bone

Length: 6.5"

Additional Information: cup varies in size from 3.2 mm to 10.2 mm

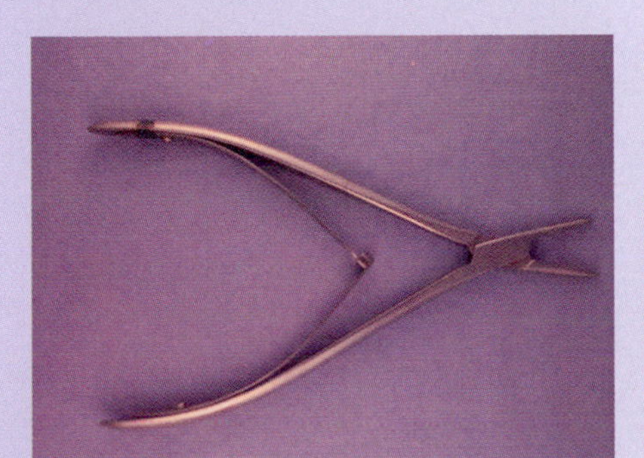
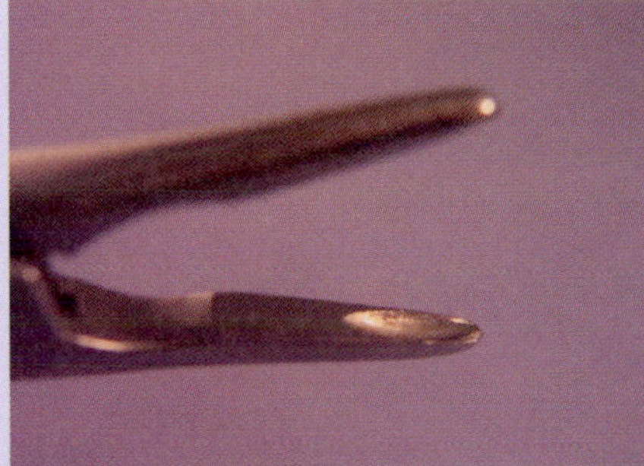

Name: Lempert rongeur

Alias: none

Category: cutting

Use: cutting away small pieces of bone

Length: 7.5"

Additional Information: 3 mm wide jaws

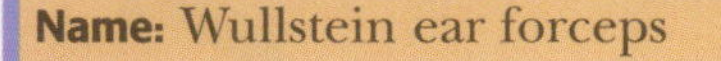

Name: Wullstein ear forceps

Alias: none

Category: grasping

Use: inserting prostheses or tubes; grasping delicate tissue or removing ossicles

Length: working length 3"

Additional Information: fine, delicate jaws

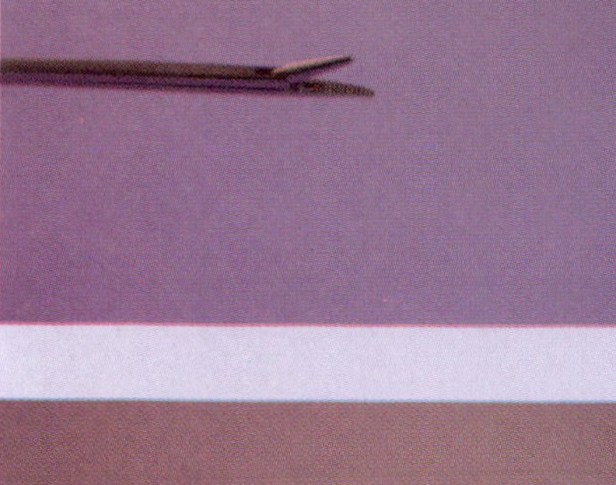

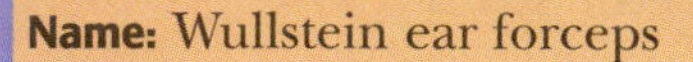

Name: Wullstein ear forceps

Alias: none

Category: grasping

Use: inserting tubes; grasping tissue

Length: working length 3"

Additional Information: serrated, heavy jaws

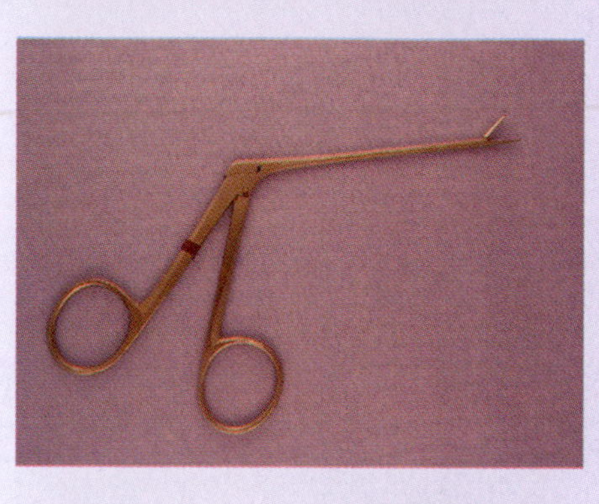

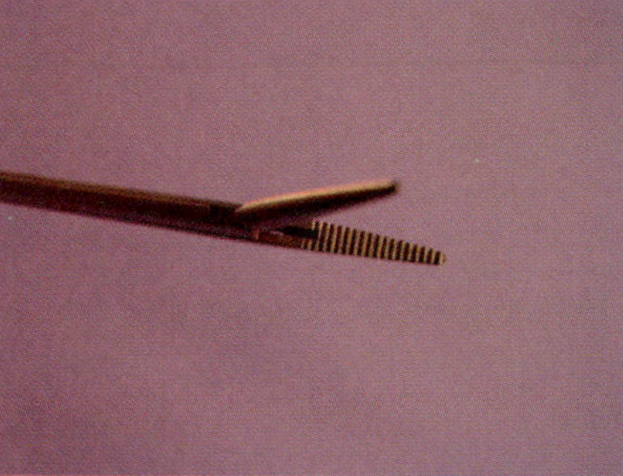

Name: McGee wire crimping forceps

Alias: none

Category: accessory

Use: crimping wire on stapes prosthesis

Length: working length 3"

Additional Information: delicate jaws

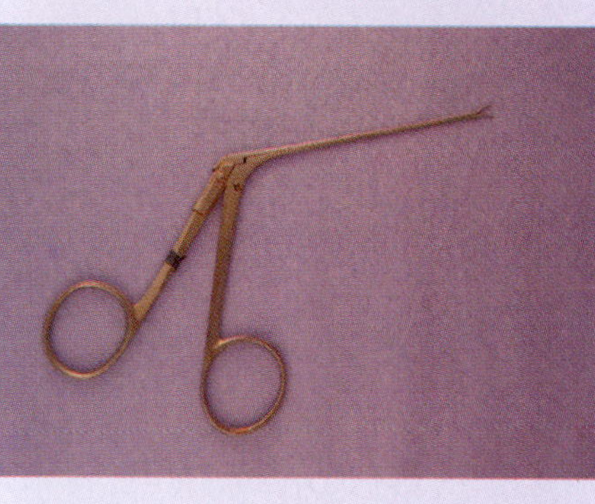

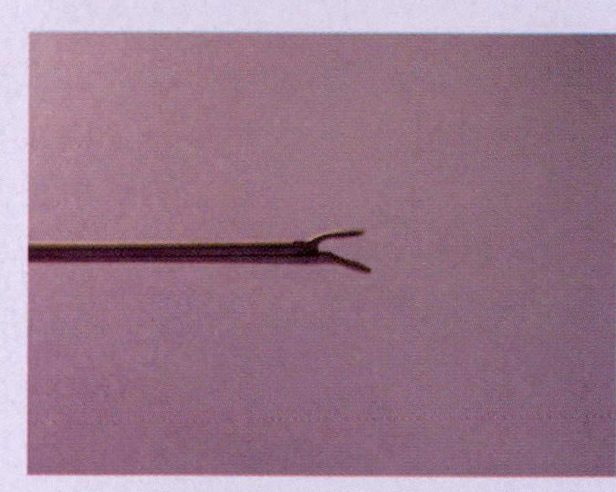

Name: House-Wullstein oval cup forceps

Alias: none

Category: grasping

Use: removing ossicles

Length: working length 3.25"

Additional Information: jaws can be bent left or right

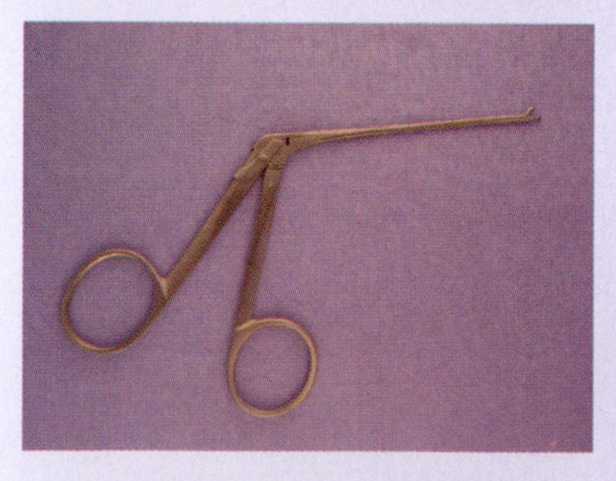

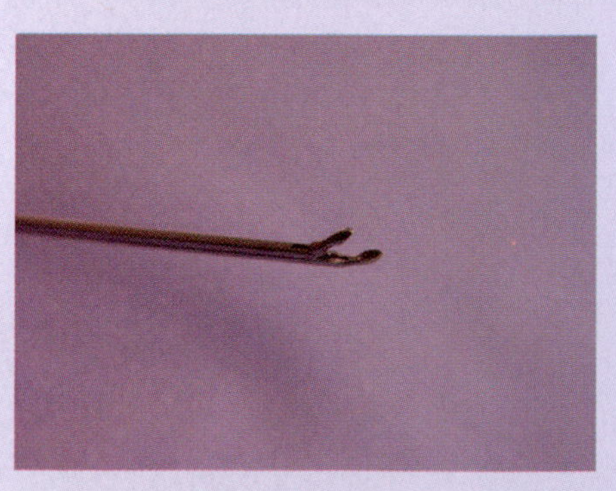

Name: cup forceps

Alias: none

Category: grasping

Use: removing ossicles

Length: working length 4"

Additional Information: cup can be 1 mm to 3 mm in diameter

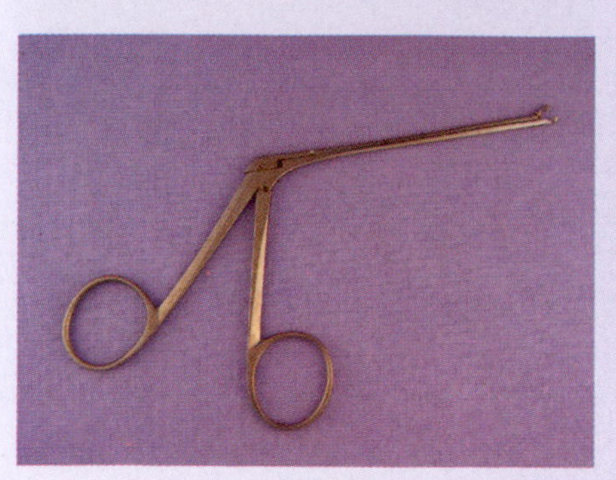

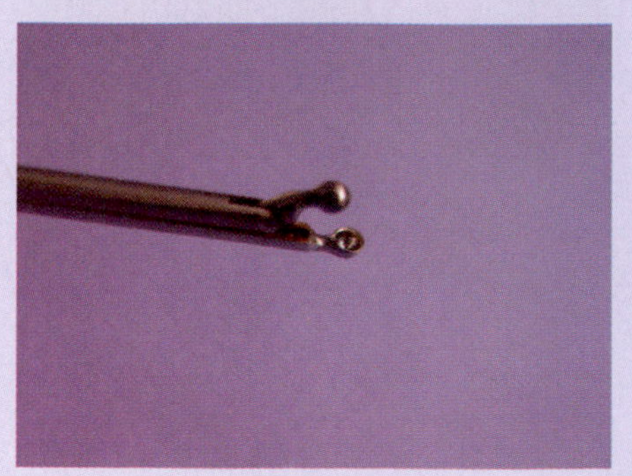

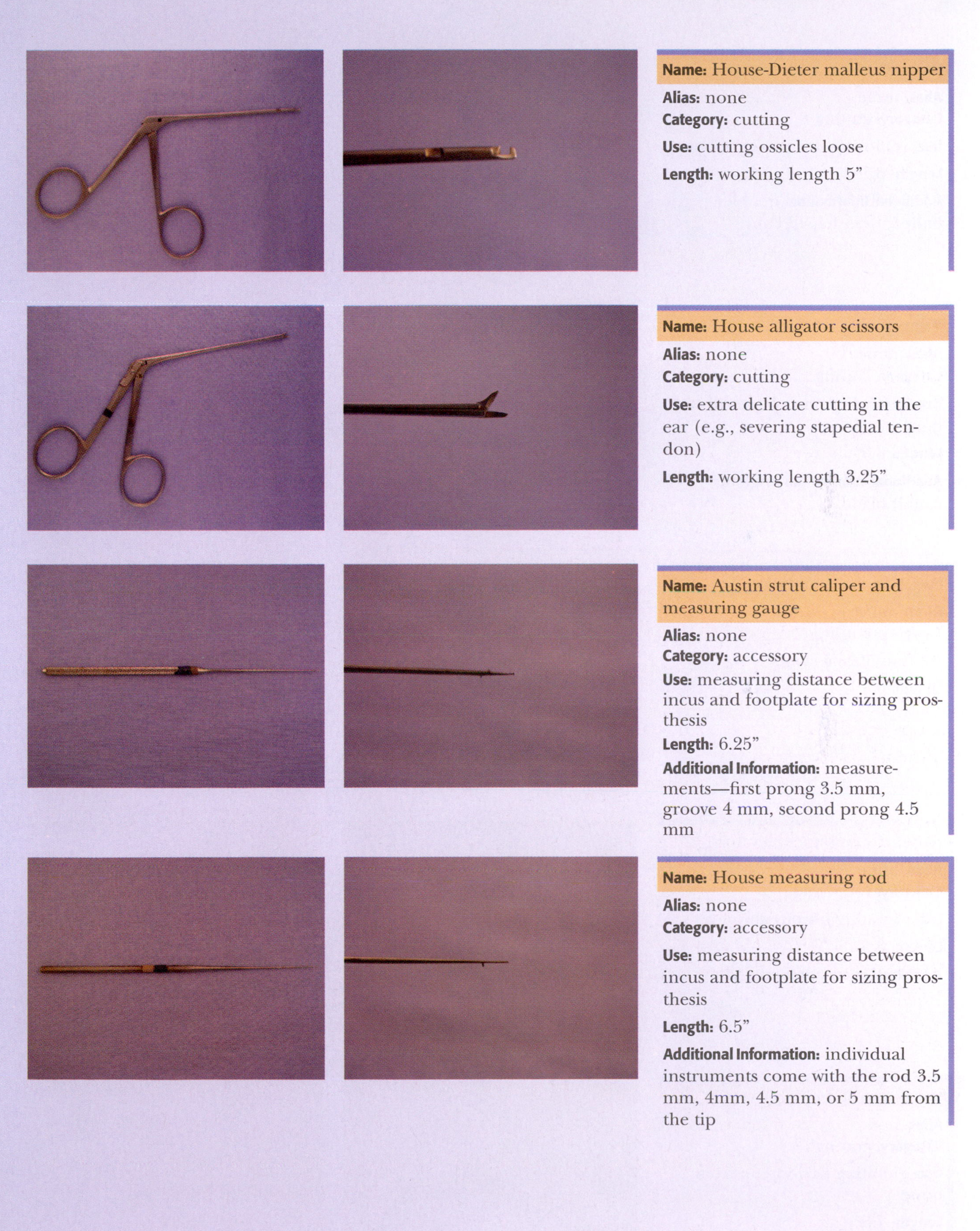

Name: House-Dieter malleus nipper

Alias: none

Category: cutting

Use: cutting ossicles loose

Length: working length 5"

Name: House alligator scissors

Alias: none

Category: cutting

Use: extra delicate cutting in the ear (e.g., severing stapedial tendon)

Length: working length 3.25"

Name: Austin strut caliper and measuring gauge

Alias: none

Category: accessory

Use: measuring distance between incus and footplate for sizing prosthesis

Length: 6.25"

Additional Information: measurements—first prong 3.5 mm, groove 4 mm, second prong 4.5 mm

Name: House measuring rod

Alias: none

Category: accessory

Use: measuring distance between incus and footplate for sizing prosthesis

Length: 6.5"

Additional Information: individual instruments come with the rod 3.5 mm, 4mm, 4.5 mm, or 5 mm from the tip

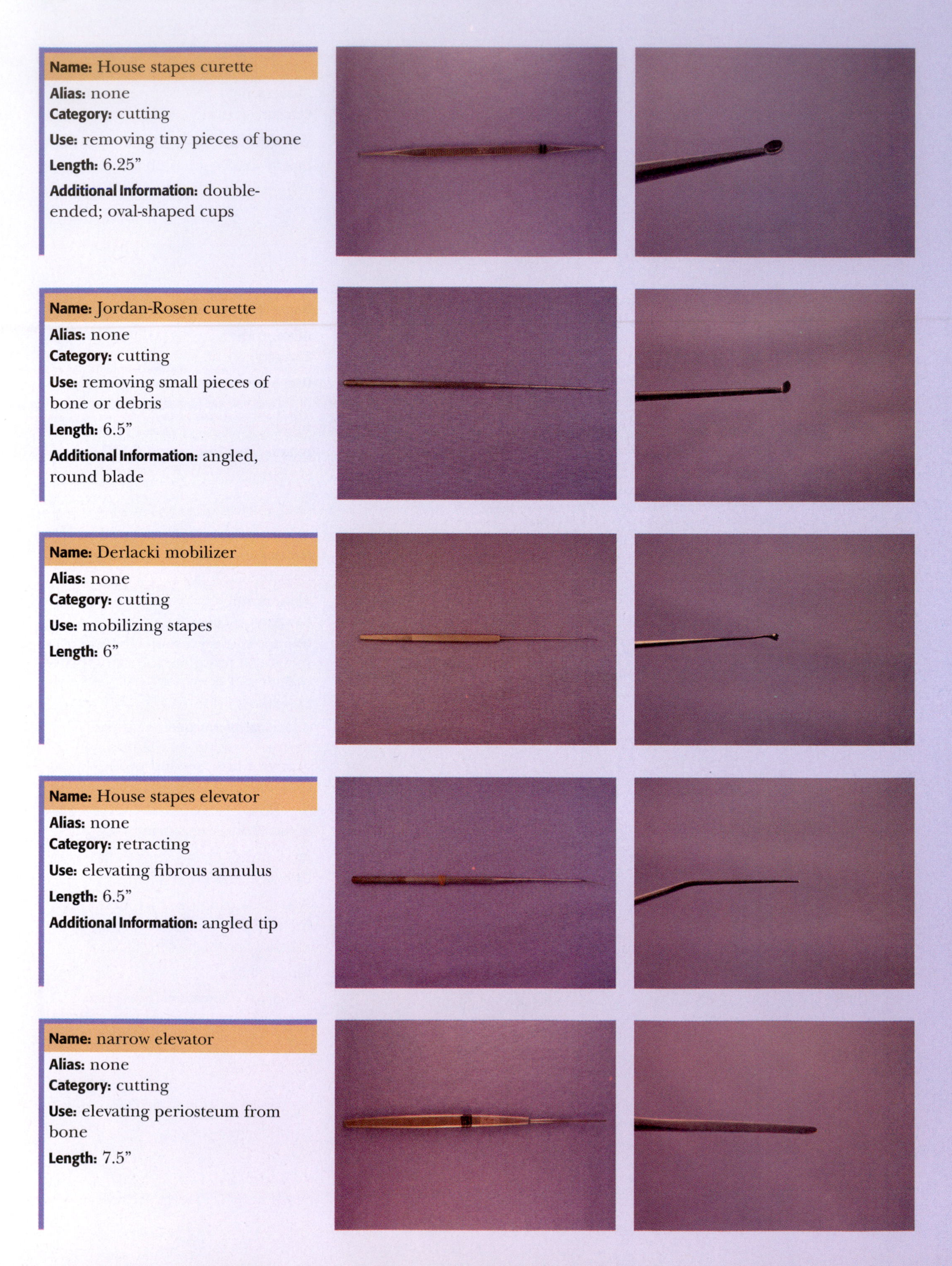

Name: House stapes curette
Alias: none
Category: cutting
Use: removing tiny pieces of bone
Length: 6.25"
Additional Information: double-ended; oval-shaped cups

Name: Jordan-Rosen curette
Alias: none
Category: cutting
Use: removing small pieces of bone or debris
Length: 6.5"
Additional Information: angled, round blade

Name: Derlacki mobilizer
Alias: none
Category: cutting
Use: mobilizing stapes
Length: 6"

Name: House stapes elevator
Alias: none
Category: retracting
Use: elevating fibrous annulus
Length: 6.5"
Additional Information: angled tip

Name: narrow elevator
Alias: none
Category: cutting
Use: elevating periosteum from bone
Length: 7.5"

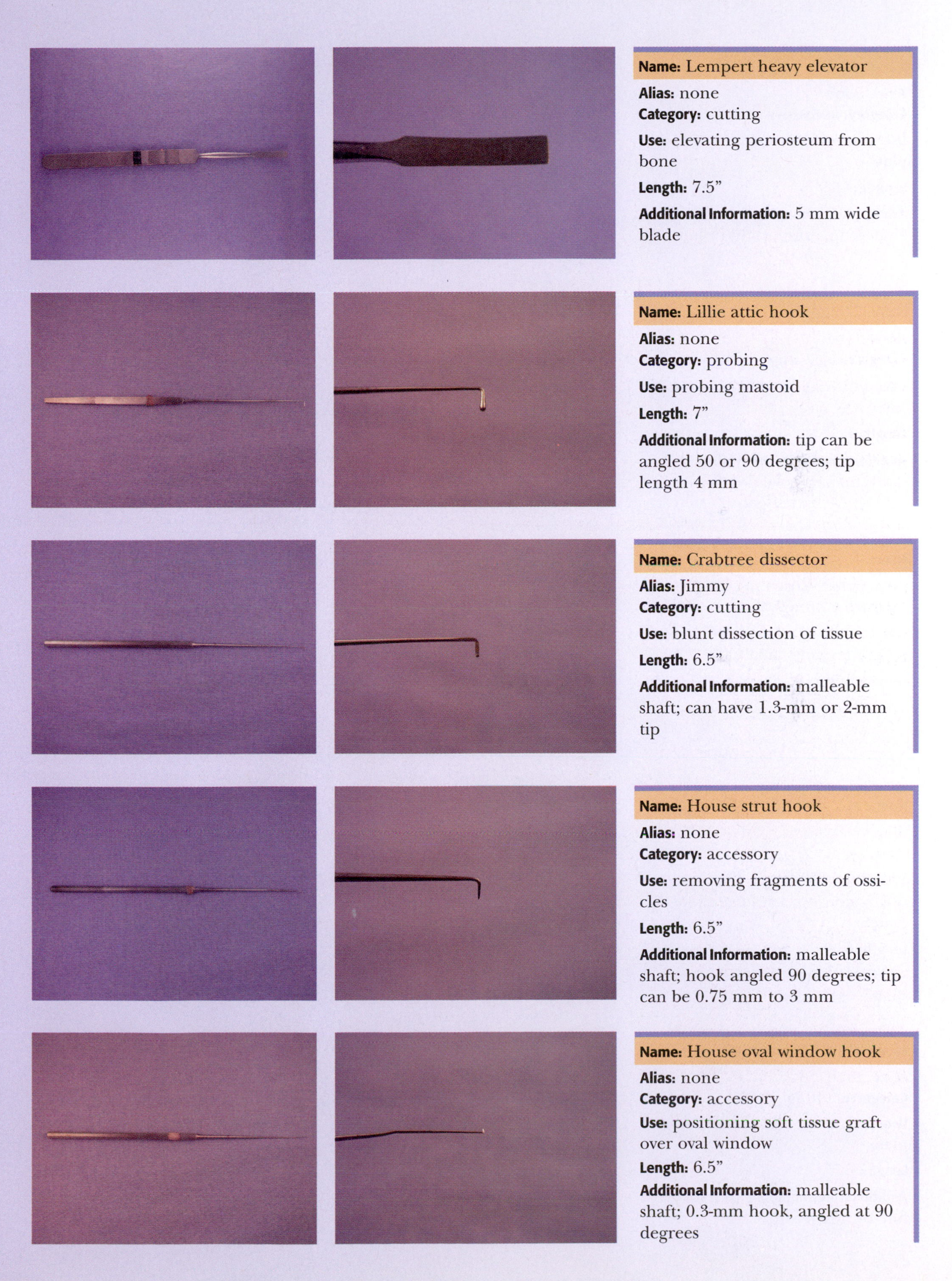

Name: Lempert heavy elevator
Alias: none
Category: cutting
Use: elevating periosteum from bone
Length: 7.5"
Additional Information: 5 mm wide blade

Name: Lillie attic hook
Alias: none
Category: probing
Use: probing mastoid
Length: 7"
Additional Information: tip can be angled 50 or 90 degrees; tip length 4 mm

Name: Crabtree dissector
Alias: Jimmy
Category: cutting
Use: blunt dissection of tissue
Length: 6.5"
Additional Information: malleable shaft; can have 1.3-mm or 2-mm tip

Name: House strut hook
Alias: none
Category: accessory
Use: removing fragments of ossicles
Length: 6.5"
Additional Information: malleable shaft; hook angled 90 degrees; tip can be 0.75 mm to 3 mm

Name: House oval window hook
Alias: none
Category: accessory
Use: positioning soft tissue graft over oval window
Length: 6.5"
Additional Information: malleable shaft; 0.3-mm hook, angled at 90 degrees

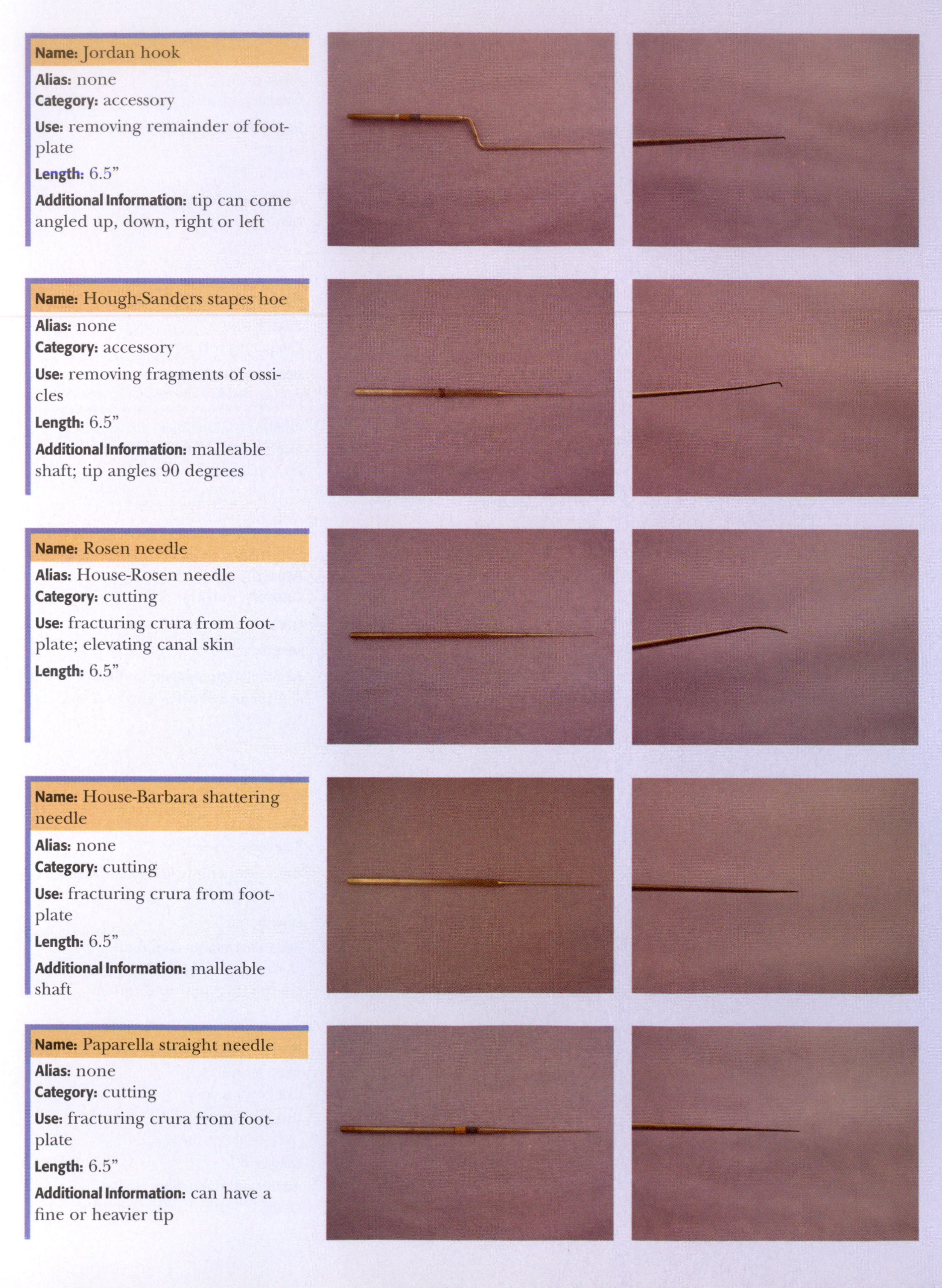

Name: Jordan hook
Alias: none
Category: accessory
Use: removing remainder of foot-plate
Length: 6.5"
Additional Information: tip can come angled up, down, right or left

Name: Hough-Sanders stapes hoe
Alias: none
Category: accessory
Use: removing fragments of ossicles
Length: 6.5"
Additional Information: malleable shaft; tip angles 90 degrees

Name: Rosen needle
Alias: House-Rosen needle
Category: cutting
Use: fracturing crura from foot-plate; elevating canal skin
Length: 6.5"

Name: House-Barbara shattering needle
Alias: none
Category: cutting
Use: fracturing crura from foot-plate
Length: 6.5"
Additional Information: malleable shaft

Name: Paparella straight needle
Alias: none
Category: cutting
Use: fracturing crura from foot-plate
Length: 6.5"
Additional Information: can have a fine or heavier tip

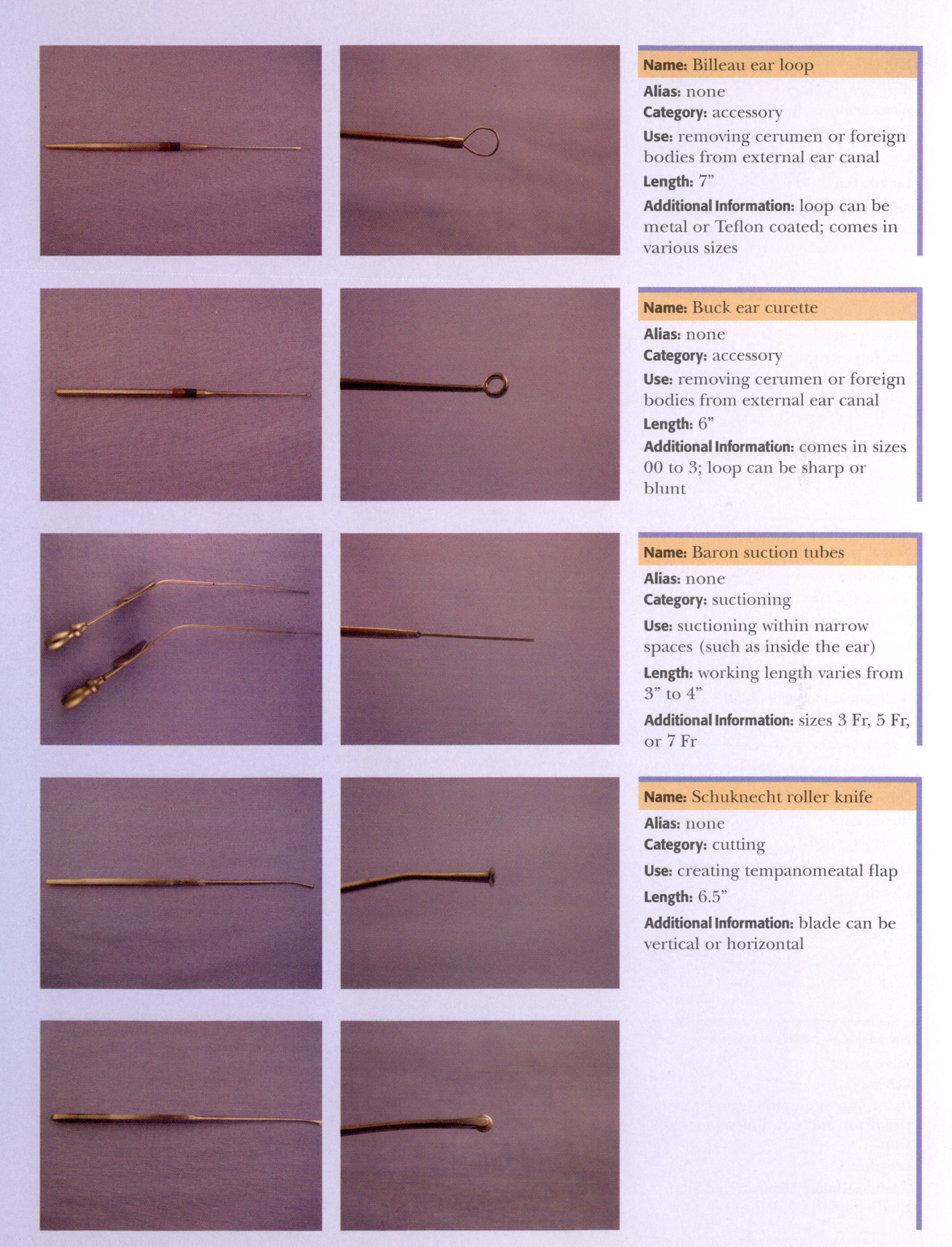

Name: Billeau ear loop

Alias: none

Category: accessory

Use: removing cerumen or foreign bodies from external ear canal

Length: 7"

Additional Information: loop can be metal or Teflon coated; comes in various sizes

Name: Buck ear curette

Alias: none

Category: accessory

Use: removing cerumen or foreign bodies from external ear canal

Length: 6"

Additional Information: comes in sizes 00 to 3; loop can be sharp or blunt

Name: Baron suction tubes

Alias: none

Category: suctioning

Use: suctioning within narrow spaces (such as inside the ear)

Length: working length varies from 3" to 4"

Additional Information: sizes 3 Fr, 5 Fr, or 7 Fr

Name: Schuknecht roller knife

Alias: none

Category: cutting

Use: creating tempanomeatal flap

Length: 6.5"

Additional Information: blade can be vertical or horizontal

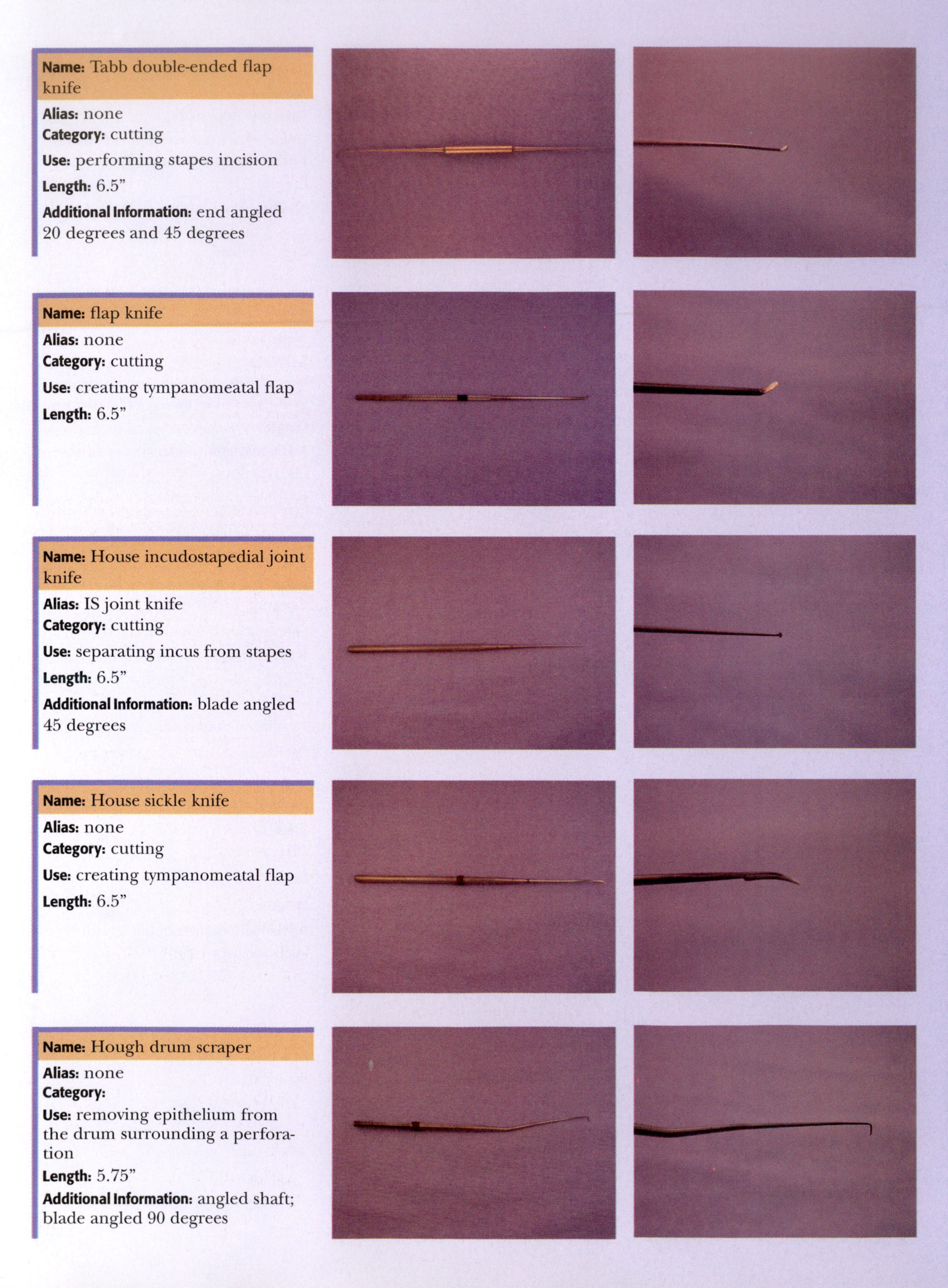

Name: Tabb double-ended flap knife

Alias: none

Category: cutting

Use: performing stapes incision

Length: 6.5”

Additional Information: end angled 20 degrees and 45 degrees

Name: flap knife

Alias: none

Category: cutting

Use: creating tympanomeatal flap

Length: 6.5”

Name: House incudostapedial joint knife

Alias: IS joint knife

Category: cutting

Use: separating incus from stapes

Length: 6.5”

Additional Information: blade angled 45 degrees

Name: House sickle knife

Alias: none

Category: cutting

Use: creating tympanomeatal flap

Length: 6.5”

Name: Hough drum scraper

Alias: none

Category:

Use: removing epithelium from the drum surrounding a perforation

Length: 5.75”

Additional Information: angled shaft; blade angled 90 degrees

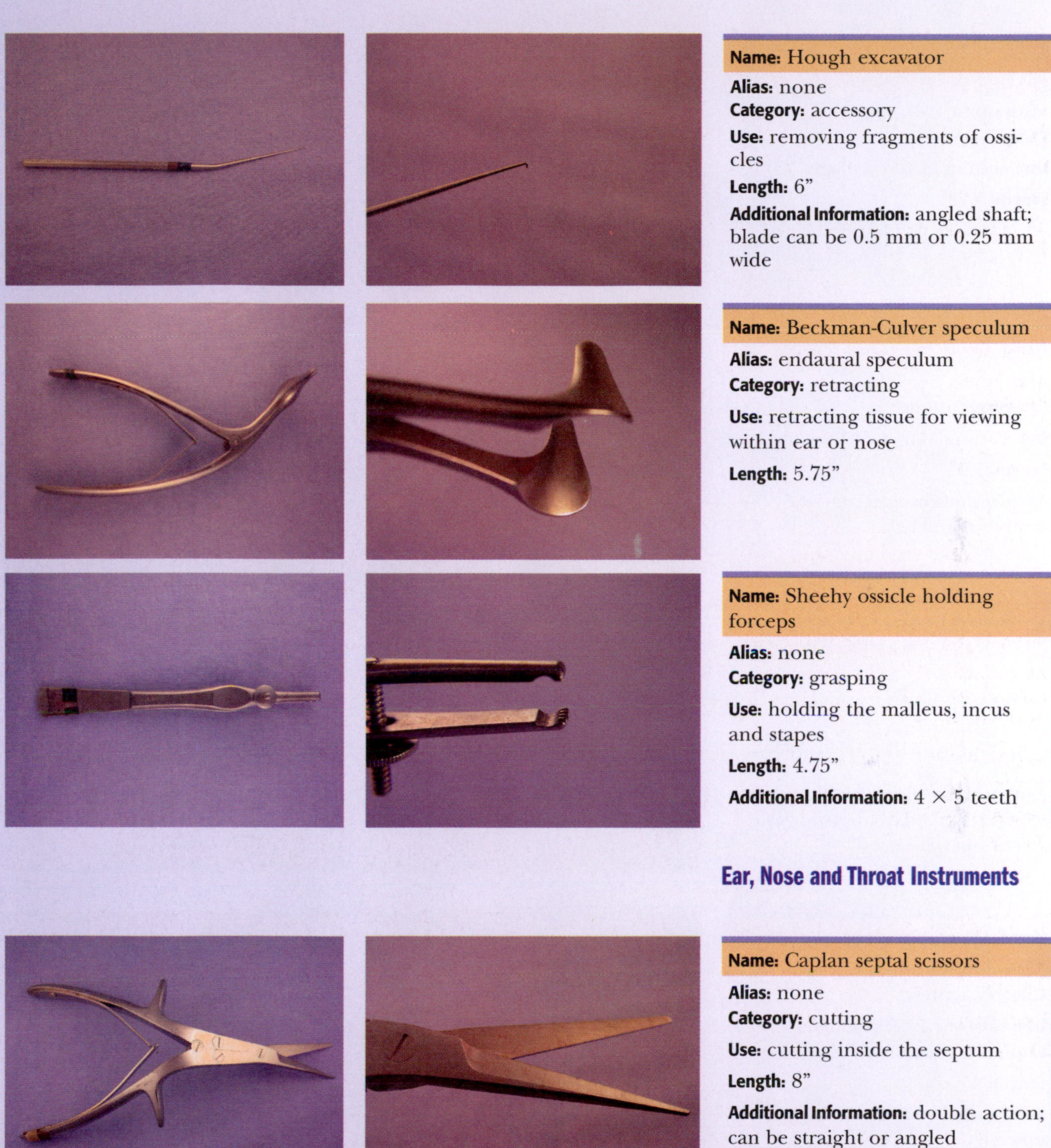

Name: Hough excavator
Alias: none
Category: accessory
Use: removing fragments of ossicles
Length: 6"
Additional Information: angled shaft; blade can be 0.5 mm or 0.25 mm wide

Name: Beckman-Culver speculum
Alias: endaural speculum
Category: retracting
Use: retracting tissue for viewing within ear or nose
Length: 5.75"

Name: Sheehy ossicle holding forceps
Alias: none
Category: grasping
Use: holding the malleus, incus and stapes
Length: 4.75"
Additional Information: 4 × 5 teeth

Ear, Nose and Throat Instruments

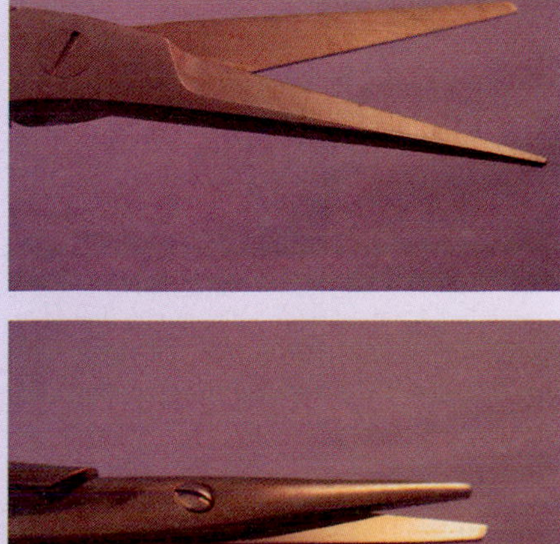

Name: Caplan septal scissors
Alias: none
Category: cutting
Use: cutting inside the septum
Length: 8"
Additional Information: double action; can be straight or angled

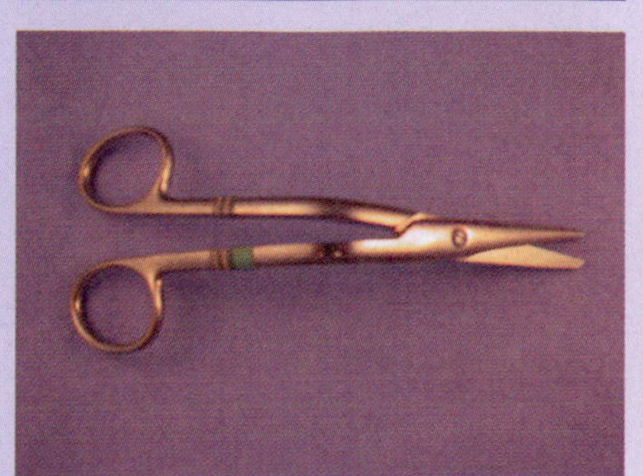

Name: Cottle angular scissors
Alias: none
Category: cutting
Use: cutting nasal cartilage
Length: 6.5"
Additional Information: heavy, rounded blades

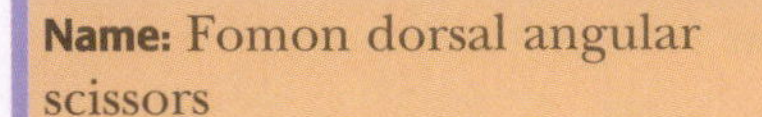

Name: Fomon dorsal angular scissors

Alias: none
Category: cutting
Use: cutting nasal cartilage
Length: 5.25"

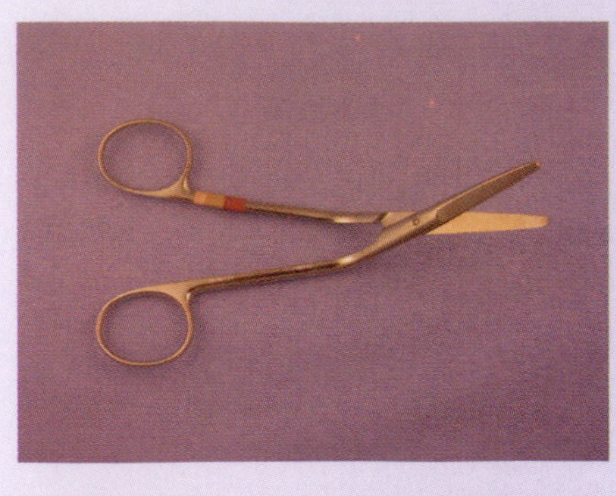

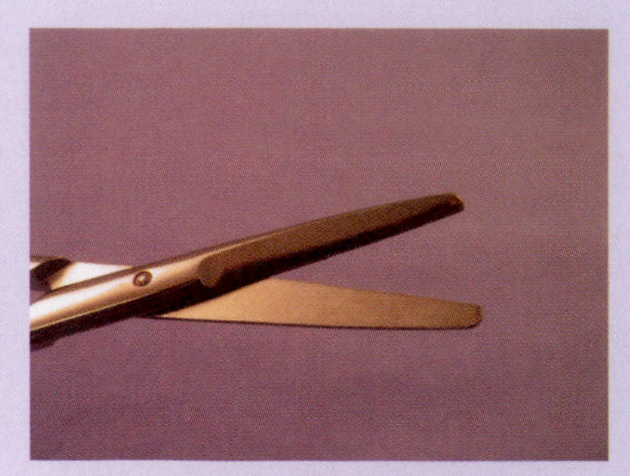

Name: Boettcher tonsil scissors

Alias: none
Category: cutting
Use: cutting away tonsil tissue
Length: 7.5"
Additional Information: curved, double-edge blades

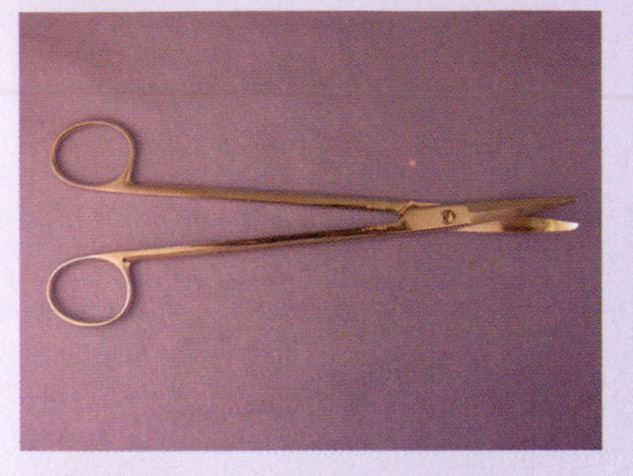

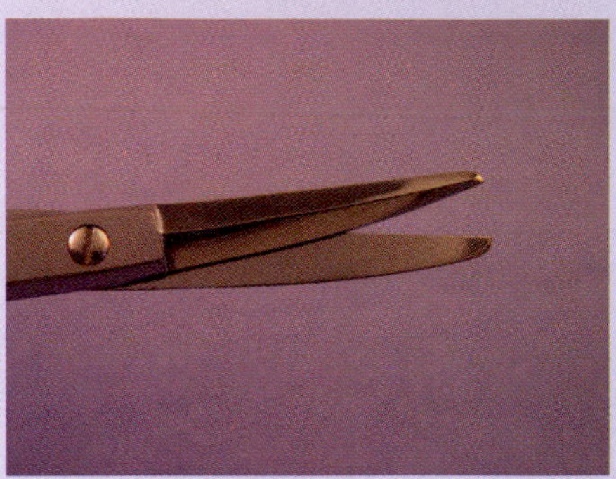

Name: Wagner scissors

Alias: none
Category: cutting
Use: cutting tissue
Length: 4.75"
Additional Information: blades can be straight, curved or angled; tips can be sharp or blunt

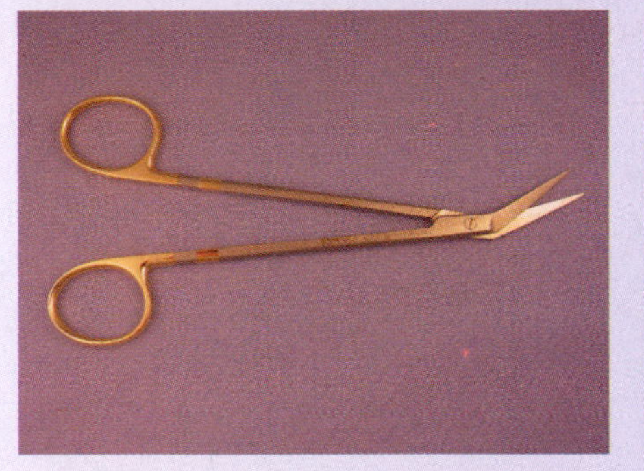

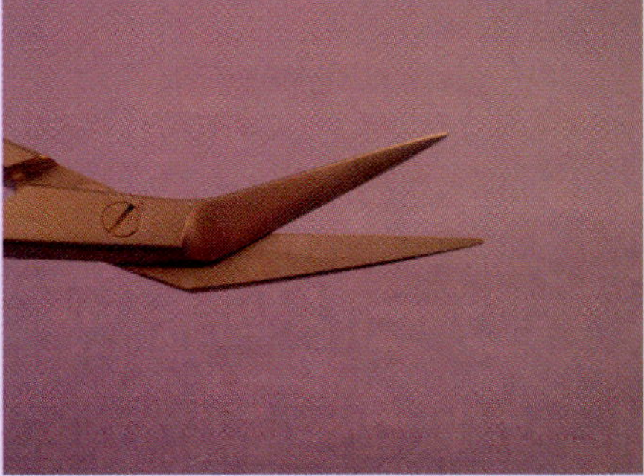

Name: Graefe scissors

Alias: none
Category: cutting
Use: dissecting delicate tissue around curved area
Length: 4"
Additional Information: blades curved upward

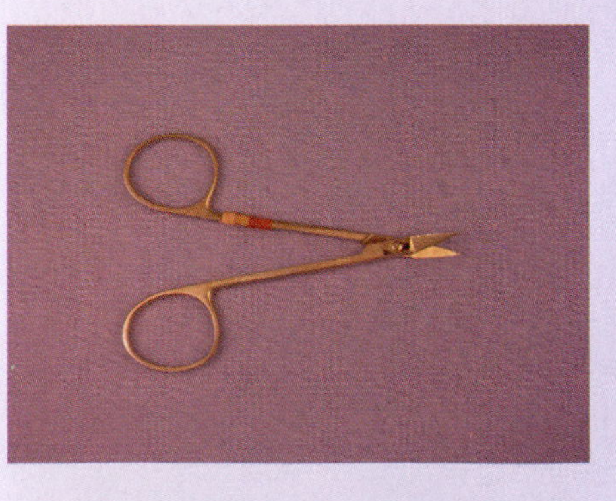

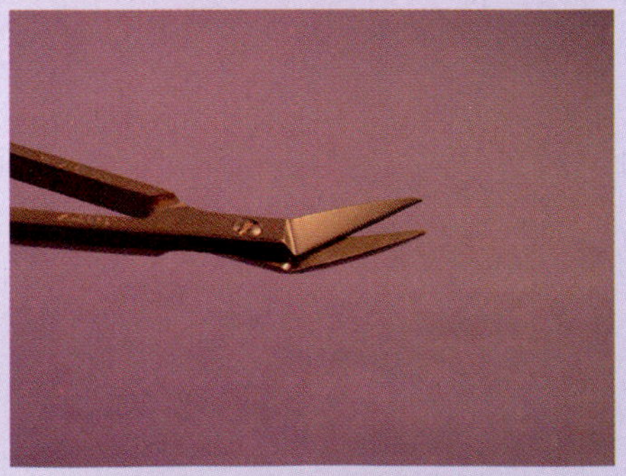

Name: Peck-Joseph scissors

Alias: none
Category: cutting
Use: cutting fine tissue or mucous membrane
Length: 5.5"
Additional Information: blades can be sharp or blunt, straight or curved

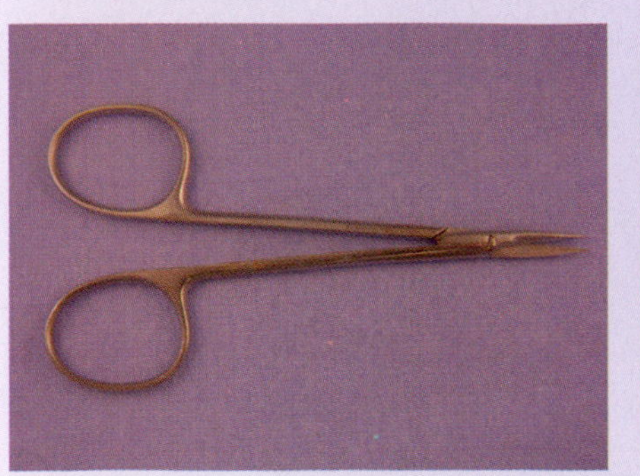

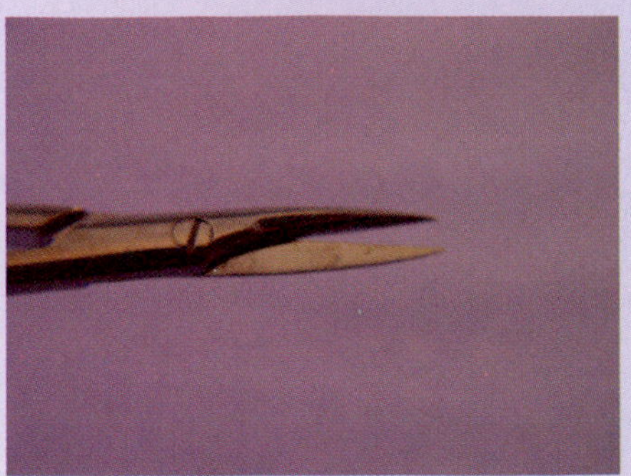

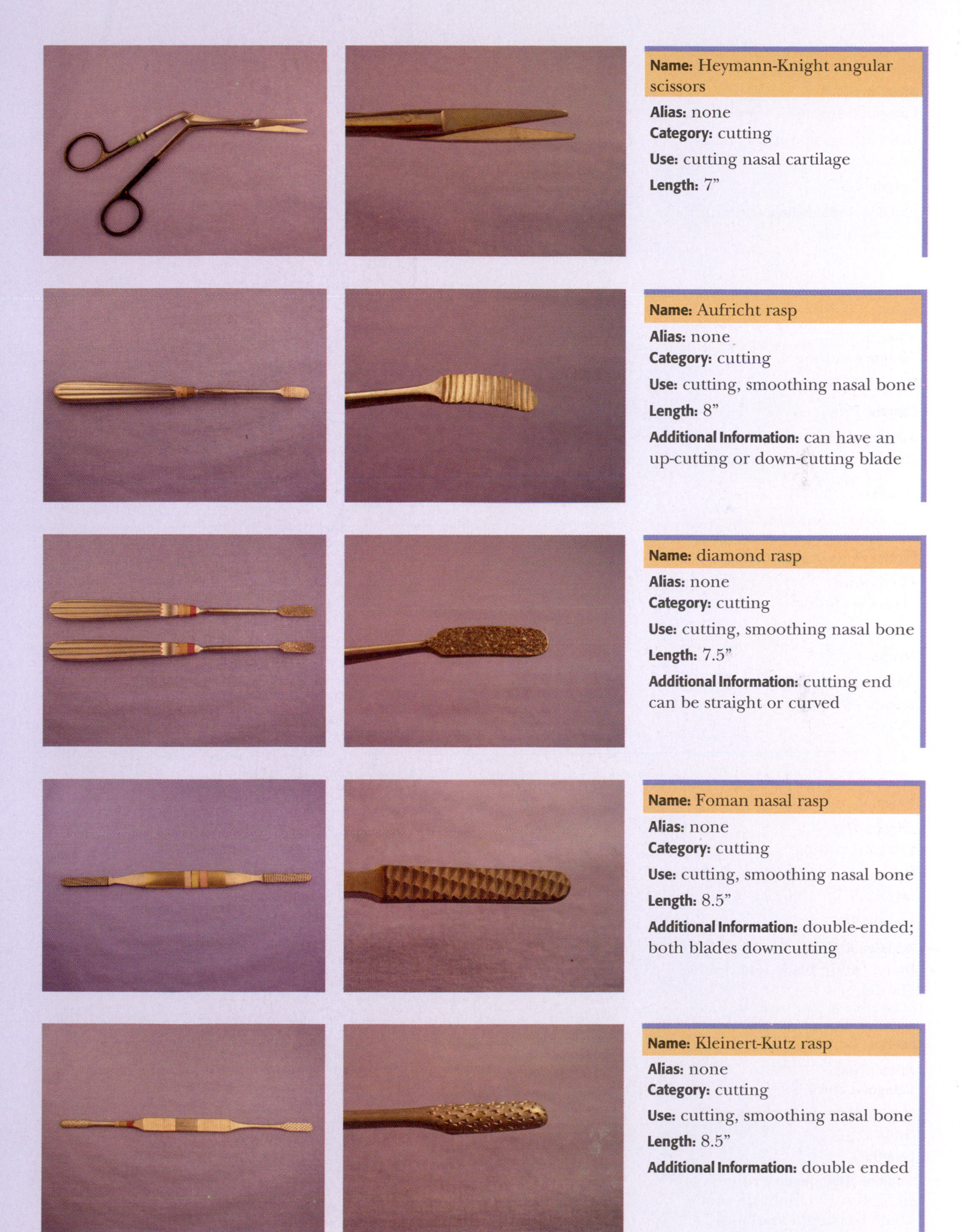

Name: Heymann-Knight angular scissors

Alias: none

Category: cutting

Use: cutting nasal cartilage

Length: 7"

Name: Aufricht rasp

Alias: none

Category: cutting

Use: cutting, smoothing nasal bone

Length: 8"

Additional Information: can have an up-cutting or down-cutting blade

Name: diamond rasp

Alias: none

Category: cutting

Use: cutting, smoothing nasal bone

Length: 7.5"

Additional Information: cutting end can be straight or curved

Name: Foman nasal rasp

Alias: none

Category: cutting

Use: cutting, smoothing nasal bone

Length: 8.5"

Additional Information: double-ended; both blades downcutting

Name: Kleinert-Kutz rasp

Alias: none

Category: cutting

Use: cutting, smoothing nasal bone

Length: 8.5"

Additional Information: double ended

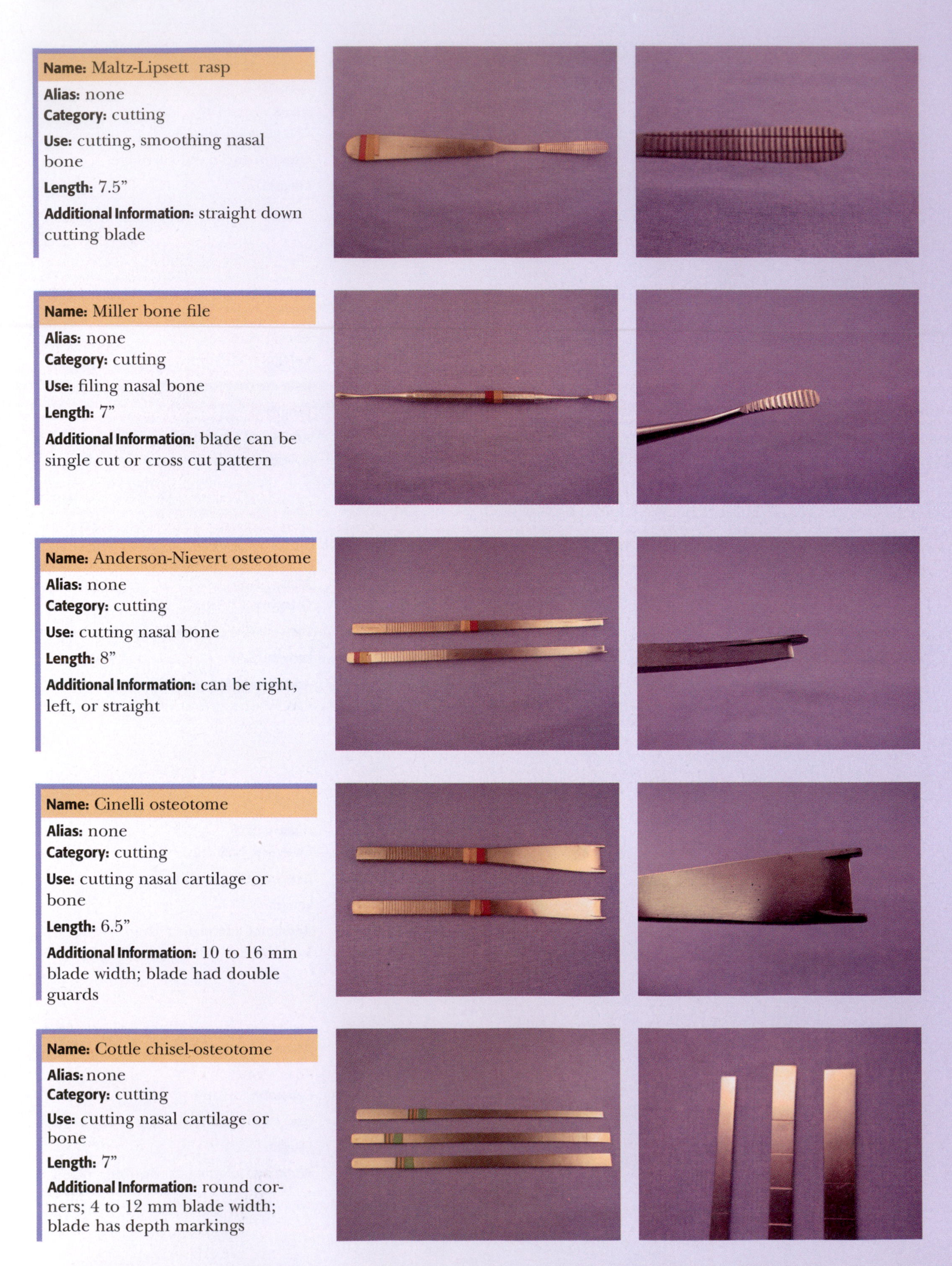

Name: Maltz-Lipsett rasp
Alias: none
Category: cutting
Use: cutting, smoothing nasal bone
Length: 7.5"
Additional Information: straight down cutting blade

Name: Miller bone file
Alias: none
Category: cutting
Use: filing nasal bone
Length: 7"
Additional Information: blade can be single cut or cross cut pattern

Name: Anderson-Nievert osteotome
Alias: none
Category: cutting
Use: cutting nasal bone
Length: 8"
Additional Information: can be right, left, or straight

Name: Cinelli osteotome
Alias: none
Category: cutting
Use: cutting nasal cartilage or bone
Length: 6.5"
Additional Information: 10 to 16 mm blade width; blade had double guards

Name: Cottle chisel-osteotome
Alias: none
Category: cutting
Use: cutting nasal cartilage or bone
Length: 7"
Additional Information: round corners; 4 to 12 mm blade width; blade has depth markings

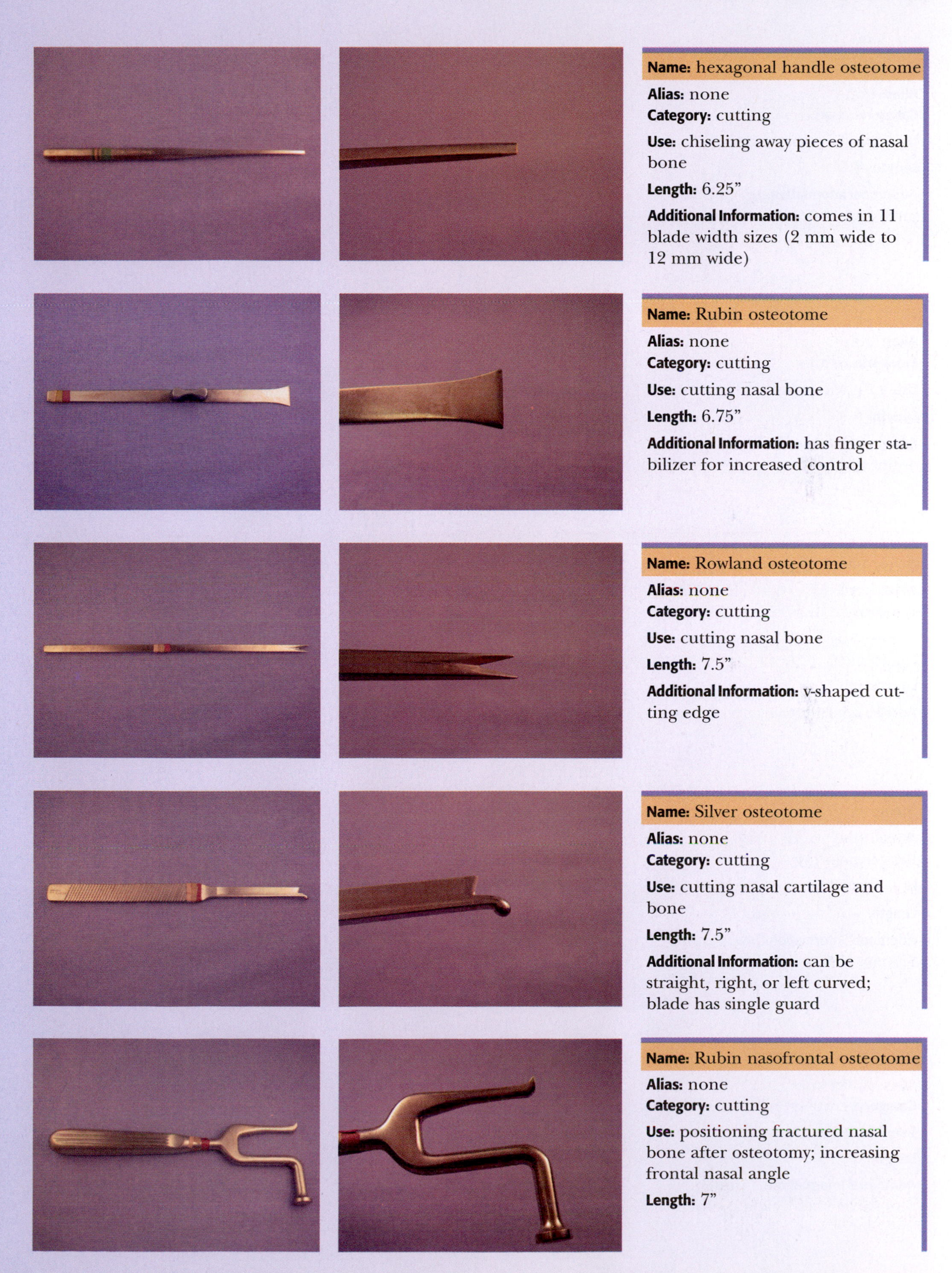

Name: hexagonal handle osteotome
Alias: none
Category: cutting
Use: chiseling away pieces of nasal bone
Length: 6.25"
Additional Information: comes in 11 blade width sizes (2 mm wide to 12 mm wide)

Name: Rubin osteotome
Alias: none
Category: cutting
Use: cutting nasal bone
Length: 6.75"
Additional Information: has finger stabilizer for increased control

Name: Rowland osteotome
Alias: none
Category: cutting
Use: cutting nasal bone
Length: 7.5"
Additional Information: v-shaped cutting edge

Name: Silver osteotome
Alias: none
Category: cutting
Use: cutting nasal cartilage and bone
Length: 7.5"
Additional Information: can be straight, right, or left curved; blade has single guard

Name: Rubin nasofrontal osteotome
Alias: none
Category: cutting
Use: positioning fractured nasal bone after osteotomy; increasing frontal nasal angle
Length: 7"

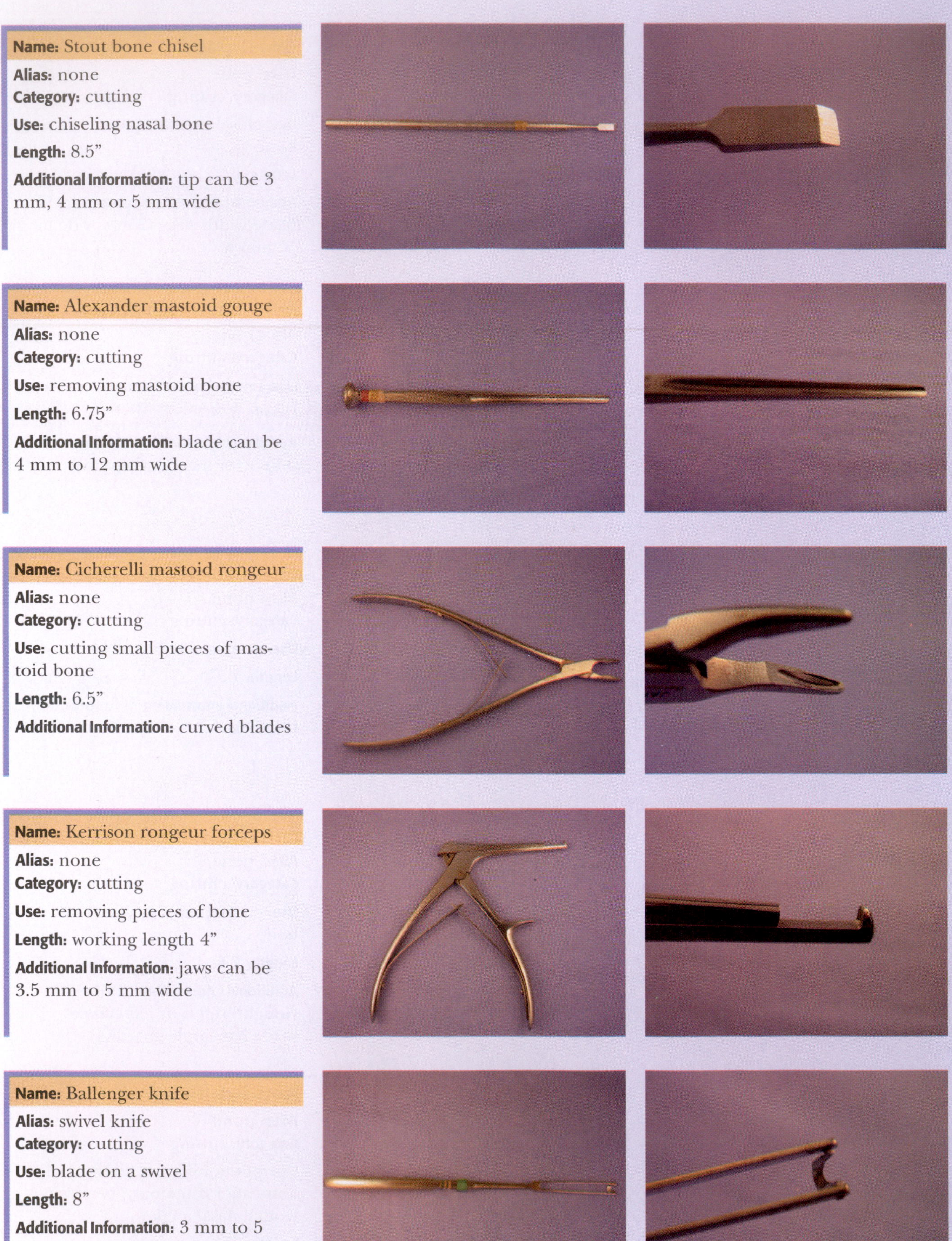

Name: Stout bone chisel
Alias: none
Category: cutting
Use: chiseling nasal bone
Length: 8.5"
Additional Information: tip can be 3 mm, 4 mm or 5 mm wide

Name: Alexander mastoid gouge
Alias: none
Category: cutting
Use: removing mastoid bone
Length: 6.75"
Additional Information: blade can be 4 mm to 12 mm wide

Name: Cicherelli mastoid rongeur
Alias: none
Category: cutting
Use: cutting small pieces of mastoid bone
Length: 6.5"
Additional Information: curved blades

Name: Kerrison rongeur forceps
Alias: none
Category: cutting
Use: removing pieces of bone
Length: working length 4"
Additional Information: jaws can be 3.5 mm to 5 mm wide

Name: Ballenger knife
Alias: swivel knife
Category: cutting
Use: blade on a swivel
Length: 8"
Additional Information: 3 mm to 5 mm swivel blade; can be straight or bayonet style

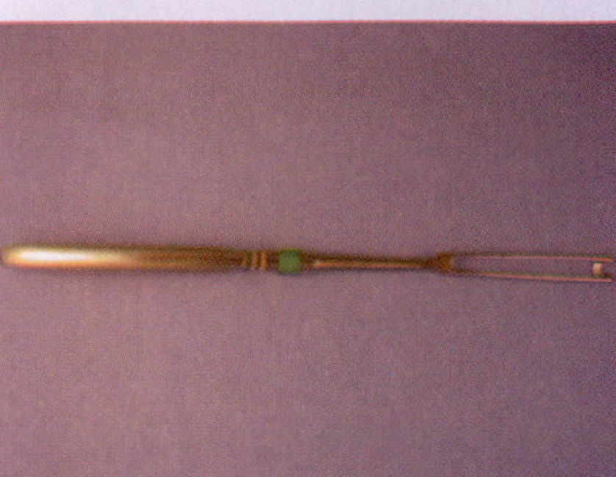

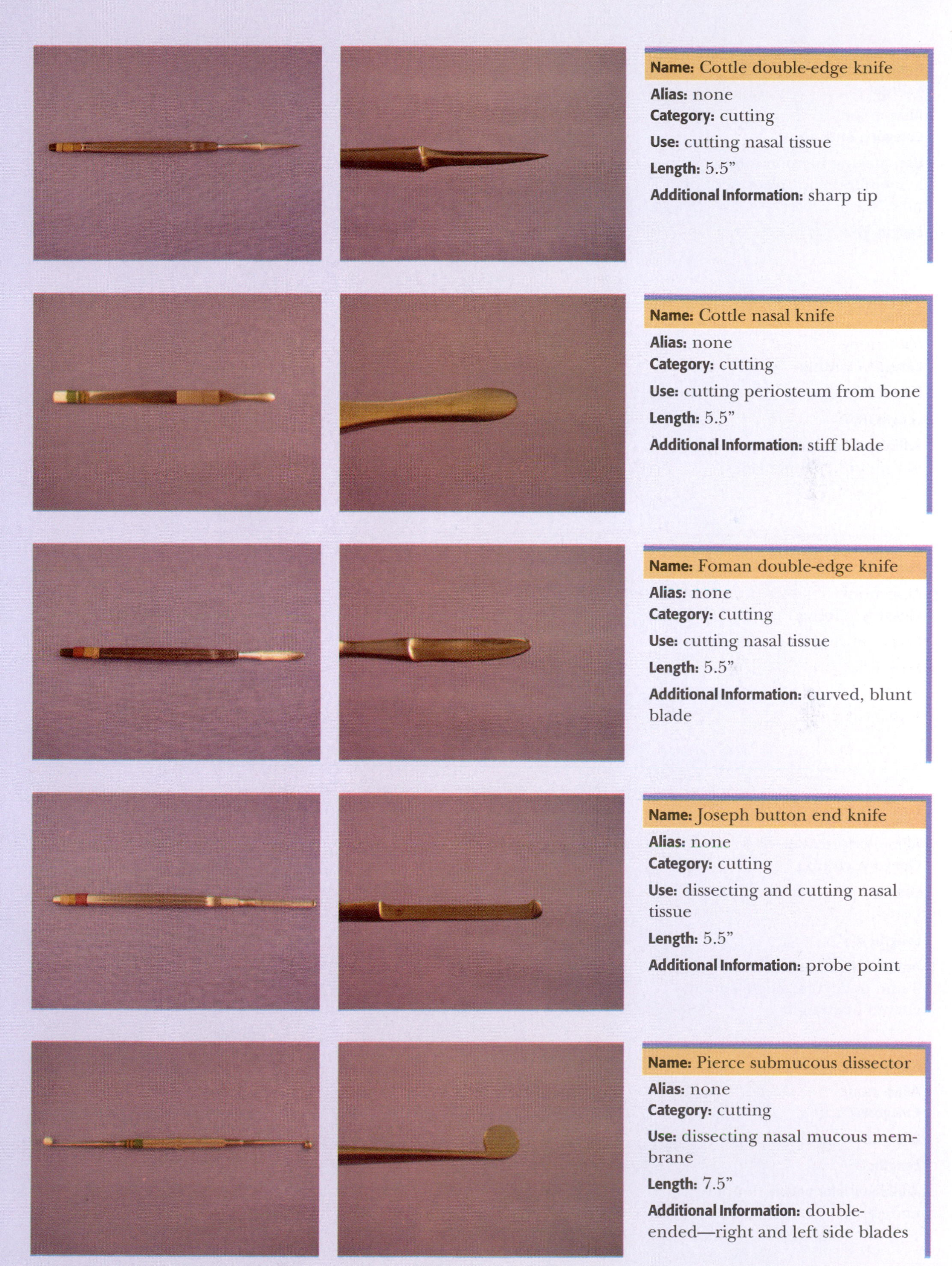

Name: Cottle double-edge knife
Alias: none
Category: cutting
Use: cutting nasal tissue
Length: 5.5"
Additional Information: sharp tip

Name: Cottle nasal knife
Alias: none
Category: cutting
Use: cutting periosteum from bone
Length: 5.5"
Additional Information: stiff blade

Name: Foman double-edge knife
Alias: none
Category: cutting
Use: cutting nasal tissue
Length: 5.5"
Additional Information: curved, blunt blade

Name: Joseph button end knife
Alias: none
Category: cutting
Use: dissecting and cutting nasal tissue
Length: 5.5"
Additional Information: probe point

Name: Pierce submucous dissector
Alias: none
Category: cutting
Use: dissecting nasal mucous membrane
Length: 7.5"
Additional Information: double-ended—right and left side blades

Name: myringotomy knife (alligator)

Alias: none

Category: cutting

Use: making incision into tympanic membrane for placement of tube

Length: n/a

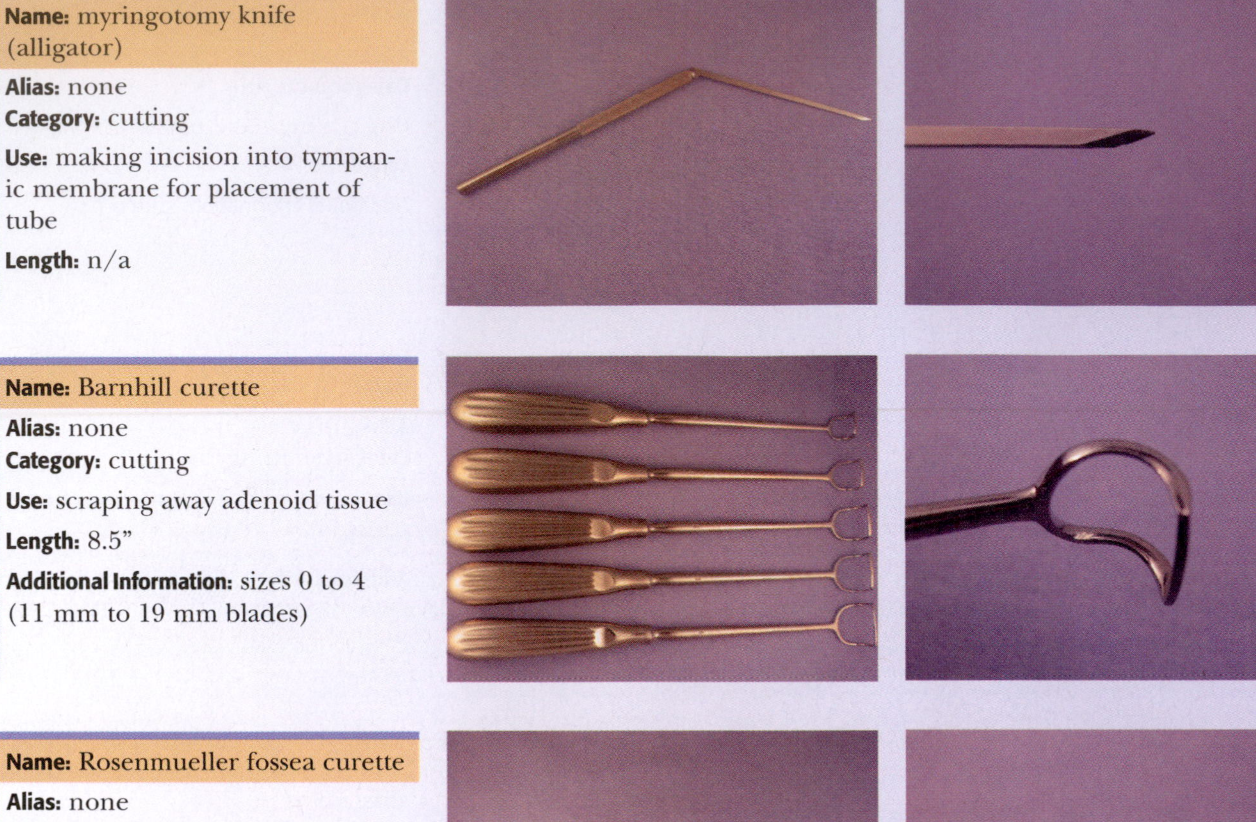

Name: Barnhill curette

Alias: none

Category: cutting

Use: scraping away adenoid tissue

Length: 8.5"

Additional Information: sizes 0 to 4 (11 mm to 19 mm blades)

Name: Rosenmueller fossea curette

Alias: none

Category: cutting

Use: removing adenoid tissue

Length: 9"

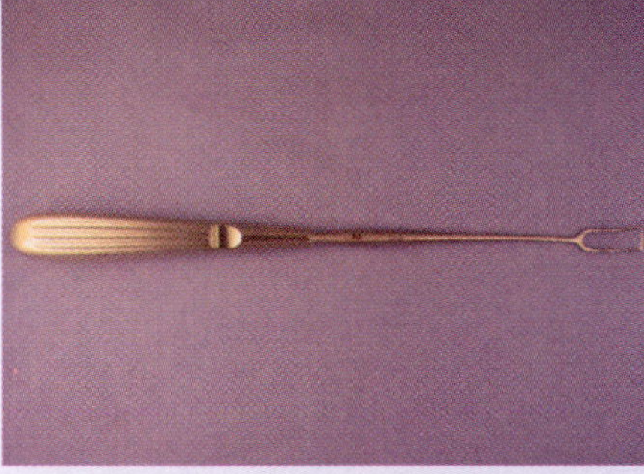

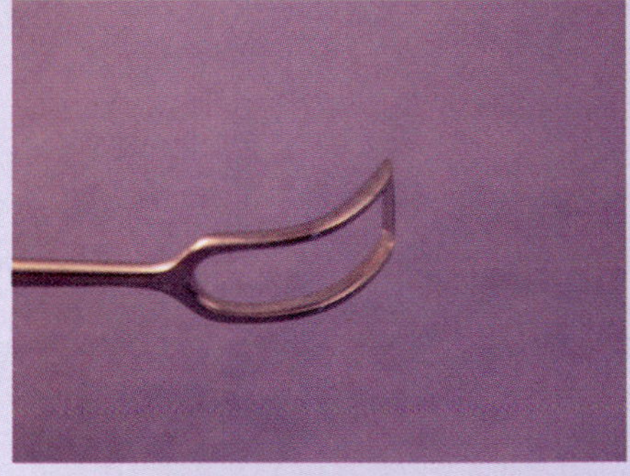

Name: Key elevator

Alias: Periosteal elevator

Category: cutting

Use: scraping periosteum from bone

Length: 6.5"

Additional Information: blade widths 3 mm to 2.5 cm; single ended; curved or straight

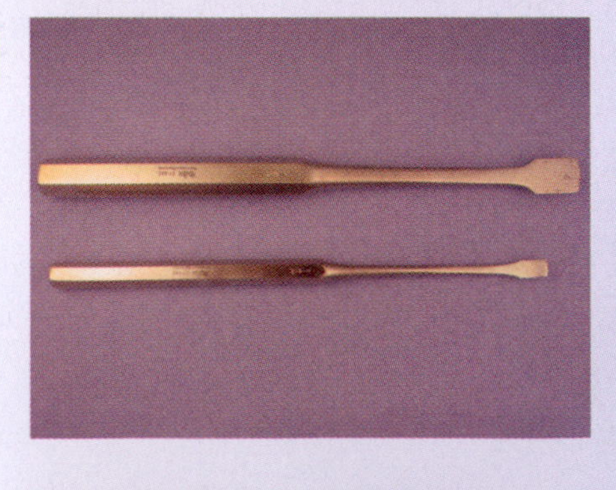

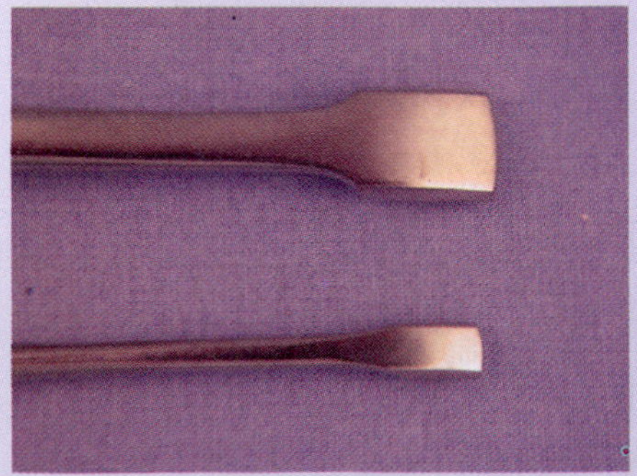

Name: Freer elevator

Alias: none

Category: cutting

Use: elevating the septum

Length: 8"

Additional Information: double ended

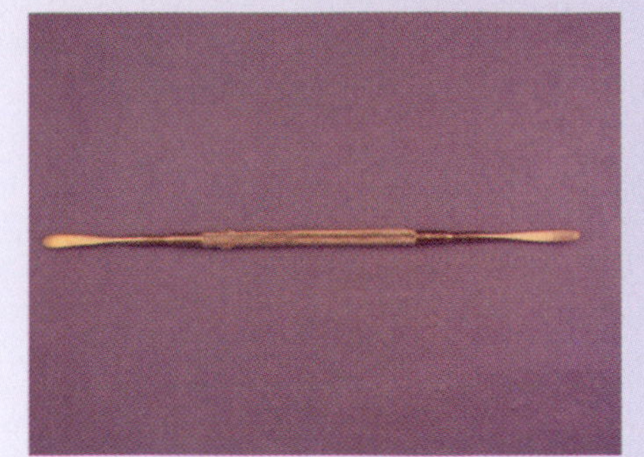

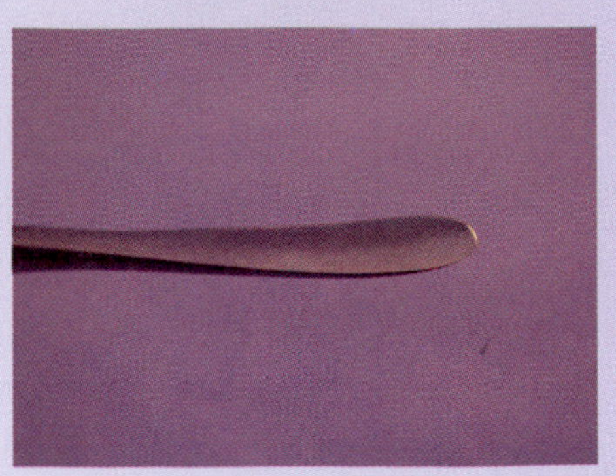

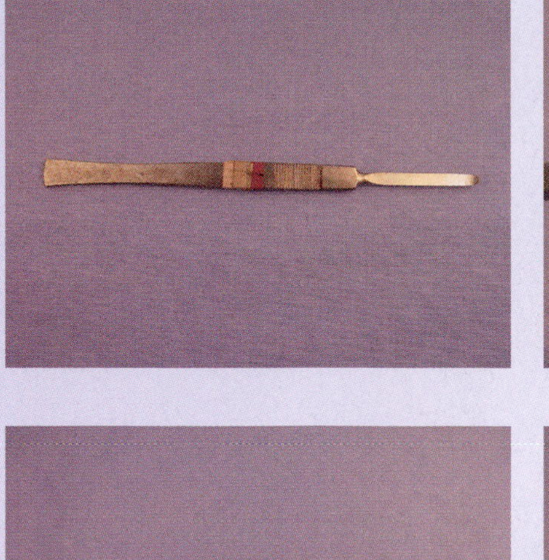

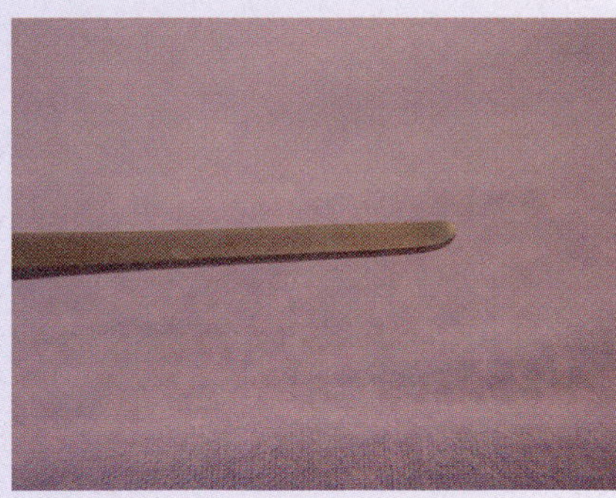

Name: MacKenty septum elevator

Alias: none

Category: cutting

Use: elevating periosteum from nasal bone

Length: 5.75"

Additional Information: flat, curved blade

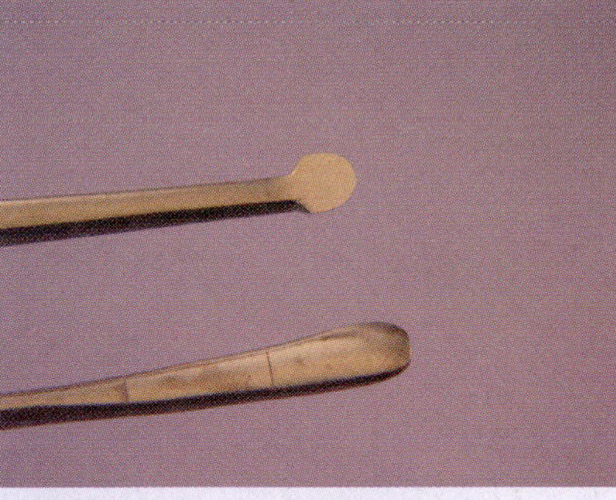

Name: Cottle elevator-feeler

Alias: none

Category: cutting

Use: measuring depth; elevating periosteum from septal bone

Length: 9"

Additional Information: double ended; graduated in centimeters

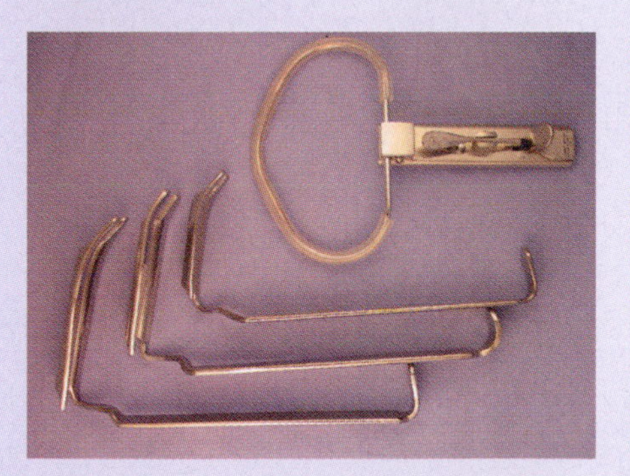

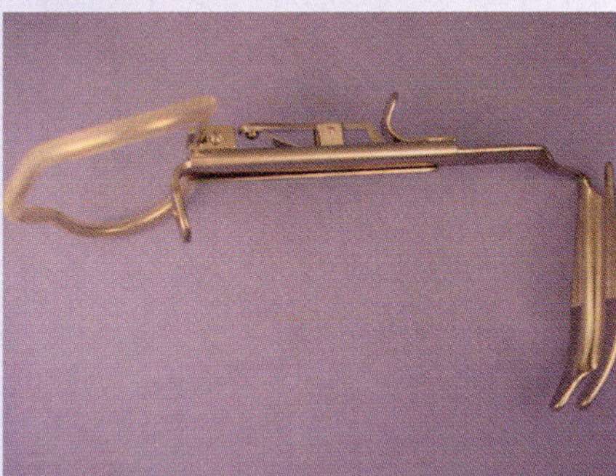

Name: Mc Ivor mouth gag

Alias: none

Category: retracting

Use: keeping mouth open during surgery

Length: n/a

Additional Information: blade width 2.5" to 4"

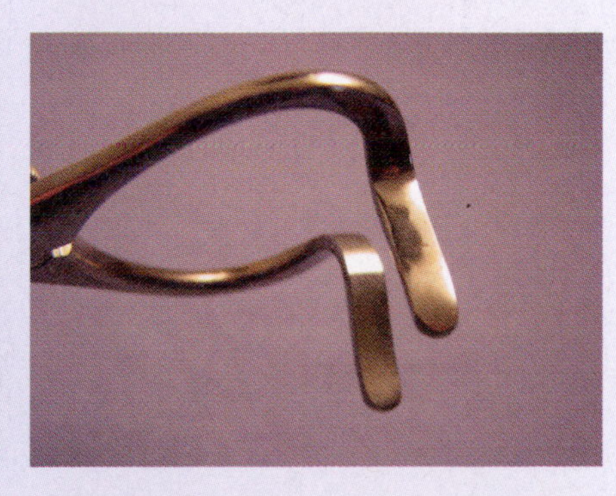

Name: Sludder-Jansen mouth gag

Alias: none

Category: retracting

Use: retracting walls of mouth

Length: 5"

Additional Information: self-retaining; arms curved to fit the face

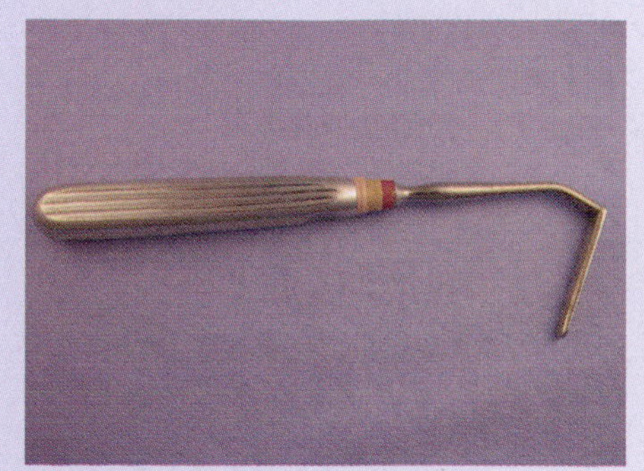

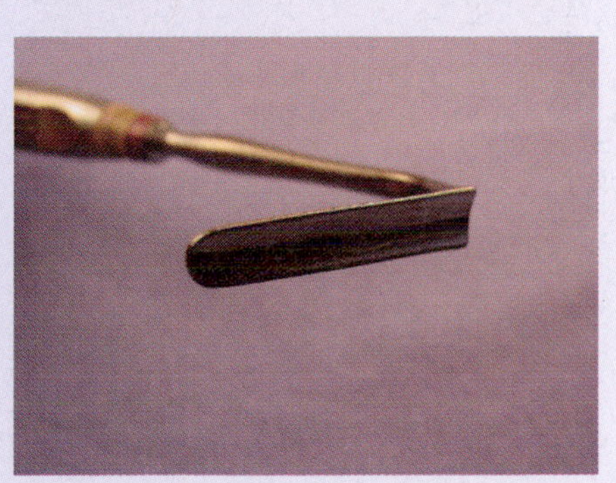

Name: Aufricht nasal retractor-speculum

Alias: none

Category: retracting

Use: retracting nasal walls; visualizing nasal passage

Length: 7.5"

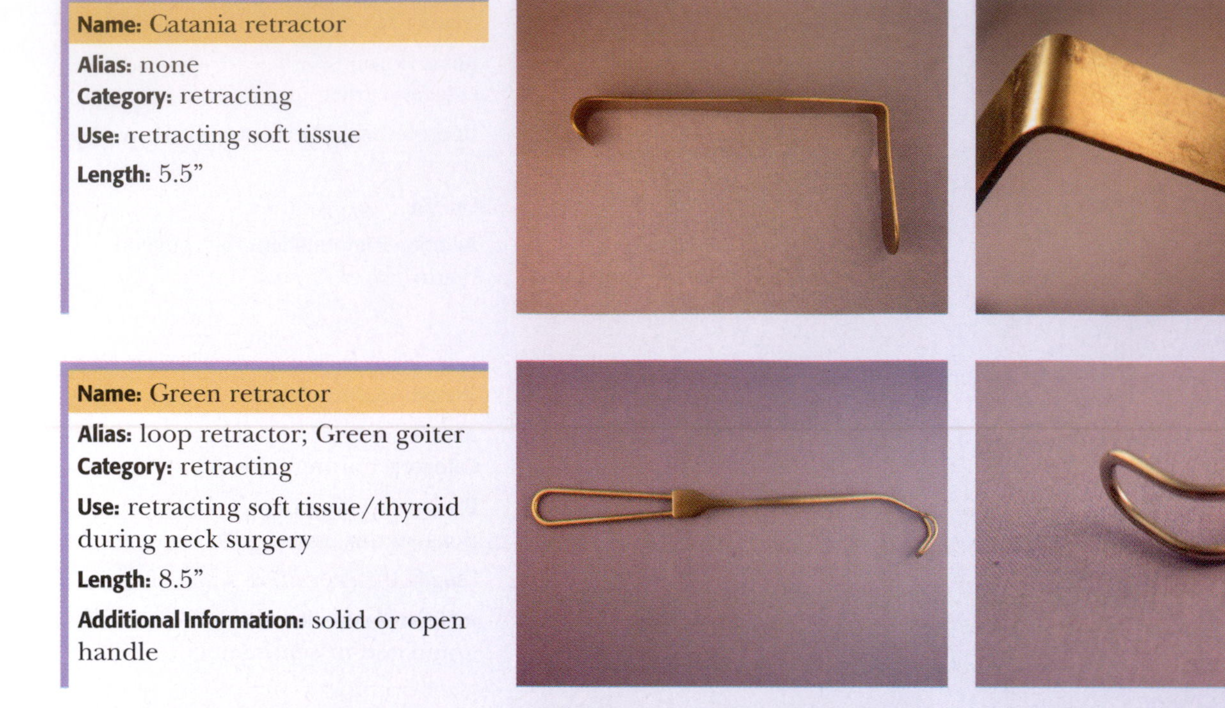

Name: Catania retractor
Alias: none
Category: retracting
Use: retracting soft tissue
Length: 5.5"

Name: Green retractor
Alias: loop retractor; Green goiter
Category: retracting
Use: retracting soft tissue/thyroid during neck surgery
Length: 8.5"
Additional Information: solid or open handle

Name: Jansen retractor
Alias: Gifford; Allport; mastoid
Category: retracting
Use: retracting mastoid or scalp
Length: 4" or 4.5"
Additional Information: blunt; 3 × 3 or 4 × 4 prongs; self-retaining

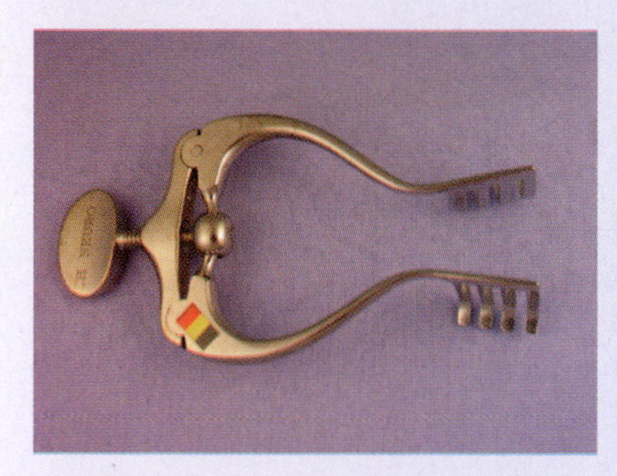

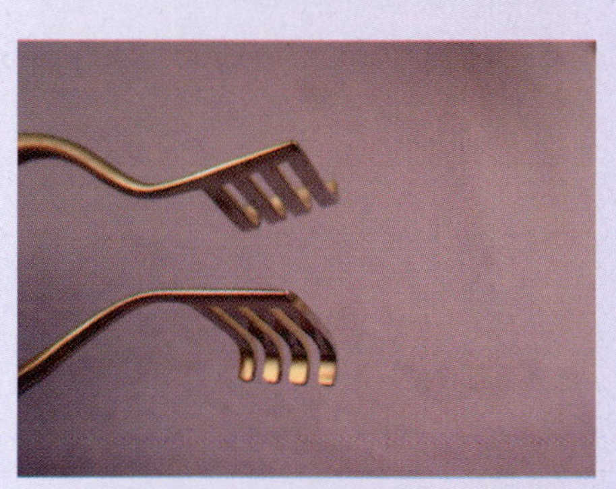

Name: Love nasopharyngeal retractor
Alias: none
Category: retracting
Use: retracting soft tissue in nasopharyngeal area
Length: n/a
Additional Information: blade width comes in sizes from 18 to 25 mm

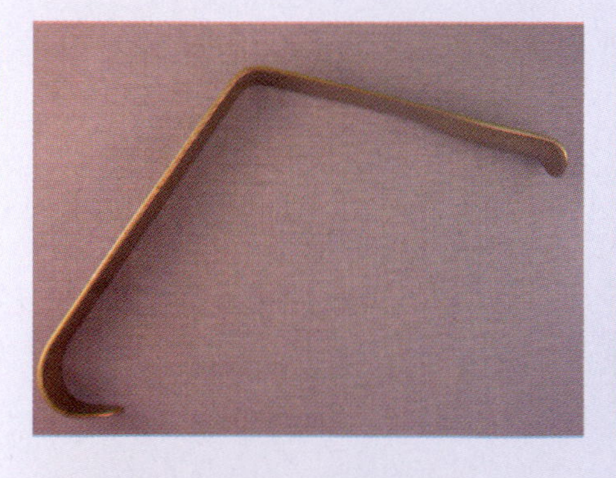

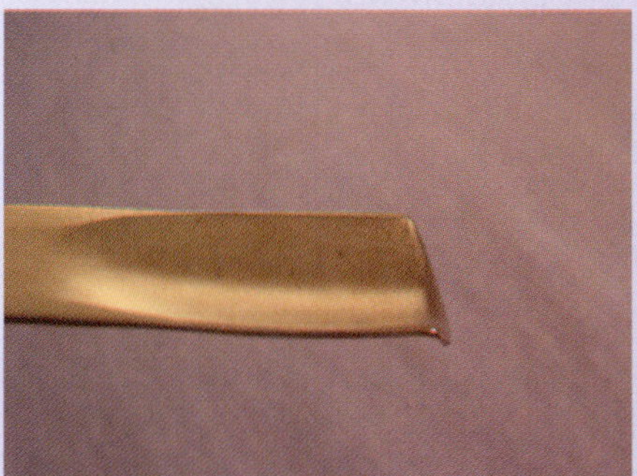

Name: Love-Gruenwald forcep
Alias: none
Category: cutting
Use: cutting and removing small bits of nasal bone
Length: 5"
Additional Information: cup-style jaw; jaw can be 2 mm × 10 mm or 3 mm × 10 mm

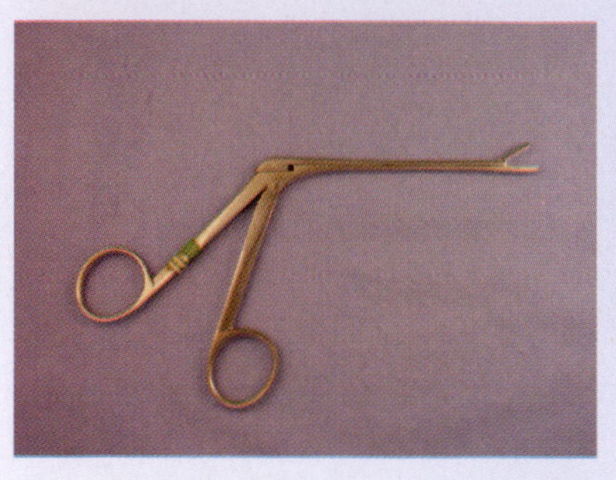

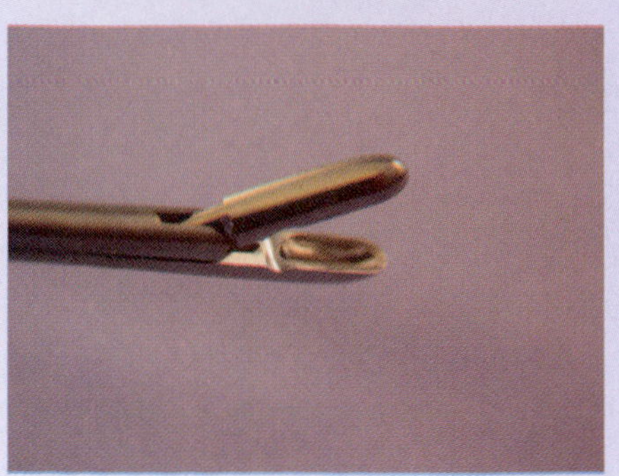

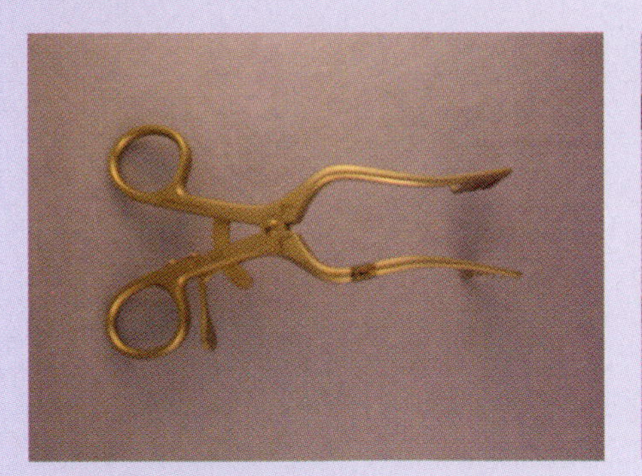
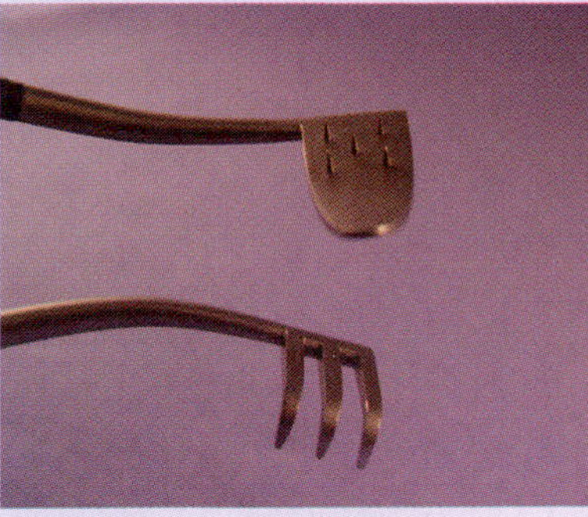

Name: mastoid retractor
Alias: none
Category: retracting
Use: retracting mastoid tissue
Length: n/a
Additional Information: 3 prong and blade jaws

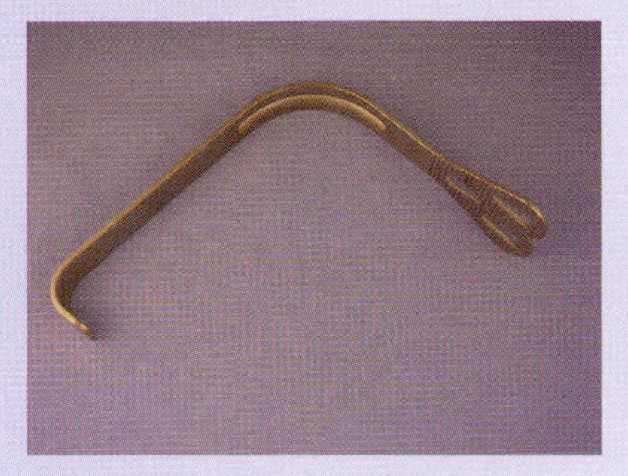
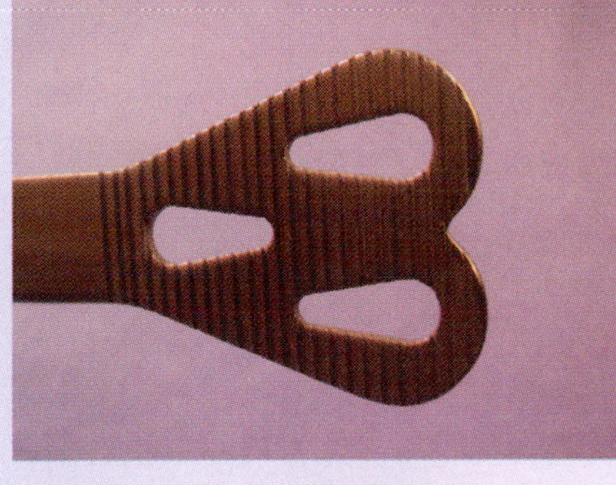

Name: Weder tongue blade
Alias: none
Category: retracting tongue downward
Length: n/a
Additional Information: small (2.8-cm wide) or large (3.5-cm wide) sizes

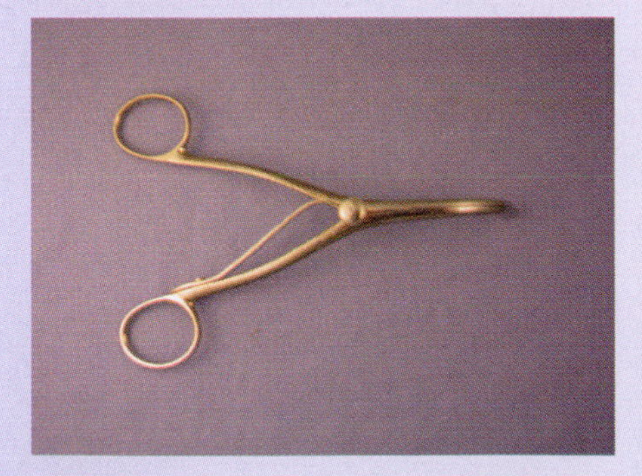
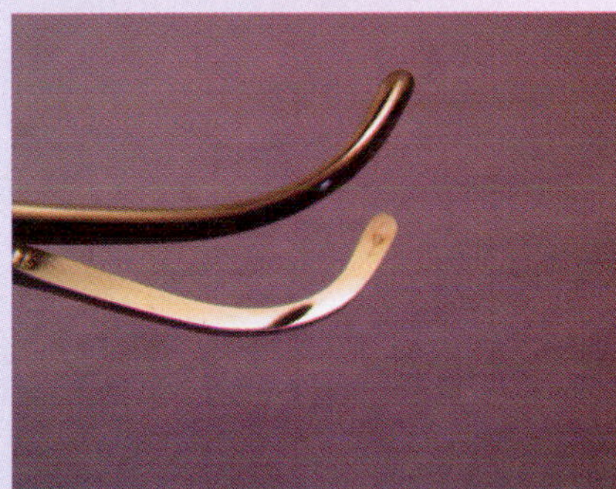

Name: Trousseau tracheal dilator
Alias: none
Category: dilating
Use: dilating tracheal stoma
Length: 5.5"
Additional Information: jaw width can be 3 mm or 6 mm

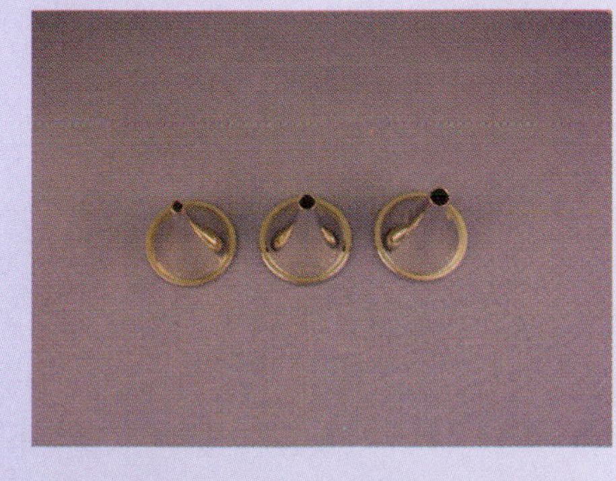
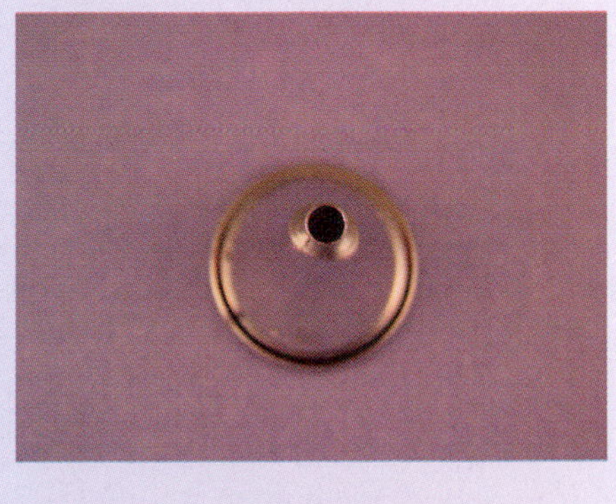

Name: Boucheron ear speculum
Alias: none
Category: accessory
Use: allow visualizing of ear canal
Length: n/a
Additional Information: comes in 8 sizes

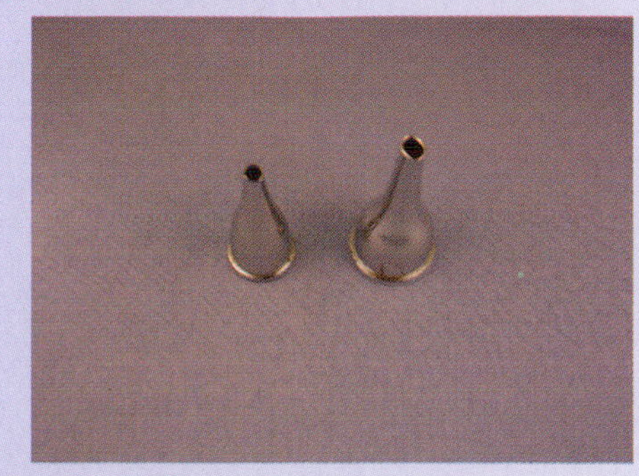
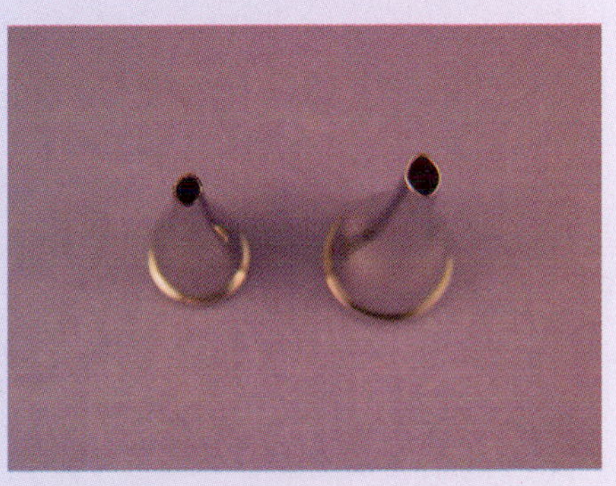

Name: Gruber ear speculum
Alias: none
Category: accessory
Use: allow visualizing of ear canal
Length: n/a
Additional Information: comes in 8 sizes

Name: microscope handle covers

Alias: none

Category: accessory

Use: placing on microscope handles to allow surgeon to manipulate the microscope:

Length: n/a

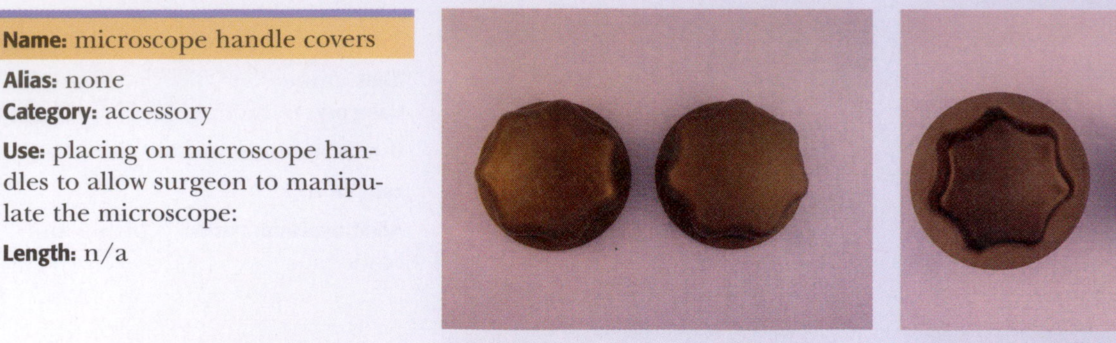

Name: Cottle narrow speculum

Alias: none

Category: retracting

Use: retracting nasal walls to allow visualization of nasal passage

Length: 5.75"

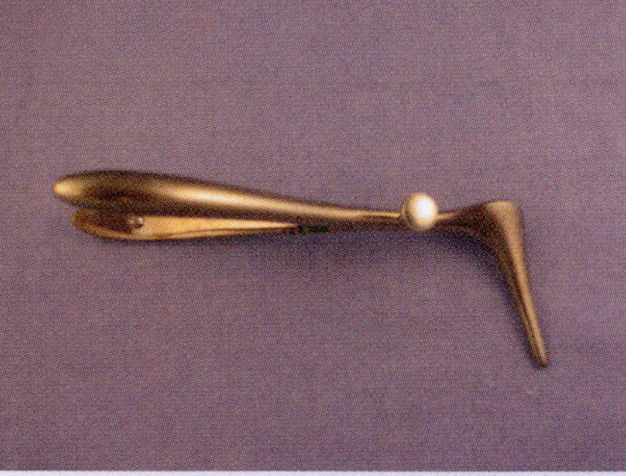

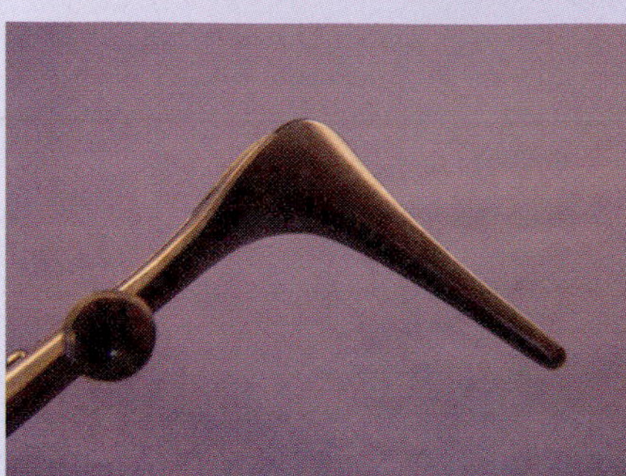

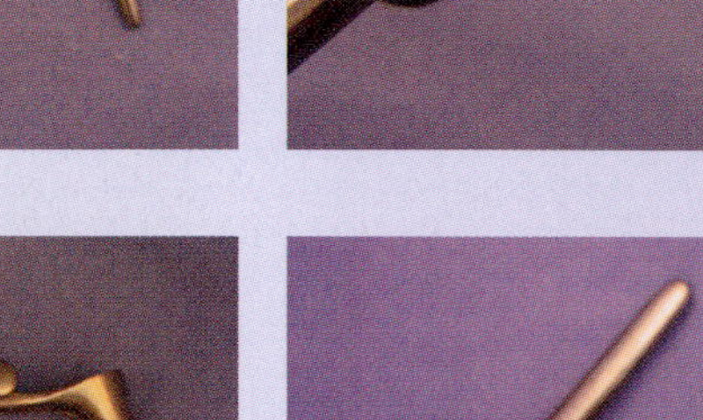

Name: Cottle nasal speculum

Alias: none

Category: retracting

Use: retracting of nasal walls to allow visualization of nasal passage

Length: 5.25"

Additional Information: blades come in short, medium, long, and extra-long lengths; blade width tapers

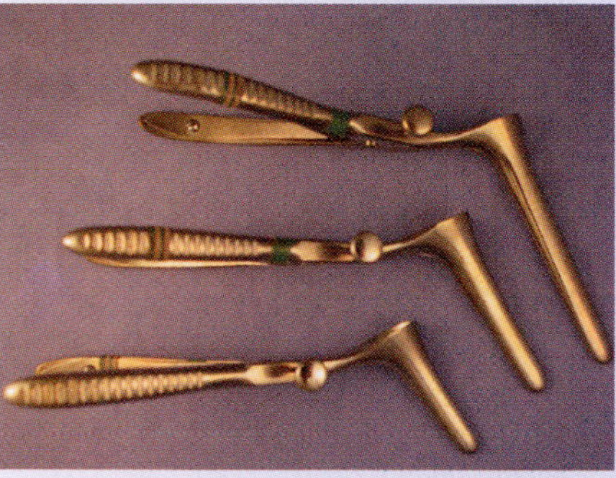

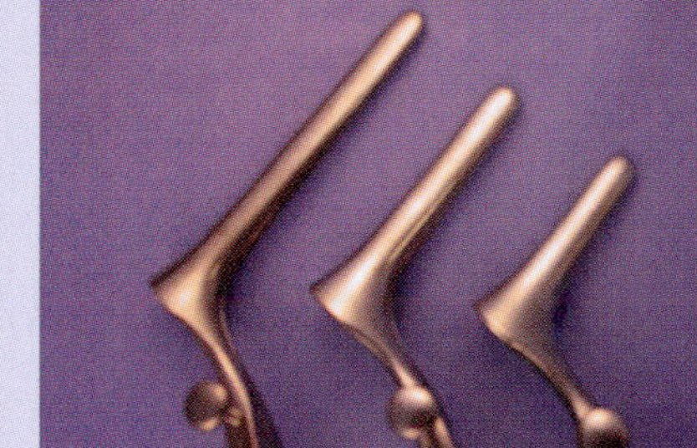

Name: Vienna nasal speculum

Alias: none

Category: retracting

Use: retracting of nasal walls to allow visualization of nasal passage

Length: 5.5"

Additional Information: blades can be small (9.5 mm × 27 mm), medium (11 mm × 30 mm) or large (13 mm × 32 mm)

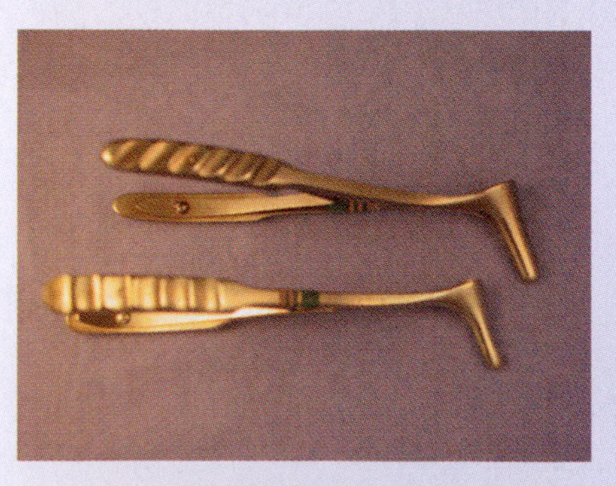

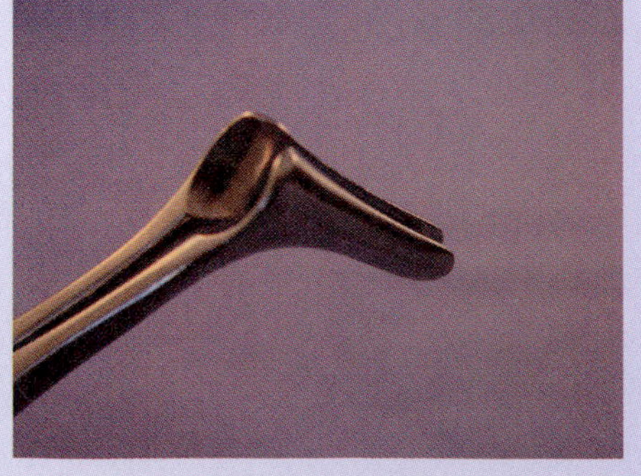

Name: Cushing bayonet forceps

Alias: none

Category: grasping

Use: grasping tissue or inserting packing into nose or ears

Length: 7"

Additional Information: serrated tips or 1 × 2 teeth

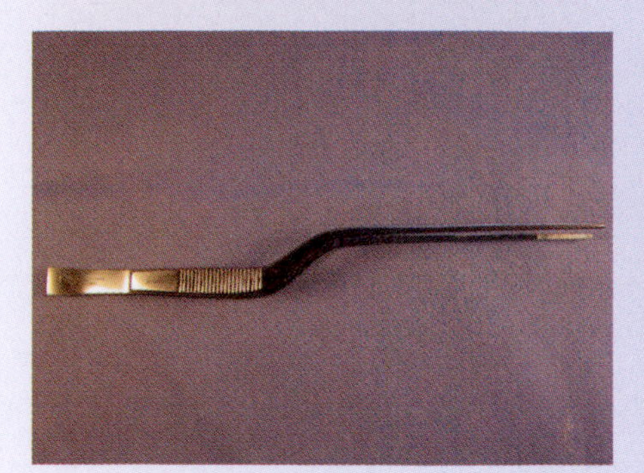

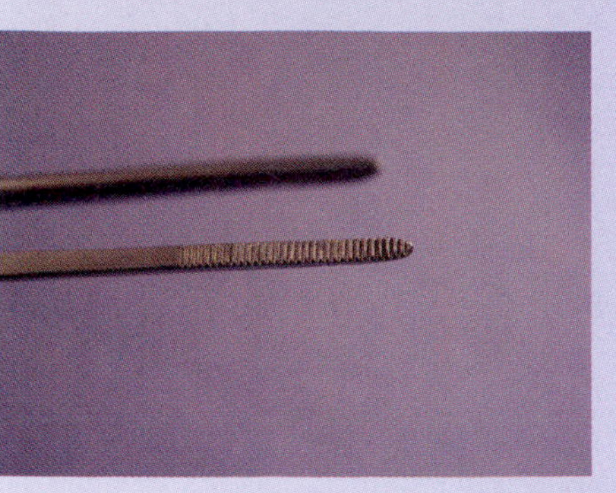

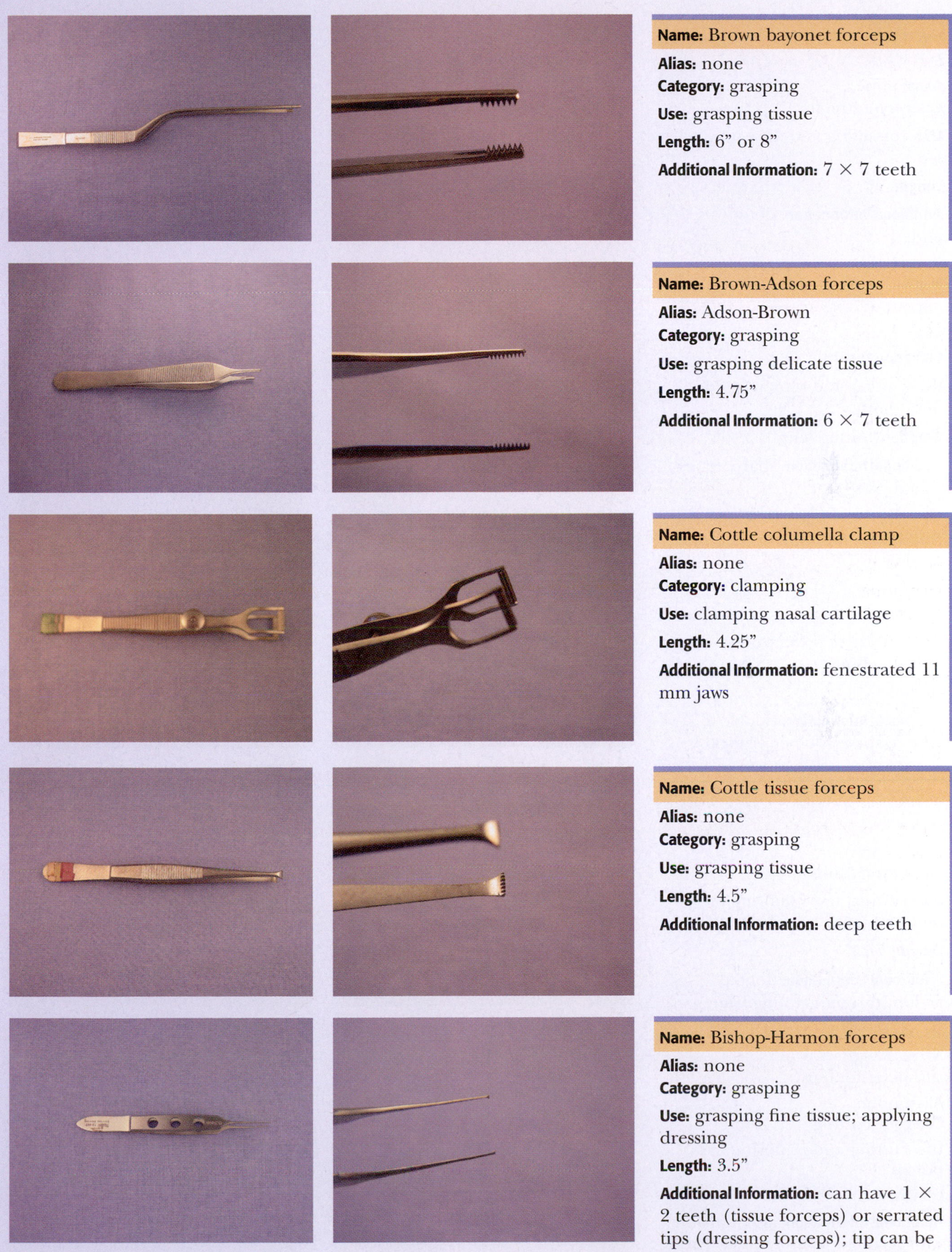

Name: Brown bayonet forceps
Alias: none
Category: grasping
Use: grasping tissue
Length: 6" or 8"
Additional Information: 7 × 7 teeth

Name: Brown-Adson forceps
Alias: Adson-Brown
Category: grasping
Use: grasping delicate tissue
Length: 4.75"
Additional Information: 6 × 7 teeth

Name: Cottle columella clamp
Alias: none
Category: clamping
Use: clamping nasal cartilage
Length: 4.25"
Additional Information: fenestrated 11 mm jaws

Name: Cottle tissue forceps
Alias: none
Category: grasping
Use: grasping tissue
Length: 4.5"
Additional Information: deep teeth

Name: Bishop-Harmon forceps
Alias: none
Category: grasping
Use: grasping fine tissue; applying dressing
Length: 3.5"
Additional Information: can have 1 × 2 teeth (tissue forceps) or serrated tips (dressing forceps); tip can be delicate (0.3 mm) or standard (0.5 mm)

Name: Hurd dissector and pillar retractor

Alias: none

Category: retractor

Use: retracting and dissecting pillae

Length: 9"

Additional Information: double ended

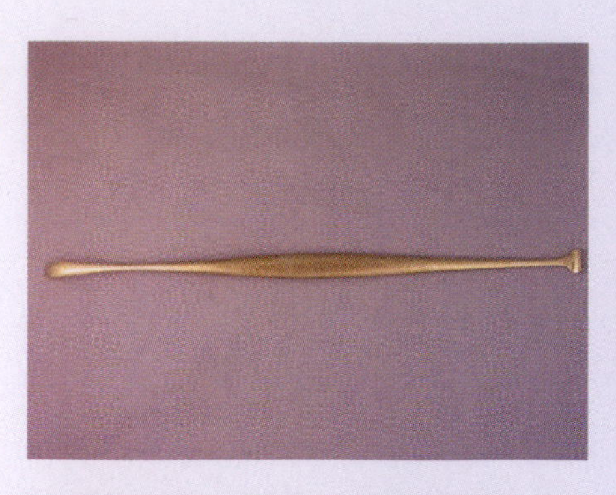

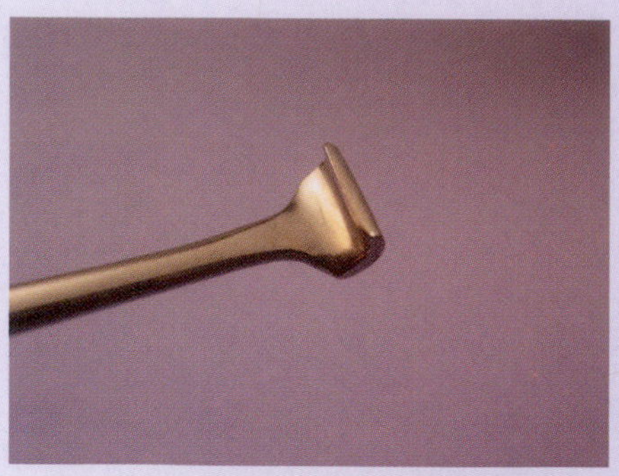

Name: Bruening ethmoid exenteration forceps

Alias: none

Category: cutting

Use: cutting and removing ethmoid bone

Length: working length 2"

Additional Information: sharp, fenestrated jaws

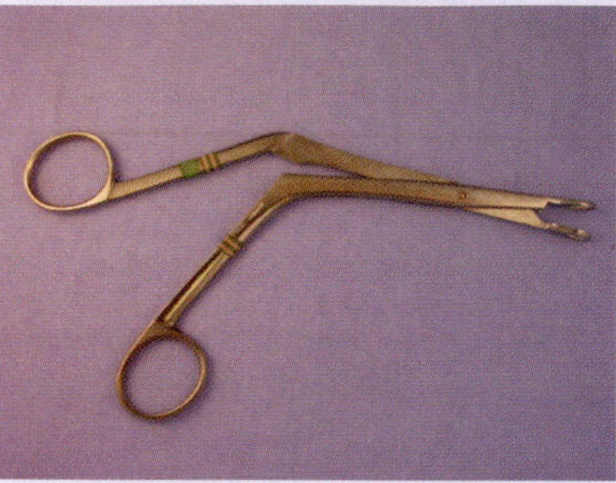

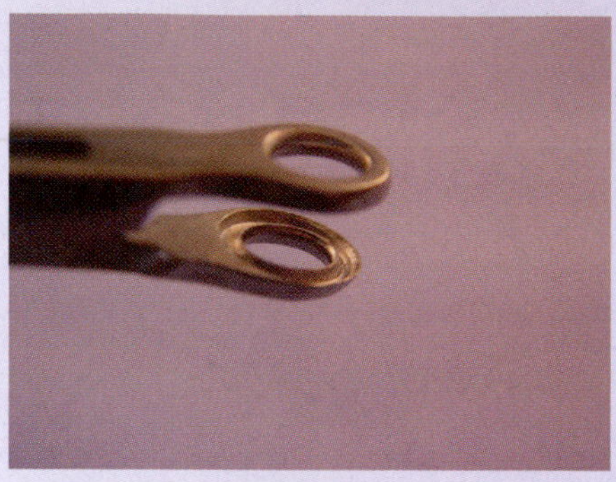

Name: Jansen-Middleton septum forceps

Alias: none

Category: cutting

Use: cutting and removing pieces of septal bone

Length: 8"

Additional Information: double action; spoon-shaped blades

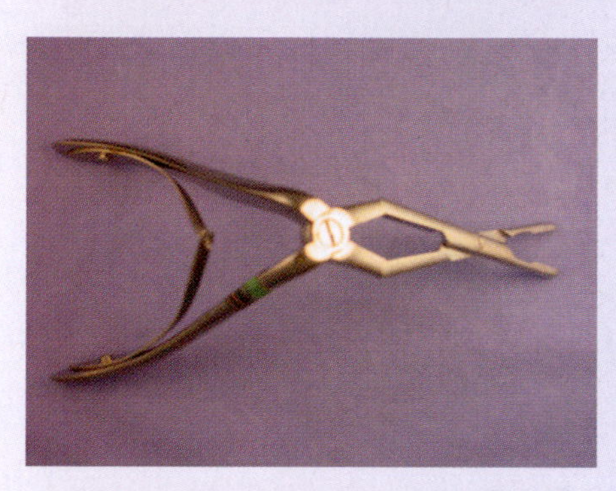

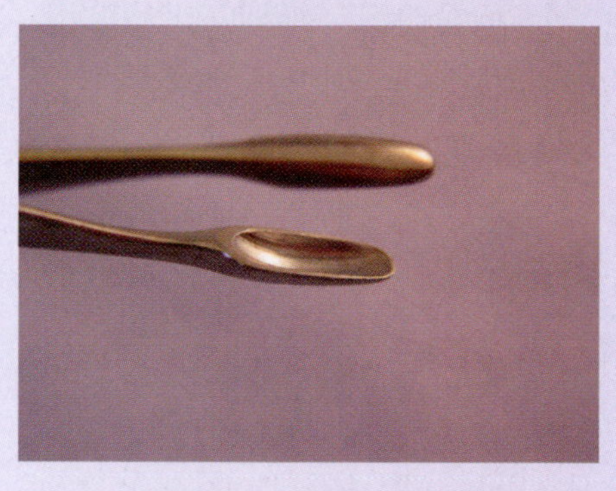

Name: Jansen-Struycken septum forceps

Alias: none

Category: cutting

Use: cutting and removing pieces of septal bone

Length: 7.75"

Additional Information: double action; through-cutting blades

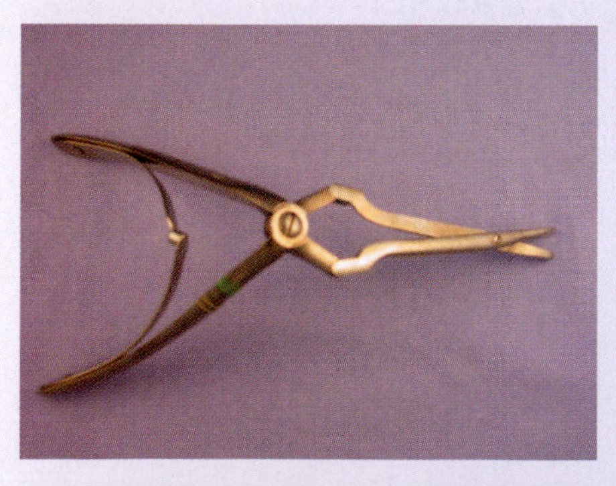

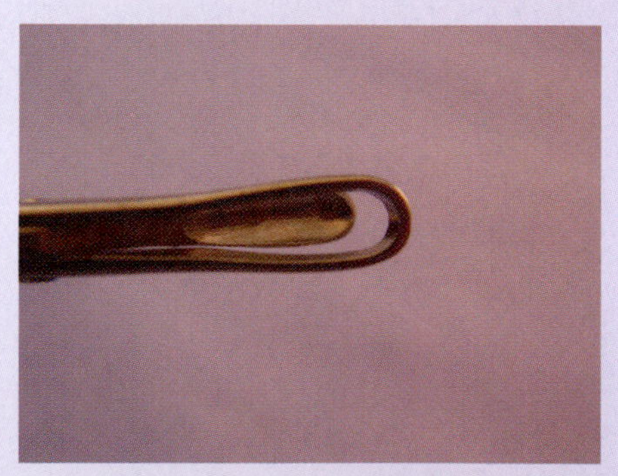

Name: Knight polypus and turbinate forceps

Alias: none

Category: cutting

Use: cutting and removing nasal polyps

Length: 6.75"

Additional Information: also available with serrated jaws; serrated style can be used as nasal dressing forceps

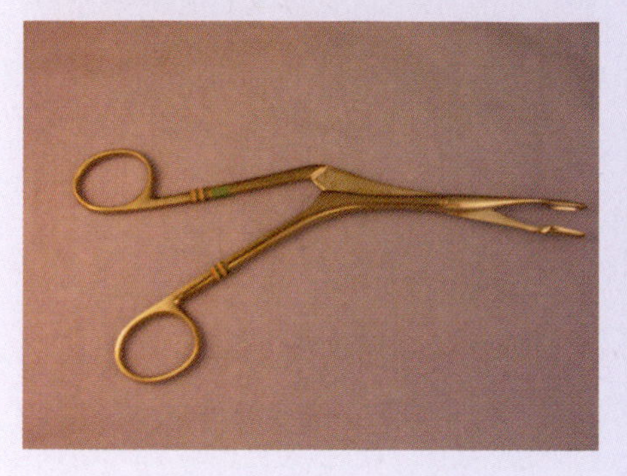

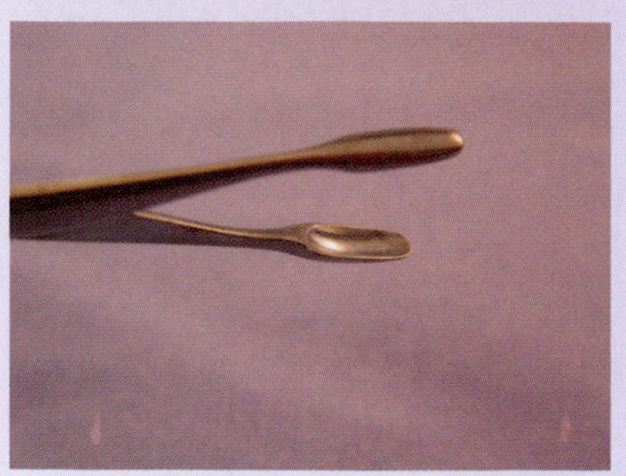

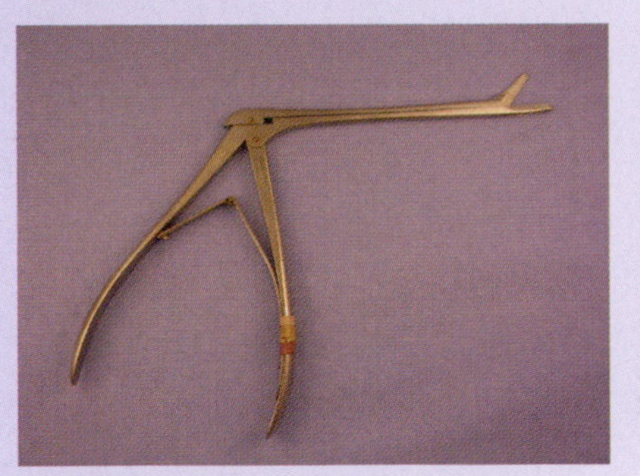
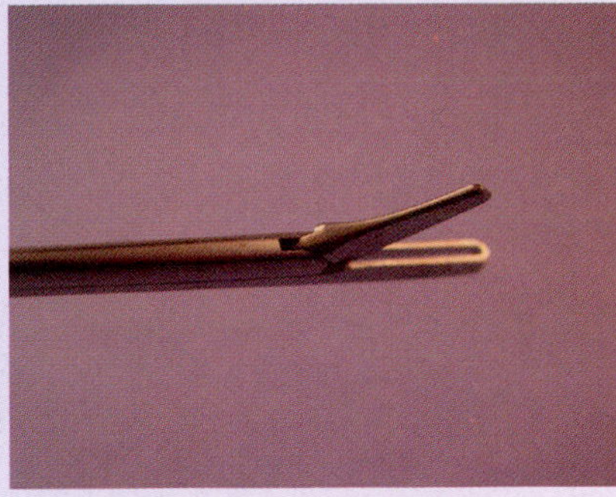

Name: Takahashi nasal punch
Alias: none
Category: cutting
Use: removing small bits of nasal tissue
Length: working length 5.5”
Additional Information: 2-mm wide bite

Name: Schmeden tonsil punch
Alias: none
Category: cutting
Use: cutting small pieces of tonsil tissue
Length: working length 5.5”
Additional Information: triangular jaws

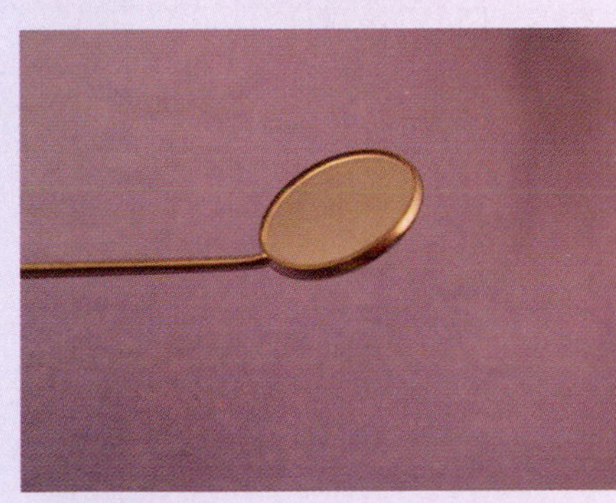

Name: laryngeal mirror
Alias: dental mirror
Category: accessory
Use: visualizing mouth or larynx
Length:
Additional Information: sizes 1 to 6 (mirror diameters range 14 mm to 24 mm)

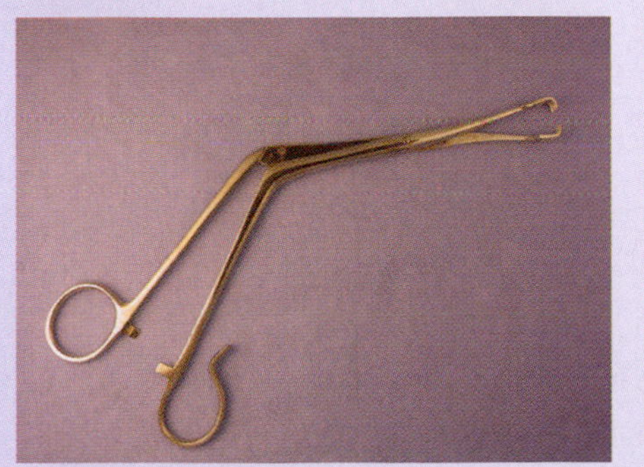
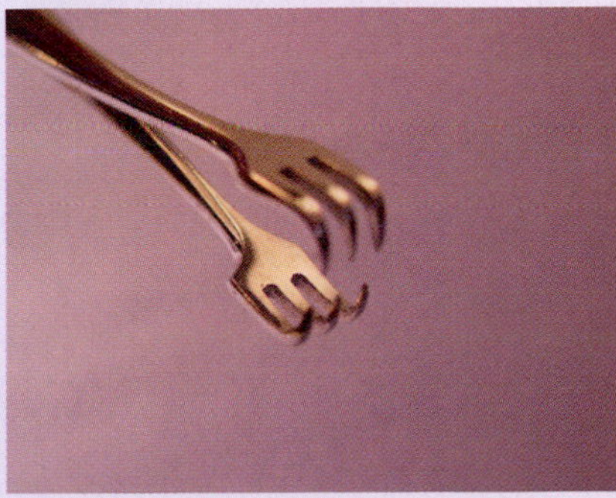

Name: Tivnen tonsil-seizing forceps
Alias: none
Category: grasping
Use: grasping tonsils for removal
Length: 8.5”
Additional Information: jaws have 3 × 3 prongs

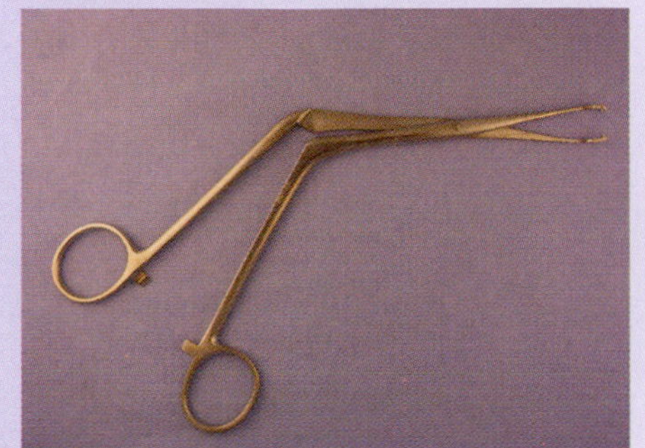
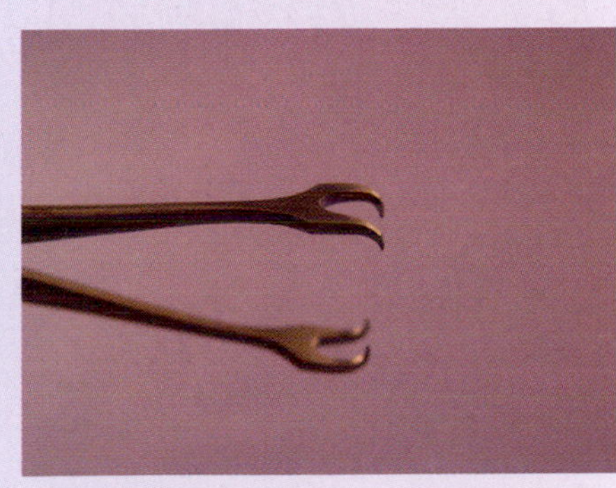

Name: Tydings tonsil-seizing forceps
Alias: none
Category: grasping
Use: removing tonsil
Length: 7.25”
Additional Information: two-prong jaws

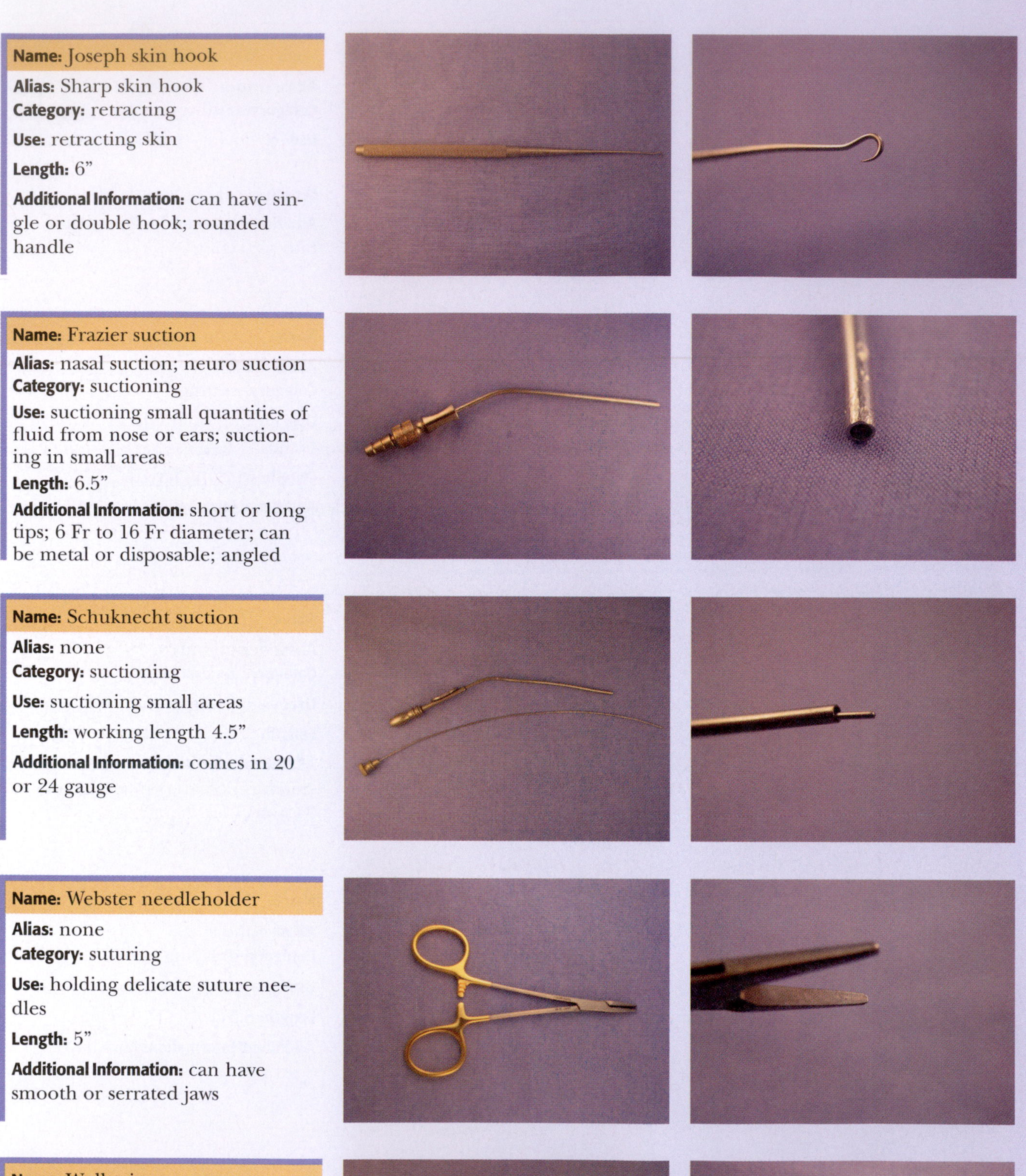

Name: Joseph skin hook
Alias: Sharp skin hook
Category: retracting
Use: retracting skin
Length: 6"
Additional Information: can have single or double hook; rounded handle

Name: Frazier suction
Alias: nasal suction; neuro suction
Category: suctioning
Use: suctioning small quantities of fluid from nose or ears; suctioning in small areas
Length: 6.5"
Additional Information: short or long tips; 6 Fr to 16 Fr diameter; can be metal or disposable; angled

Name: Schuknecht suction
Alias: none
Category: suctioning
Use: suctioning small areas
Length: working length 4.5"
Additional Information: comes in 20 or 24 gauge

Name: Webster needleholder
Alias: none
Category: suturing
Use: holding delicate suture needles
Length: 5"
Additional Information: can have smooth or serrated jaws

Name: Wullstein ear currette
Alias: none
Category: accessory
Use: removing wax or foreign bodies from ear
Length: 5.75"
Additional Information: ring tip diameter 1.3 mm to 2.3 mm

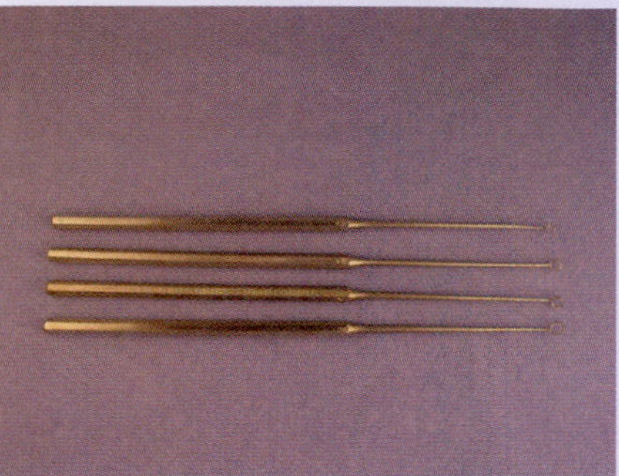

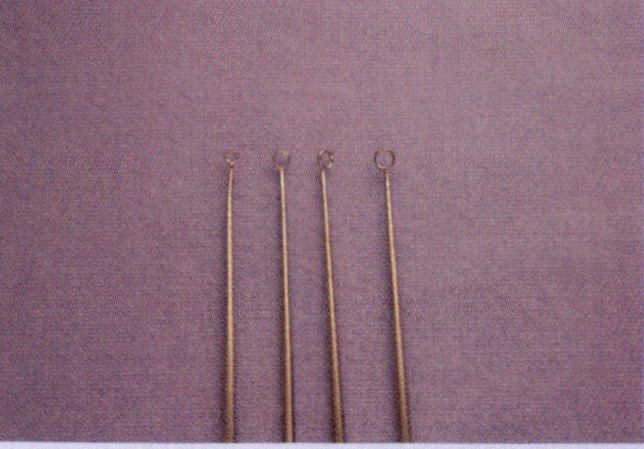

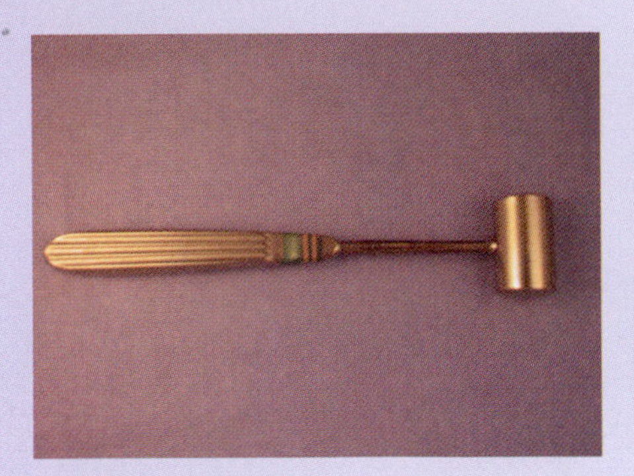
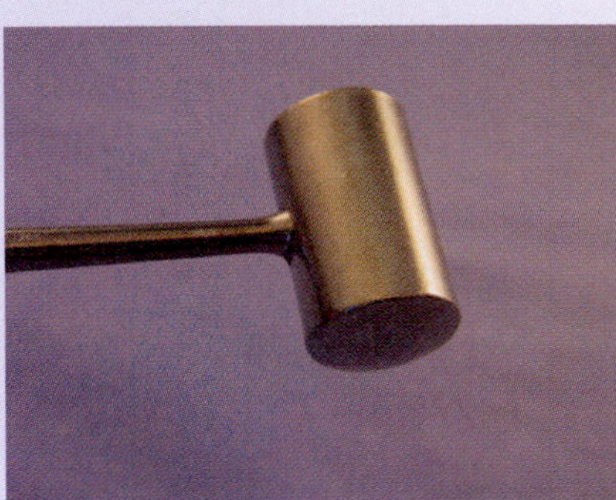

Name: Cottle mallet

Alias: none

Category: accessory

Use: exerting force on an object (such as an osteotome or chisel)

Length: 7.5"

Additional Information: flat face is used with chisels or osteotomes; round face is used with Cottle bone crusher to prepare cartilage implant material

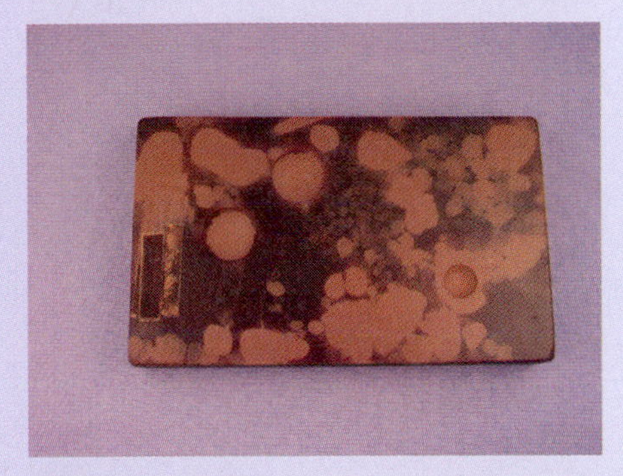

Name: Cartilage cutting board

Alias: Teflon block

Category: accessory

Use: providing a flat, hard surface to reshape cartilage or grafts

Length: 3" × 5"

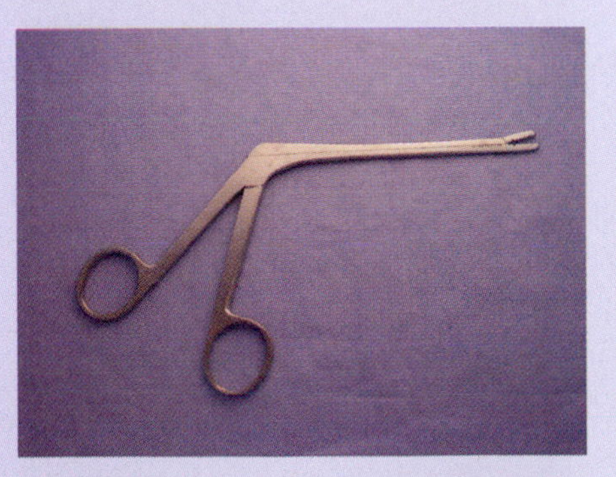

Name: Takahashi

Alias: pituitary forceps

Category: cutting

Use: removing small tissue fragments and polyps

Length: 5"

Additional Information: comes in 2 mm or 3 mm bite size

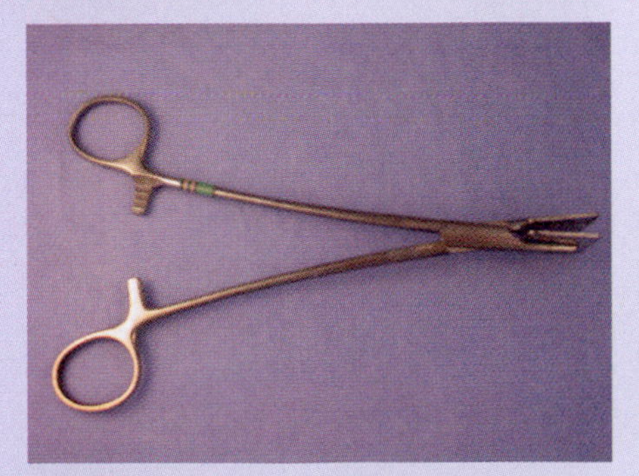
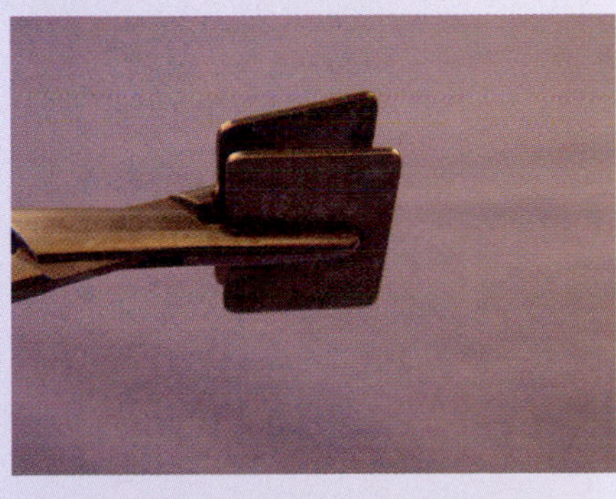

Name: House gelfoam pressure forceps

Alias: none

Category: clamping

Use: compressing gelfoam; thinning fascia grafts

Length: 6"

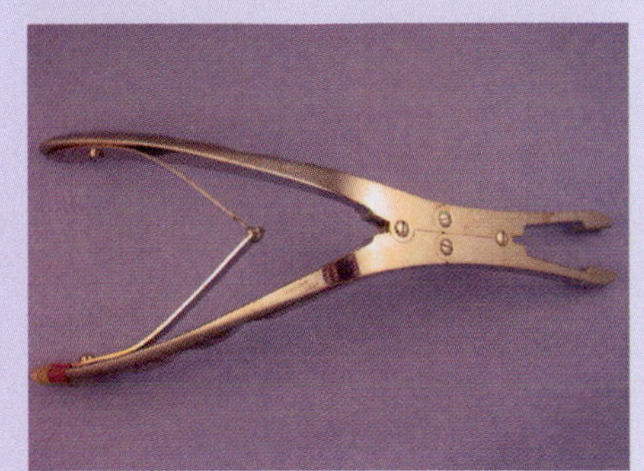
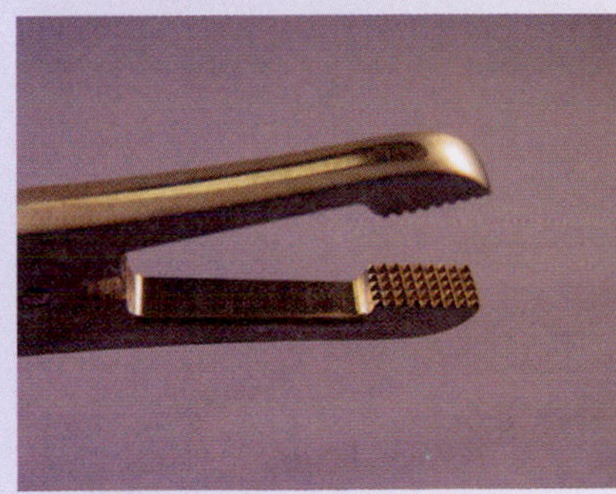

Name: Rubin morselizer

Alias: none

Category: cutting

Use: crushing nasal cartilage, enabling repositioning of the septum to midline

Length: 10"

Additional Information: jaws 15 mm × 5.5 mm

Name: Hajek septum chisel

Alias: none

Category: cutting

Use: chiseling away pieces of nasal bone

Length: 6"

Additional Information: v-shaped cutting blade; blade can be 4 mm, 6 mm, or 8 mm wide

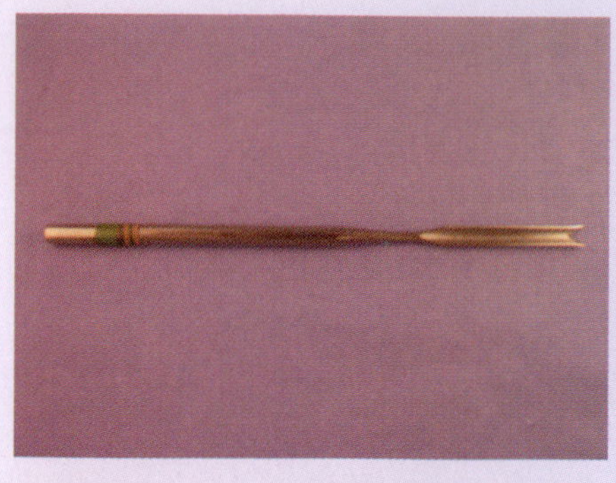

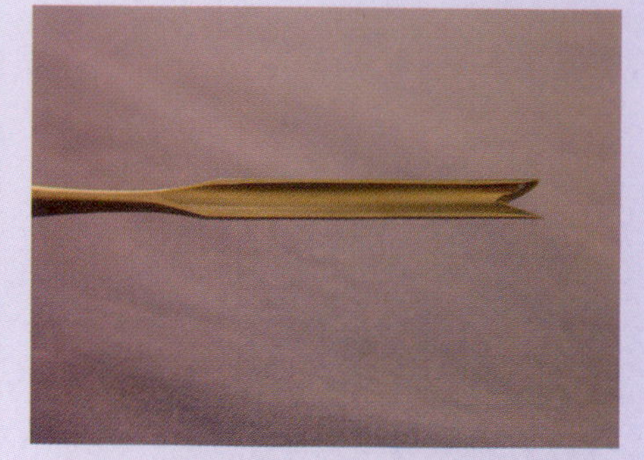

Name: Latrobe soft palate retractor

Alias: none

Category: retracting

Use: retracting soft palate

Length: working length 5.5"

Additional Information: open handle

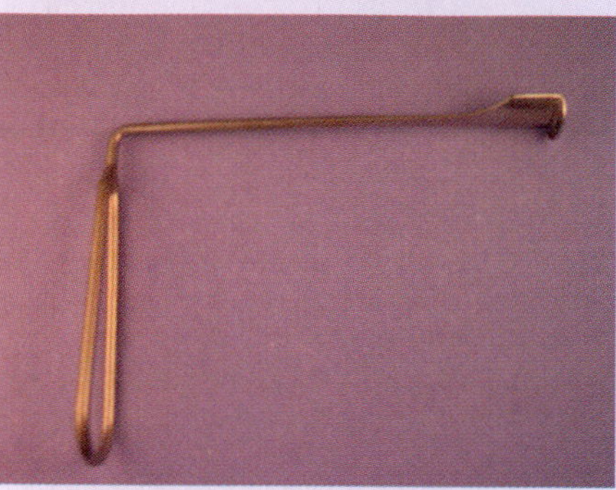

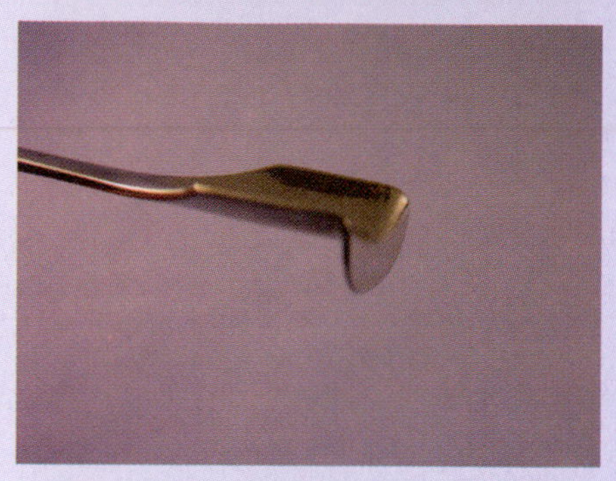

Name: Skeeter drill

Alias: none

Category: accessory

Use: drilling in small places (mastoid, ear)

Length: n/a

Additional Information: bits come in a variety of point diameters

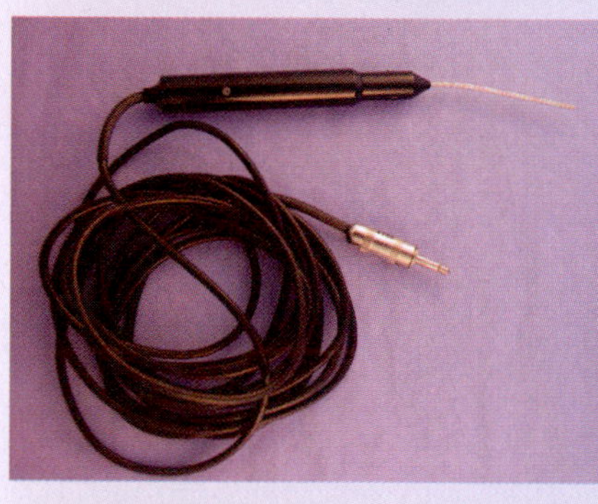

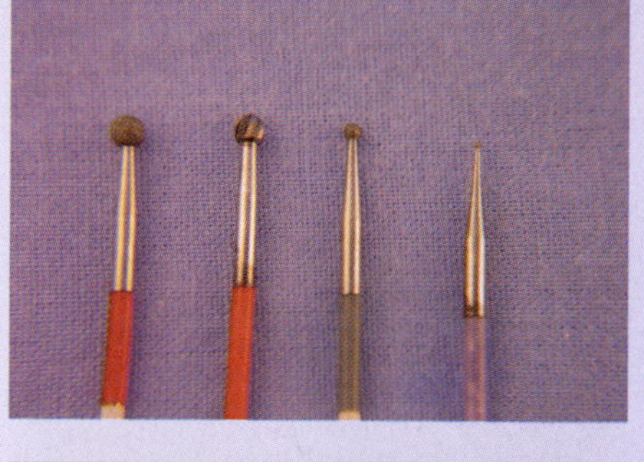

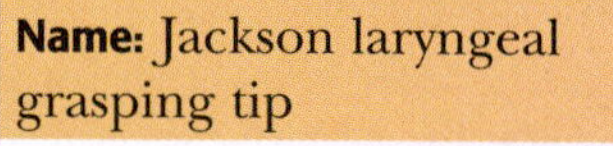

Name: Jackson laryngeal grasping tip

Alias: none

Category: grasping

Use: grasping heavy laryngeal tissue during laryngoscopy

Length: working length varies

Additional Information: toothed

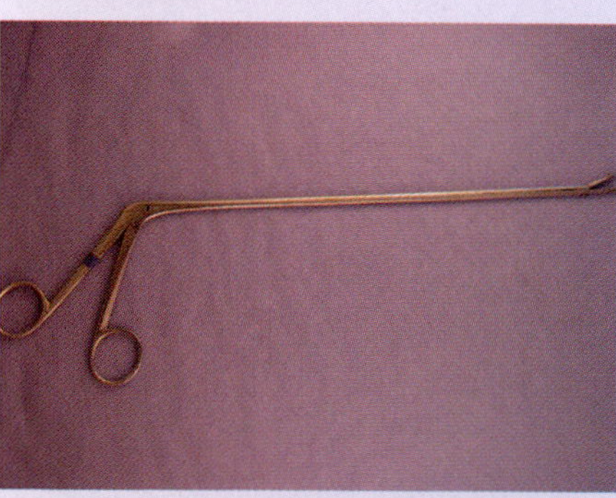

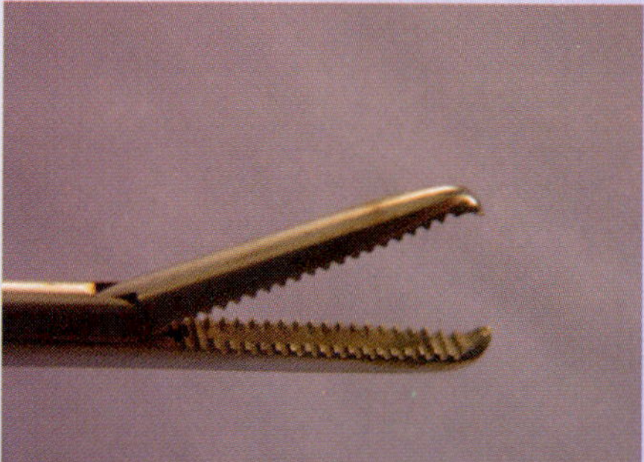

Name: Jako microlaryngeal grasping forceps

Alias: none

Category: grasping

Use: grasping very delicate or small pieces of tissue during layngoscopy

Length: working length 9.5"

Additional Information: jaws can be straight, angled left, or angled right

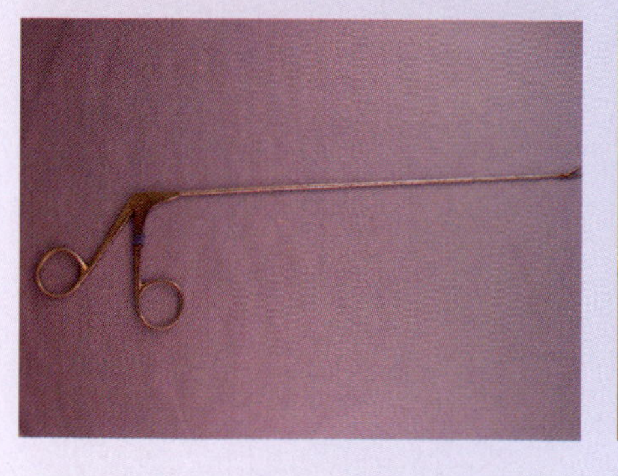

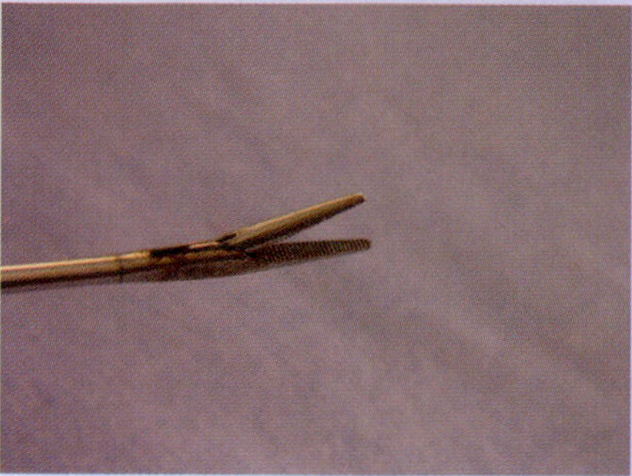

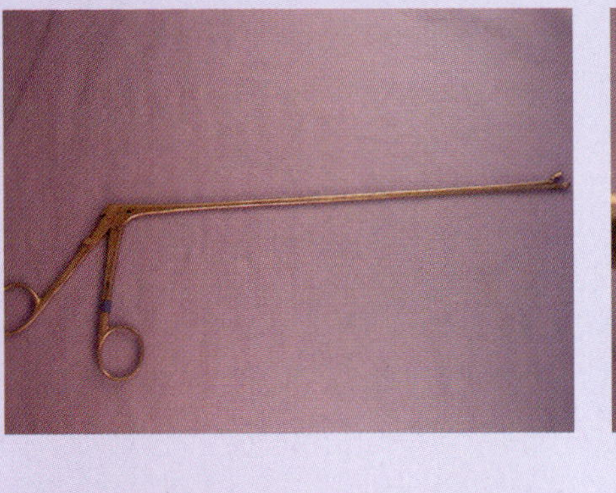

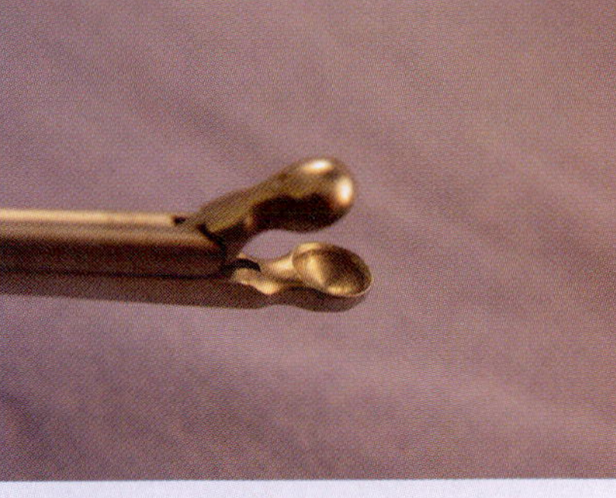

Name: cup forceps

Alias: none

Category: cutting

Use: removing small bits of tissue (sometimes for biopsy)

Length: varies

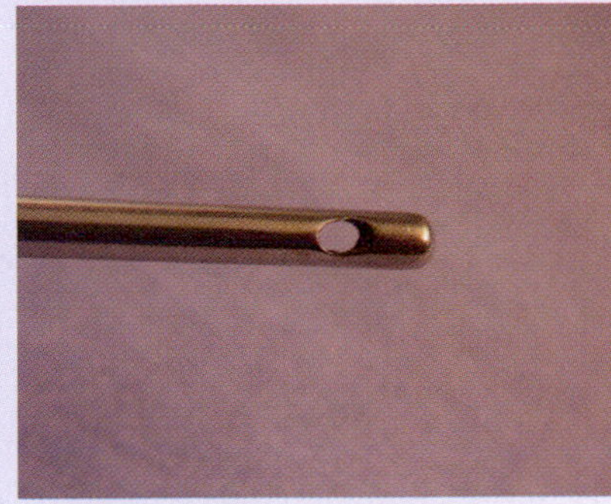

Name: Jackson velvet eye aspirating tube

Alias: none

Category: suctioning

Use: suctioning the larynx during laryngoscopy

Length: comes in 10" to 26" lengths

Additional Information: 4 mm diameter

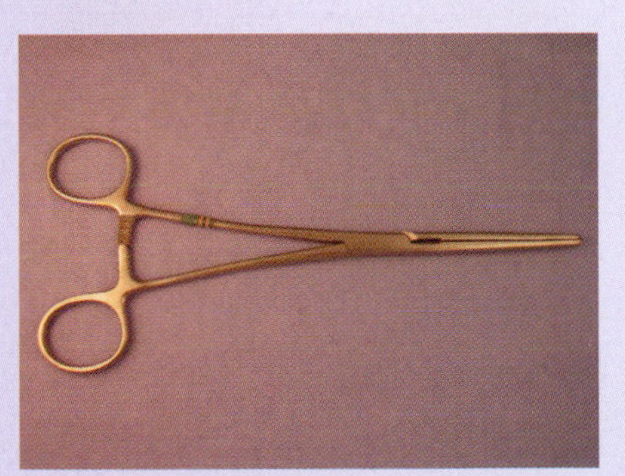

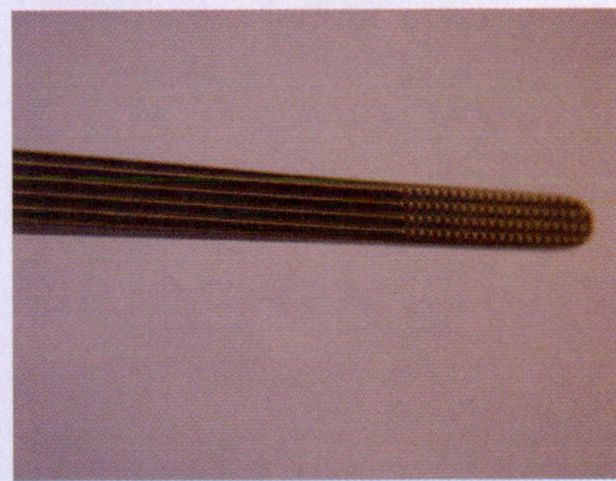

Name: Carmalt artery forcep

Alias: none

Category: clamping

Use: clamping tissue or blood vessels

Length: 6.5" or 8"

Additional Information: jaws can be straight or curved

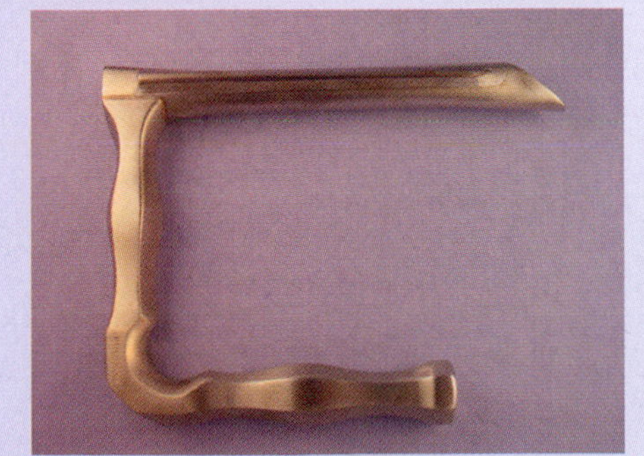

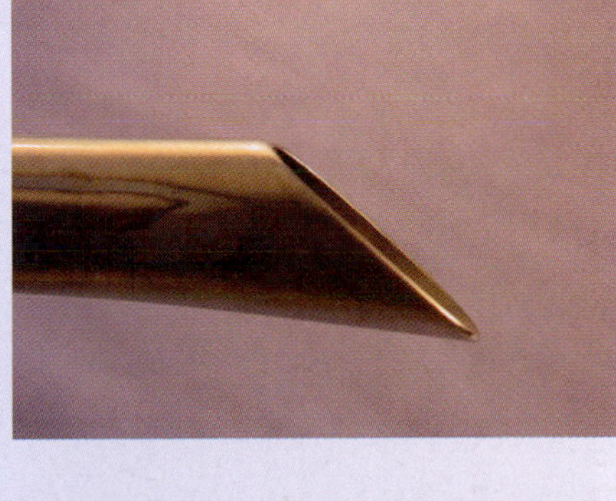

Name: rigid laryngoscope

Alias: none

Category: accessory

Use: viewing of the adult larynx to look for masses or tumors

Length: n/a

Additional Information: this is one example of a rigid laryngoscope

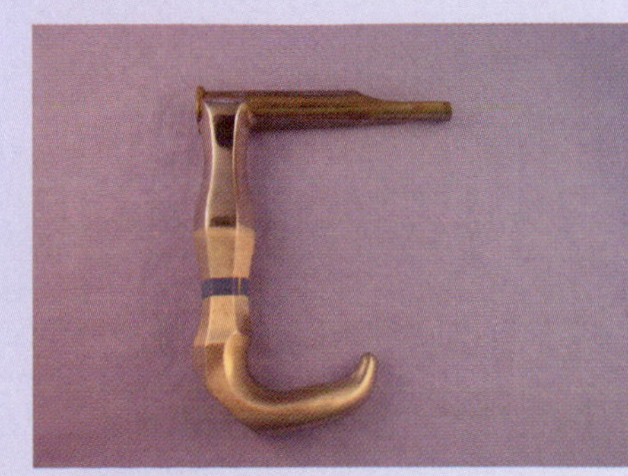

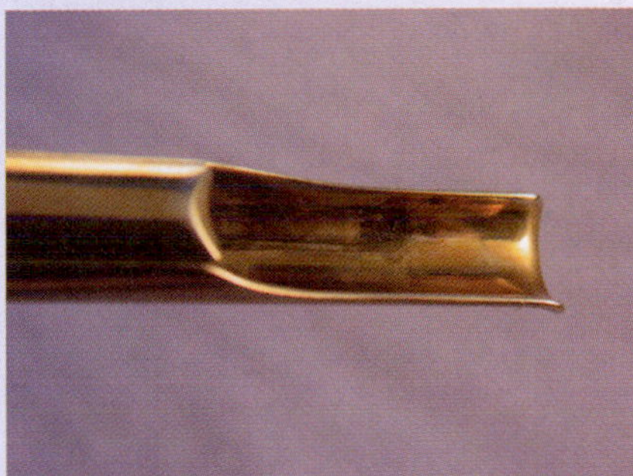

Name: rigid pediatric laryngoscope

Alias: none

Category: accessory

Use: viewing of the pediatric larynx to look for masses or tumors

Length: n/a

Additional Information: this is one example of a rigid laryngoscope

Name: Takahashi nasal forceps

Alias: none

Category: cutting

Use: removal of small pieces of tissue or bone

Length: 5" shaft

Additional Information: 2 to 4 mm wide bite

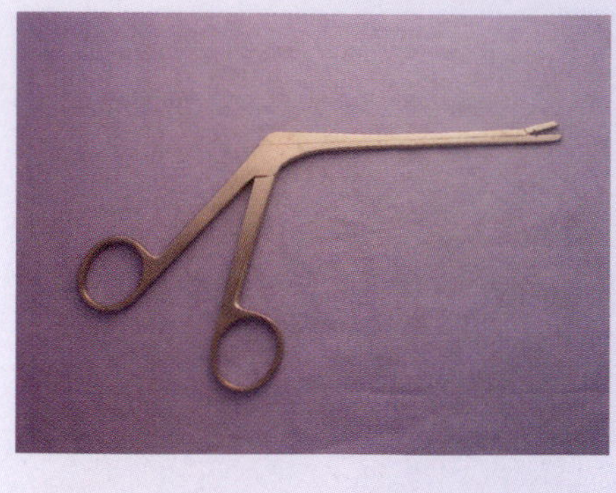

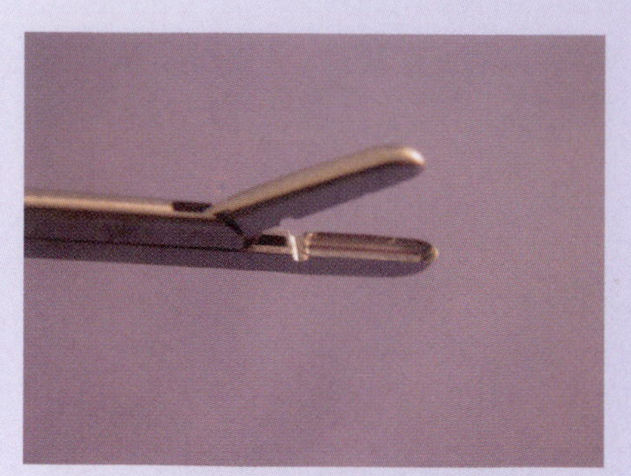

Name: Tydings tonsil snare

Alias: snare

Category: grasping

Use: grasping and removal of tonsil tissue

Length: n/a

Additional Information: wire is replaceable

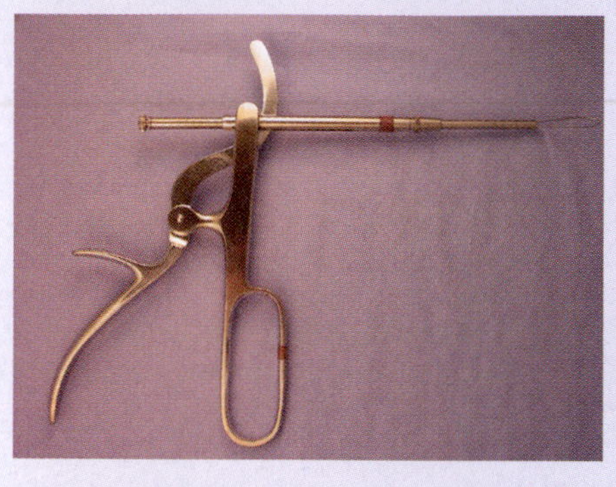

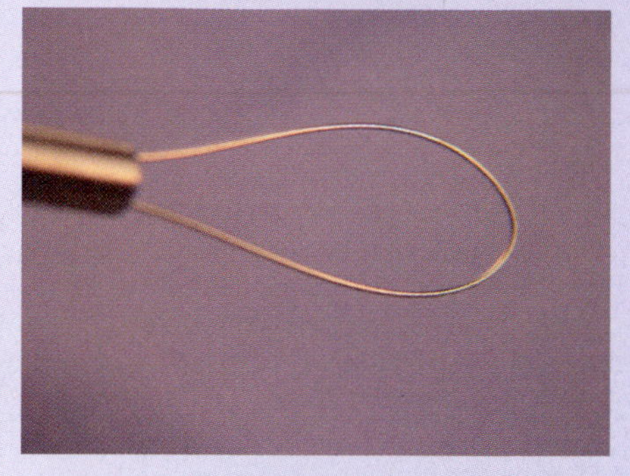

Name: Walsham septal straightener

Alias: none

Category: accessory

Use: straightening the septal cartilage during nasal surgery

Length: 9"

Additional Information: come available for left- or right-sided use

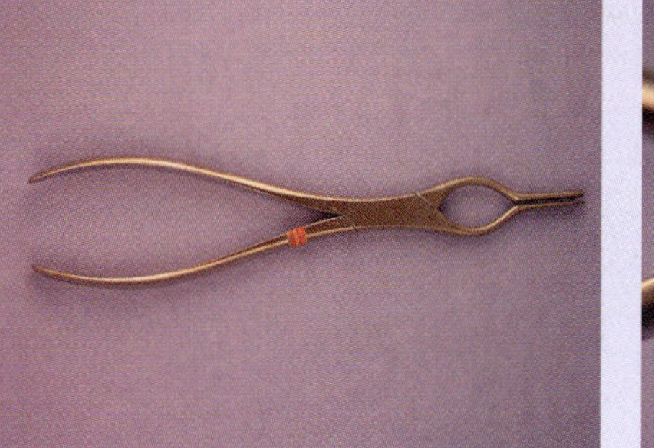

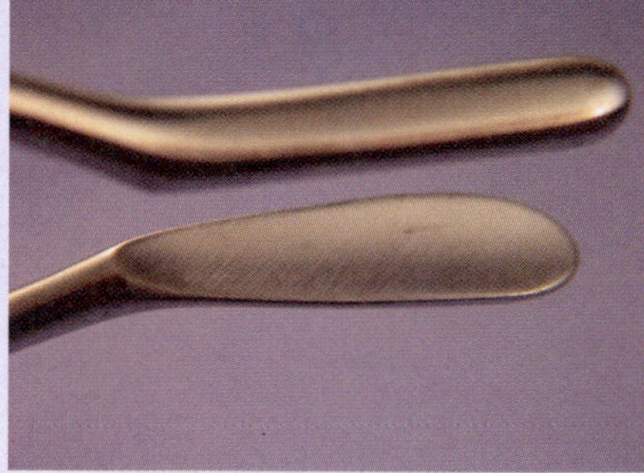

Q&A

Surgical Session—Ear, Nose, and Throat Instruments

1) Before performing a septoplasty, the surgeon needs to remove the preoperative packing and visualize the nasal passage. You would hand him/her bayonet forceps and a:
   a. Vienna nasal speculum
   b. Freer/elevator
   c. Cottle nasal knife
   d. Cottle angular scissors
2) Which of the following could be used to remove wax or foreign bodies from the ear?
   a. Knight
   b. Wullstein
   c. Weder
   d. Latrobe
3) You are scrubbed in on a tracheotomy. The surgeon asks for a tracheal dilator. You hand him/her a:
   a. Knight
   b. Weder
   c. Peck-Joseph
   d. Trousseau
4) The surgeon has freed the tonsil from the tonsil bed and now is ready to remove it. Which of the following is (are) tonsil-seizing forceps?
   a. Tivnen
   b. Tydings
   c. Love
   d. both a & b

5) All of the following are grasping instruments *except* a:
   a. Bishop-Harmon
   b. Tydings
   c. Frasier
   d. Brown-Adson

6) Before performing a tonsillectomy, the surgeon asks for a mouth gag. You could hand him/her:
   a. Cottle
   b. Hurd
   c. McIver
   d. Joseph

7) The surgeon is performing a myringotomy. You anticipate needing suction once the incision is made. Which of the following would you have ready to hand him/her?
   a. Frasier
   b. Hurd
   c. Brown-Adson
   d. Jansen

8) All of the following are cutting instruments *except* a:
   a. Maltz nasal rasp
   b. Takahashi
   c. Rubin morselizer
   d. Catania

9) All of the following are scissors *except*:
   a. Foman
   b. Barnhill
   c. Cottle angular
   d. Caplan

10) The surgeon needs to retract the tongue downwards, you hand him/her a:
   a. Weder
   b. Jansen
   c. Gruber
   d. Wullstein

11) All of the following are osteotomes *except*:
   a. Cottle
   b. Silver
   c. Cinelli
   d. MacKenty

12) A__________ is a morselizer.
   a. Hurd
   b. Jennings
   c. Rubin
   d. Peck-Joseph

13) __________ is a type of soft palate retractor.
   a. Carmalt
   b. Latrobe
   c. Brown
   d. House

14) The surgeon needs to mobilize the stapes. A __________ is a stapes mobilizer.
   a. Derlacki
   b. Crabtree
   c. Rosen
   d. Jordan

15) You are scrubbed on a stapedectomy. The surgeon requests an ossicle holding forceps. You would hand him/her a:
   a. Crabtree
   b. Sheehy
   c. Lampert
   d. Spratt

16) The surgeon will need both hands free to perform part of the ear surgery. You anticipate having to assemble and hook the ____________ speculum holder to the OR bed.
   a. House
   b. Rosen
   c. Shea
   d. Lillie

Ophthalmologic Instruments 7

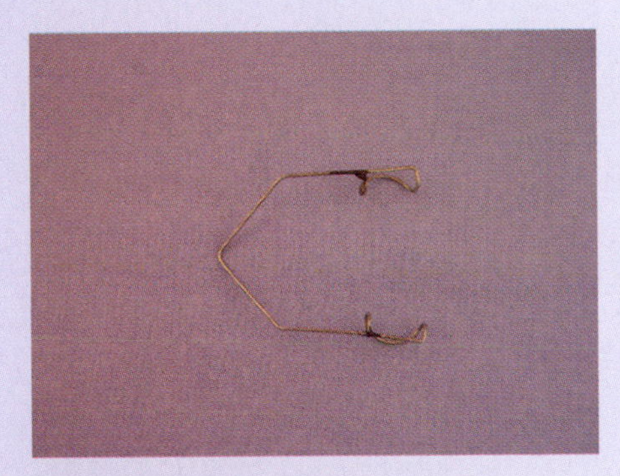

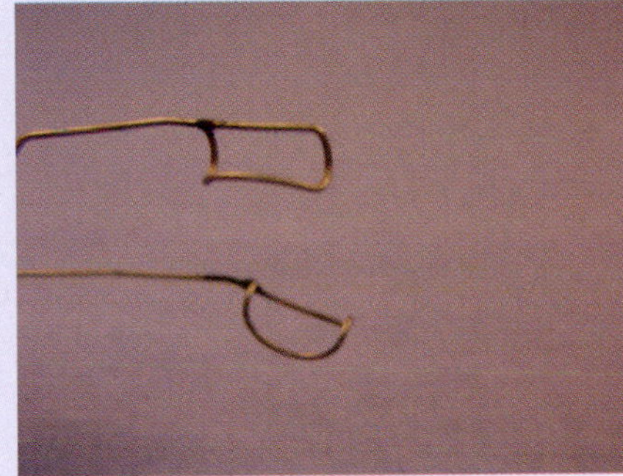

Name: Barraquer eye speculum

Alias: none

Category: retracting

Use: keeping eyelids open during surgery

Length: 1.3" or 1.6"

Additional Information: blades can be solid or fenestrated

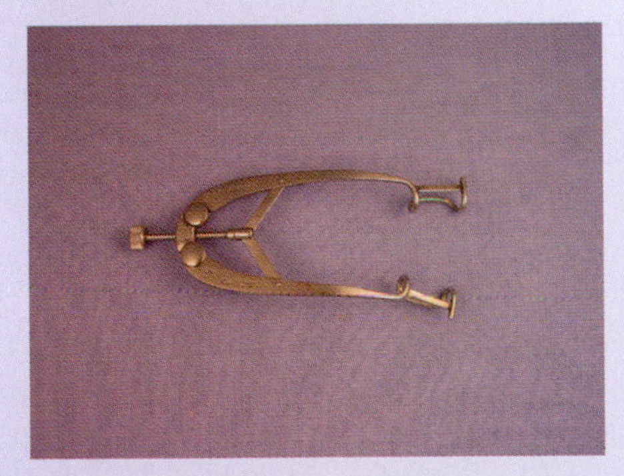

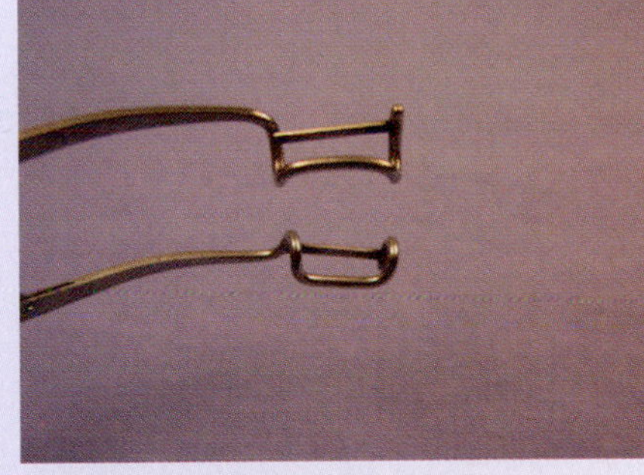

Name: Castroviejo eye speculum

Alias: none

Category: retracting

Use: keeping eyelids open during surgery

Length: 3" (15 mm blades) or 3.2" (16 mm blades)

Additional Information: fenestrated blades in 15 mm or 16 mm sizes

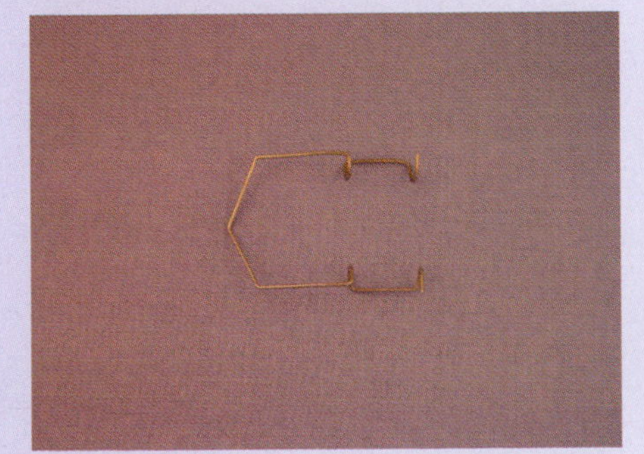

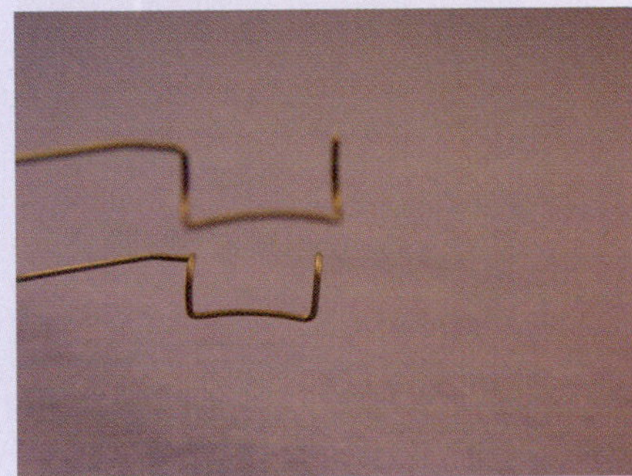

Name: Kratz Berraquer eye speculum

Alias: none

Category: retracting

Use: keeping eyelids open during surgery

Length: 1.6"

Additional Information: open blades

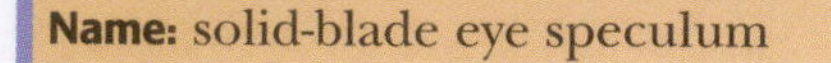

Name: solid-blade eye speculum

Alias: none

Category: retracting

Use: keeping eyelids open during surgery

Length: 3.5"

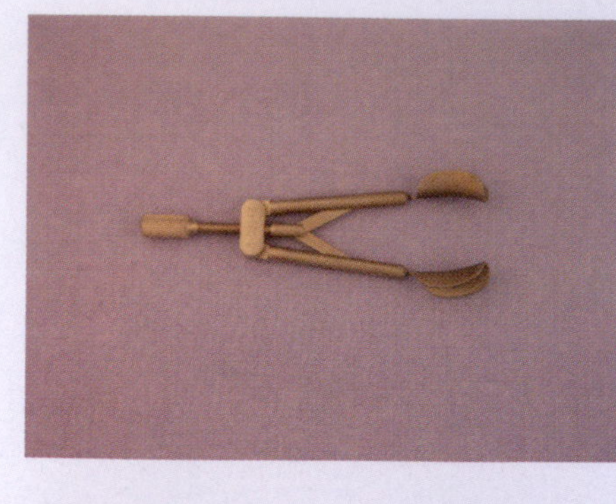

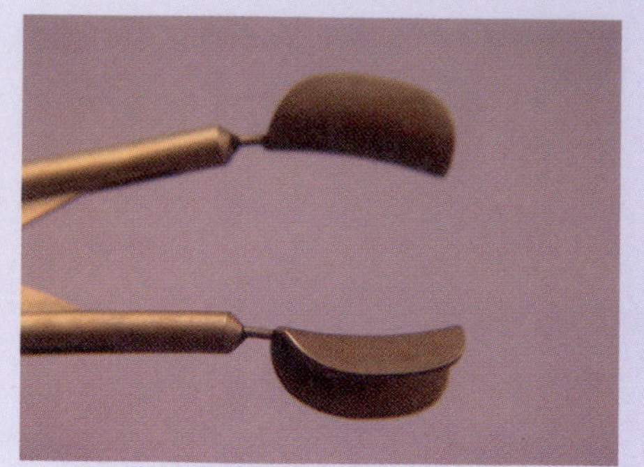

Name: Williams eye speculum

Alias: none

Category: retracting

Use: keeping eyelids open during surgery

Length: 2.7" (pediatric) or 3.4" (adult)

Additional Information: fenestrated blades; pediatric size has 11 mm blades, adult size has 14 mm blades

Name: Bowman lacrimal probe

Alias: none

Category: probing

Use: probing lacrimal ducts

Length: 5.9"

Additional Information: come in sizes 0000 to 8

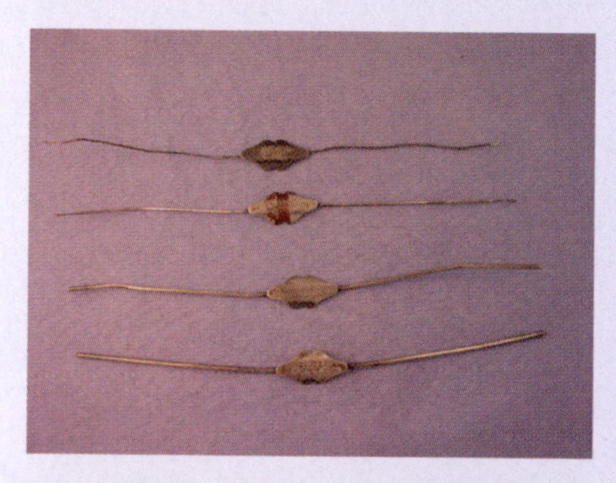

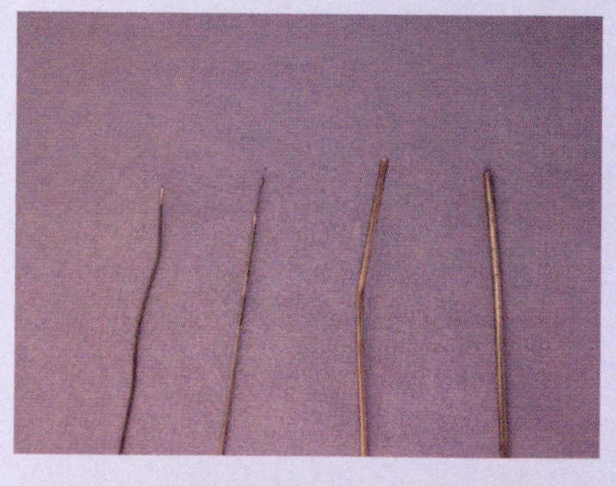

Name: strabismus retractor

Alias: none

Category: retracting

Use: retracting conjunctiva during strabismus surgery

Length: 5.5"

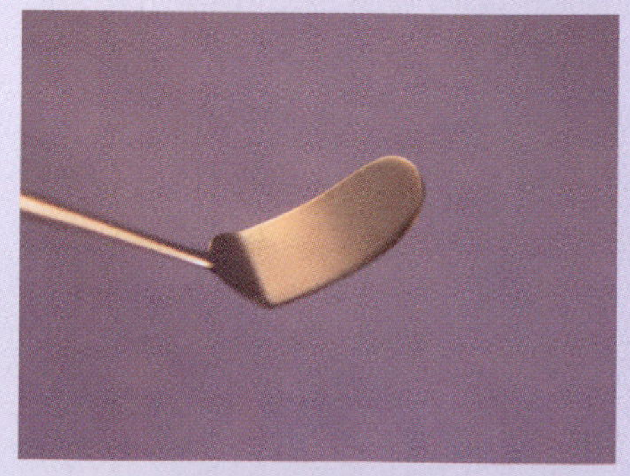

Name: Schepens orbital retractor

Alias: none

Category: retracting

Use: retracting orbit

Length: 5.75"

Additional Information: 4.5 mm notch in the blade

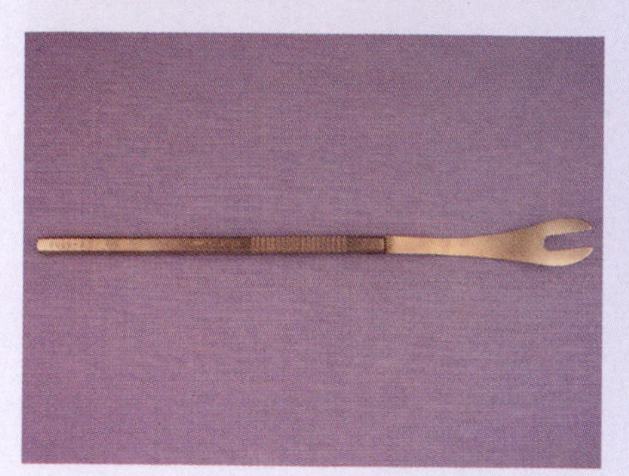

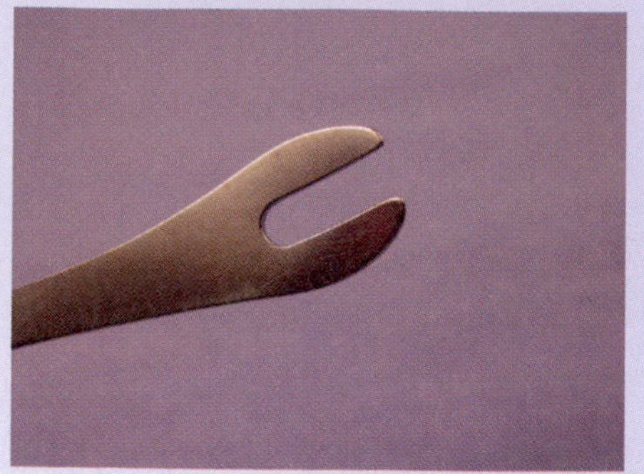

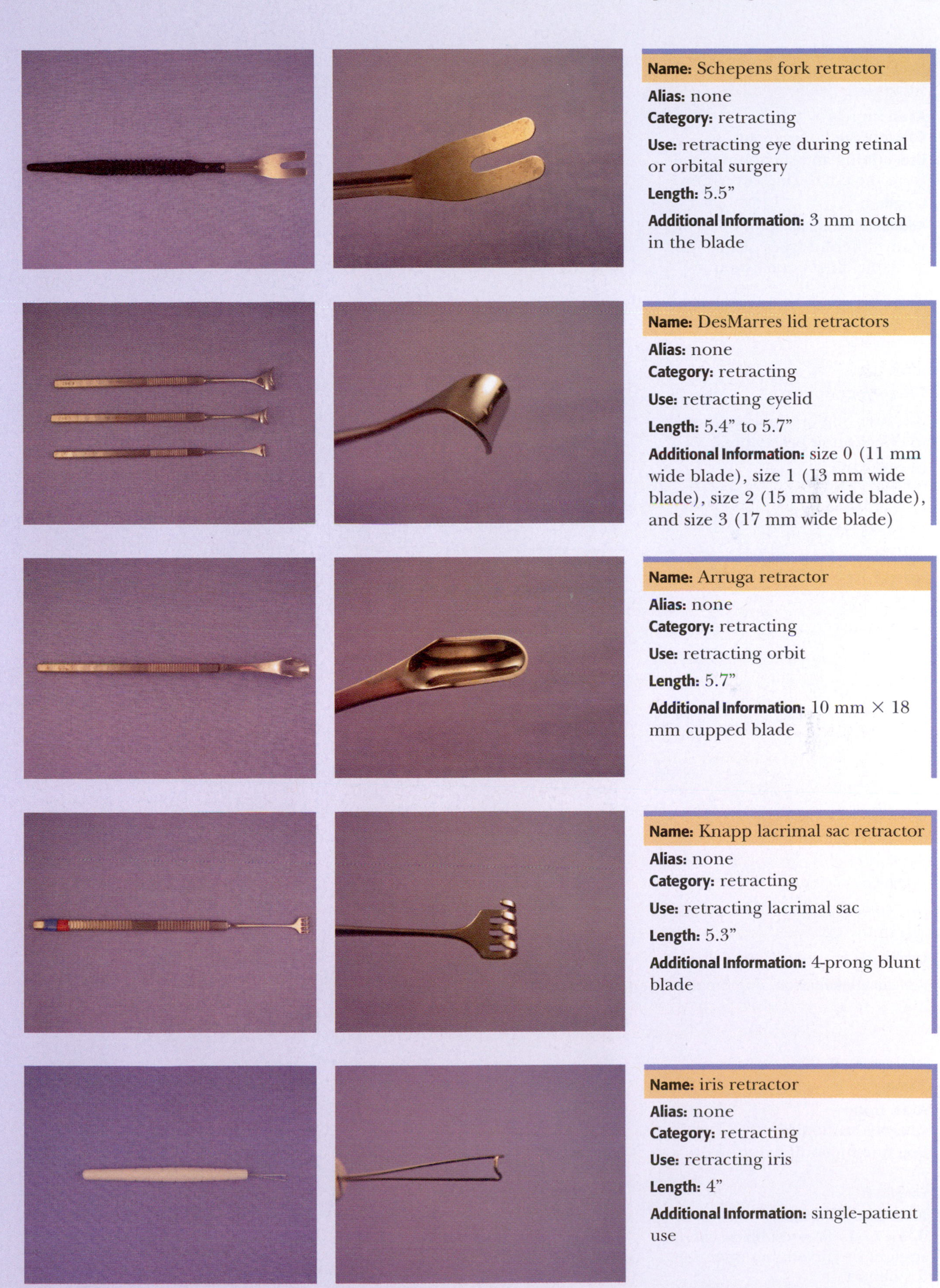

Name: Schepens fork retractor
Alias: none
Category: retracting
Use: retracting eye during retinal or orbital surgery
Length: 5.5"
Additional Information: 3 mm notch in the blade

Name: DesMarres lid retractors
Alias: none
Category: retracting
Use: retracting eyelid
Length: 5.4" to 5.7"
Additional Information: size 0 (11 mm wide blade), size 1 (13 mm wide blade), size 2 (15 mm wide blade), and size 3 (17 mm wide blade)

Name: Arruga retractor
Alias: none
Category: retracting
Use: retracting orbit
Length: 5.7"
Additional Information: 10 mm × 18 mm cupped blade

Name: Knapp lacrimal sac retractor
Alias: none
Category: retracting
Use: retracting lacrimal sac
Length: 5.3"
Additional Information: 4-prong blunt blade

Name: iris retractor
Alias: none
Category: retracting
Use: retracting iris
Length: 4"
Additional Information: single-patient use

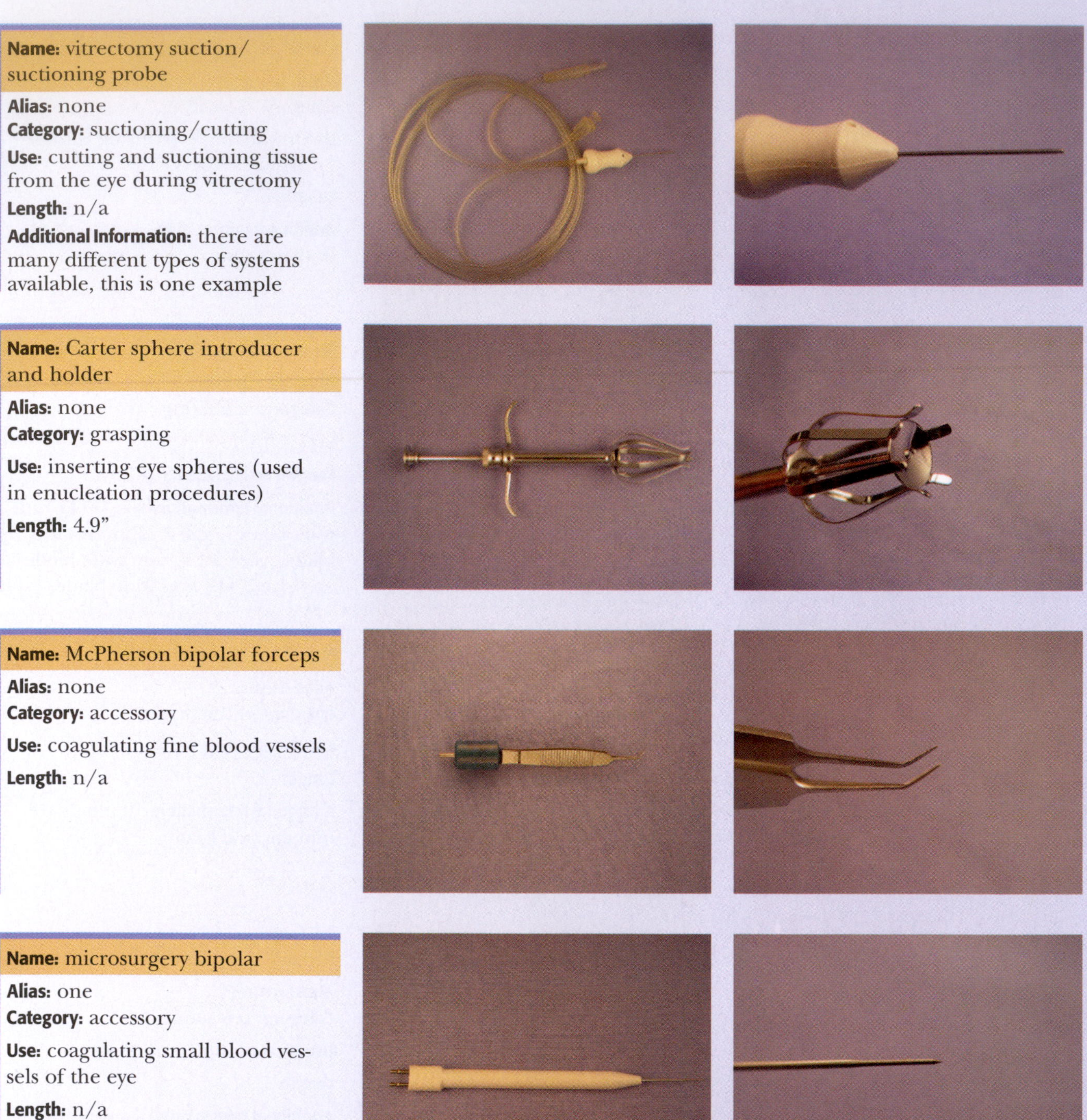

Name: vitrectomy suction/ suctioning probe

Alias: none

Category: suctioning/cutting

Use: cutting and suctioning tissue from the eye during vitrectomy

Length: n/a

Additional Information: there are many different types of systems available, this is one example

Name: Carter sphere introducer and holder

Alias: none

Category: grasping

Use: inserting eye spheres (used in enucleation procedures)

Length: 4.9"

Name: McPherson bipolar forceps

Alias: none

Category: accessory

Use: coagulating fine blood vessels

Length: n/a

Name: microsurgery bipolar

Alias: one

Category: accessory

Use: coagulating small blood vessels of the eye

Length: n/a

Additional Information: single-patient use

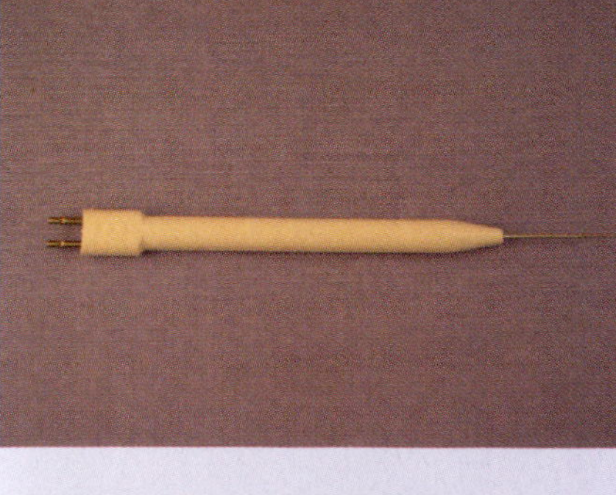

Name: Adson suction

Alias: none

Category: suctioning

Use: fine suctioning during eye surgery

Length: 6"

Additional Information: comes in 5, 7, 9, 11, or 15 Fr sizes; blade can be straight or curved; has opening for obturator

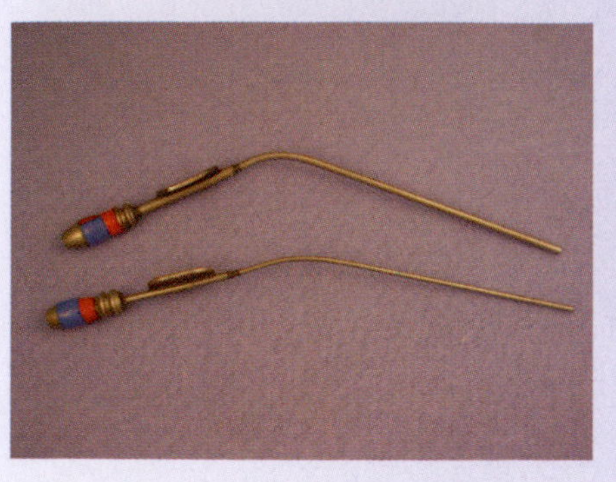

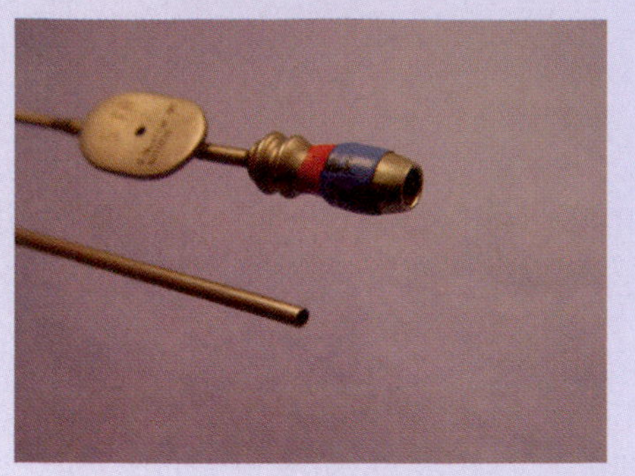

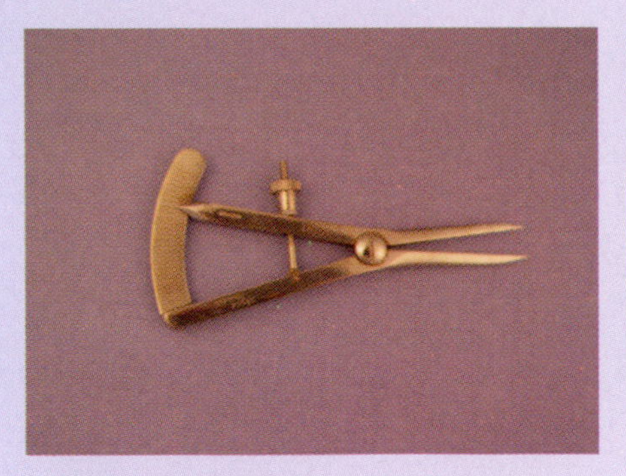

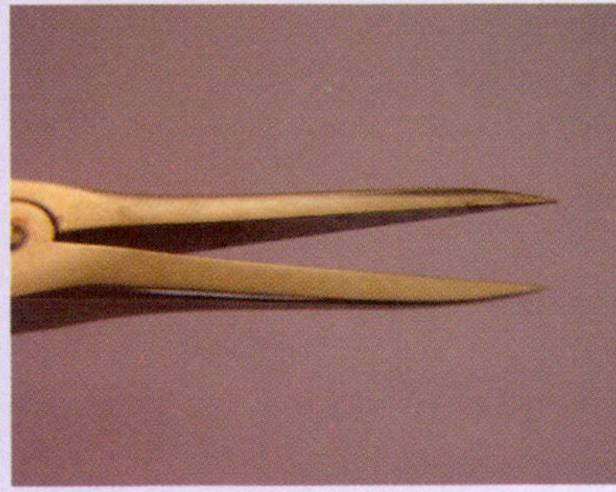

Name: Castroviejo caliper

Alias: none

Category: accessory

Length: 3.5"

Use: measuring and marking

Additional Information: measures in mm; can be straight or curved; thumbscrew holds tips apart

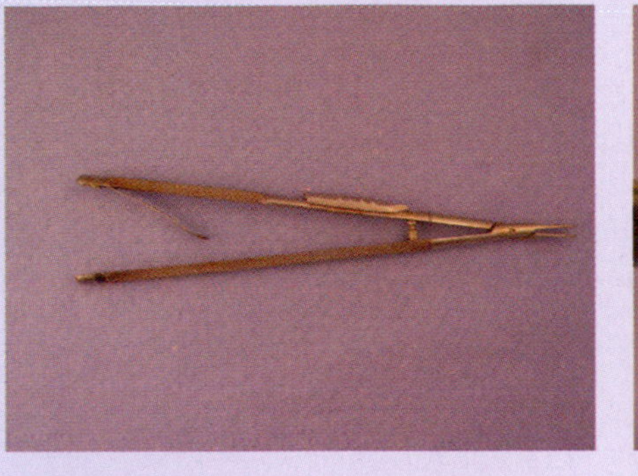

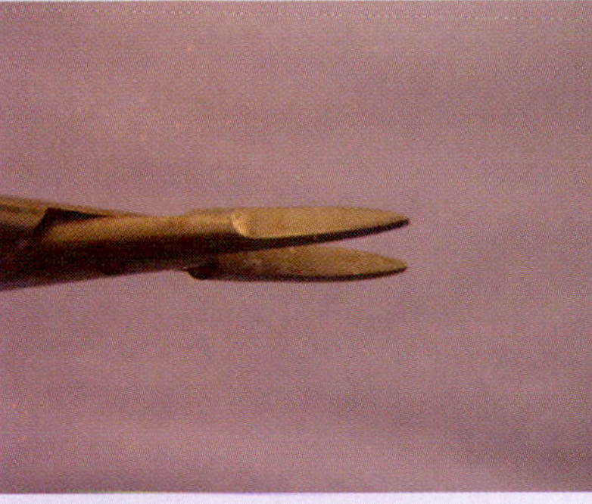

Name: Castroviejo blade breaker and holder

Alias: none

Category: grasping

Use: holding and/or breaking stainless-steel breakable blades

Length: 5.5"

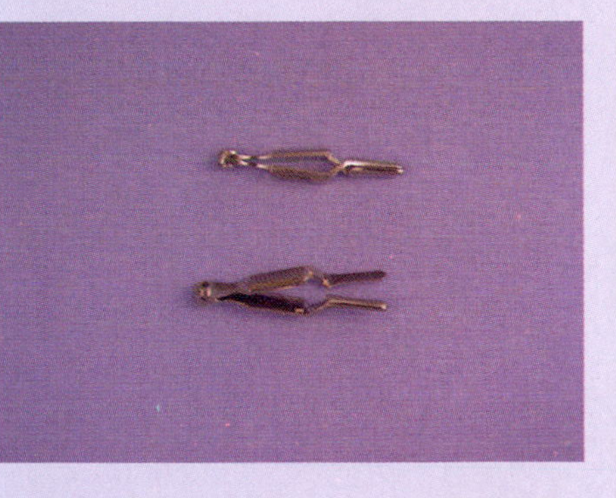

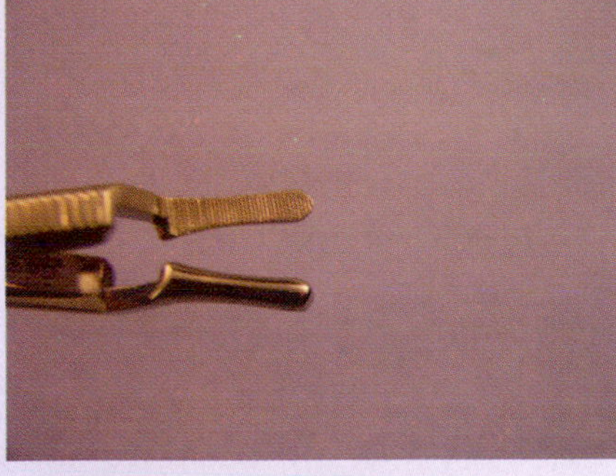

Name: Serrefine clamps

Alias: none

Category: clamping

Use: holding sutures out of the field

Length: 1.5"

Name: Hanna trephine system

Alias: none

Category: cutting

Use: cutting graft from donor cornea

Length: n/a

Additional Information: requires insertion of single-use trephine blade

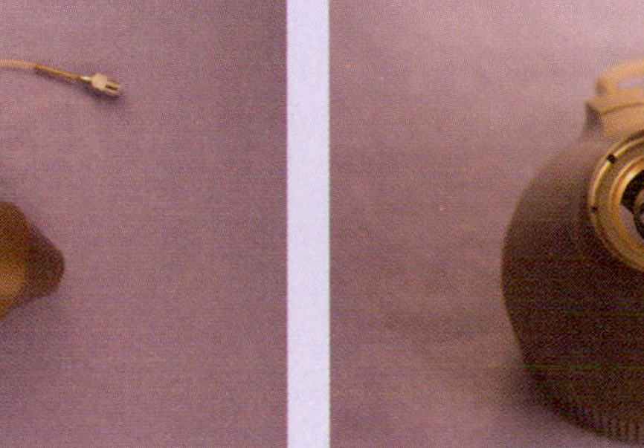

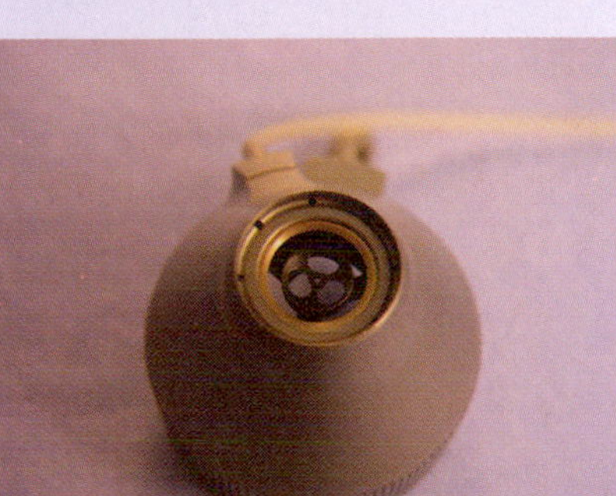

Name: Hanna trephine system

Alias: none

Category: cutting

Use: cutting patient's diseased cornea for removal

Length: n/a

Additional Information: requires insertion of single-use trephine blade

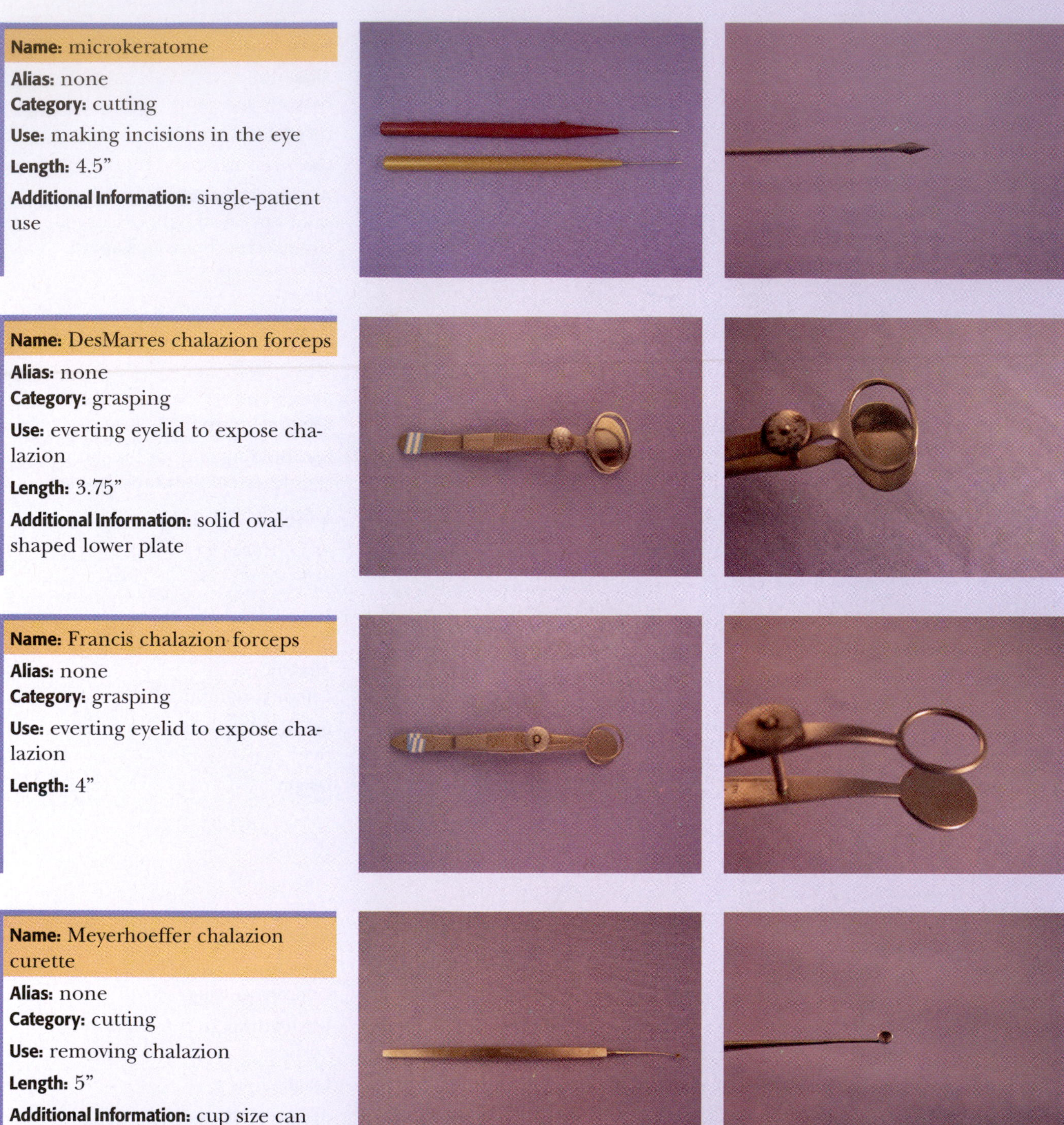

Name: microkeratome
Alias: none
Category: cutting
Use: making incisions in the eye
Length: 4.5"
Additional Information: single-patient use

Name: DesMarres chalazion forceps
Alias: none
Category: grasping
Use: everting eyelid to expose chalazion
Length: 3.75"
Additional Information: solid oval-shaped lower plate

Name: Francis chalazion forceps
Alias: none
Category: grasping
Use: everting eyelid to expose chalazion
Length: 4"

Name: Meyerhoeffer chalazion curette
Alias: none
Category: cutting
Use: removing chalazion
Length: 5"
Additional Information: cup size can be 1.5 mm to 3.5 mm

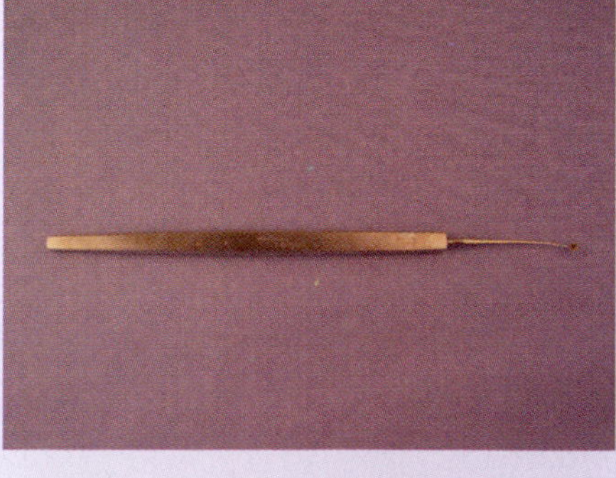

Name: Gills-Welch curette
Alias: none
Category: cutting
Use: removing chalazion
Length: 5"

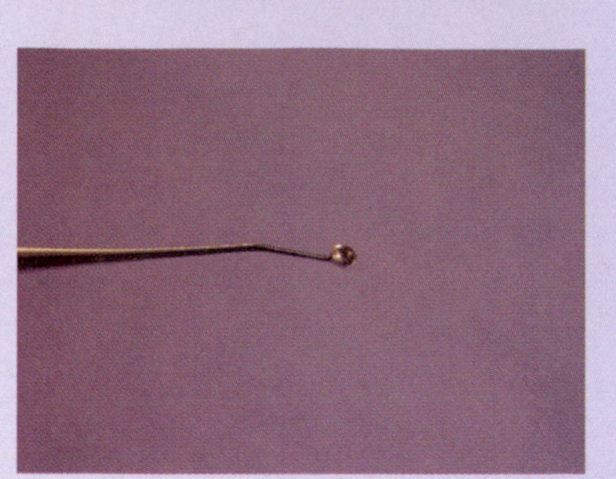

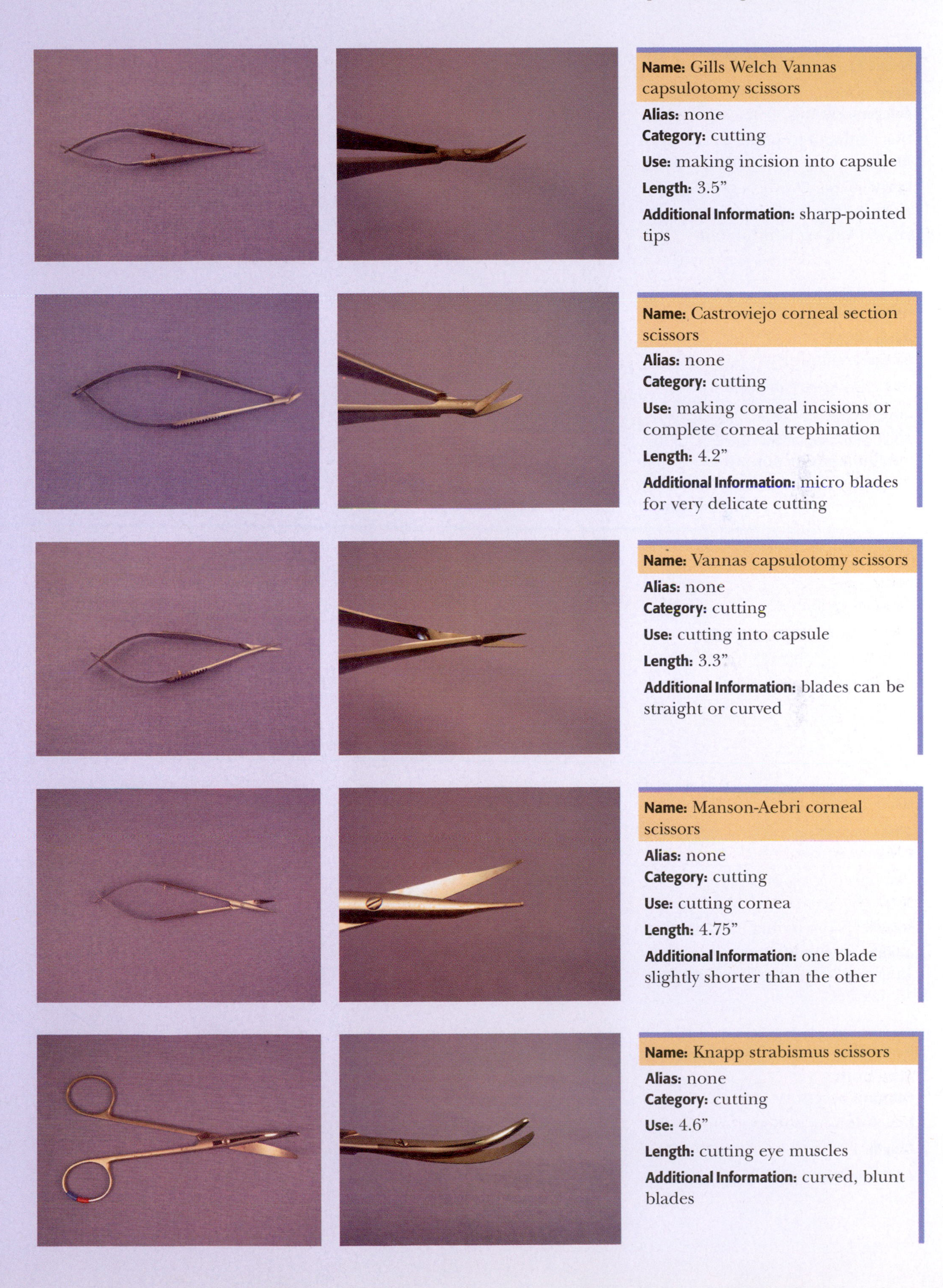

Name: Gills Welch Vannas capsulotomy scissors
Alias: none
Category: cutting
Use: making incision into capsule
Length: 3.5"
Additional Information: sharp-pointed tips

Name: Castroviejo corneal section scissors
Alias: none
Category: cutting
Use: making corneal incisions or complete corneal trephination
Length: 4.2"
Additional Information: micro blades for very delicate cutting

Name: Vannas capsulotomy scissors
Alias: none
Category: cutting
Use: cutting into capsule
Length: 3.3"
Additional Information: blades can be straight or curved

Name: Manson-Aebri corneal scissors
Alias: none
Category: cutting
Use: cutting cornea
Length: 4.75"
Additional Information: one blade slightly shorter than the other

Name: Knapp strabismus scissors
Alias: none
Category: cutting
Use: 4.6"
Length: cutting eye muscles
Additional Information: curved, blunt blades

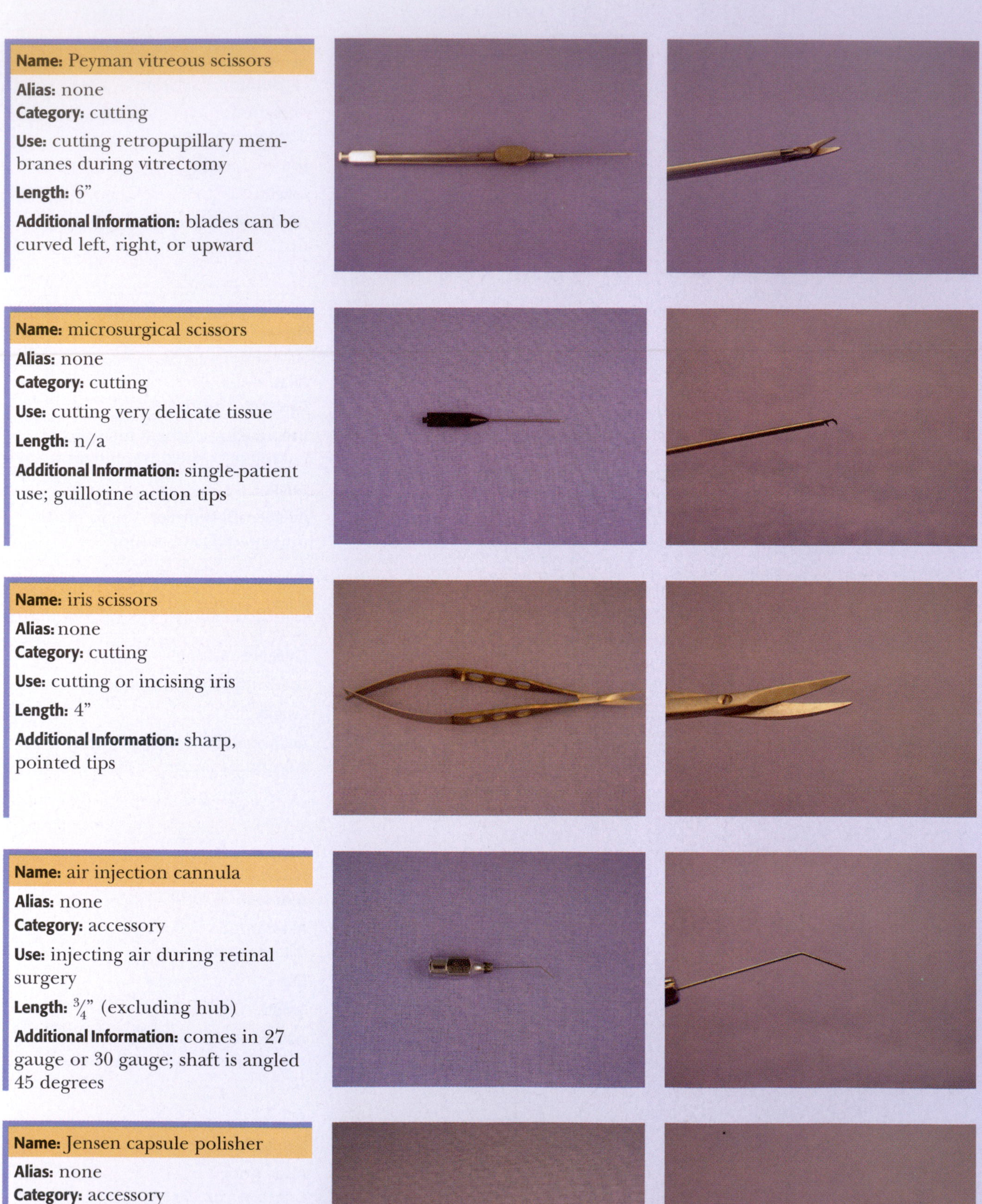

Name: Peyman vitreous scissors
Alias: none
Category: cutting
Use: cutting retropupillary membranes during vitrectomy
Length: 6"
Additional Information: blades can be curved left, right, or upward

Name: microsurgical scissors
Alias: none
Category: cutting
Use: cutting very delicate tissue
Length: n/a
Additional Information: single-patient use; guillotine action tips

Name: iris scissors
Alias: none
Category: cutting
Use: cutting or incising iris
Length: 4"
Additional Information: sharp, pointed tips

Name: air injection cannula
Alias: none
Category: accessory
Use: injecting air during retinal surgery
Length: $\frac{3}{4}$" (excluding hub)
Additional Information: comes in 27 gauge or 30 gauge; shaft is angled 45 degrees

Name: Jensen capsule polisher
Alias: none
Category: accessory
Use: polishing posterior capsule
Length: 1"
Additional Information: 27-gauge cannula

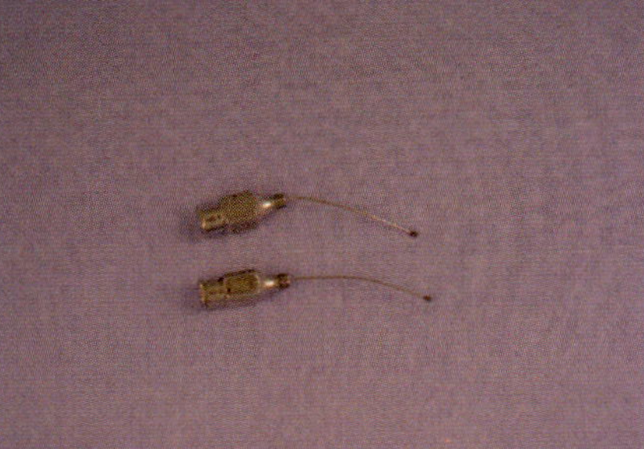

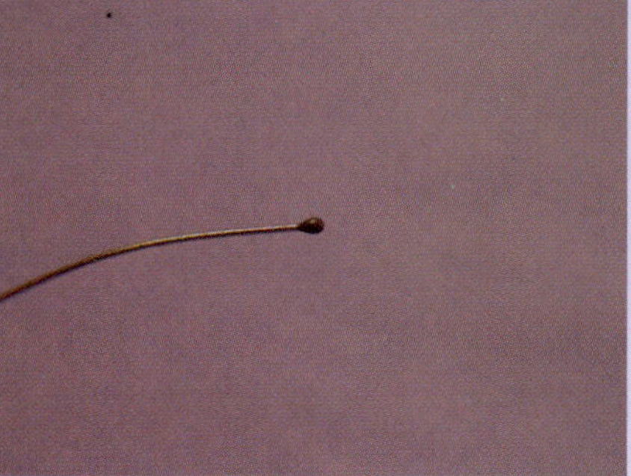

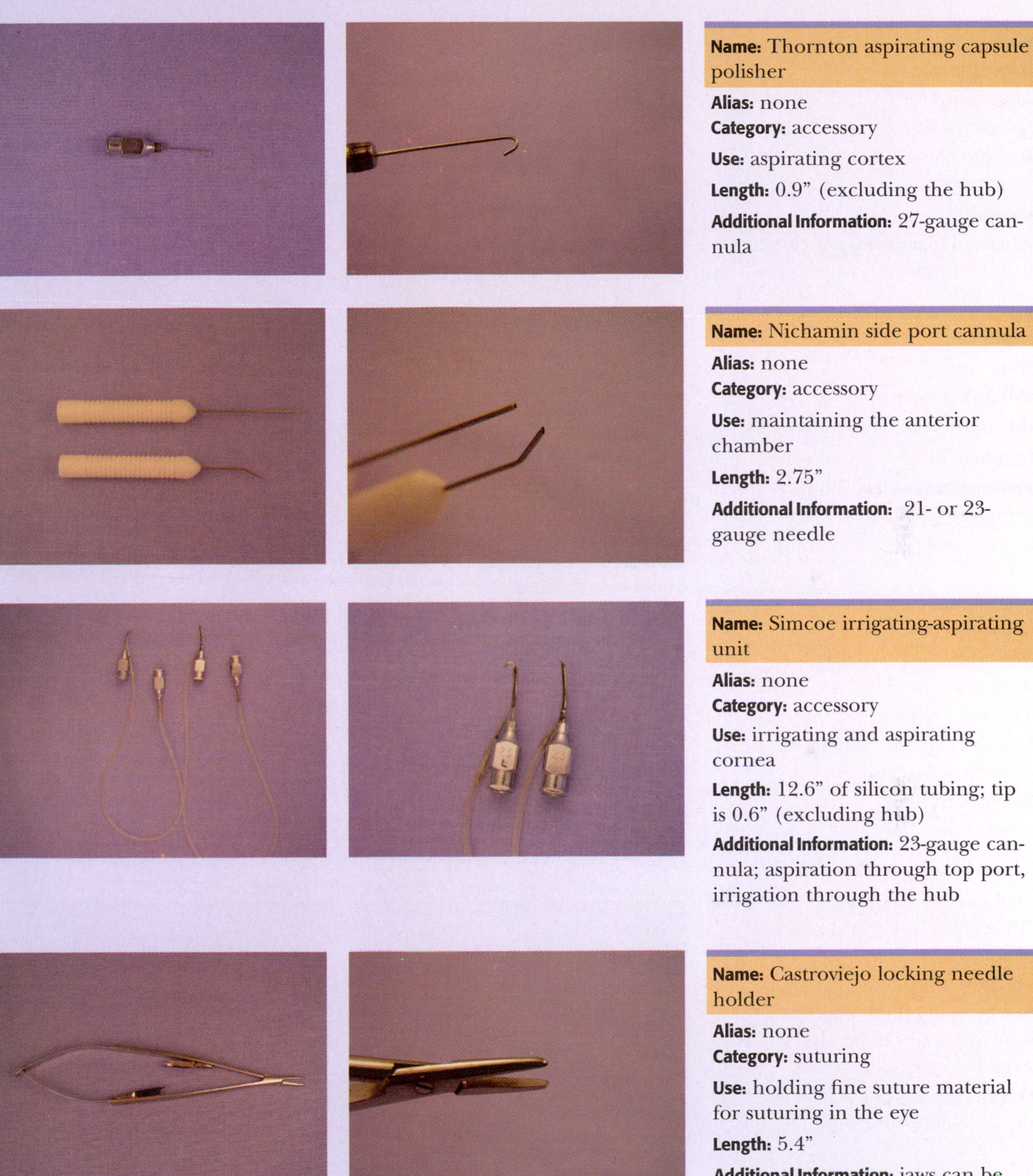

Name: Thornton aspirating capsule polisher

Alias: none

Category: accessory

Use: aspirating cortex

Length: 0.9" (excluding the hub)

Additional Information: 27-gauge cannula

Name: Nichamin side port cannula

Alias: none

Category: accessory

Use: maintaining the anterior chamber

Length: 2.75"

Additional Information: 21- or 23-gauge needle

Name: Simcoe irrigating-aspirating unit

Alias: none

Category: accessory

Use: irrigating and aspirating cornea

Length: 12.6" of silicon tubing; tip is 0.6" (excluding hub)

Additional Information: 23-gauge cannula; aspiration through top port, irrigation through the hub

Name: Castroviejo locking needle holder

Alias: none

Category: suturing

Use: holding fine suture material for suturing in the eye

Length: 5.4"

Additional Information: jaws can be straight or curved; jaws can be fine (for more delicate sutures) or medium

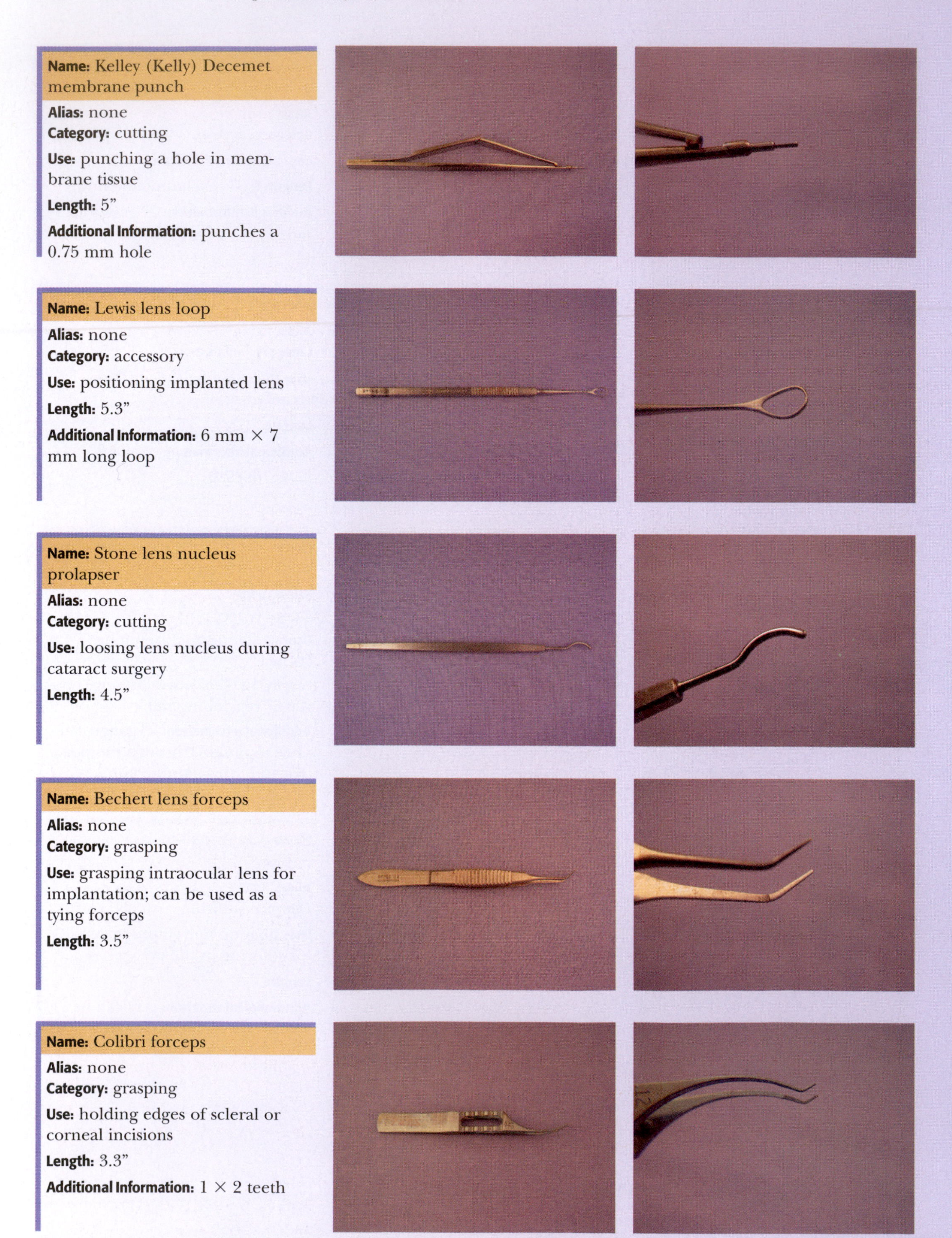

Name: Kelley (Kelly) Decemet membrane punch

Alias: none

Category: cutting

Use: punching a hole in membrane tissue

Length: 5"

Additional Information: punches a 0.75 mm hole

Name: Lewis lens loop

Alias: none

Category: accessory

Use: positioning implanted lens

Length: 5.3"

Additional Information: 6 mm × 7 mm long loop

Name: Stone lens nucleus prolapser

Alias: none

Category: cutting

Use: loosing lens nucleus during cataract surgery

Length: 4.5"

Name: Bechert lens forceps

Alias: none

Category: grasping

Use: grasping intraocular lens for implantation; can be used as a tying forceps

Length: 3.5"

Name: Colibri forceps

Alias: none

Category: grasping

Use: holding edges of scleral or corneal incisions

Length: 3.3"

Additional Information: 1 × 2 teeth

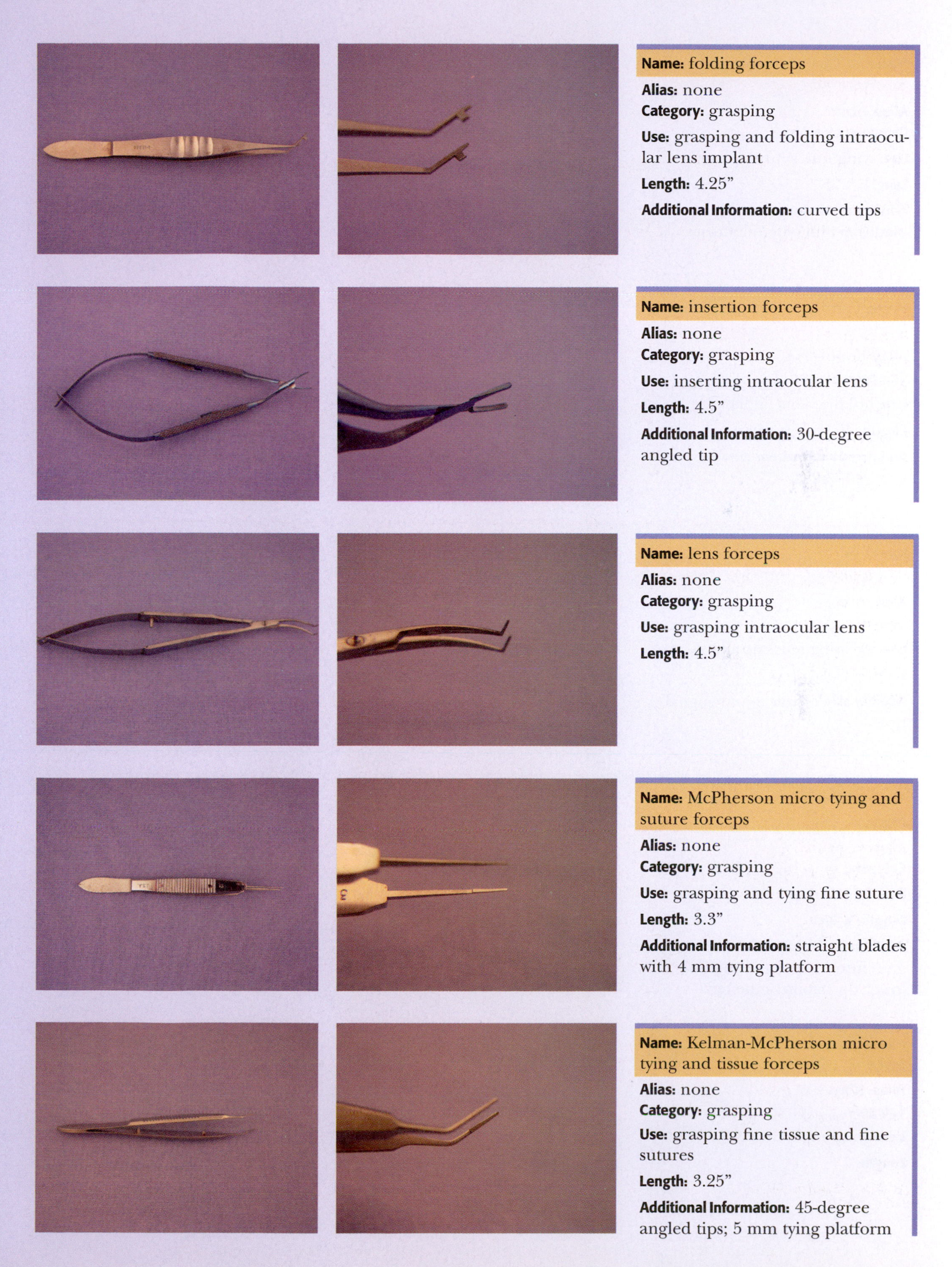

Name: folding forceps
Alias: none
Category: grasping
Use: grasping and folding intraocular lens implant
Length: 4.25"
Additional Information: curved tips

Name: insertion forceps
Alias: none
Category: grasping
Use: inserting intraocular lens
Length: 4.5"
Additional Information: 30-degree angled tip

Name: lens forceps
Alias: none
Category: grasping
Use: grasping intraocular lens
Length: 4.5"

Name: McPherson micro tying and suture forceps
Alias: none
Category: grasping
Use: grasping and tying fine suture
Length: 3.3"
Additional Information: straight blades with 4 mm tying platform

Name: Kelman-McPherson micro tying and tissue forceps
Alias: none
Category: grasping
Use: grasping fine tissue and fine sutures
Length: 3.25"
Additional Information: 45-degree angled tips; 5 mm tying platform

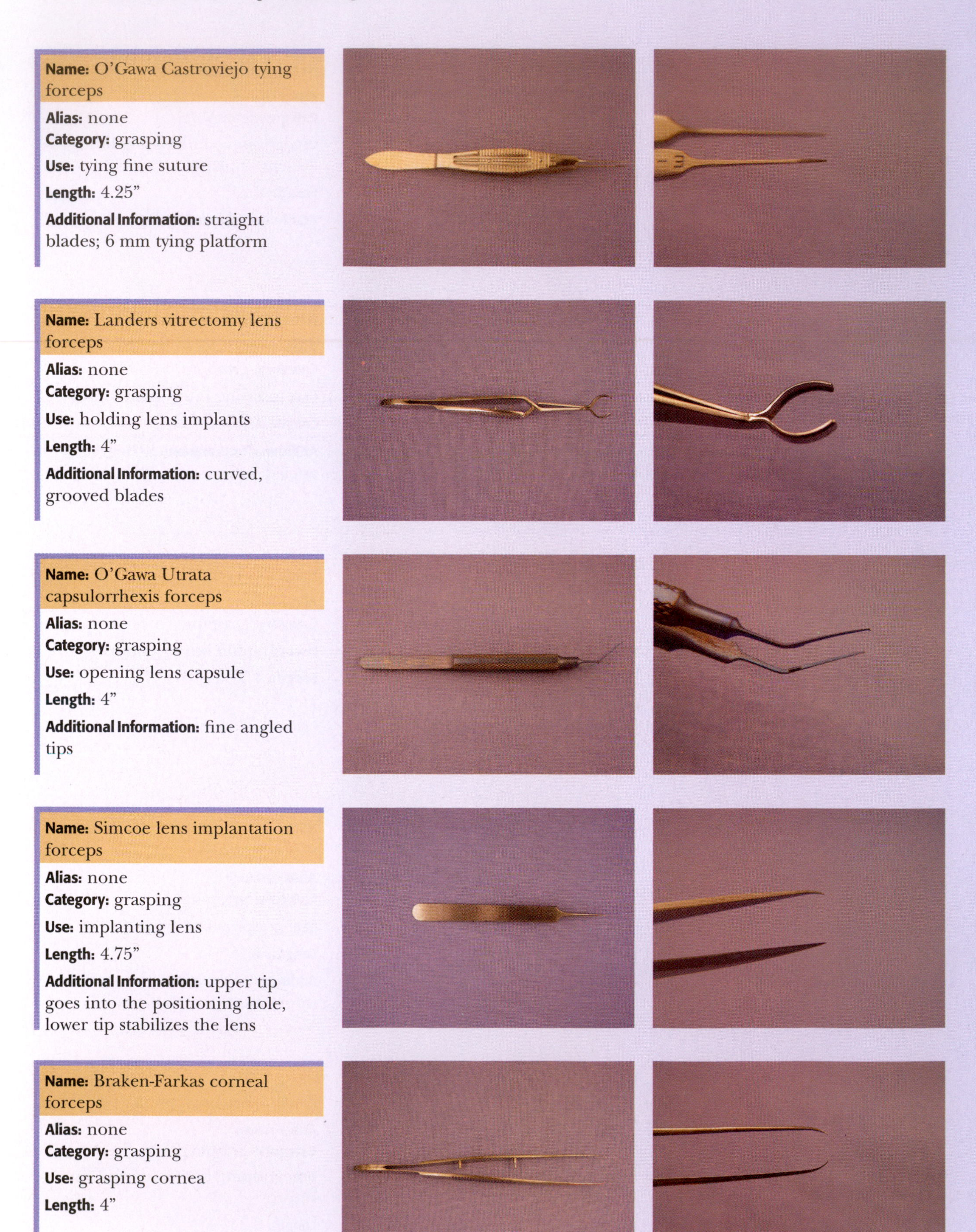

Name: O'Gawa Castroviejo tying forceps

Alias: none

Category: grasping

Use: tying fine suture

Length: 4.25"

Additional Information: straight blades; 6 mm tying platform

Name: Landers vitrectomy lens forceps

Alias: none

Category: grasping

Use: holding lens implants

Length: 4"

Additional Information: curved, grooved blades

Name: O'Gawa Utrata capsulorrhexis forceps

Alias: none

Category: grasping

Use: opening lens capsule

Length: 4"

Additional Information: fine angled tips

Name: Simcoe lens implantation forceps

Alias: none

Category: grasping

Use: implanting lens

Length: 4.75"

Additional Information: upper tip goes into the positioning hole, lower tip stabilizes the lens

Name: Braken-Farkas corneal forceps

Alias: none

Category: grasping

Use: grasping cornea

Length: 4"

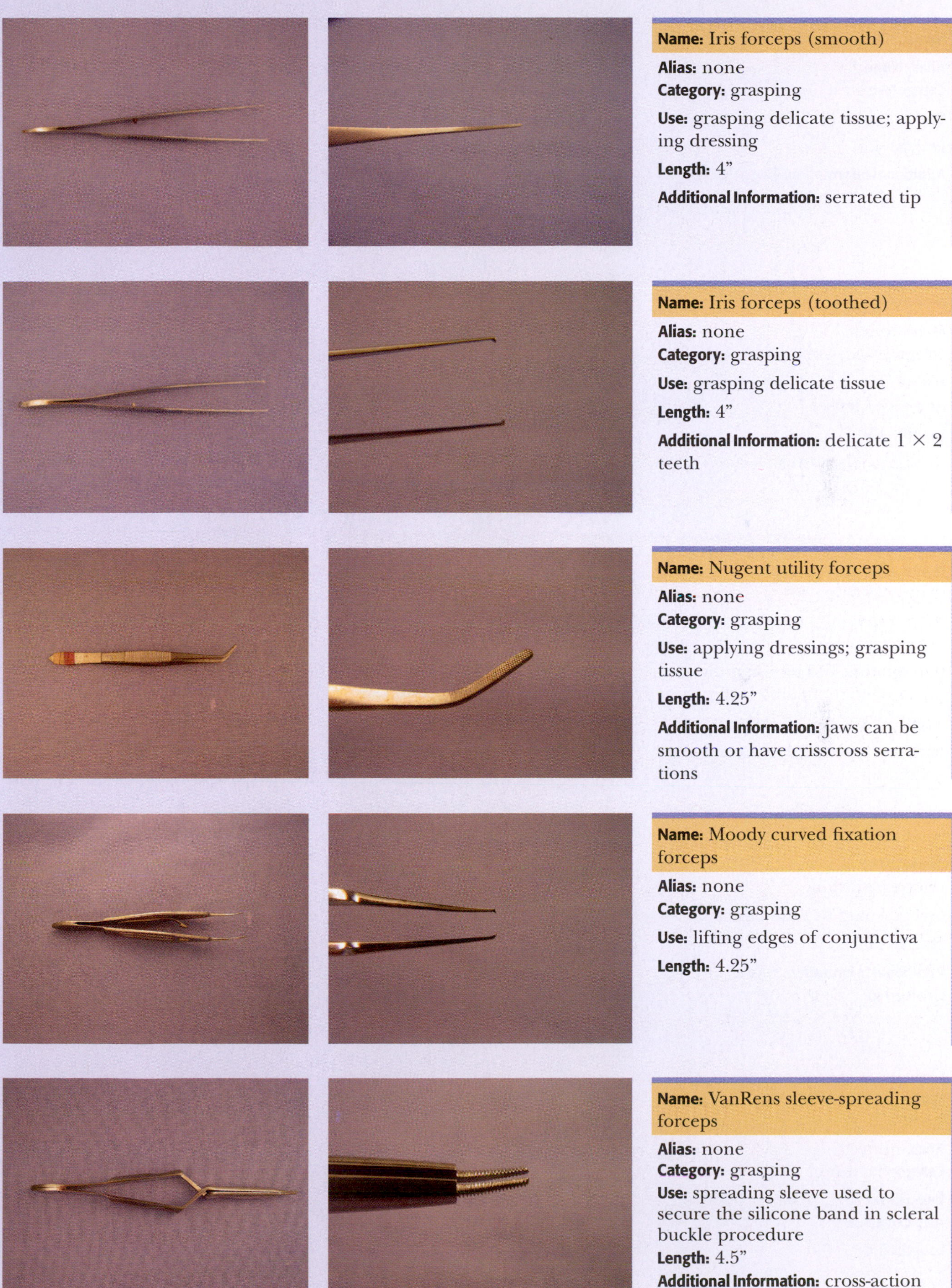

Name: Iris forceps (smooth)

Alias: none

Category: grasping

Use: grasping delicate tissue; applying dressing

Length: 4"

Additional Information: serrated tip

Name: Iris forceps (toothed)

Alias: none

Category: grasping

Use: grasping delicate tissue

Length: 4"

Additional Information: delicate 1 × 2 teeth

Name: Nugent utility forceps

Alias: none

Category: grasping

Use: applying dressings; grasping tissue

Length: 4.25"

Additional Information: jaws can be smooth or have crisscross serrations

Name: Moody curved fixation forceps

Alias: none

Category: grasping

Use: lifting edges of conjunctiva

Length: 4.25"

Name: VanRens sleeve-spreading forceps

Alias: none

Category: grasping

Use: spreading sleeve used to secure the silicone band in scleral buckle procedure

Length: 4.5"

Additional Information: cross-action handle

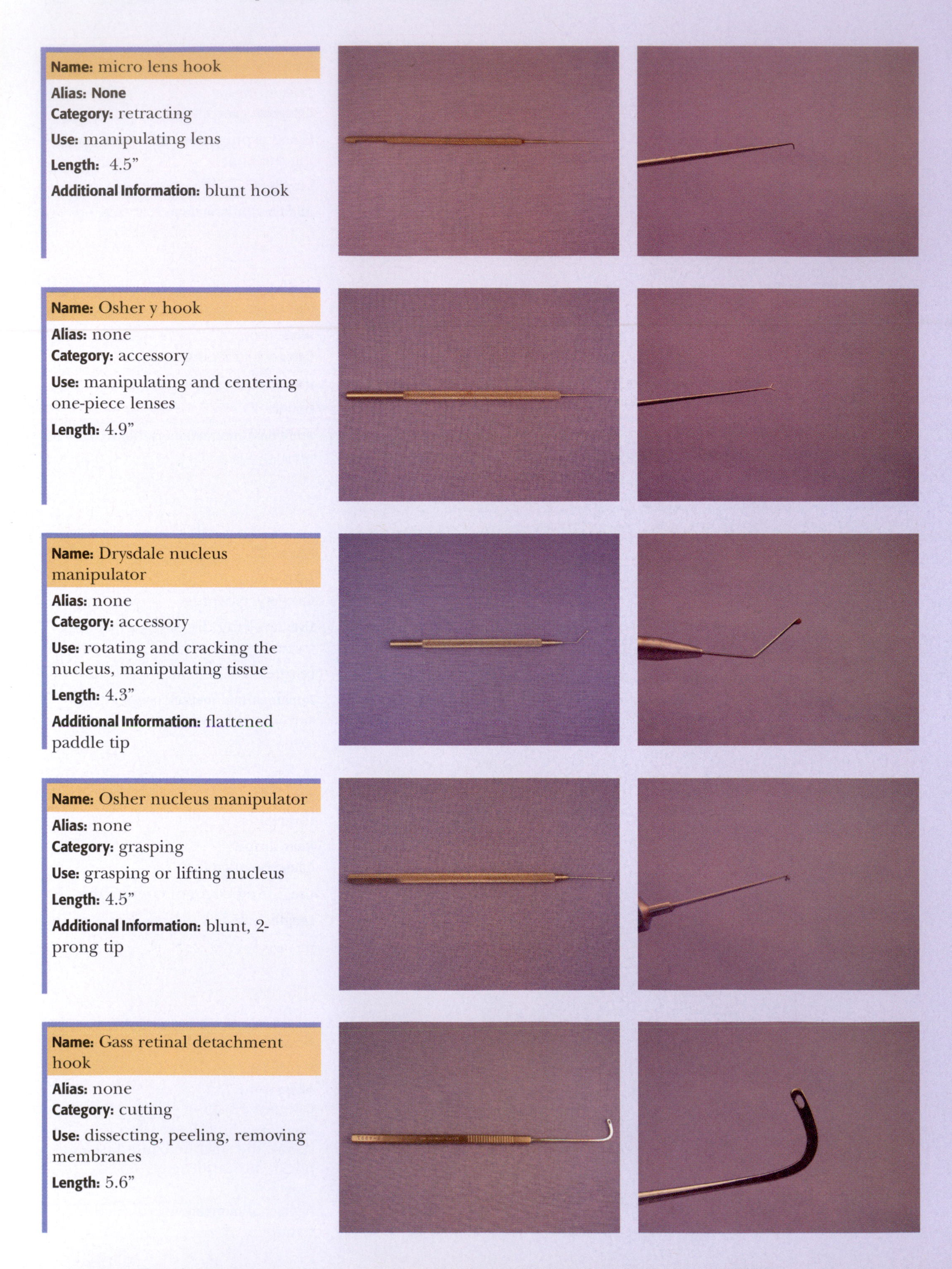

Name: micro lens hook
Alias: None
Category: retracting
Use: manipulating lens
Length: 4.5"
Additional Information: blunt hook

Name: Osher y hook
Alias: none
Category: accessory
Use: manipulating and centering one-piece lenses
Length: 4.9"

Name: Drysdale nucleus manipulator
Alias: none
Category: accessory
Use: rotating and cracking the nucleus, manipulating tissue
Length: 4.3"
Additional Information: flattened paddle tip

Name: Osher nucleus manipulator
Alias: none
Category: grasping
Use: grasping or lifting nucleus
Length: 4.5"
Additional Information: blunt, 2-prong tip

Name: Gass retinal detachment hook
Alias: none
Category: cutting
Use: dissecting, peeling, removing membranes
Length: 5.6"

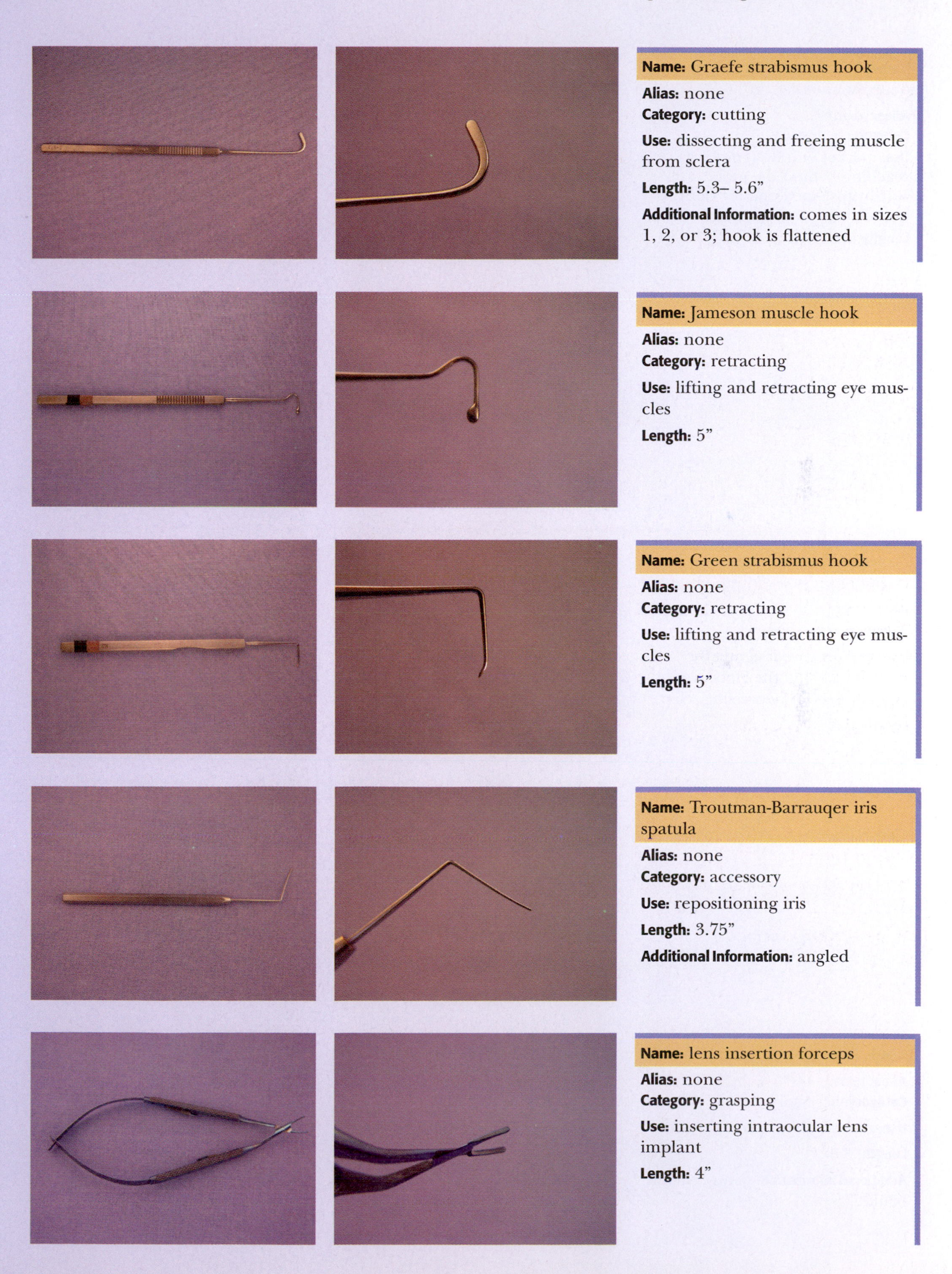

Name: Graefe strabismus hook

Alias: none

Category: cutting

Use: dissecting and freeing muscle from sclera

Length: 5.3– 5.6"

Additional Information: comes in sizes 1, 2, or 3; hook is flattened

Name: Jameson muscle hook

Alias: none

Category: retracting

Use: lifting and retracting eye muscles

Length: 5"

Name: Green strabismus hook

Alias: none

Category: retracting

Use: lifting and retracting eye muscles

Length: 5"

Name: Troutman-Barrauqer iris spatula

Alias: none

Category: accessory

Use: repositioning iris

Length: 3.75"

Additional Information: angled

Name: lens insertion forceps

Alias: none

Category: grasping

Use: inserting intraocular lens implant

Length: 4"

Name: O'Connor scleral depressor-marker

Alias: none

Category: accessory

Use: marker end designed for reaching behind the globe, teardrop shaped end for depressing sclera

Length: 5.25"

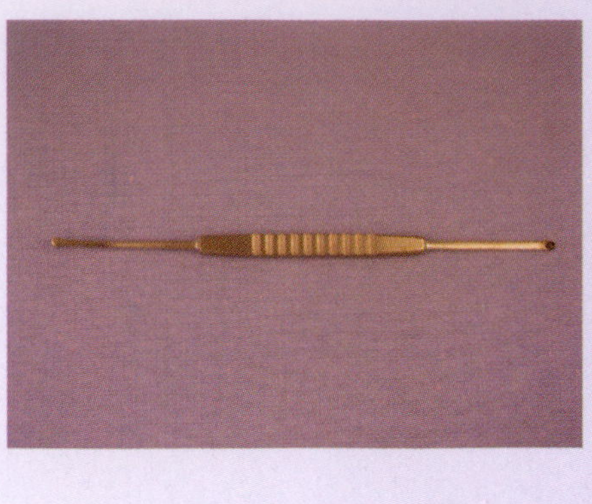

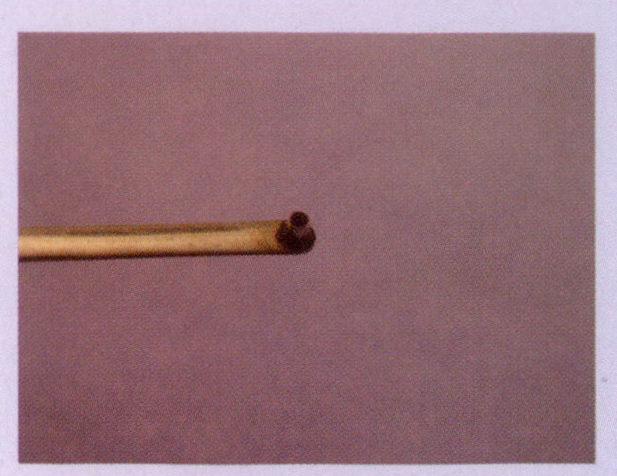

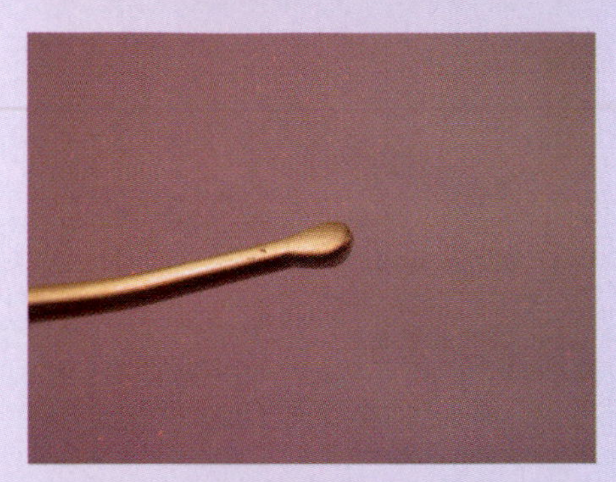

Name: Schocket double-ended scleral depressor

Alias: none

Category: accessory

Use: marker end designed for reaching behind the globe, rounded end used for depressing sclera

Length: 5.3"

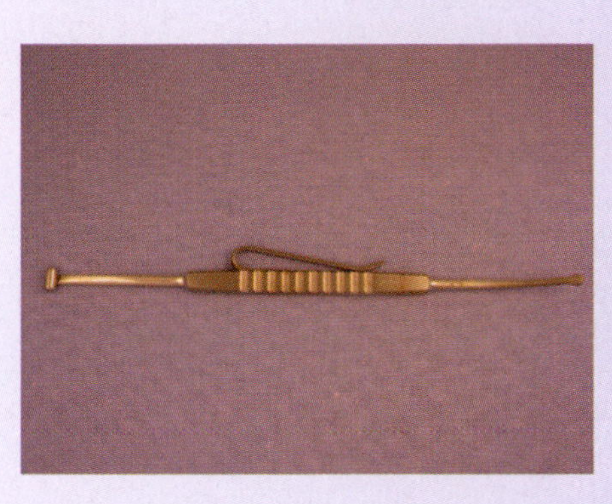

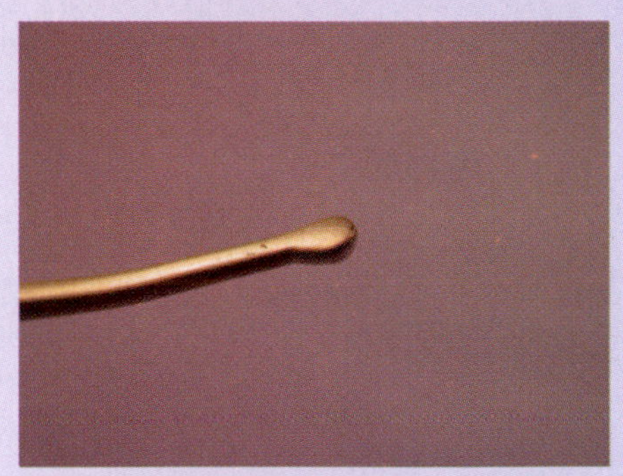

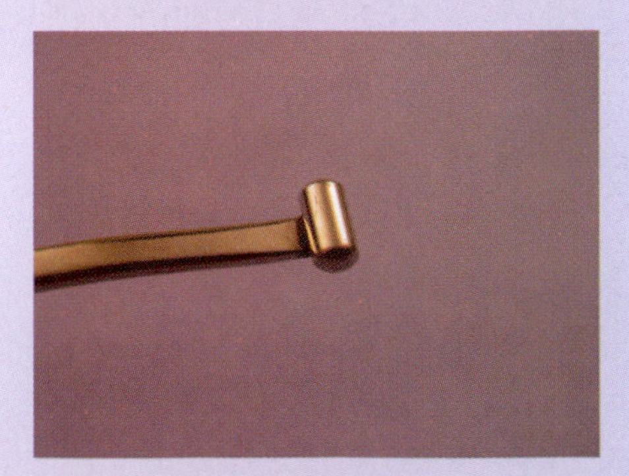

Name: Barraquer iris spatula

Alias: none

Category: accessory

Use: repositioning iris

Length: 3.5"

Additional Information: gently curved blade

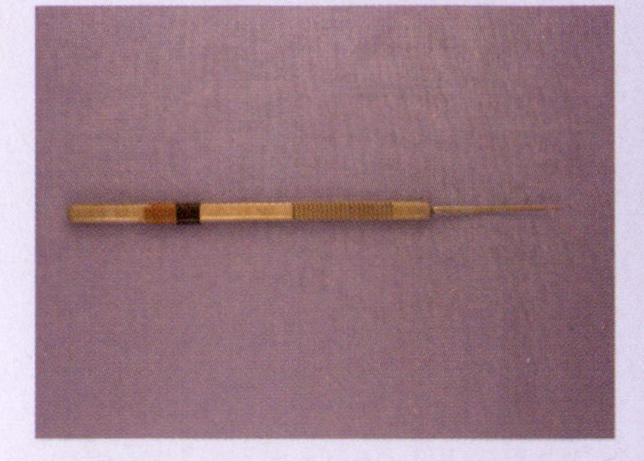

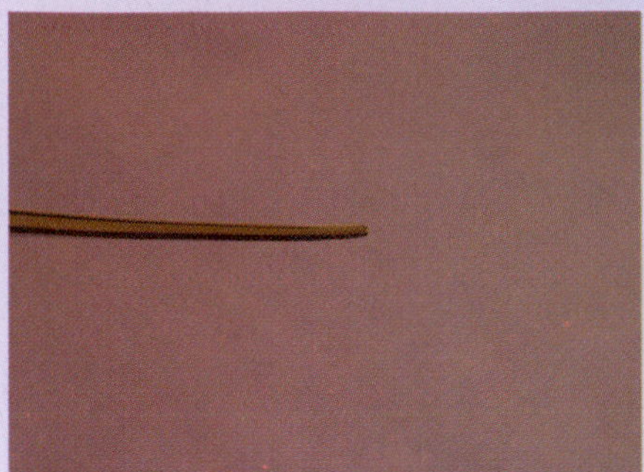

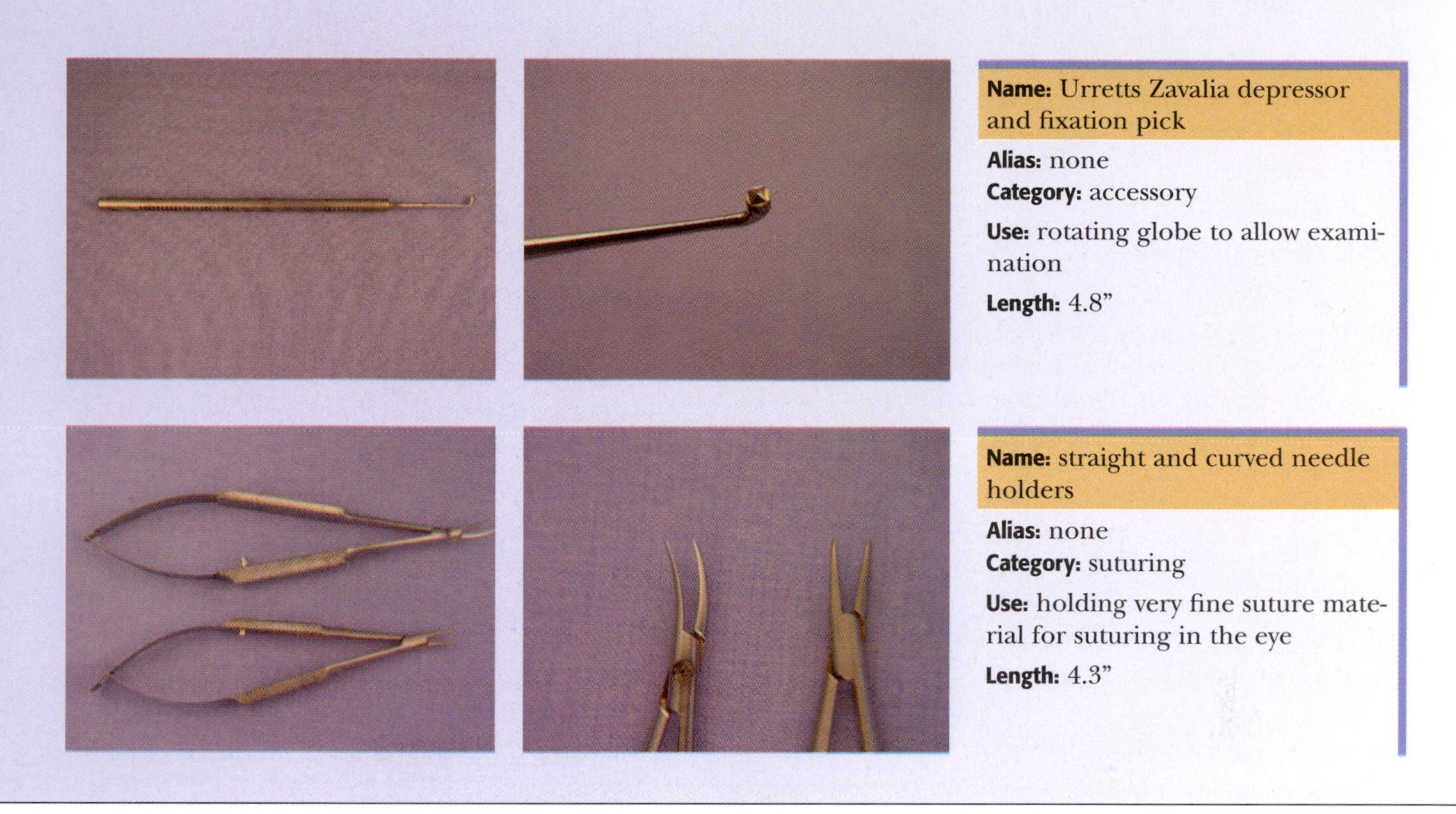

Name: Urretts Zavalia depressor and fixation pick

Alias: none

Category: accessory

Use: rotating globe to allow examination

Length: 4.8"

Name: straight and curved needle holders

Alias: none

Category: suturing

Use: holding very fine suture material for suturing in the eye

Length: 4.3"

Q&A

Surgical Session—Ophthalmologic Surgery

1) The surgeon asks for an eye speculum. You could hand him/her any of the following *except* a:
   a. Williams
   b. Barraquer
   c. Schepens
   d. Kratz-Berraquer

2) The next step in the surgery requires the use of lacrimal probes. You need to have the __________ probes ready.
   a. Bowman
   b. Adson
   c. Gills-Welch
   d. Peyman

3) The Y hook used to manipulate and center lenses is a(n):
   a. Gass
   b. Osher
   c. Williams
   d. Green

4) A(n) ____________ is a type of strabismus hook.
   a. Graefe
   b. Barraquer
   c. Adson
   d. Castroviejo

5) You are scrubbed on a corneal transplant. The surgeon is preparing to cut the donor cornea. You need to have the ____________ trephine ready.
   a. Williams
   b. DeMerres
   c. Francis
   d. Hanna

6) Which of the following instruments is likely *not* to be found on the set-up for chalazion surgery?
   a. Francis forceps
   b. DeMerres forceps
   c. Meyerhoeffer curette
   d. Peyman scissors

7) A __________ is a type of lens loop.
   a. Lewis
   b. Bechert
   c. McPherson
   d. Landers

8) During eye surgery many different lens forceps may be used. Which of the following is *not* a lens forceps?
 a. Landers
 b. Simcoe
 c. Kelley Decemet
 d. Bechert

9) You are scrubbed on a scleral buckle procedure. The surgeon requests a sleeve-spreading forceps to aid in securing the silicone sleeve. You would hand him/her a(n):
 a. Nugent
 b. VanRens
 c. Iris
 d. Drysdale

10) A __________ is a fork retractor used mainly during retinal and orbital surgery.
 a. Bowman
 b. Schepens
 c. Serrefine
 d. DeMerres

11) The surgeon is performing an enucleation for cancer. The instrument used to insert the sphere is a:
 a. Carter
 b. Knapp
 c. Gass
 d. Greene

12) The surgeon requests a lacrimal sac retractor. You would hand him/her a(n):
 a. Arruga
 b. Moody
 c. Nugent
 d. Knapp

13) The surgeon is suturing and requests a tying forceps. You could hand him/her any of the following *except* a(n):
 a. McPherson
 b. Jameson
 c. Kelman-McPherson
 d. O'Gawa Castroviejo

14) You are scrubbed on cataract surgery. You know that the surgeon will need a lens nucleus prolapser next. In anticipation, you have the __________ ready to hand to him/her.
 a. Stone
 b. Lewis
 c. Colibri
 d. Schocket

15) A(n) ______________ is a type of capsulorrhexis forceps.
 a. Simcoe
 b. O'Gawa-Catroviejo
 c. O'Gawa-Utrata
 d. Braken-Farkas

16) The surgeon requests a capsule polisher. You would hand him/her a(n):
 a. Colibri
 b. Thornton
 c. Arruga
 d. Gills-Welch

8 Cardiothoracic and Vascular Instruments

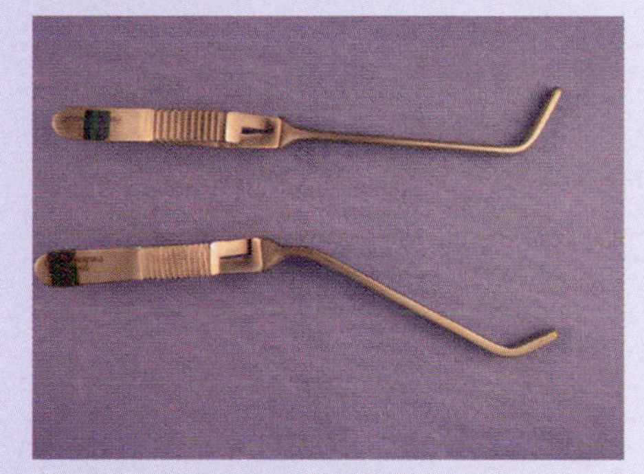

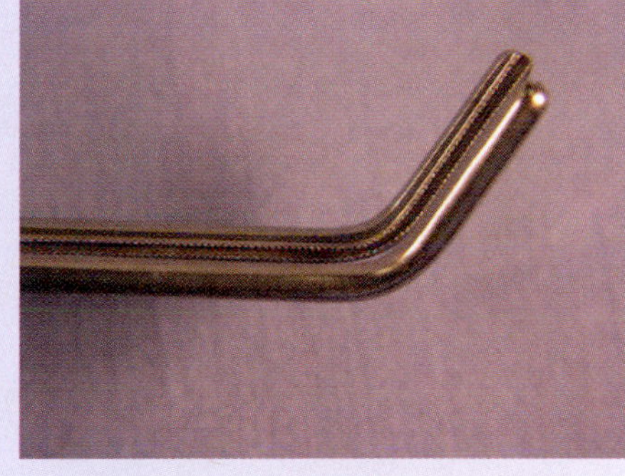

Name: DeBakey bulldog clamp

Alias: none

Category: clamping

Use: temporary occlusion of peripheral blood vessels

Length: 3"to 4.5"

Additional Information: atraumatic jaws; jaws can be 20 mm, 30 mm, 45 mm, or 60 mm long; can be reusable or disposable

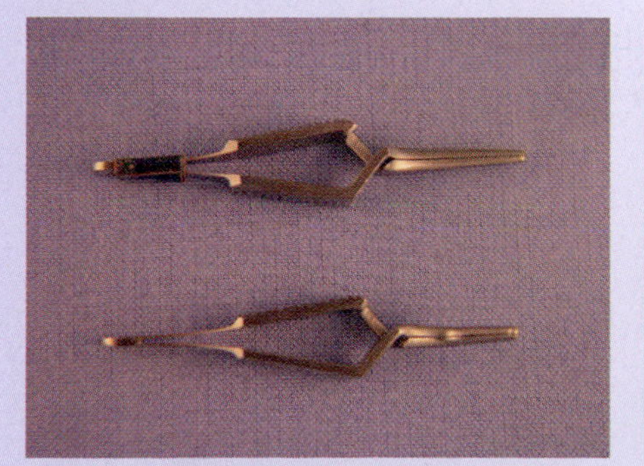

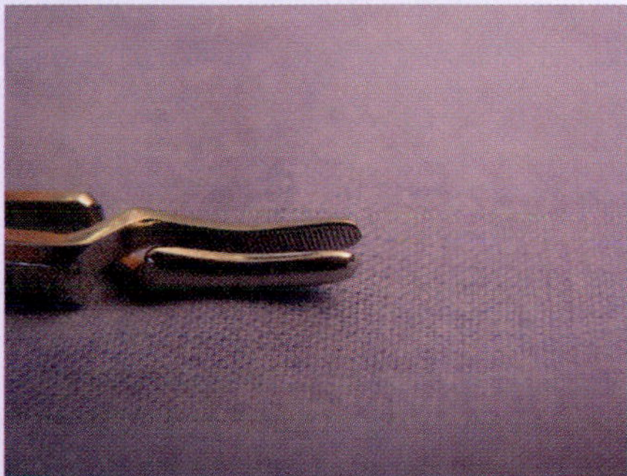

Name: Diethrich bulldog clamp

Alias: none

Category: clamping

Use: temporary occlusion of small peripheral blood vessels; can be used as a suture tag

Length: 2"

Additional Information: straight or curved jaws; jaws can be 8 mm, 12 mm, or 20 mm long

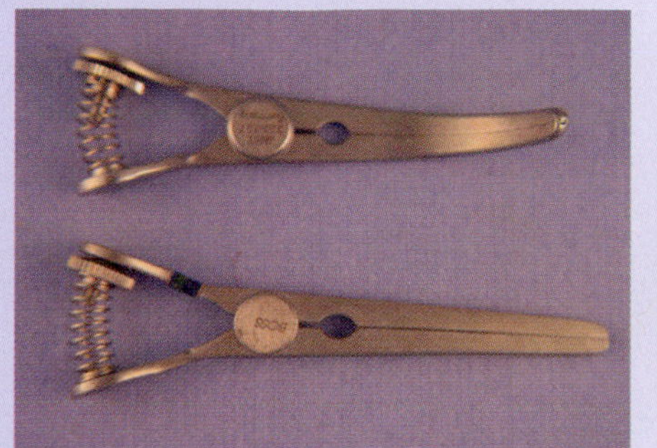

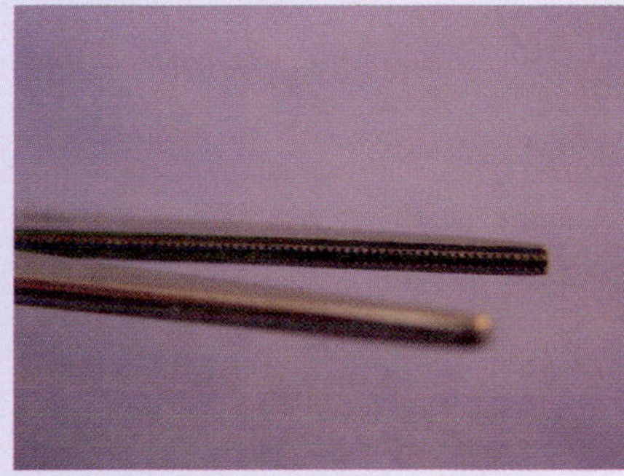

Name: Glover bulldog clamp

Alias: none

Category: clamping

Use: temporary occlusion of peripheral blood vessels

Length: 2" to 4.75"

Additional Information: straight or curved jaws; jaw length 1.8 cm to 6cm

Name: Cooley ring-handled bulldog clamp

Alias: none

Category: clamping

Use: clamping medium size blood vessels

Length: 5.75"

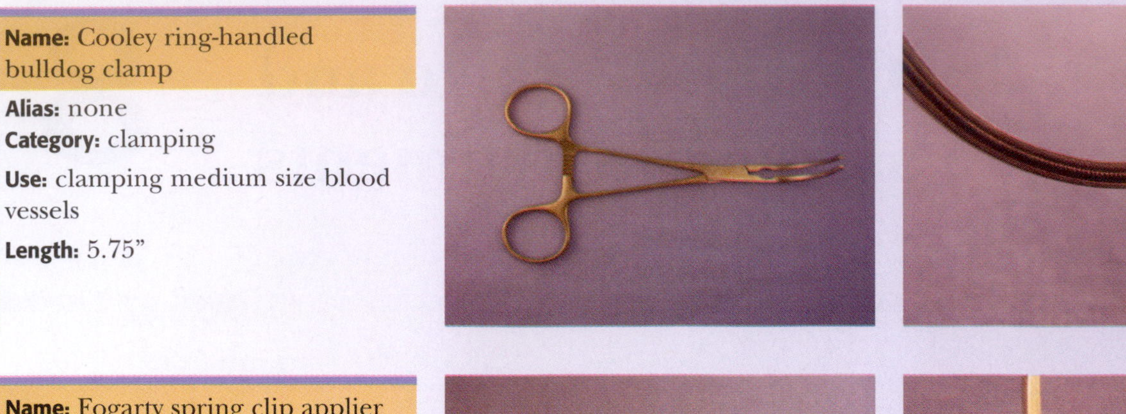

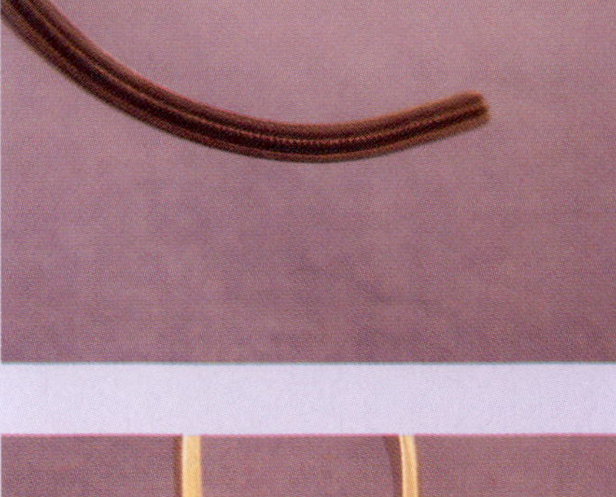

Name: Fogarty spring clip applier

Alias: bulldog applier

Category: clamping

Use: applying single use spring clips (bulldogs)

Length: 7"

Additional Information: come in sizes to apply 6 mm or 12 mm clips

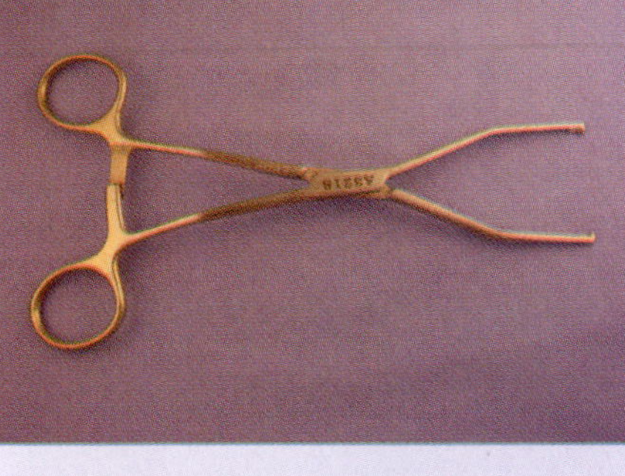

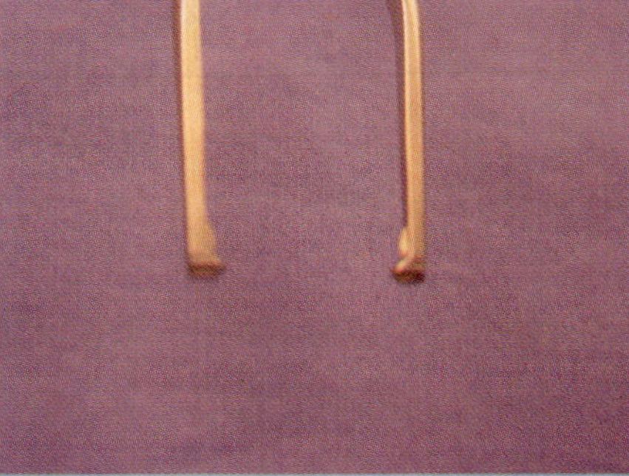

Name: Bulldog applying forceps

Alias: none

Category: grasping

Use: applying bulldog clamps during cardiac/vascular procedures

Length: 9"

Additional Information: angled tips

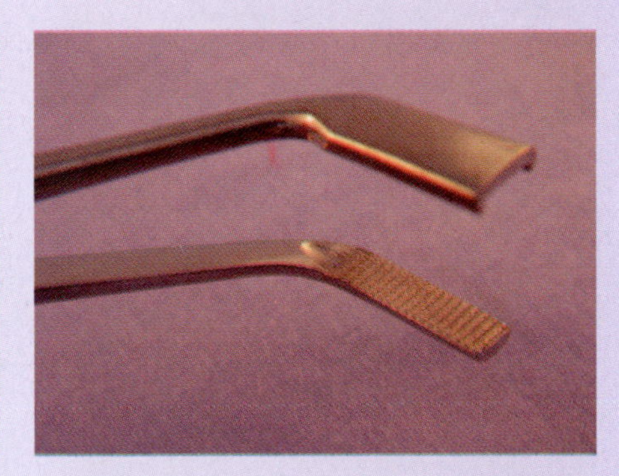

Name: Javid carotid graft clamp

Alias: carotid shunt clamp

Category: clamping

Use: holding temporary bypass graft in place

Length: 6.25" or 7"

Additional Information: angled jaws 4 mm or 6 mm

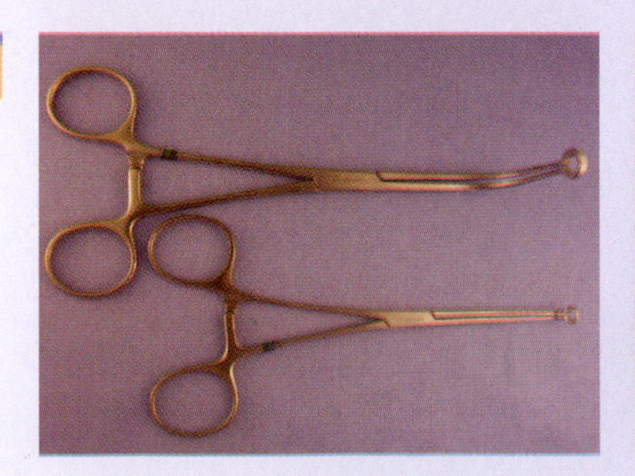

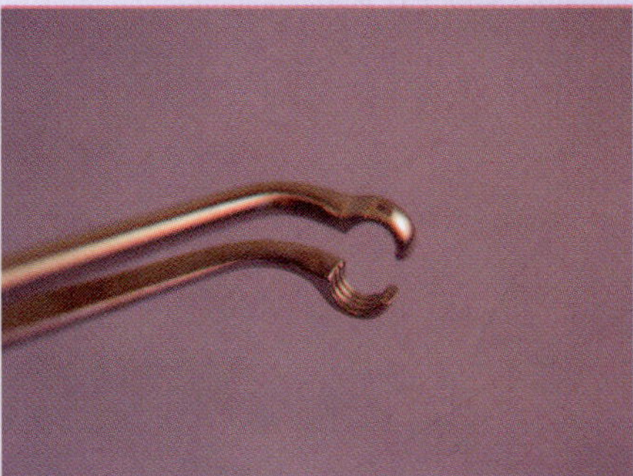

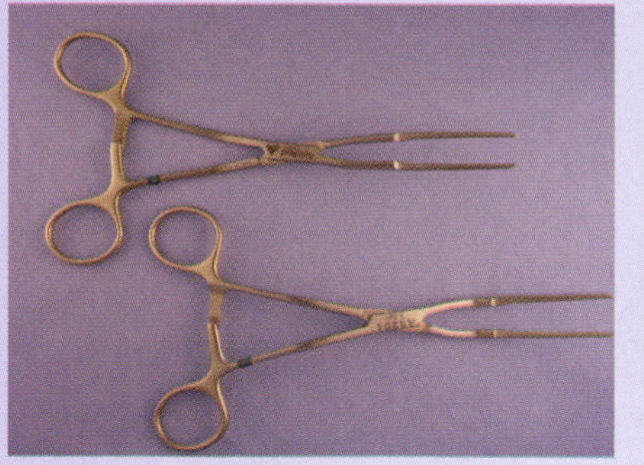

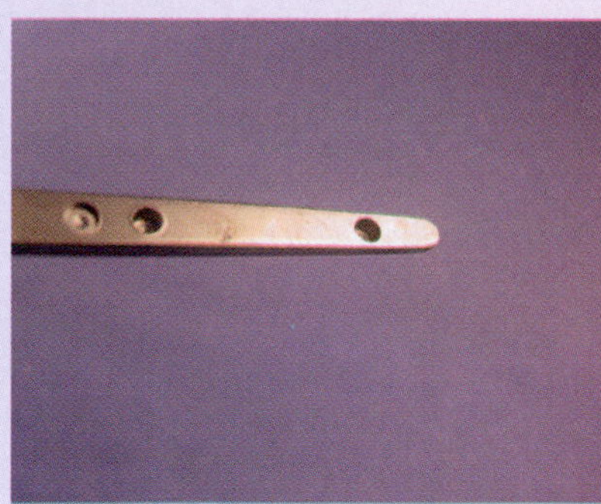

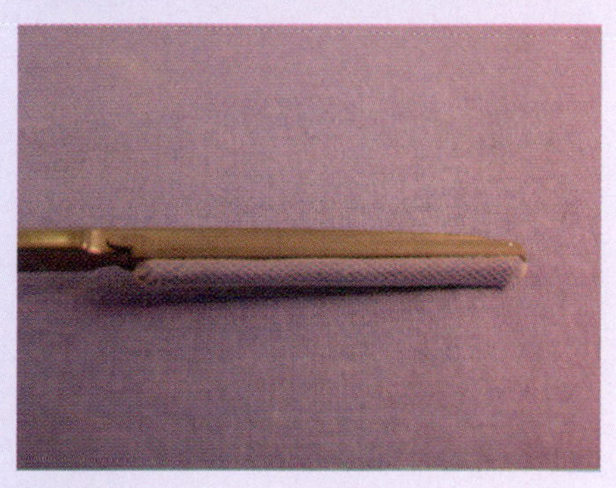

Name: Fogarty hydragrip clamp

Alias: none

Category: clamping

Use: occluding arteries

Length: 4.5" (curved); 6.5" (straight)

Additional Information: replaceable jaw inserts permit occlusion with minimal trauma to blood vessel

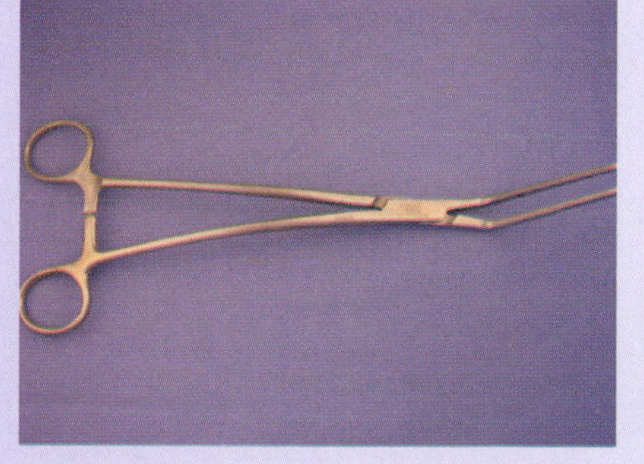

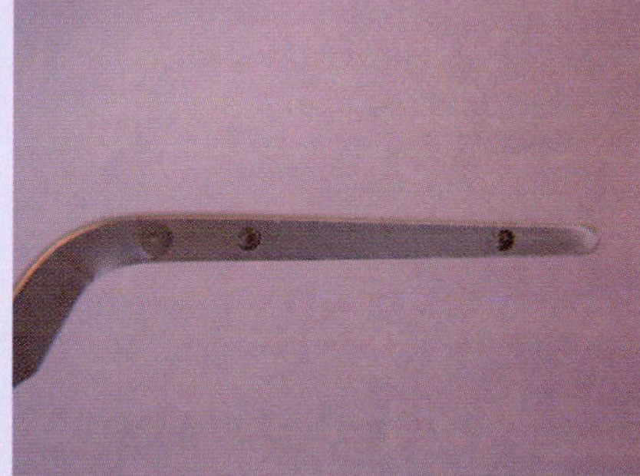

Name: Fogarty aortic cross clamp

Alias: none

Category: clamping

Use: cross clamping the aorta

Length: 8.5"

Additional Information: jaws use 61 mm inserts

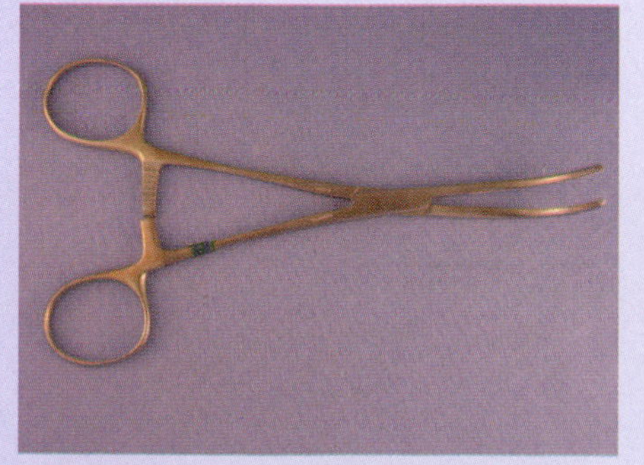

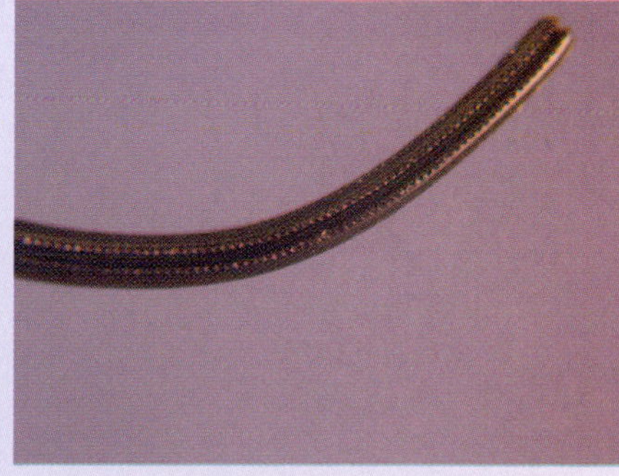

Name: DeBakey aorta clamp

Alias: none

Category: clamping

Use: total occlusion of blood flow in the aorta

Length: 7.25"

Additional Information: curved shanks; atraumatic jaws

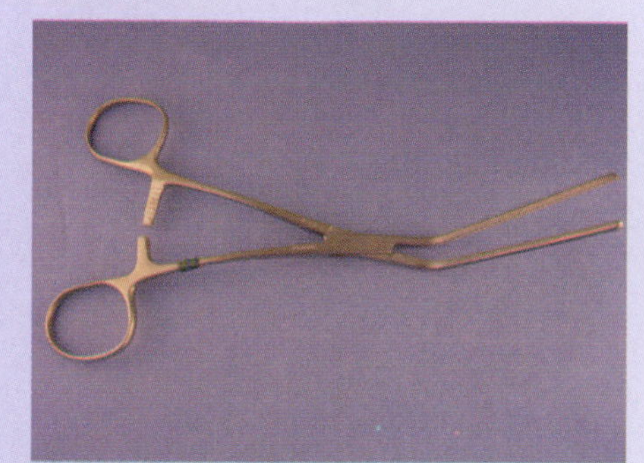

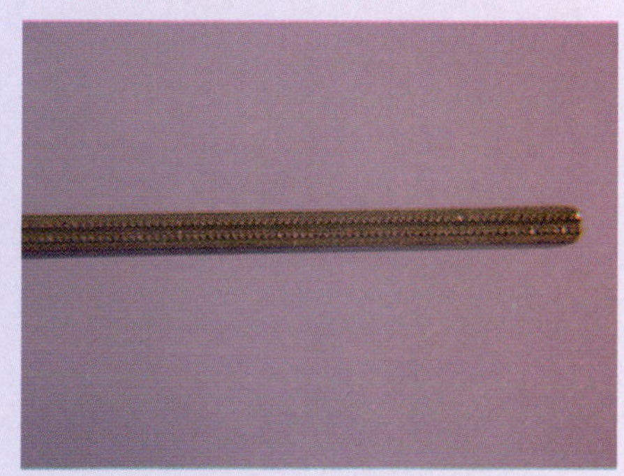

Name: DeBakey peripheral vascular clamp

Alias: DeBakey multi-purpose clamp

Category: clamping

Use: occluding blood vessels

Length: 8.25", 9", or 12"

Additional Information: atraumatic jaws; jaws angled 60 degrees

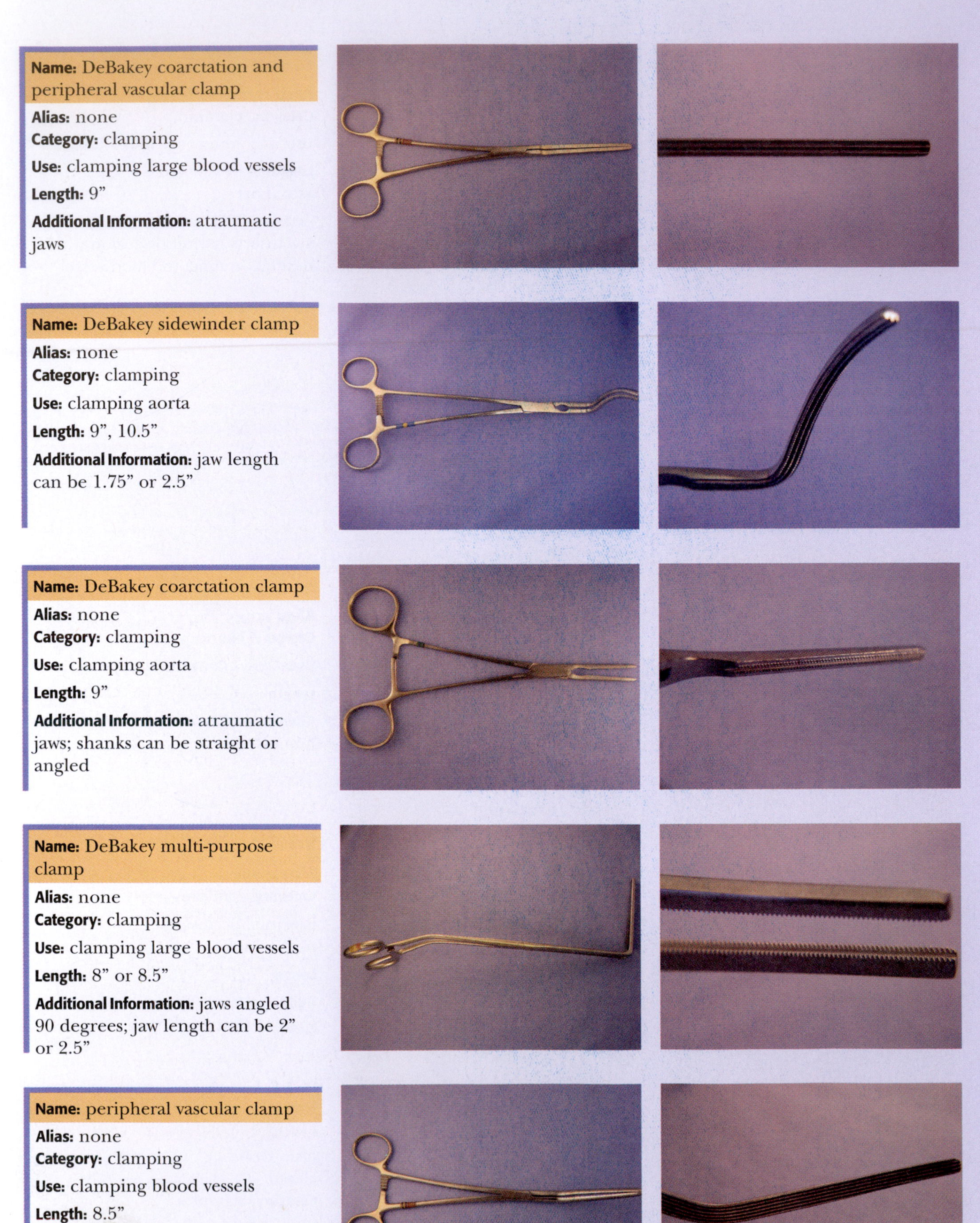

Name: DeBakey coarctation and peripheral vascular clamp

Alias: none

Category: clamping

Use: clamping large blood vessels

Length: 9"

Additional Information: atraumatic jaws

Name: DeBakey sidewinder clamp

Alias: none

Category: clamping

Use: clamping aorta

Length: 9", 10.5"

Additional Information: jaw length can be 1.75" or 2.5"

Name: DeBakey coarctation clamp

Alias: none

Category: clamping

Use: clamping aorta

Length: 9"

Additional Information: atraumatic jaws; shanks can be straight or angled

Name: DeBakey multi-purpose clamp

Alias: none

Category: clamping

Use: clamping large blood vessels

Length: 8" or 8.5"

Additional Information: jaws angled 90 degrees; jaw length can be 2" or 2.5"

Name: peripheral vascular clamp

Alias: none

Category: clamping

Use: clamping blood vessels

Length: 8.5"

Additional Information: vertical serrations

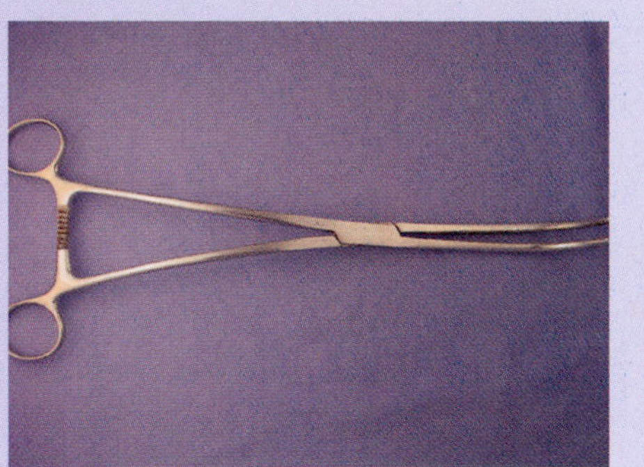
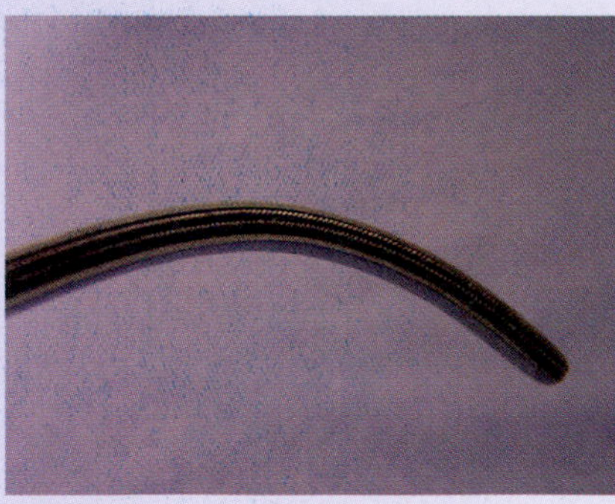

Name: Cooley cardiovascular clamp
Alias: none
Category: clamping
Use: temporary occlusion of the iliac artery during aortic aneurysm repair
Length: 10.75"
Additional Information: jaw length can be 7 cm or 7.3 cm

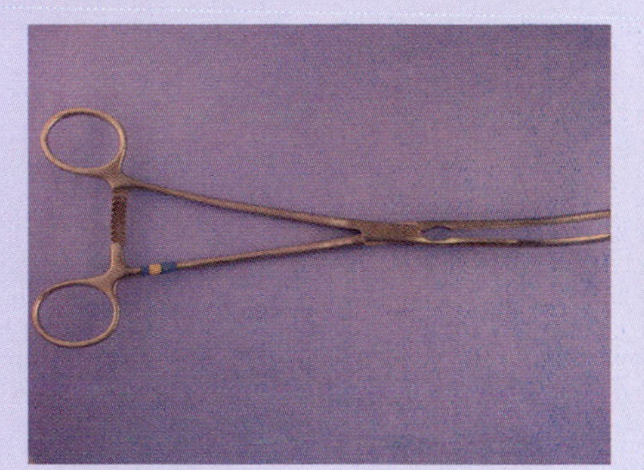
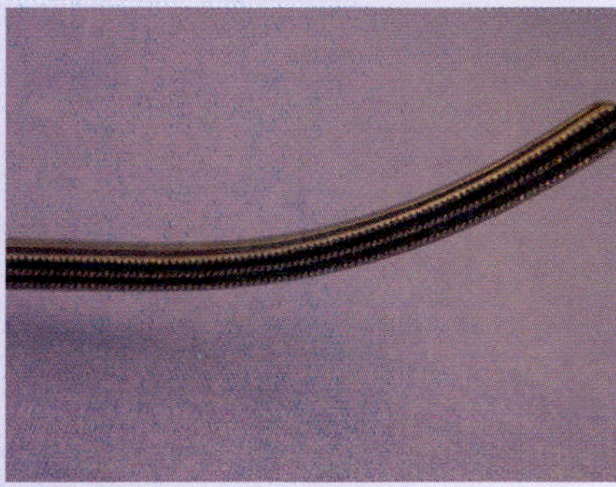

Name: Cooley coarctation clamp
Alias: none
Category: clamping
Use: clamping aorta
Length: 10.5"

Name: Satinsky clamp
Alias: Debakey partial occlusion clamp
Category: clamping
Use: partial occlusion of blood vessel—occludes blood flow to area clamped off but allows flow to continue through the rest of the vessel
Length: 9.5" or 10"
Additional Information: atraumatic jaws; jaw length 3.5 cm to 7.5 cm

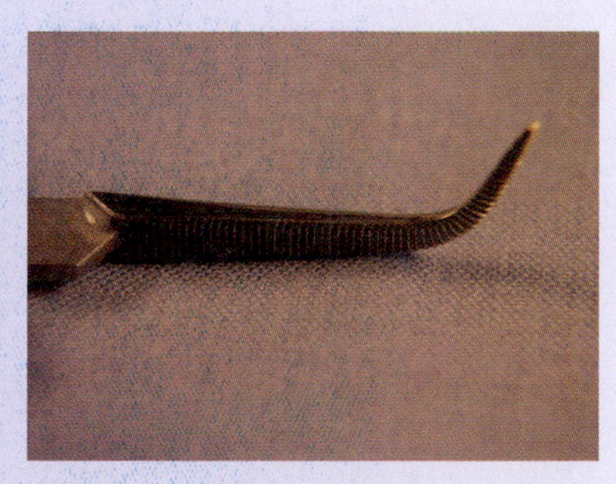

Name: Gemini artery forceps
Alias: right angle; mixter
Category: clamping
Use: clamping fine peripheral arteries; passing tie or loop underneath a vessel
Length: 5.5" to 11"
Additional Information: fully serrated jaws; jaws have fine "J" curve

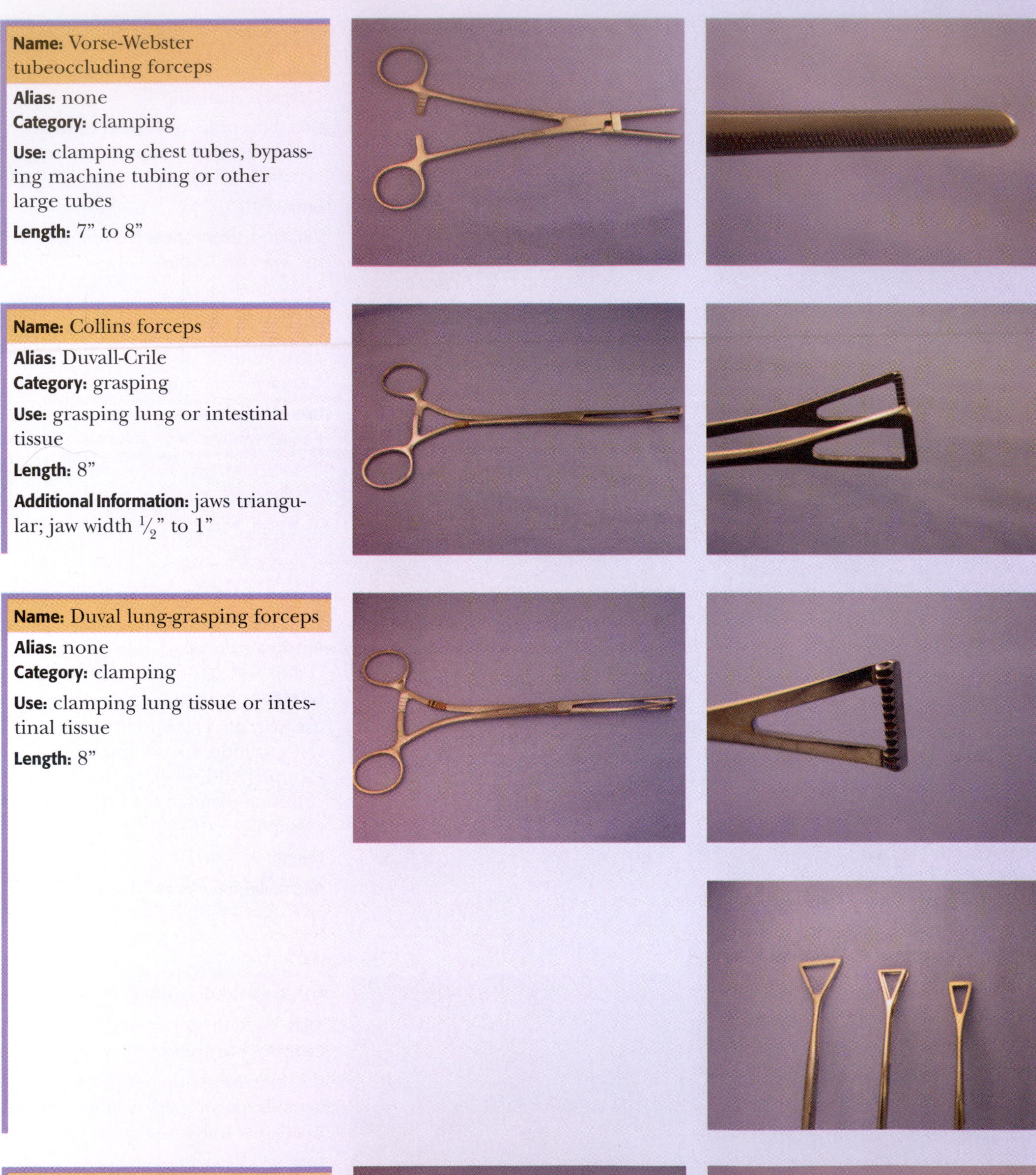

Name: Vorse-Webster tubeoccluding forceps

Alias: none

Category: clamping

Use: clamping chest tubes, bypassing machine tubing or other large tubes

Length: 7" to 8"

Name: Collins forceps

Alias: Duvall-Crile

Category: grasping

Use: grasping lung or intestinal tissue

Length: 8"

Additional Information: jaws triangular; jaw width $\frac{1}{2}$" to 1"

Name: Duval lung-grasping forceps

Alias: none

Category: clamping

Use: clamping lung tissue or intestinal tissue

Length: 8"

Name: Sarot bronchus clamp

Alias: none

Category: clamping

Use: clamping bronchus during lung surgery

Length: 9"

Additional Information: comes in right- and left-side styles

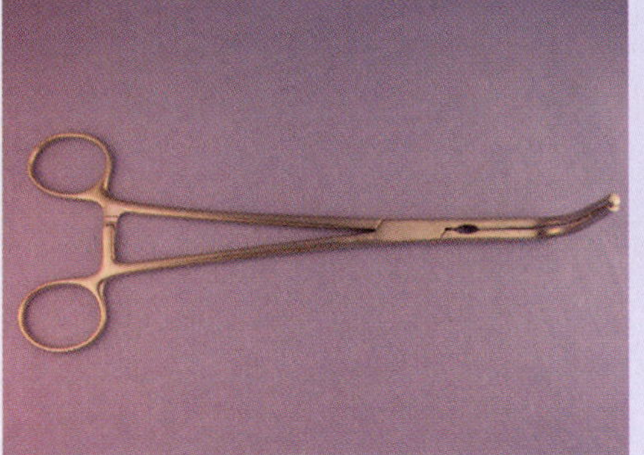

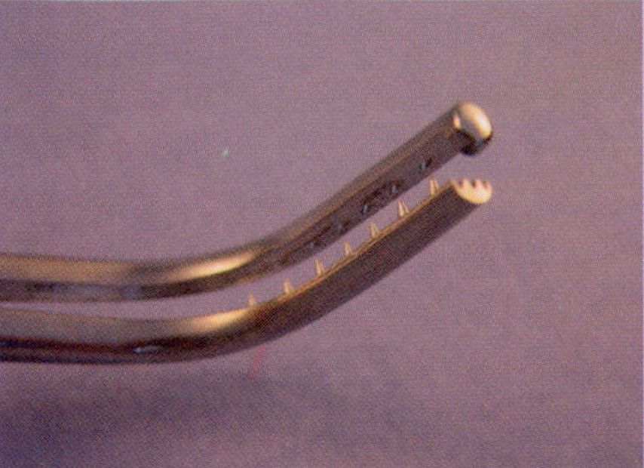

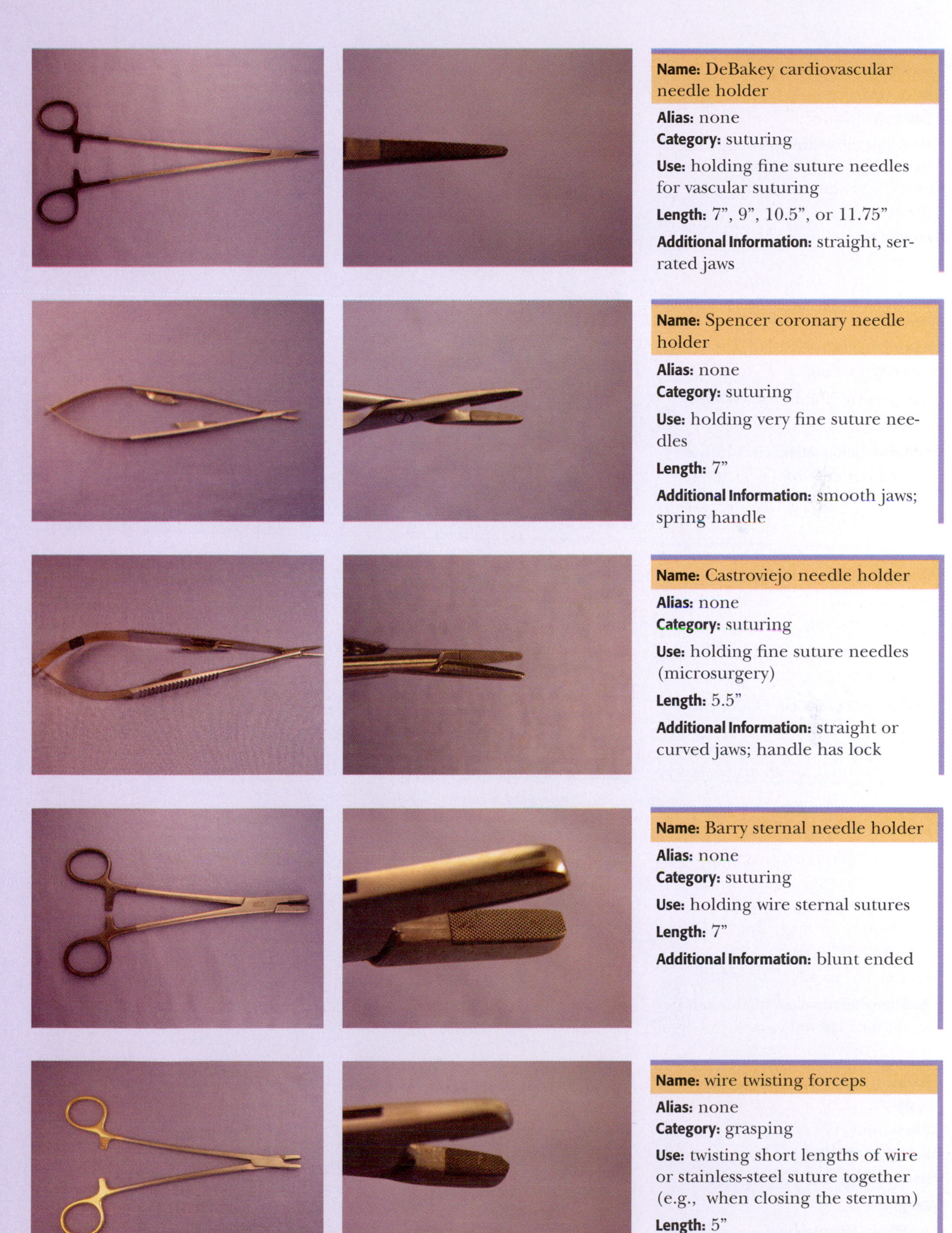

Name: DeBakey cardiovascular needle holder

Alias: none

Category: suturing

Use: holding fine suture needles for vascular suturing

Length: 7", 9", 10.5", or 11.75"

Additional Information: straight, serrated jaws

Name: Spencer coronary needle holder

Alias: none

Category: suturing

Use: holding very fine suture needles

Length: 7"

Additional Information: smooth jaws; spring handle

Name: Castroviejo needle holder

Alias: none

Category: suturing

Use: holding fine suture needles (microsurgery)

Length: 5.5"

Additional Information: straight or curved jaws; handle has lock

Name: Barry sternal needle holder

Alias: none

Category: suturing

Use: holding wire sternal sutures

Length: 7"

Additional Information: blunt ended

Name: wire twisting forceps

Alias: none

Category: grasping

Use: twisting short lengths of wire or stainless-steel suture together (e.g., when closing the sternum)

Length: 5"

Name: Rummel stylet

Alias: none

Category: suture

Use: pulling suture through rubber choker (chokers used to hold aortic and venous cannulas in place)

Length: 8"

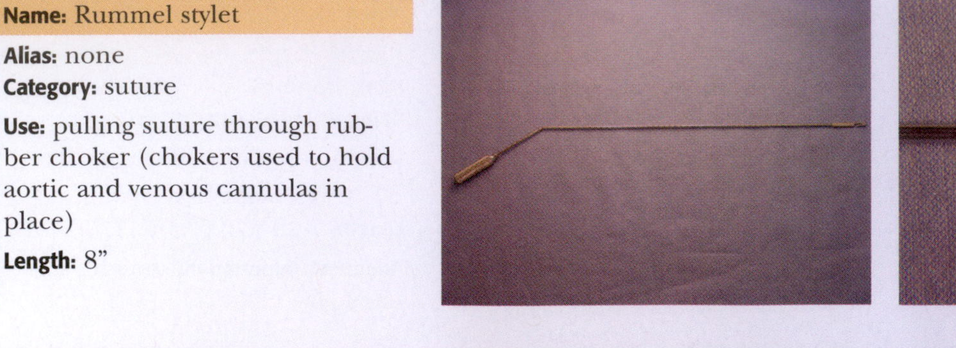

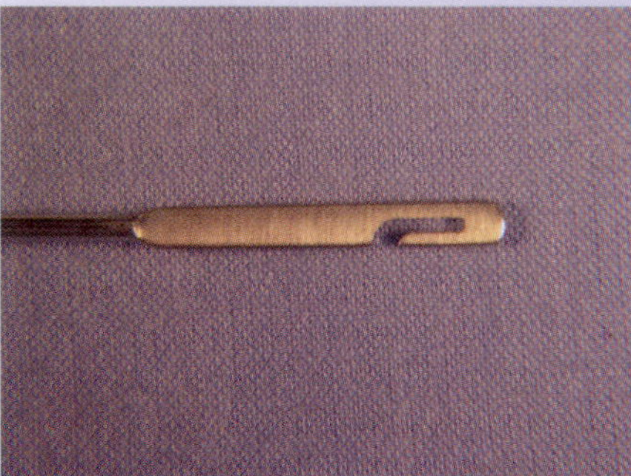

Name: Lawrie scissors

Alias: Duckbill scissors

Category: cutting

Use: cutting fine blood vessels

Length: 7"

Additional Information: circumflex jaws

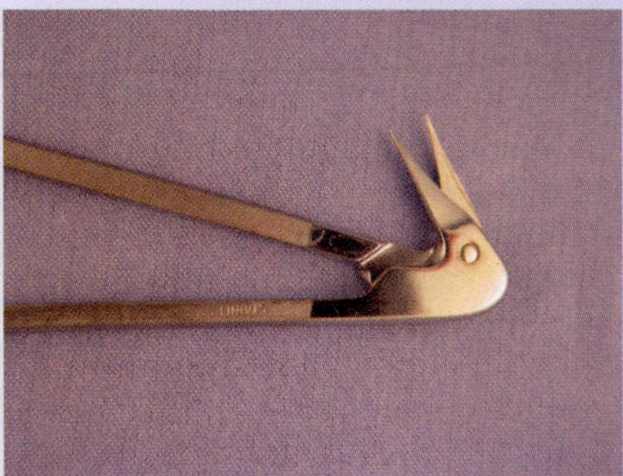

Name: Potts-Smith scissors

Alias: none

Category: cutting

Use: cutting fine blood vessels

Length: 5.25" to 7"

Additional Information: blades can have 25-, 45-, or 60-degree angle; blades can be delicate or standard; essential for an arteriotomy

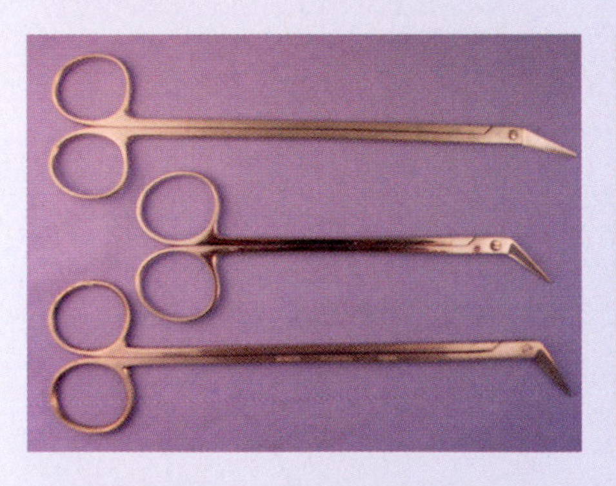

Name: Tenotomy scissors

Alias: dolphin-nose scissors; Stevens scissors

Category: cutting

Use: cutting or dissecting fine tissue or blood vessels

Length: 3.5" to 4.5"

Additional Information: blades can be straight or curved

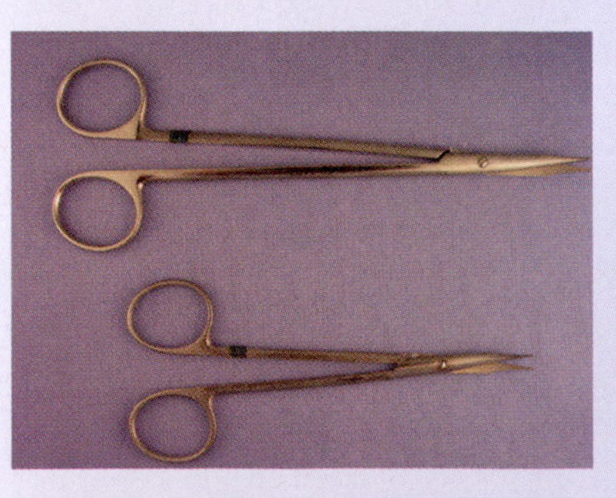

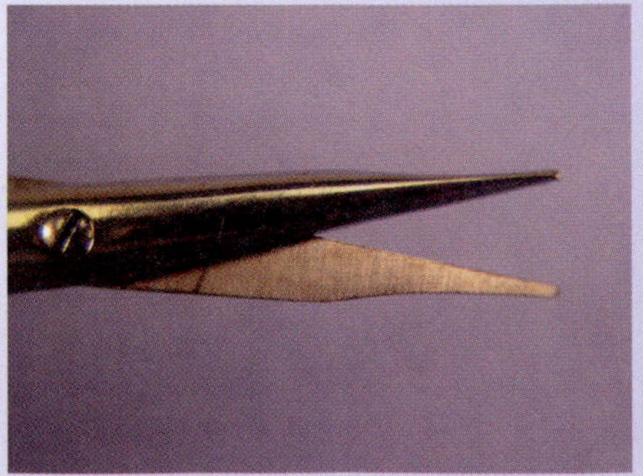

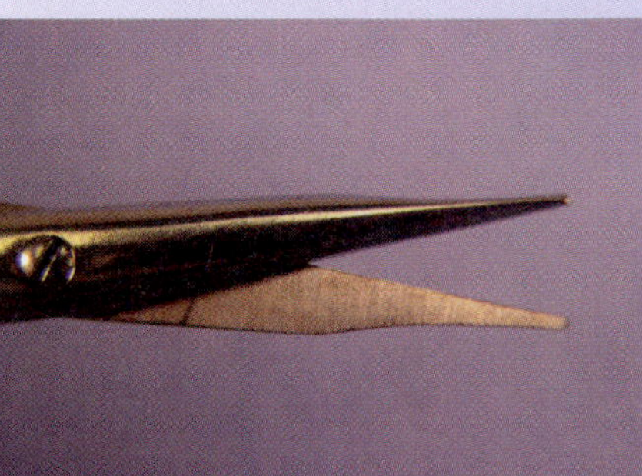

Name: Castroviejo microcorneal scissors

Alias: none

Category: cutting

Use: cutting fine blood vessels

Length: 4"

Additional Information: curved blades

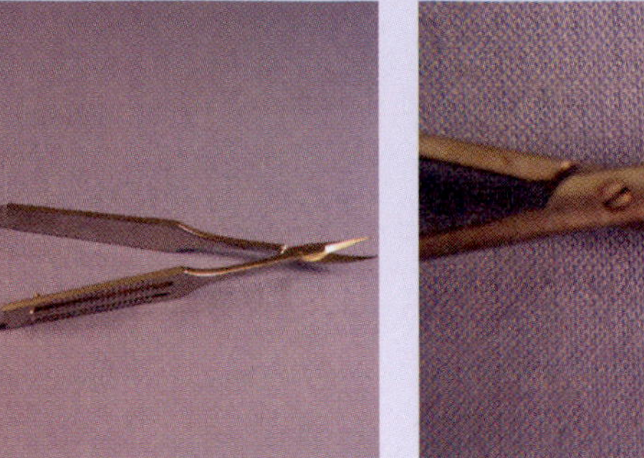

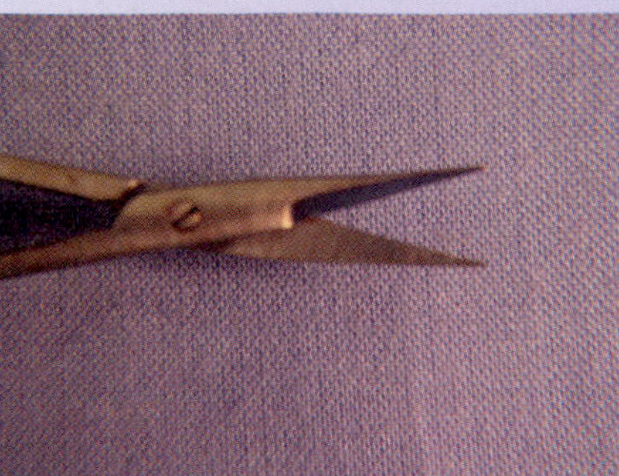

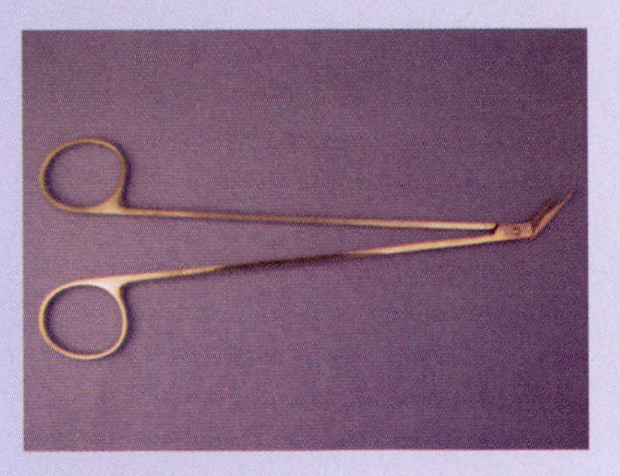
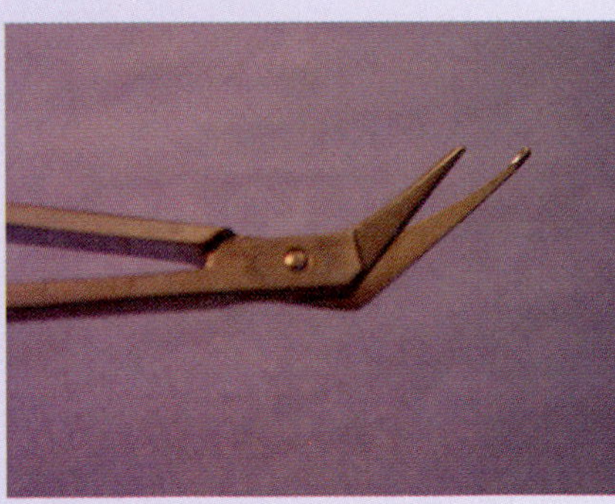

Name: Cooley vascular scissors

Alias: none

Category: cutting

Use: cutting small blood vessels

Length: 7.25"

Additional Information: 1 mm or 1.5 mm probe on the scissors tip

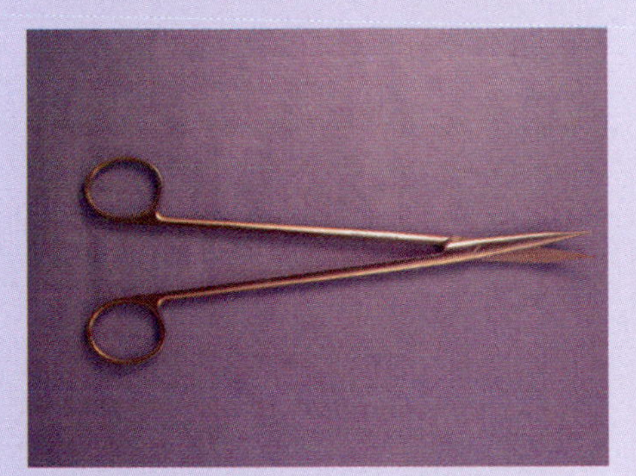
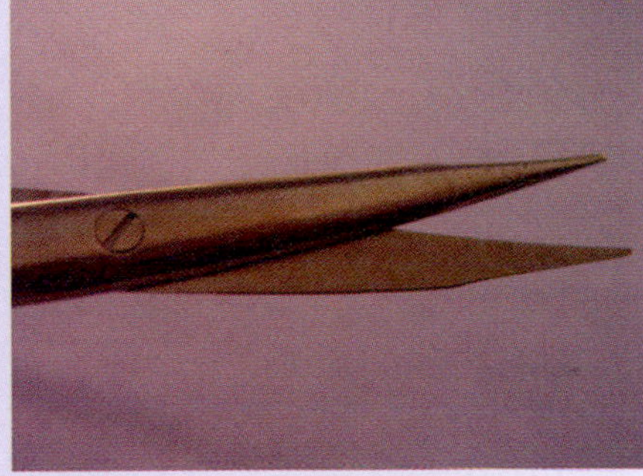

Name: Jameson scissors

Alias: none

Category: cutting

Use: tissue dissection

Length: 5.5" or 7"

Additional Information: curved blades

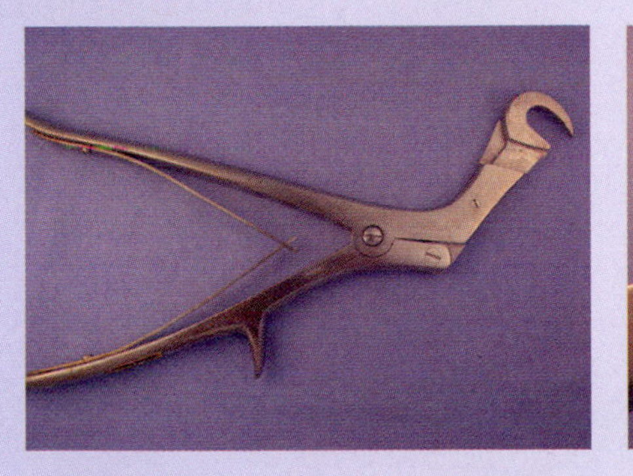
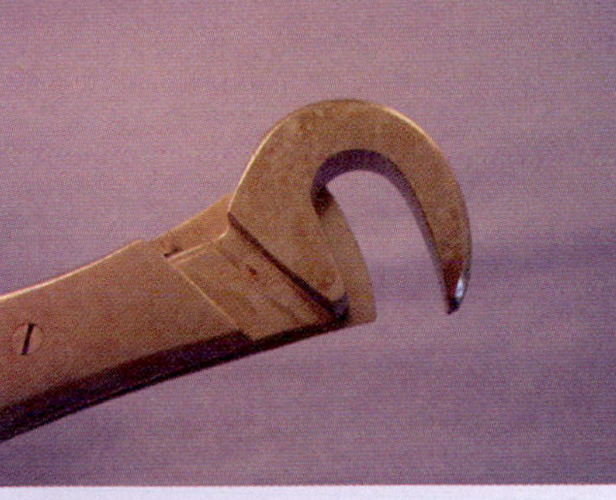

Name: Giertz-Shoemaker rib shears

Alias: none

Category: cutting

Use: cutting ribs

Length: 9.75"

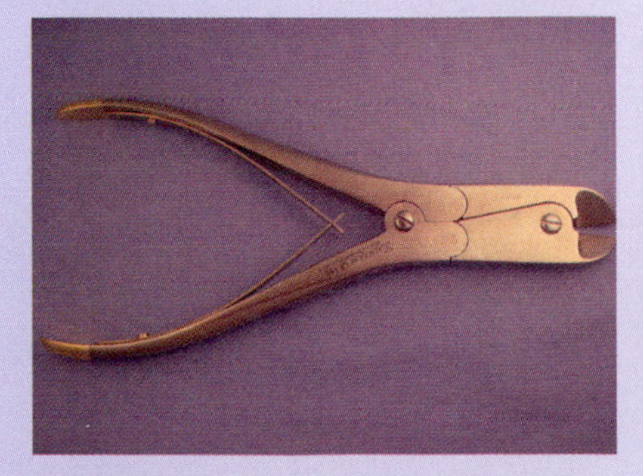
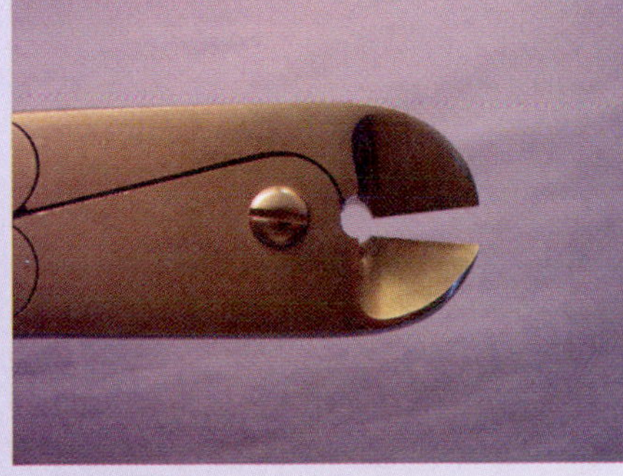

Name: wire-cutting pliers

Alias: double-action parallel pliers

Category: cutting

Use: cutting wire or stainless-steel suture

Length: n/a

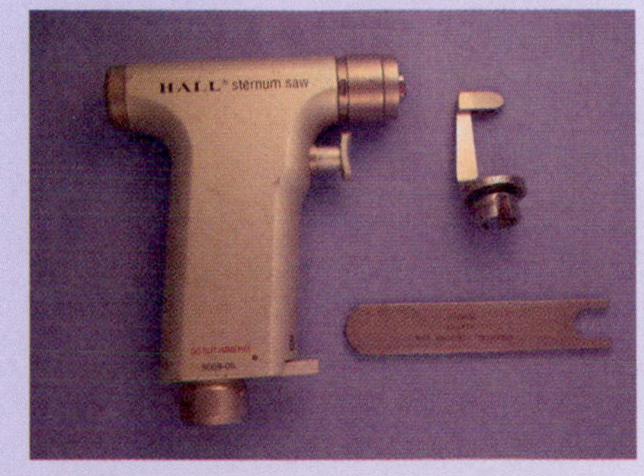

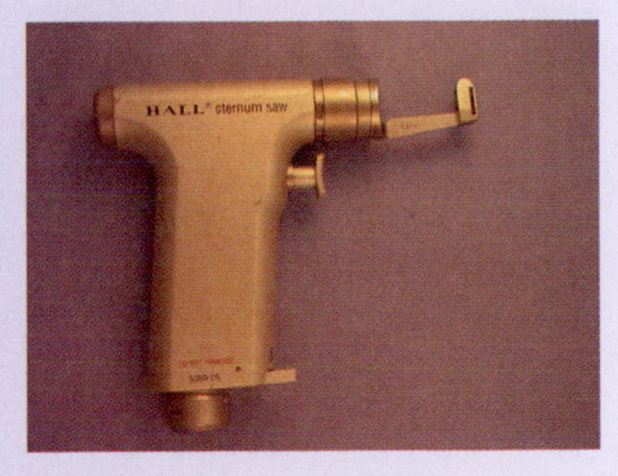

Name: Hall sternal saw

Alias: none

Category: cutting

Use: cutting through sternum

Length: n/a

Additional Information: attaches to a nitrogen source for power

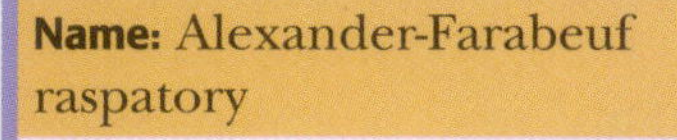

Name: Alexander-Farabeuf raspatory

Alias: Alexander double-ended costal periosteotome
Category: cutting

Use: removing cartilage and tissue from bone

Length: 8.5"

Additional Information: double ended

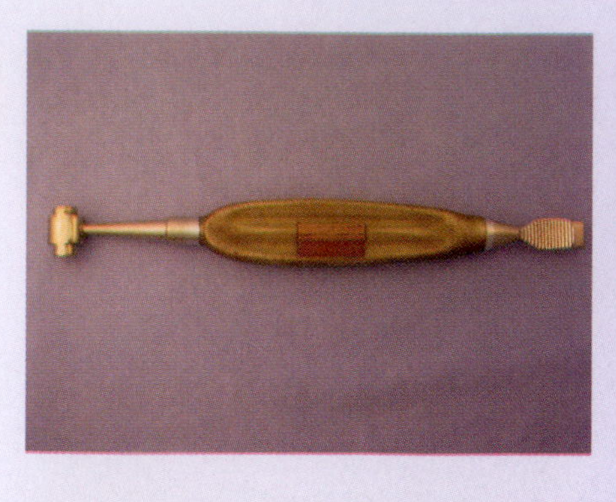

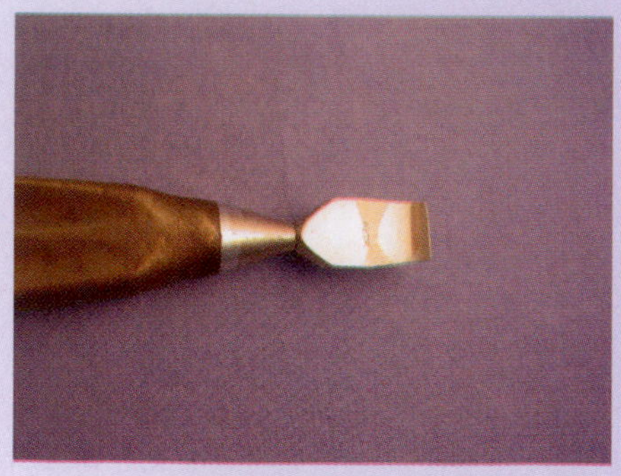

Name: Doyen rib raspatory

Alias: rib stripper and elevator; Doyen coastal elevators; pigtails
Category: cutting

Use: removing tissue and cartilage from ribs

Length: 7"

Additional Information: available with left or right blade

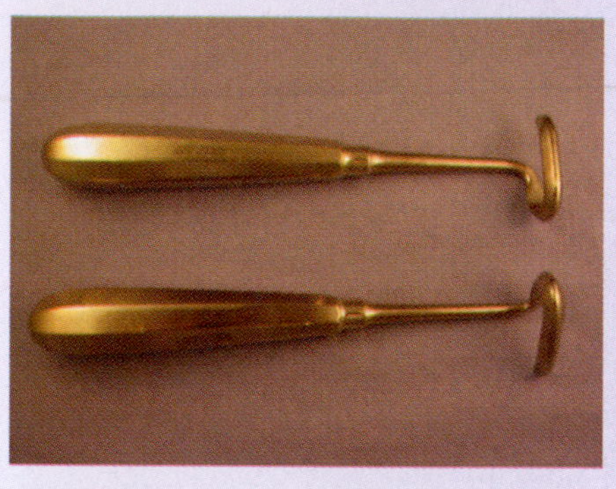

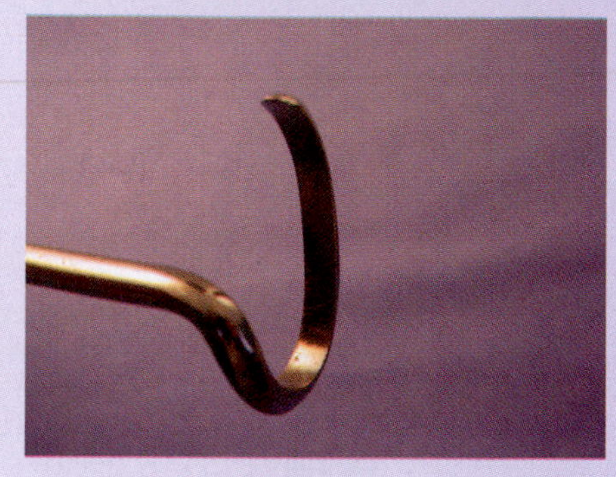

Name: Matson raspatory

Alias: Matson rib stripper
Category: cutting

Use: removing peristeum from ribs

Length: 8.75"

Additional Information: also comes in pediatric size (5.5")

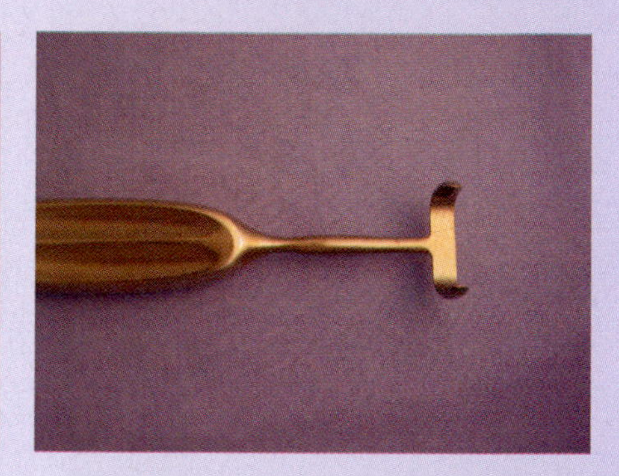

Name: Semb raspatory

Alias: none
Category: cutting

Use: removing peristeum from bone

Length: n/a

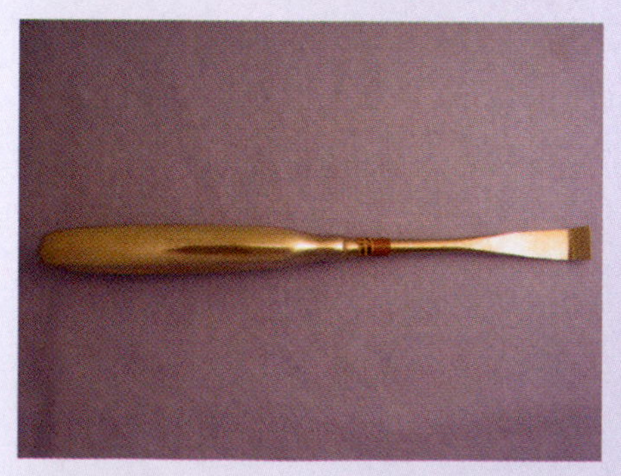

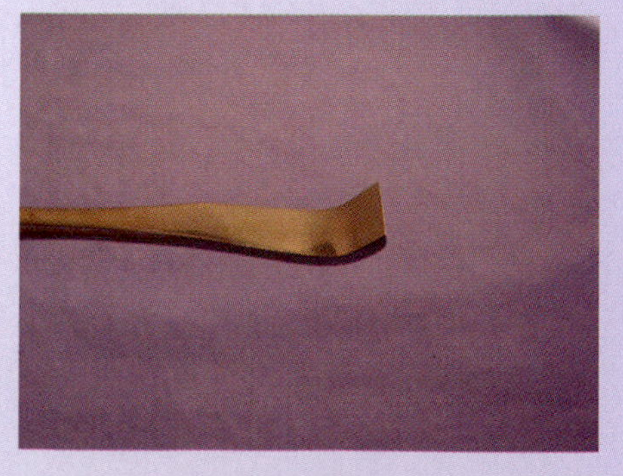

Name: Leather valvulotome

Alias: modified Mills vulvulotome
Category: cutting

Use: cutting heart valve

Length: 9.5" or 13"

Additional Information: retrograde instrument has cutting blade on the inside of the tip; antegrade instrument has cutting blade on the leading edge of the tip

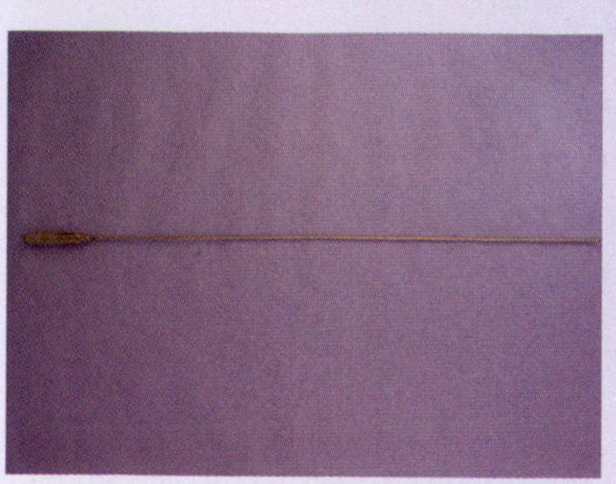

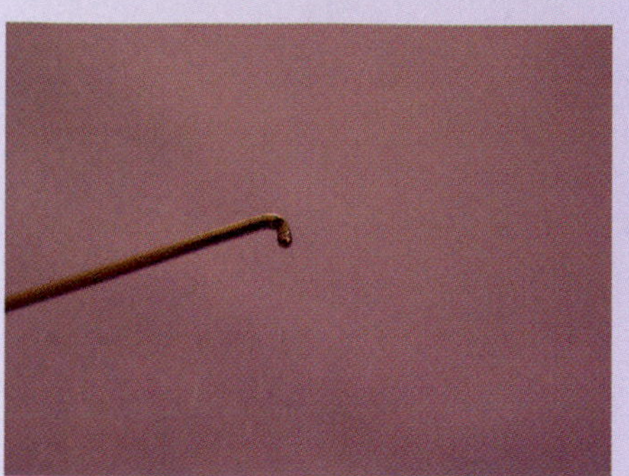

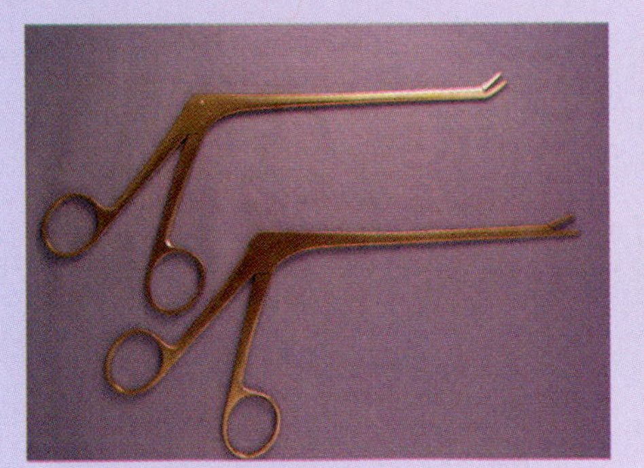

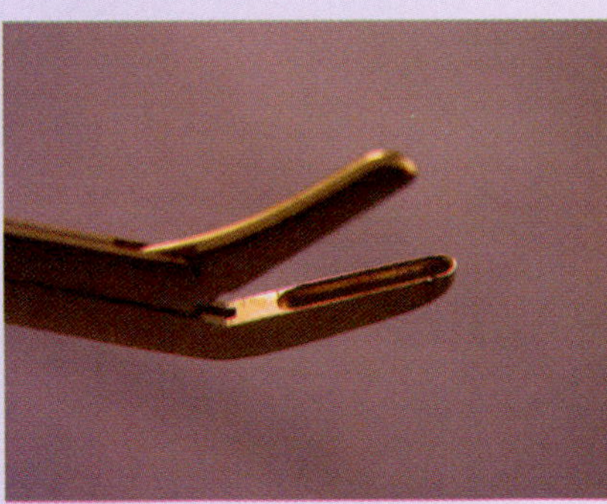

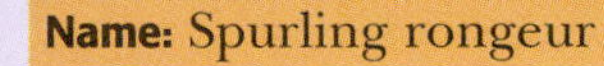

Name: Spurling rongeur

Alias: Spurling intervertebral disc rongeur

Category: cutting

Use: removing bits of tissue or calcium deposits

Length: shaft is 6” or 7”

Additional Information: jaws can be straight, up, or down

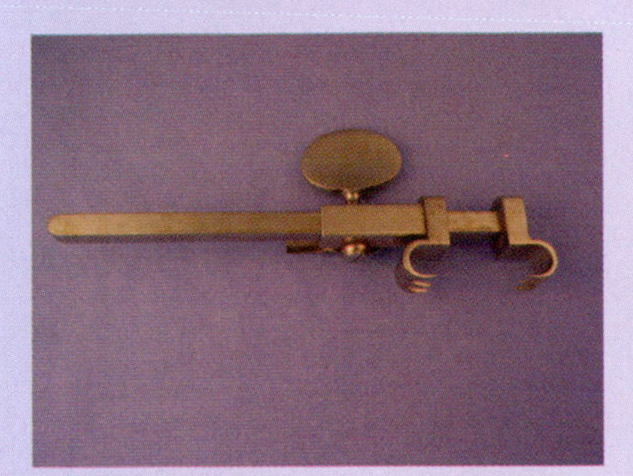

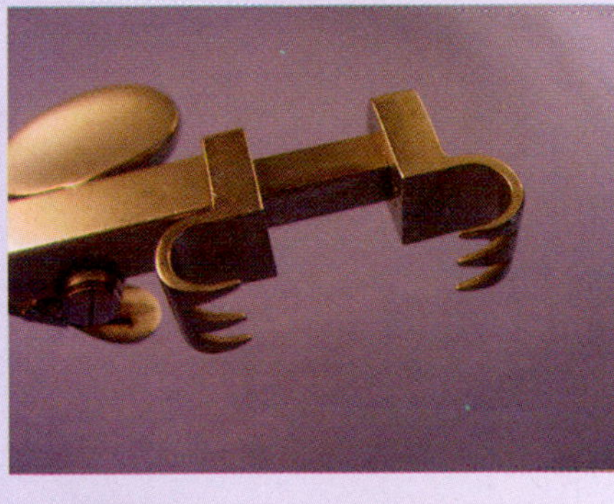

Name: Bailey-Gibbon rib contractor

Alias: Bailey rib approximator

Category: accessory

Use: contracting ribs back together

Length: 7”

Additional Information: can have ½” or 1 3/8” arms

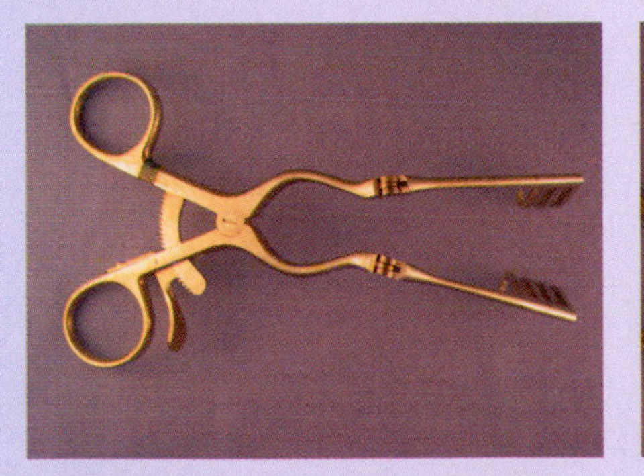

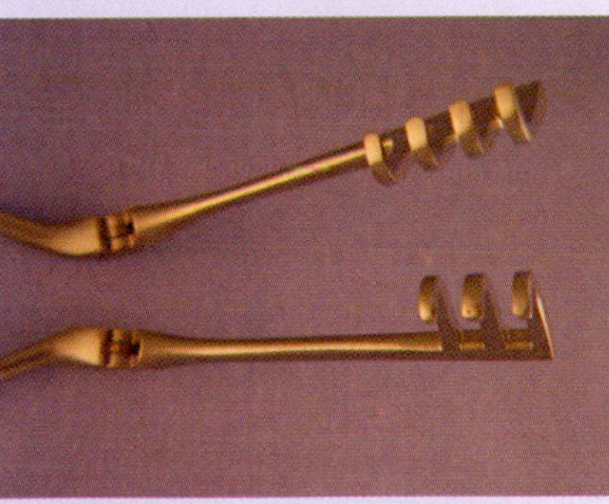

Name: Beckmann retractor

Alias: none

Category: retracting

Use: retracting tissue

Length: 6.75”

Additional Information: hinged shanks; 3 × 4 prongs

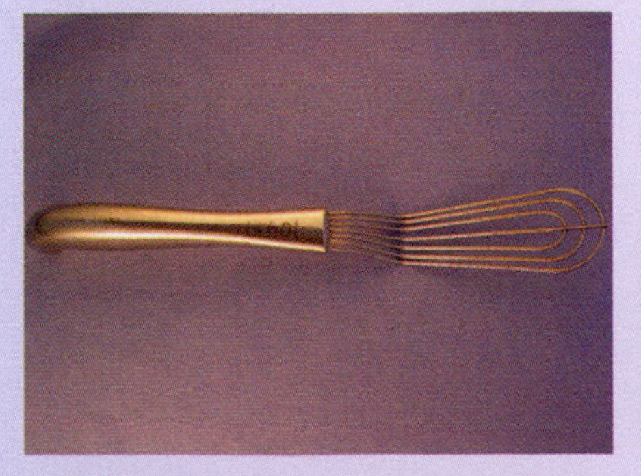

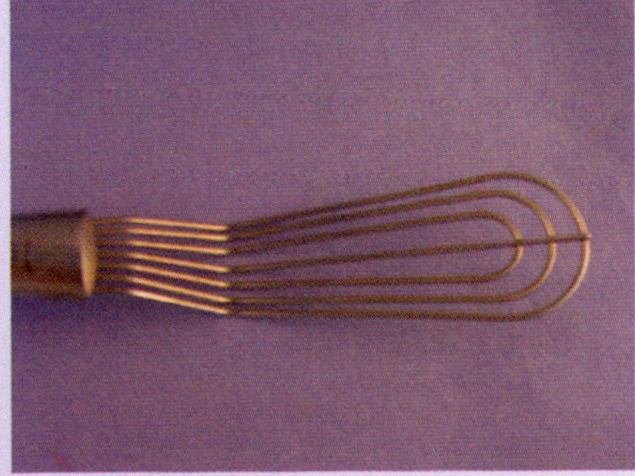

Name: Allison lung retractor

Alias: eggbeaters

Category: retracting

Use: retracting lung

Length: 10.5” or 12.5”

Additional Information: blade can be 1.5” or 2.5” wide

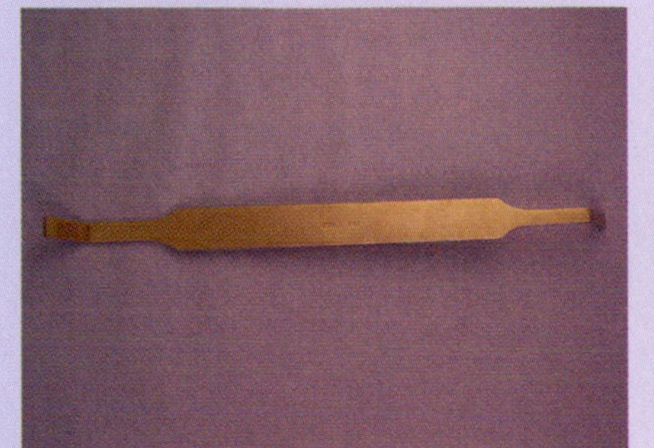

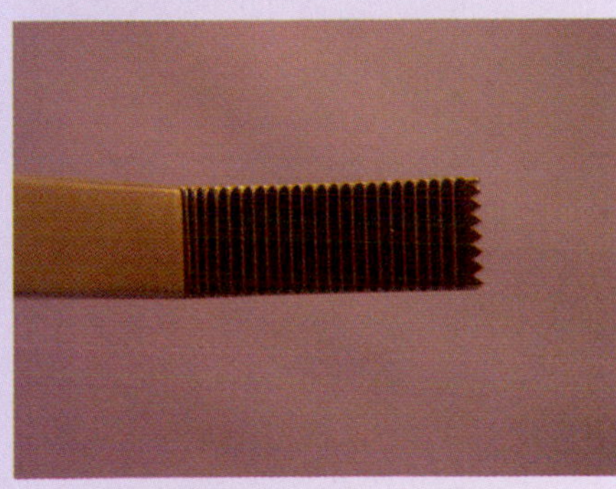

Name: atrial valve retractor

Alias: none

Category: retracting

Use: retracting atrial valve during cardiac surgery

Length: 8”

Additional Information: serrated ends with teeth

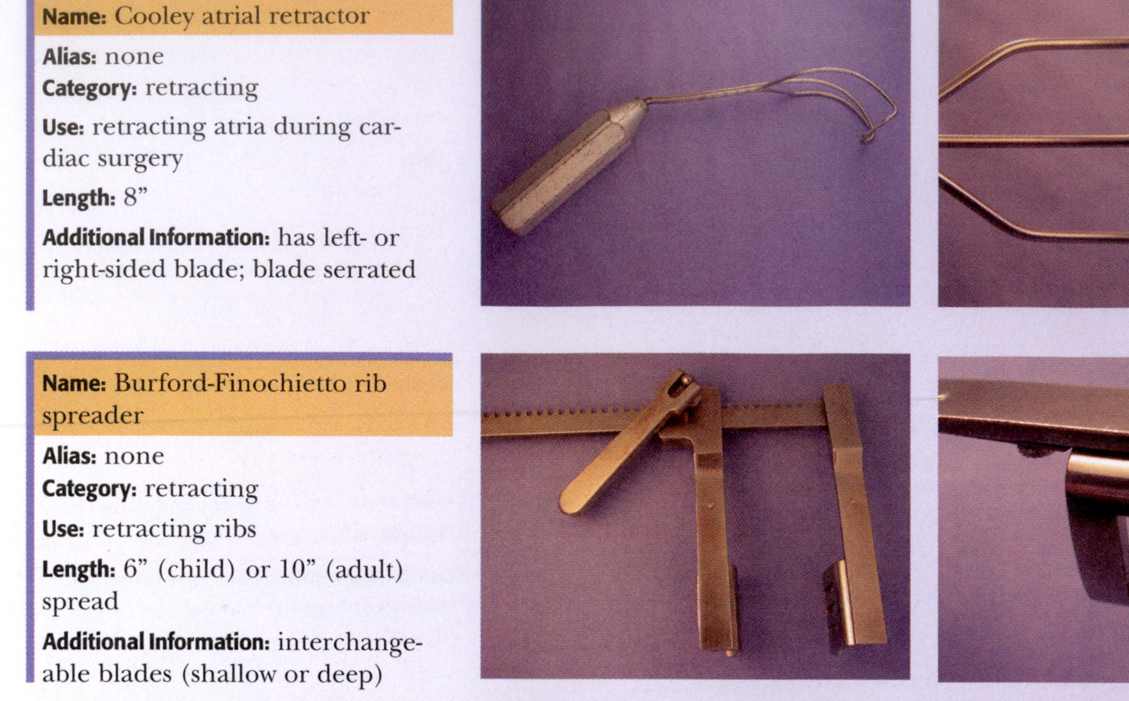

Name: Cooley atrial retractor
Alias: none
Category: retracting
Use: retracting atria during cardiac surgery
Length: 8”
Additional Information: has left- or right-sided blade; blade serrated

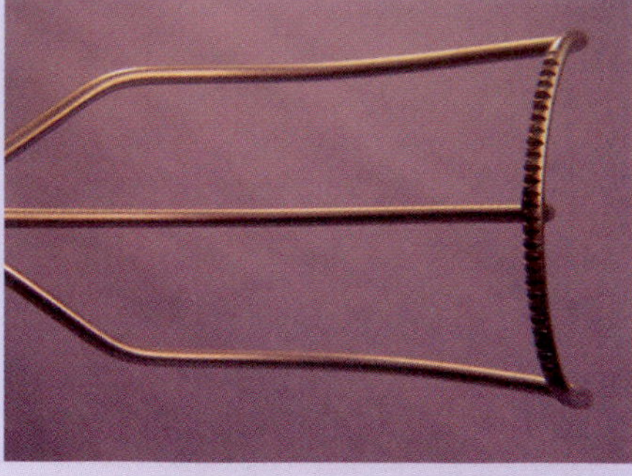

Name: Burford-Finochietto rib spreader
Alias: none
Category: retracting
Use: retracting ribs
Length: 6” (child) or 10” (adult) spread
Additional Information: interchangeable blades (shallow or deep)

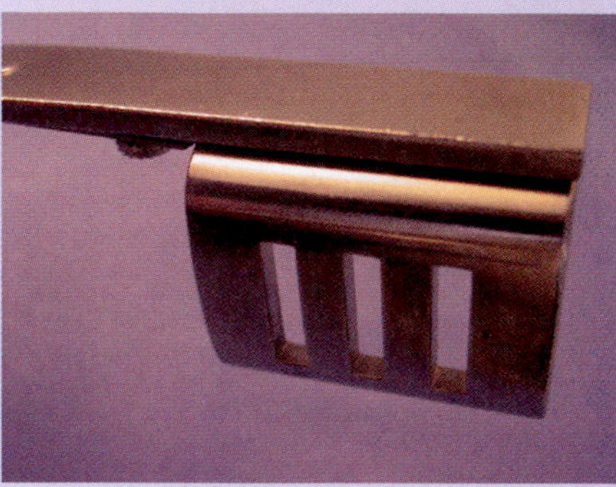

Name: Carpentier atrial retractor
Alias: none
Category: retracting
Use: retracting atria during cardiac surgery
Length: n/a
Additional Information: self-retaining; blade length varies

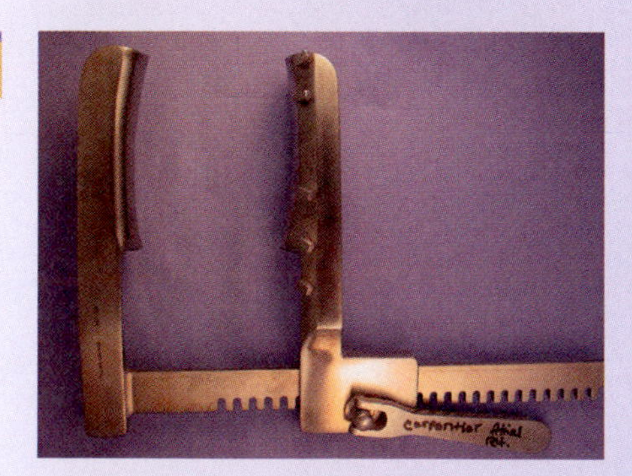

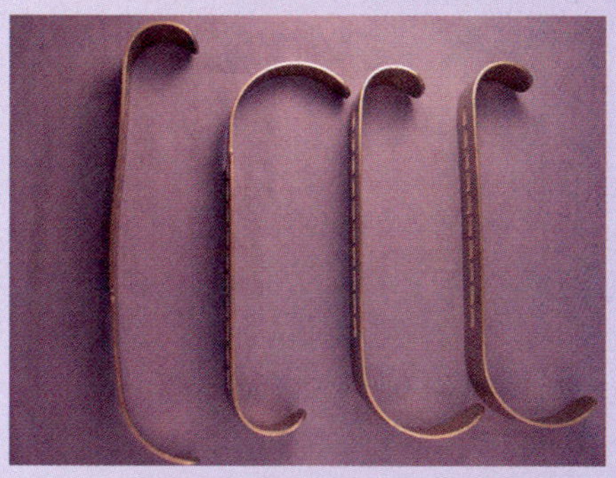

Name: Tuffier rib spreader
Alias: none
Category: retracting
Use: retracting ribs
Length: 7” spread

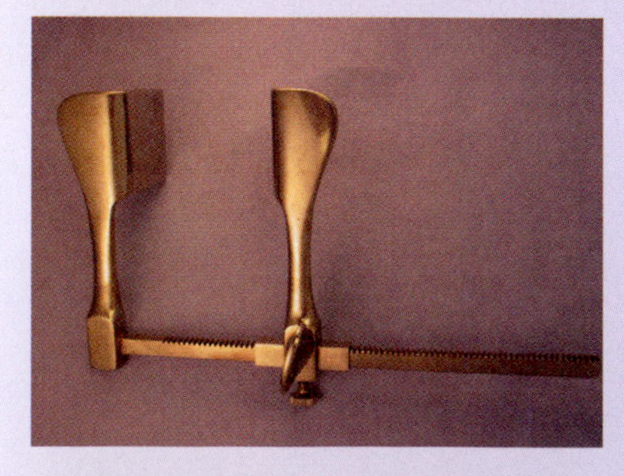

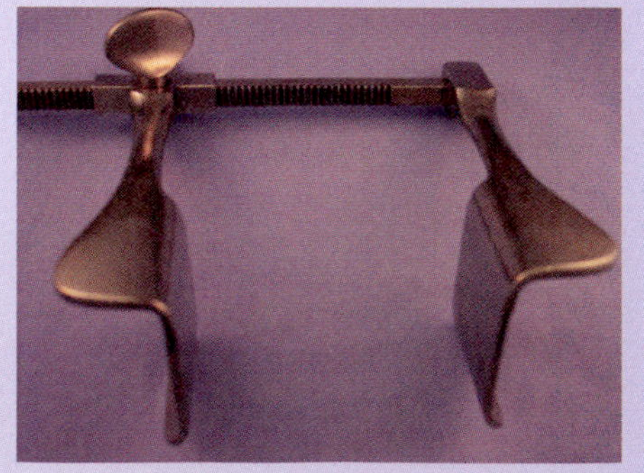

Name: Ankeney retractor
Alias: sternal retractor
Category: retracting
Use: retraction of the sternal bones after sternotomy
Length: n/a
Additional Information: comes in adult (maximum spread 180 mm) or pediatric size (maximum spread 160 mm)

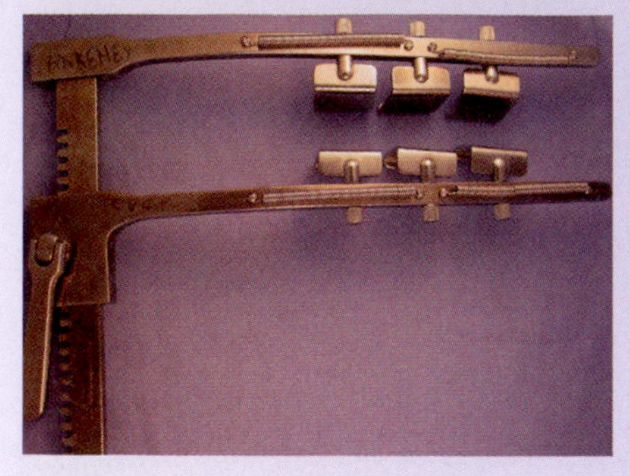

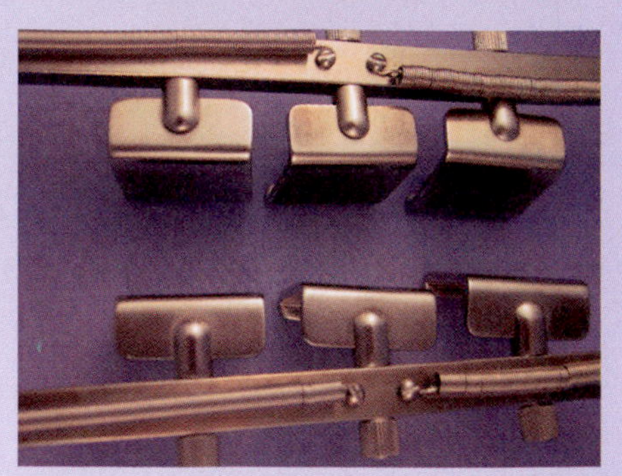

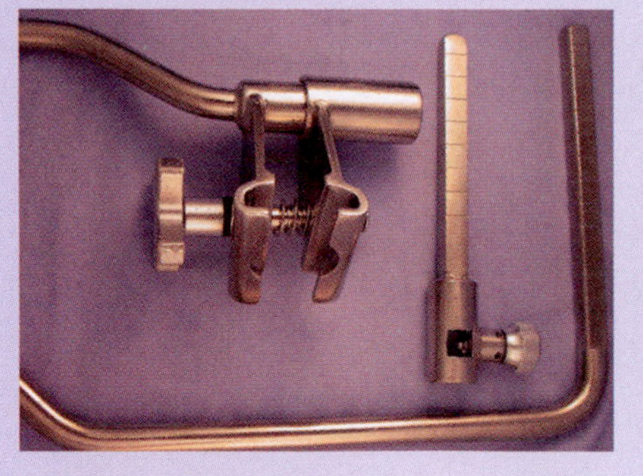

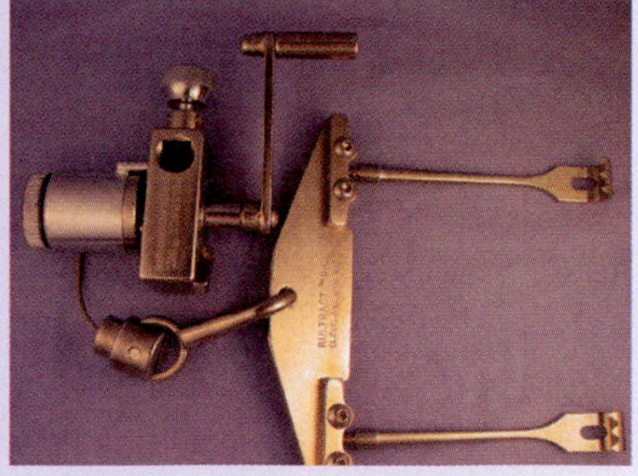

Name: Internal Mammary retractor
Alias: IM retractor
Category: retracting
Use: retraction of tissue to allow for freeing of internal mammary artery during CABG
Length: n/a
Additional Information: posts attach to the surgical bed

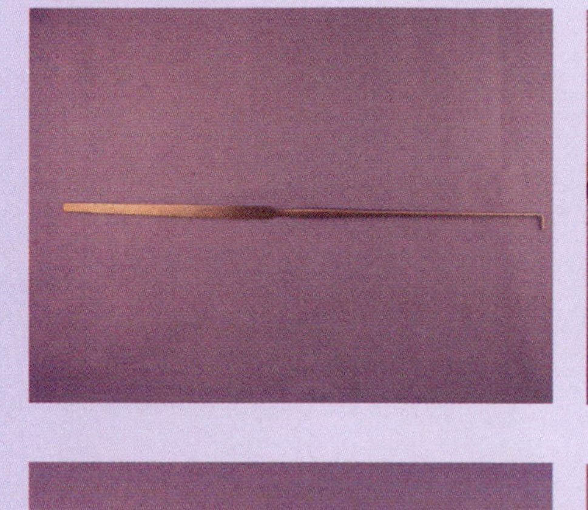

Name: Dandy nerve hook
Alias: none
Category: retracting
Use: retracting nerves
Length: 8.5"
Additional Information: blunt tip; tip can be pointed straight, left, or right

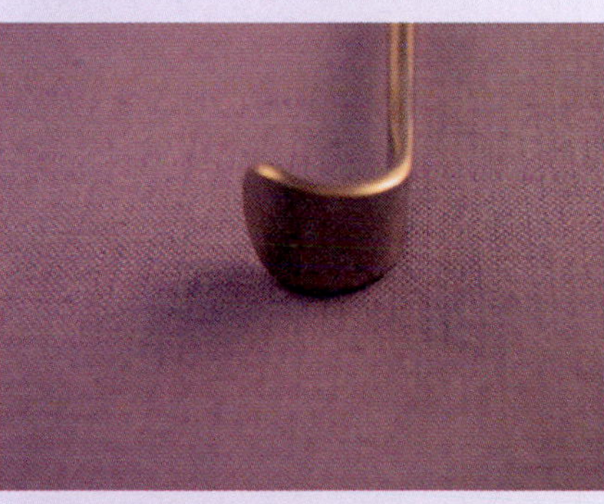

Name: Cushing vein retractor
Alias: none
Category: retracting
Use: retracting blood vessels
Length: 8" or 12"
Additional Information: open handle

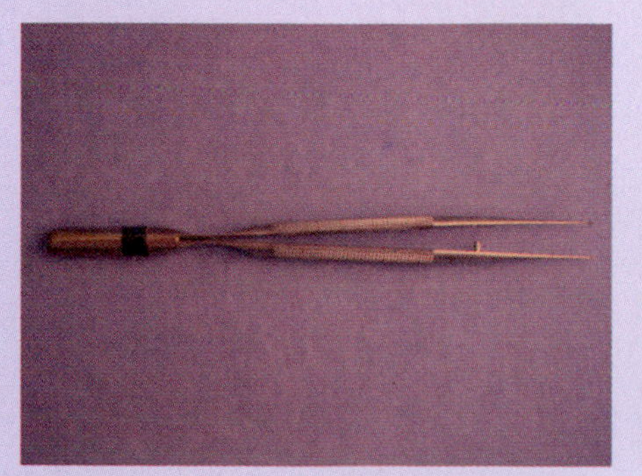

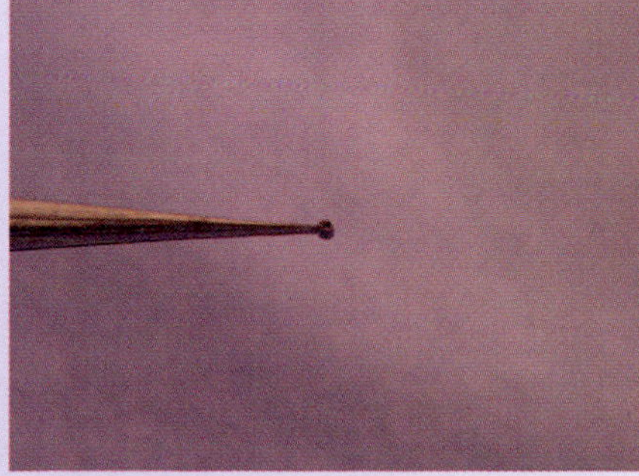

Name: Mills/Dennis micro ring forceps
Alias: none
Category: grasping
Use: grasping very fine tissue or vessels
Length: 6" to 9"
Additional Information: has 1-mm or 2-mm ring

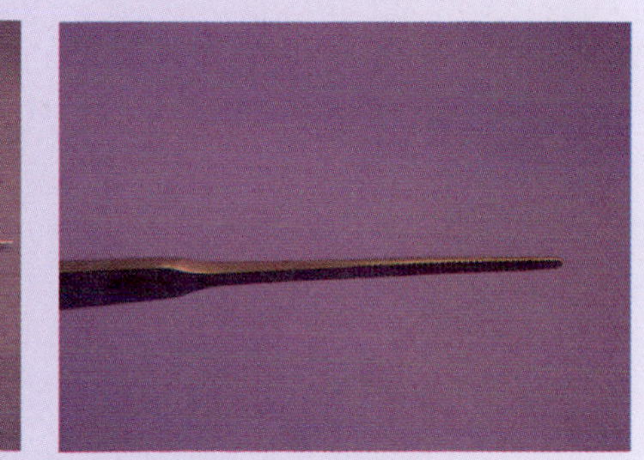

Name: Gerald forceps
Alias: none
Category: grasping
Use: grasping fine tissue
Length: 7"
Additional Information: come with 1 × 2 teeth or serrated jaws

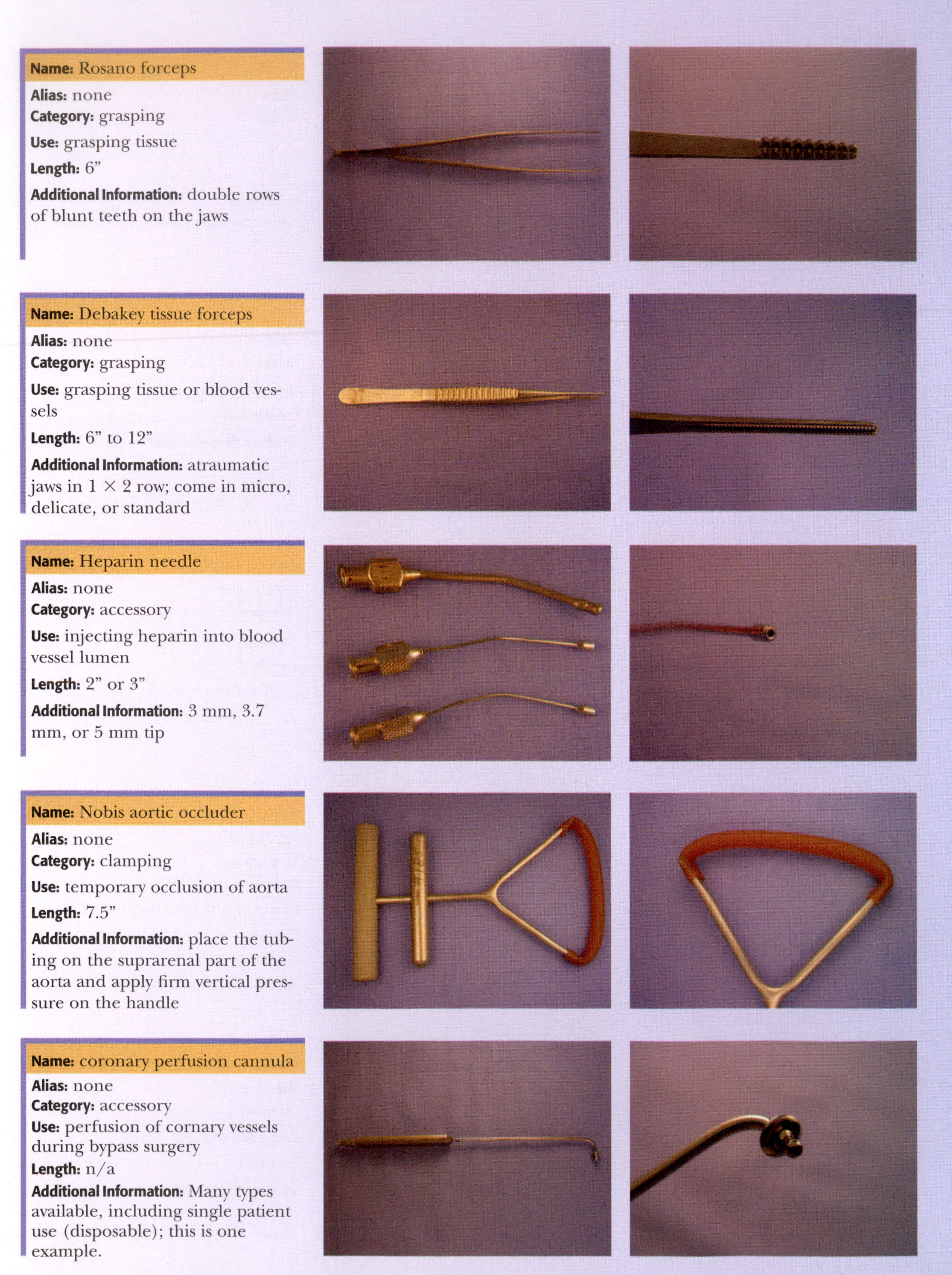

Name: Rosano forceps
Alias: none
Category: grasping
Use: grasping tissue
Length: 6”
Additional Information: double rows of blunt teeth on the jaws

Name: Debakey tissue forceps
Alias: none
Category: grasping
Use: grasping tissue or blood vessels
Length: 6” to 12”
Additional Information: atraumatic jaws in 1 × 2 row; come in micro, delicate, or standard

Name: Heparin needle
Alias: none
Category: accessory
Use: injecting heparin into blood vessel lumen
Length: 2” or 3”
Additional Information: 3 mm, 3.7 mm, or 5 mm tip

Name: Nobis aortic occluder
Alias: none
Category: clamping
Use: temporary occlusion of aorta
Length: 7.5”
Additional Information: place the tubing on the suprarenal part of the aorta and apply firm vertical pressure on the handle

Name: coronary perfusion cannula
Alias: none
Category: accessory
Use: perfusion of cornary vessels during bypass surgery
Length: n/a
Additional Information: Many types available, including single patient use (disposable); this is one example.

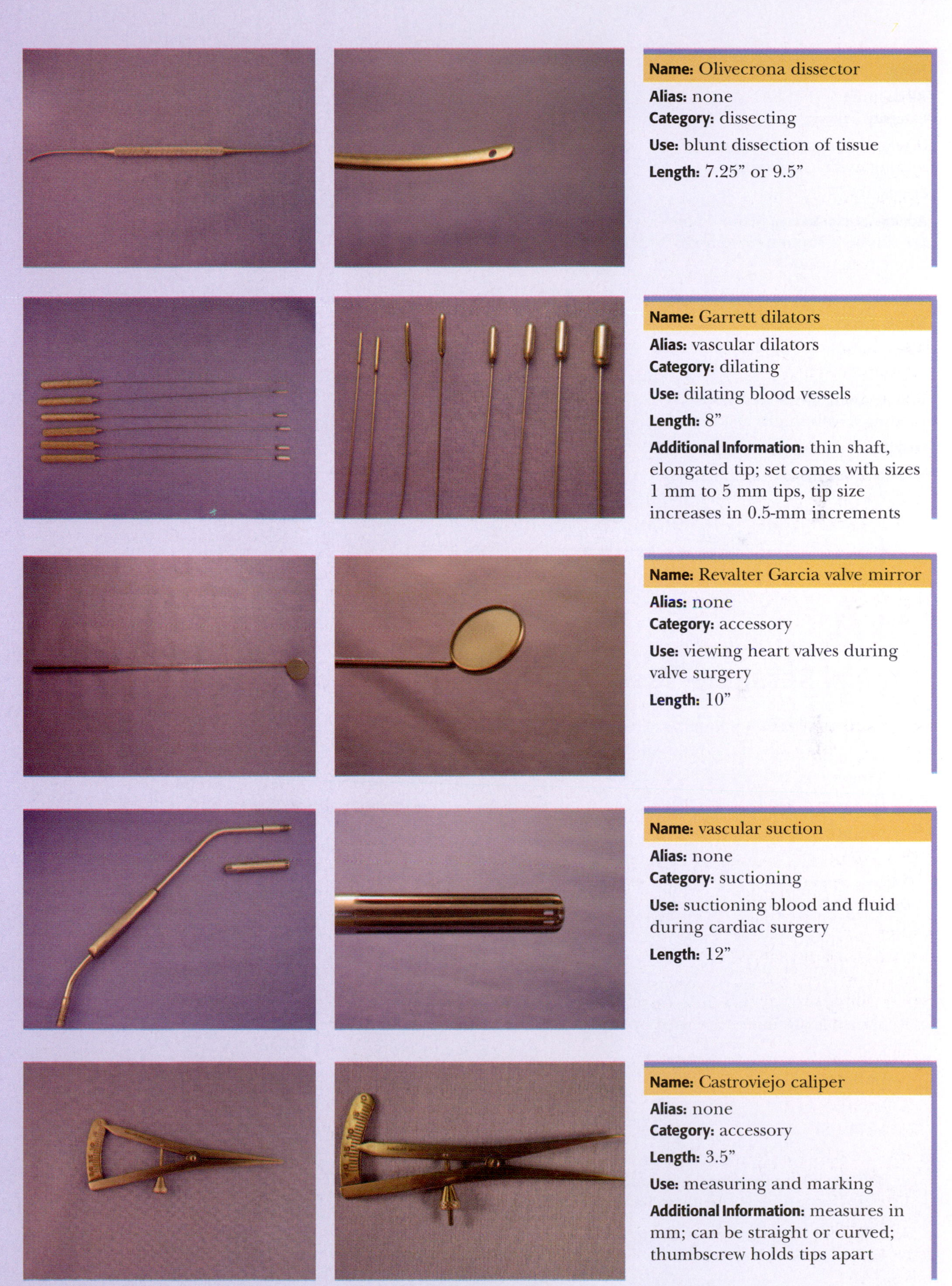

Name: Olivecrona dissector
Alias: none
Category: dissecting
Use: blunt dissection of tissue
Length: 7.25" or 9.5"

Name: Garrett dilators
Alias: vascular dilators
Category: dilating
Use: dilating blood vessels
Length: 8"
Additional Information: thin shaft, elongated tip; set comes with sizes 1 mm to 5 mm tips, tip size increases in 0.5-mm increments

Name: Revalter Garcia valve mirror
Alias: none
Category: accessory
Use: viewing heart valves during valve surgery
Length: 10"

Name: vascular suction
Alias: none
Category: suctioning
Use: suctioning blood and fluid during cardiac surgery
Length: 12"

Name: Castroviejo caliper
Alias: none
Category: accessory
Length: 3.5"
Use: measuring and marking
Additional Information: measures in mm; can be straight or curved; thumbscrew holds tips apart

Name: aortic punch

Alias: none

Category: cutting

Use: punching hole in aorta for joining cardiac bypass grafts

Length: n/a

Additional Information: blade diameter can be 2.7 mm to 5.6 mm; single-patient use

Name: Peers towel clip

Alias: none

Category: grasping

Use: holding cords to drapes; holding towels in place

Length: 5"

Additional Information: nonperforating jaws

Q&A

Surgical Session—Vascular, Thoracic, Cardiac Instruments

1) The surgeon asks for a bulldog clamp. You could hand him/her any of the following *except* a:
   a. Gregory
   b. DeBakey
   c. Diethrich
   d. Lawrie
2) A Gemini is what type of clamp?
   a. aortic cross
   b. right angle
   c. peripheral occlusion
   d. bulldog
3) Replaceable jaw inserts are used on which clamp?
   a. Fogarty
   b. DeBakey
   c. Satinsky
   d. Javid
4) The surgeon needs to contract the ribs back together before closing the chest. You anticipate this and have a ______________ ready to hand to him/her.
   a. Giertz-Stille
   b. Bailey-Gibbon
   c. Garrett
   d. Gerald
5) The surgeon asks for a lung retractor. You would hand him/her a(n):
   a. Allison
   b. Davidson
   c. Duval
   d. DeBakey
6) During a carotid endarterectomy, the surgeon requests a carotid artery bypass shunt clamp. You hand him/her a:
   a. Fogarty
   b. Javid
   c. Cooley
   d. Glover
7) Potts scissors tips can be angled at all of the following degrees *except:*
   a. 25
   b. 45
   c. 50
   d. 60

8) A ____________ is a type of rib raspatory.

a. Barry
b. Satinsky
c. Debakey
d. Doyon

9) You are scrubbed on a lung lobectomy. You know this surgeon uses a bronchus clamp with teeth. You have a ______________ clamp ready to hand him/her.

a. Sarot
b. Allison
c. Glover
d. Collin

10) The CABG surgery is almost complete. The surgeon is ready to place the stainless-steel sutures in the sternum. You would use a _________ needle holder to pass the wire sutures on.

a. Debakey
b. Coronary
c. Barry
d. Castroviejo

11) All of the following are types of scissors *except:*

a. Lawrie
b. Tenotomy
c. Jameson
d. Rummel

12) During a thoracotomy the surgeon needs to remove a rib. Which instrument would be used to cut the rib?

a. Giertz-Shoemaker
b. Doyon
c. Alexander-Ferebeuf
d. Matson

13) All of the following can be types of DeBakey clamps *except*:

a. sidewinder
b. coarctation
c. aorta
d. carotid artery bypass shunt

14) Which of the following is *not* a raspatory?

a. Bailey
b. Doyon
c. Semb
d. Matson

15) During coronary valve surgery the surgeon requests a hand-held atrial retractor. You would hand him/her a:

a. Tuffier
b. Buford-Finochietto
c. Charpentier
d. Cooley

16) During vascular surgery the surgeon needs to dilate a blood vessel. You would have the ____________ dilators ready.

a. Crane
b. Cogswell
c. Garrett
d. Javid

Dental, Plastic, and Maxillofacial Instruments

9

DENTAL/MAXILLOFACIAL INSTRUMENTS

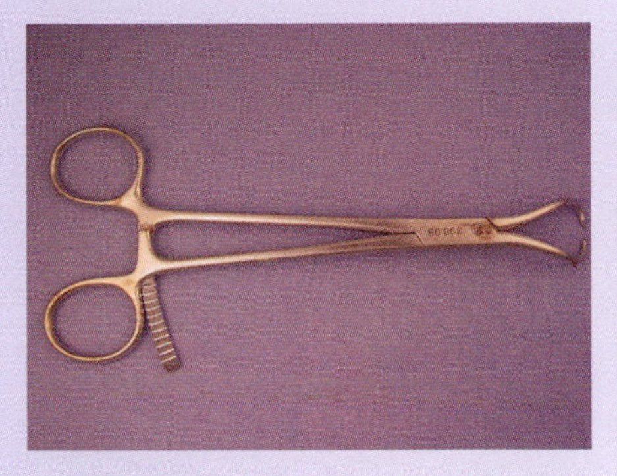

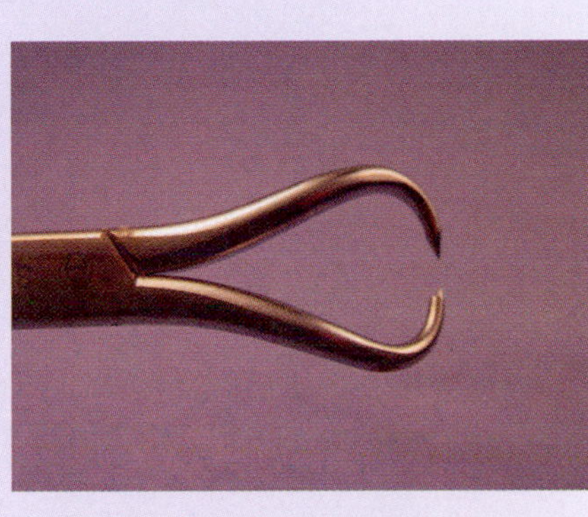

Name: bone reduction forceps

Alias: none

Category: grasping

Use: holding fractured bone segments together

Length: 5" or 6.75"

Additional Information: pointed jaw

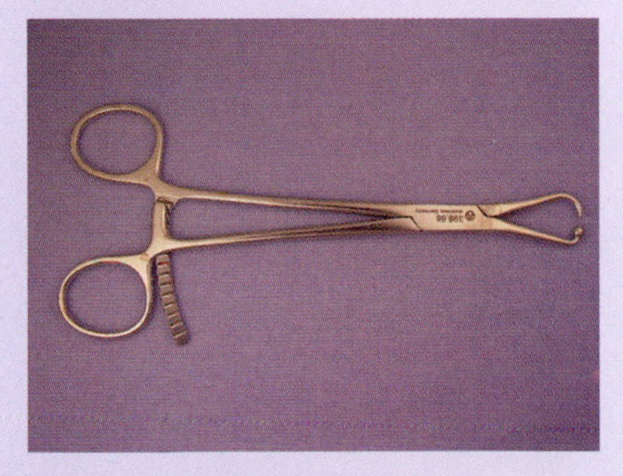

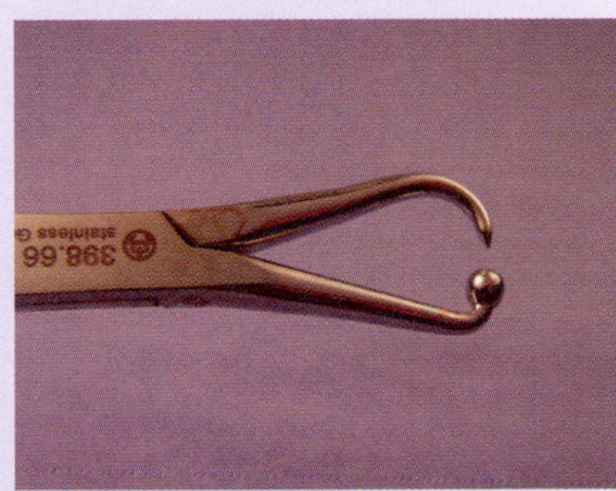

Name: plate and bone holder

Alias: none

Category: grasping

Use: holding plate and fracture site intact until it can be screwed in place

Length: n/a

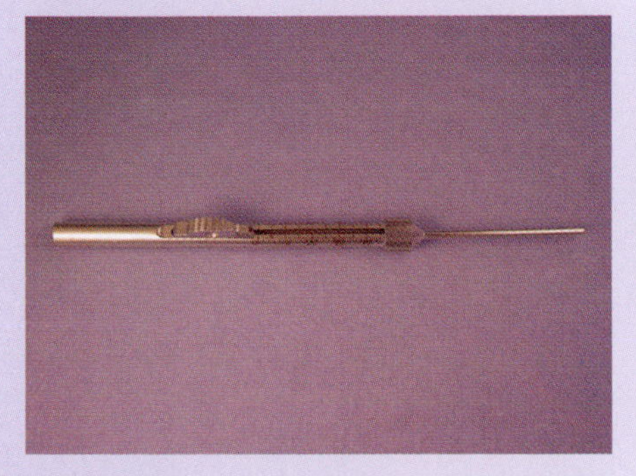

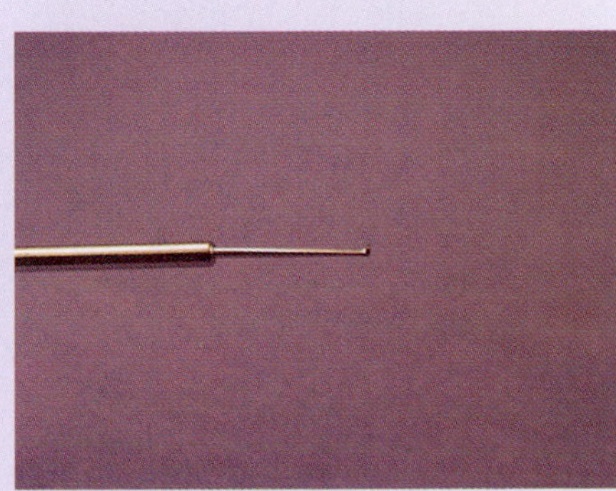

Name: depth gauge

Alias: none

Category: accessory

Use: measuring depth of drill holes

Length: 6.5"

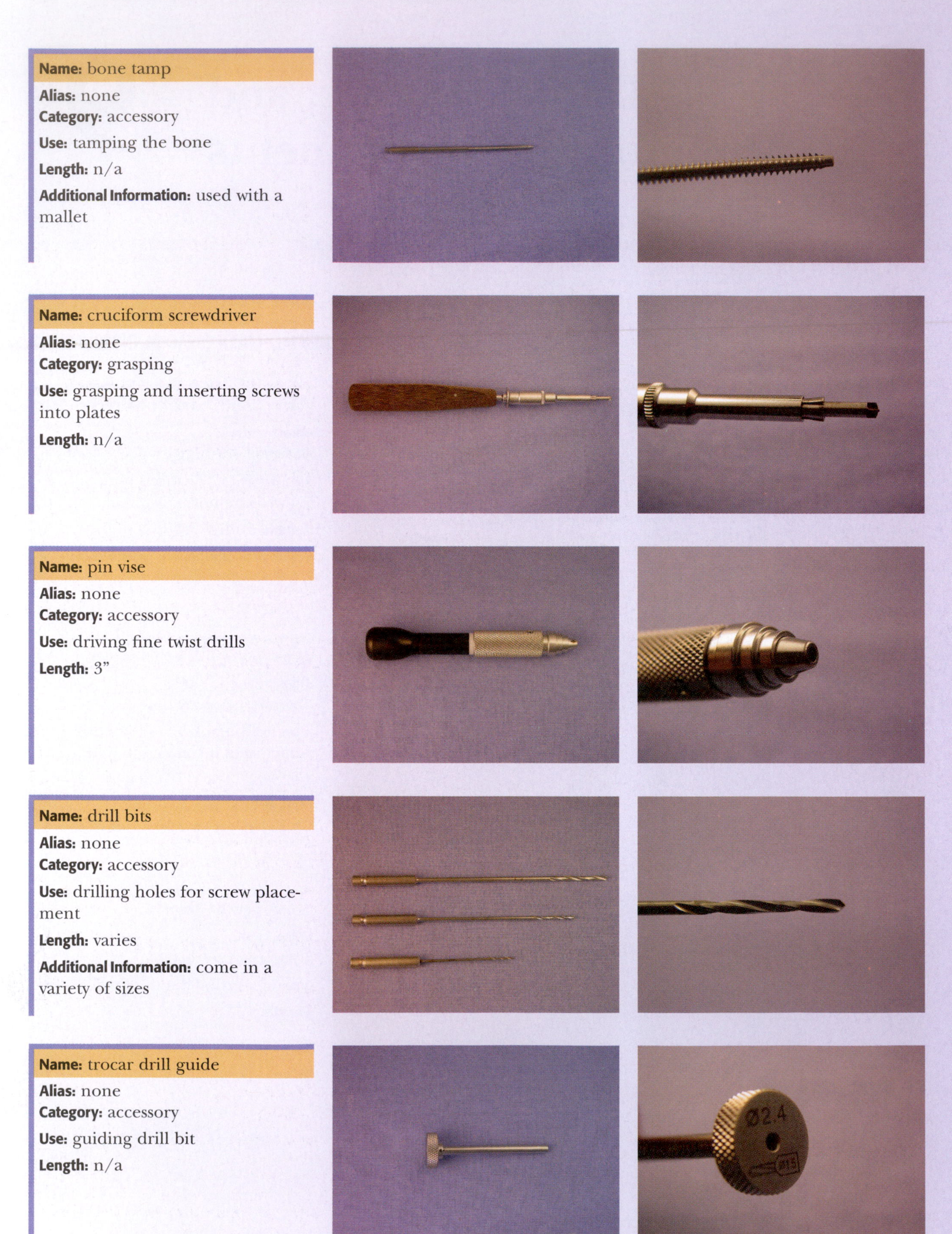

Name: bone tamp
Alias: none
Category: accessory
Use: tamping the bone
Length: n/a
Additional Information: used with a mallet

Name: cruciform screwdriver
Alias: none
Category: grasping
Use: grasping and inserting screws into plates
Length: n/a

Name: pin vise
Alias: none
Category: accessory
Use: driving fine twist drills
Length: 3"

Name: drill bits
Alias: none
Category: accessory
Use: drilling holes for screw placement
Length: varies
Additional Information: come in a variety of sizes

Name: trocar drill guide
Alias: none
Category: accessory
Use: guiding drill bit
Length: n/a

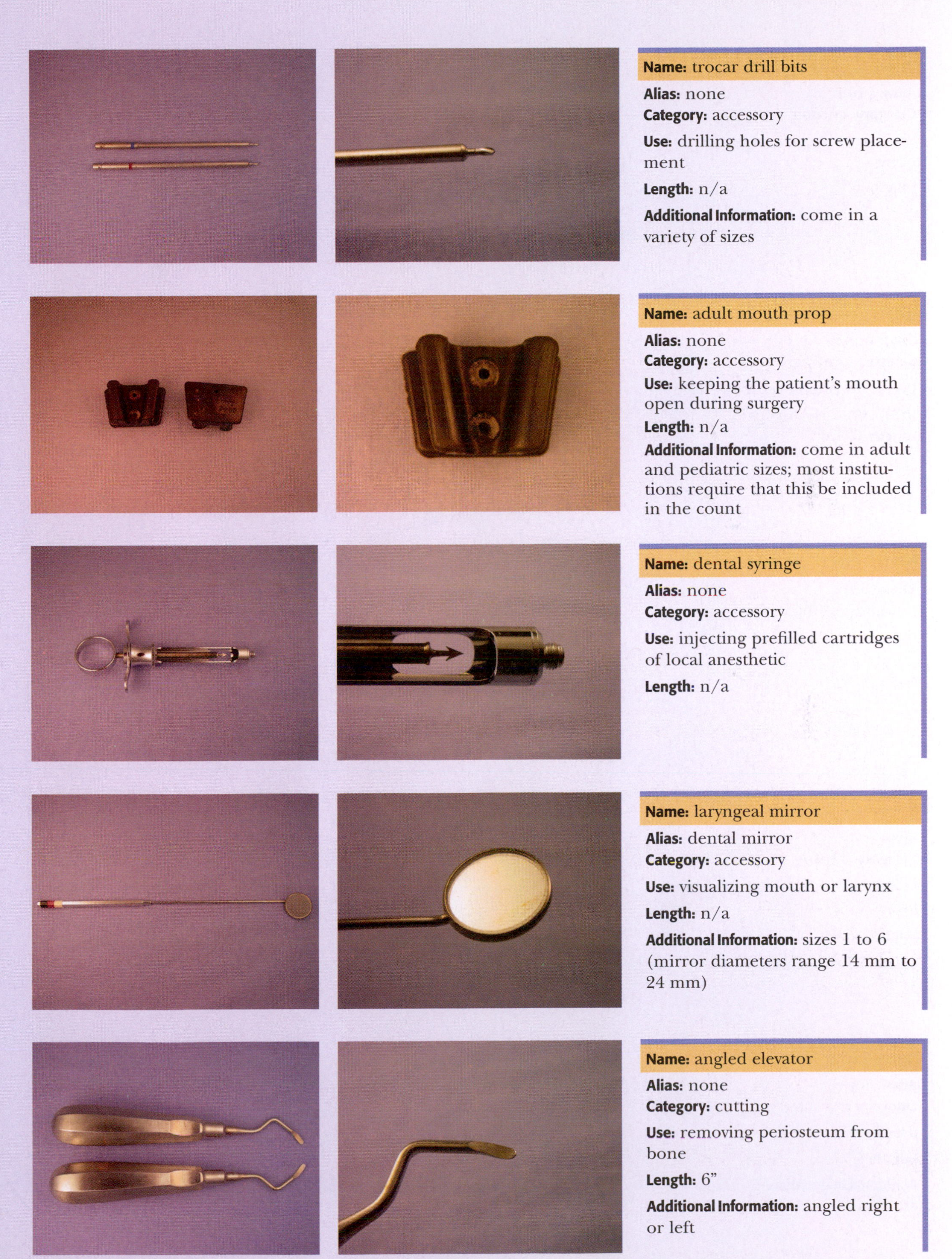

Name: trocar drill bits
Alias: none
Category: accessory
Use: drilling holes for screw placement
Length: n/a
Additional Information: come in a variety of sizes

Name: adult mouth prop
Alias: none
Category: accessory
Use: keeping the patient's mouth open during surgery
Length: n/a
Additional Information: come in adult and pediatric sizes; most institutions require that this be included in the count

Name: dental syringe
Alias: none
Category: accessory
Use: injecting prefilled cartridges of local anesthetic
Length: n/a

Name: laryngeal mirror
Alias: dental mirror
Category: accessory
Use: visualizing mouth or larynx
Length: n/a
Additional Information: sizes 1 to 6 (mirror diameters range 14 mm to 24 mm)

Name: angled elevator
Alias: none
Category: cutting
Use: removing periosteum from bone
Length: 6"
Additional Information: angled right or left

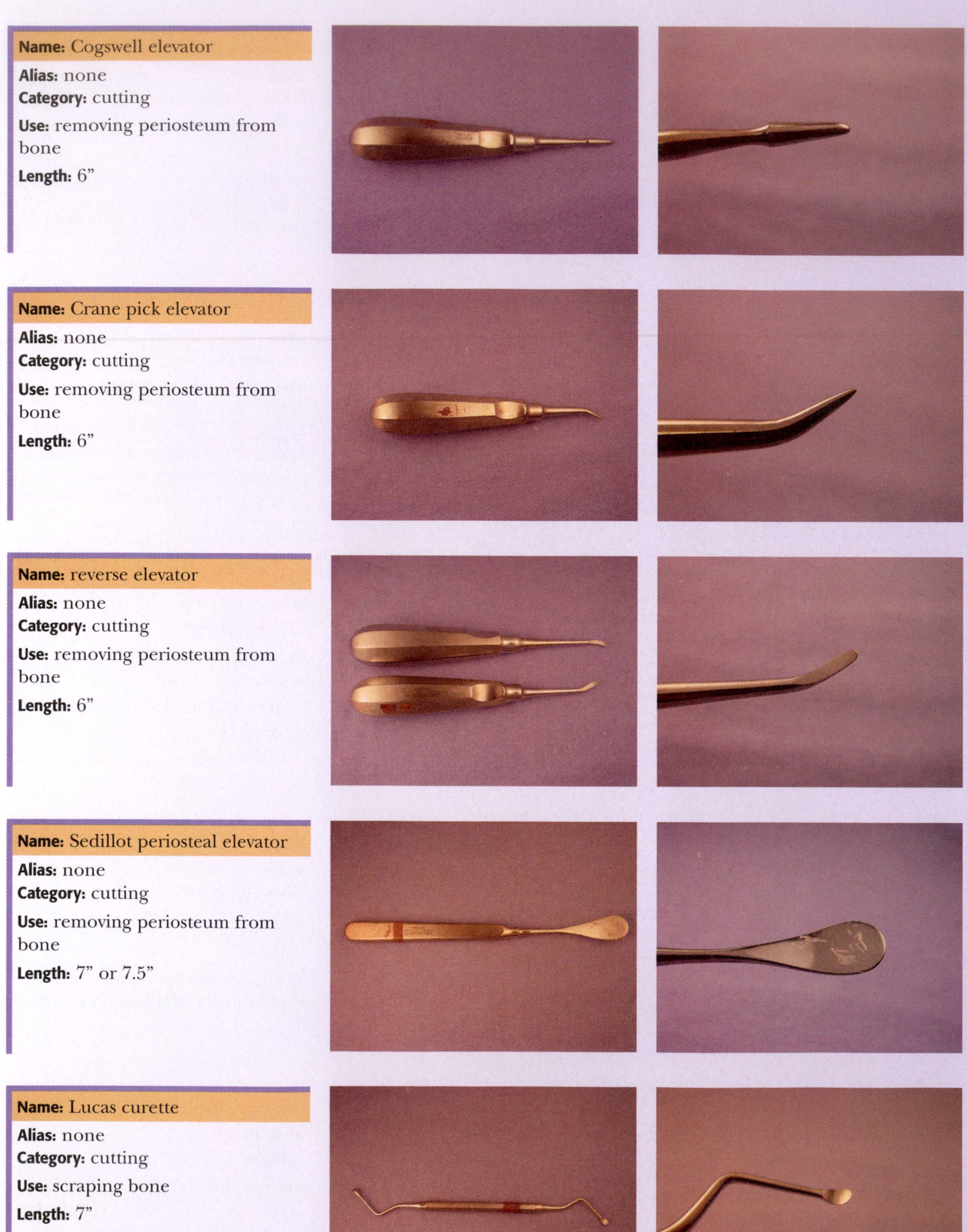

Name: Cogswell elevator
Alias: none
Category: cutting
Use: removing periosteum from bone
Length: 6"

Name: Crane pick elevator
Alias: none
Category: cutting
Use: removing periosteum from bone
Length: 6"

Name: reverse elevator
Alias: none
Category: cutting
Use: removing periosteum from bone
Length: 6"

Name: Sedillot periosteal elevator
Alias: none
Category: cutting
Use: removing periosteum from bone
Length: 7" or 7.5"

Name: Lucas curette
Alias: none
Category: cutting
Use: scraping bone
Length: 7"
Additional Information: double ended (left and right)

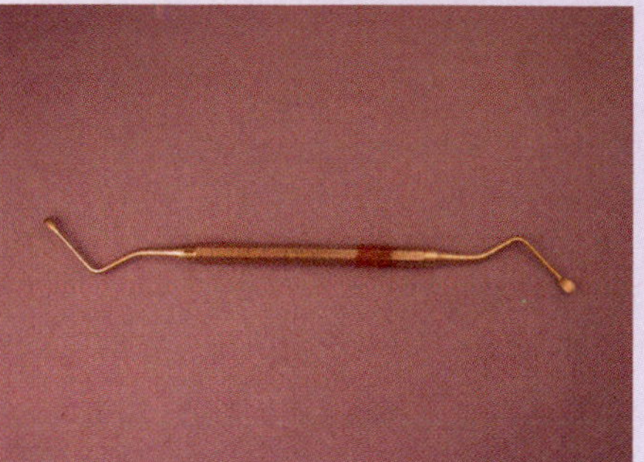

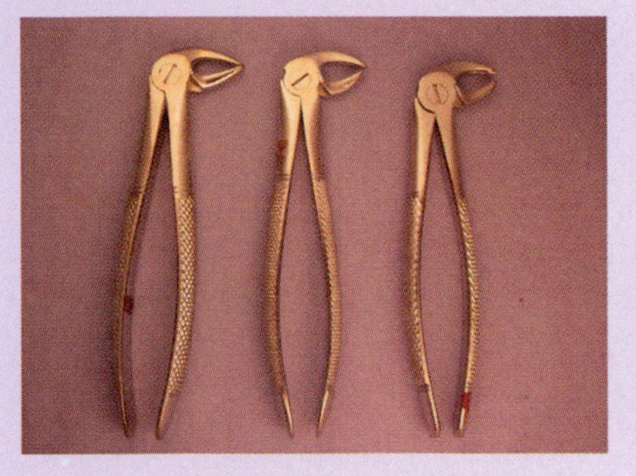

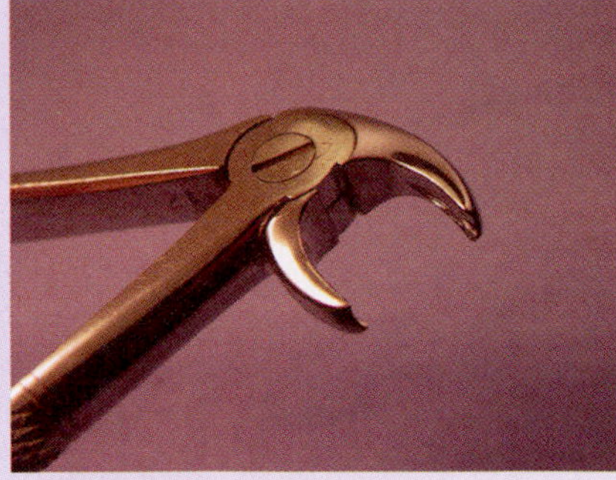

Name: molar extracting forceps
Alias: none
Category: grasping
Use: extracting molars
Length: 6”
Additional Information: English type

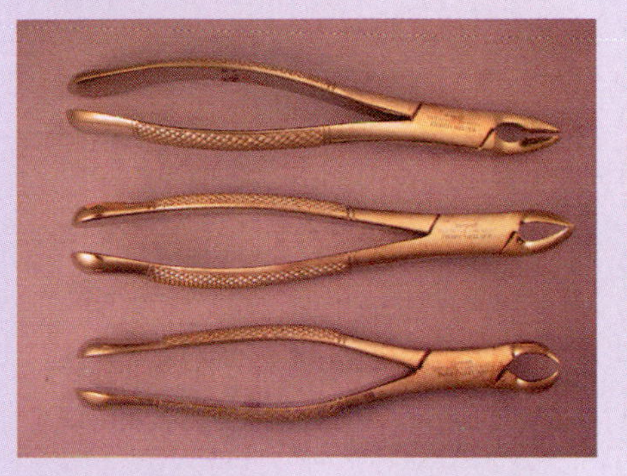

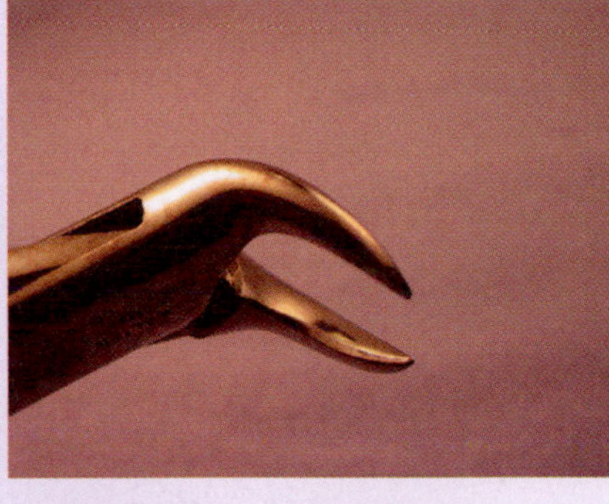

Name: extracting forceps
Alias: none
Category: grasping
Use: extracting upper or lower teeth
Length: 6.5”

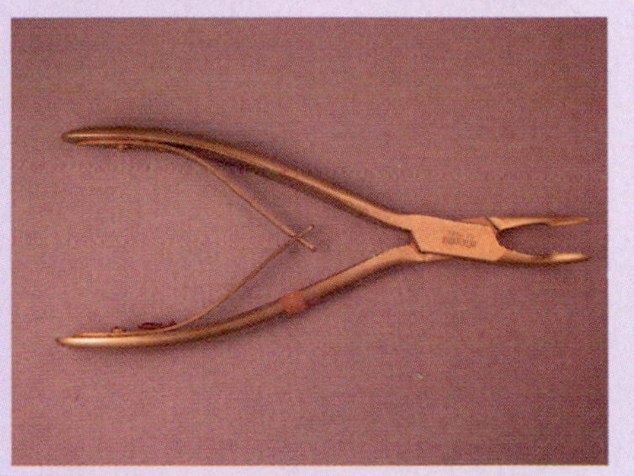

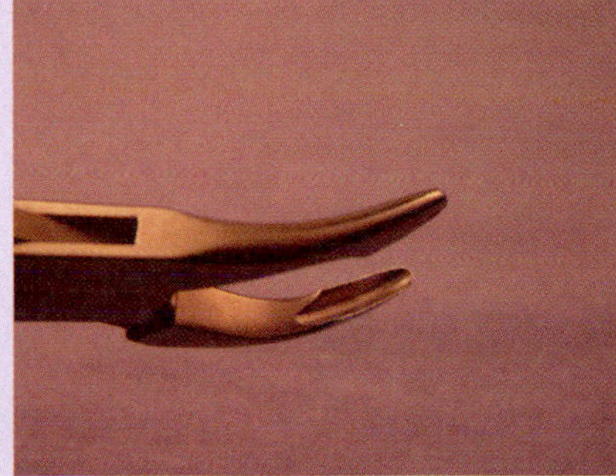

Name: Bane rongeur
Alias: none
Category: cutting
Use: cutting away pieces of bone
Length: 7”
Additional Information: curved, tapered jaws

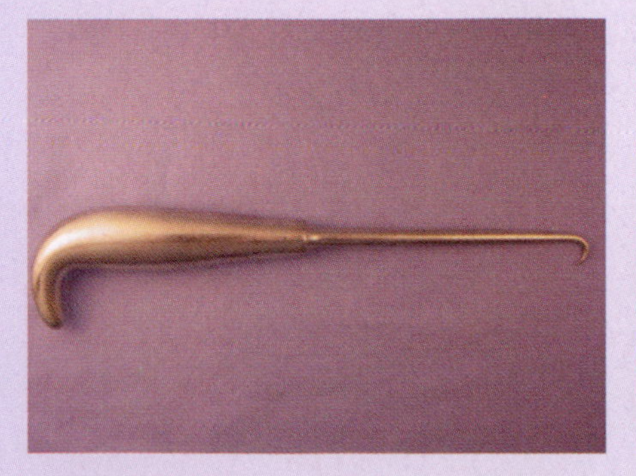

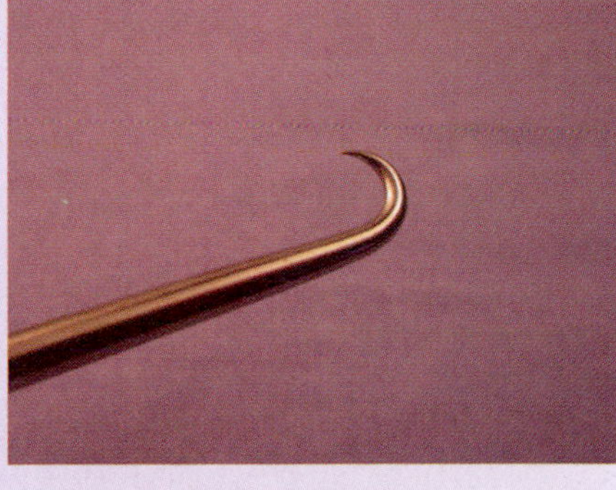

Name: Gillies bone and zygoma hook
Alias: Dingman zygoma hook
Category: retracting
Use: retracting bone
Length: 6.5” or 7.5”
Additional Information: single sharp hook

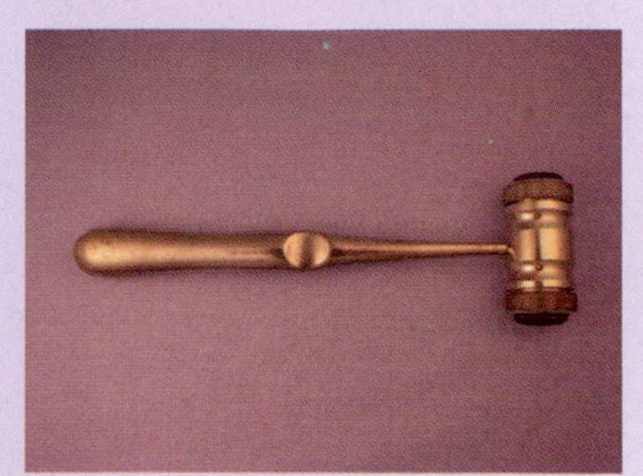

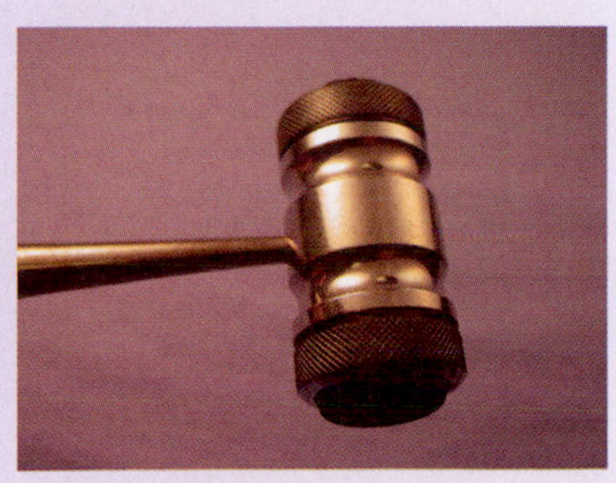

Name: Mead mallet
Alias: none
Category: accessory
Use: exerting force on an object (such as a chisel or osteotome)
Length: 7.5”
Additional Information: 1” head diameter

Name: McKesson suction

Alias: none

Category: suction

Use: suctioning blood and fluid

Length: 7"

Additional Information: tip 2 mm, 3 mm or 4 mm diameter

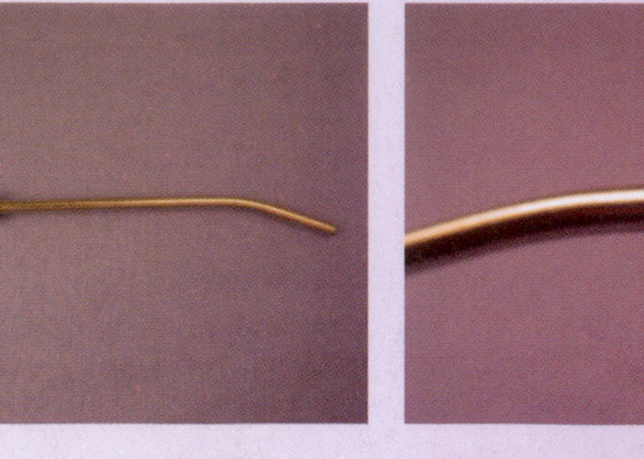

Name: Dean scissors

Alias: none

Category: cutting

Use: dissecting tissue

Length: 6.75"

Additional Information: angled blades; curved handles

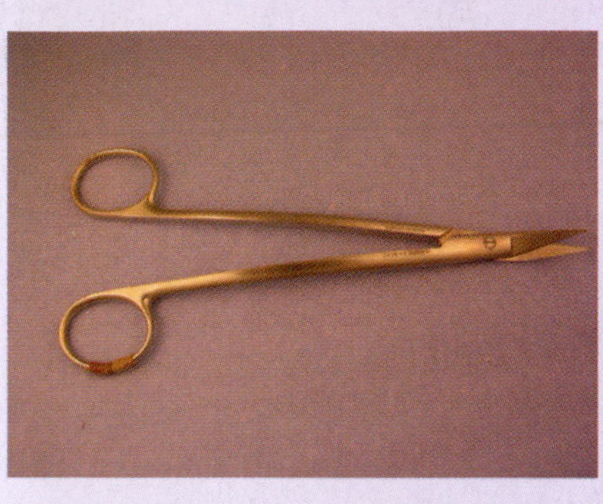

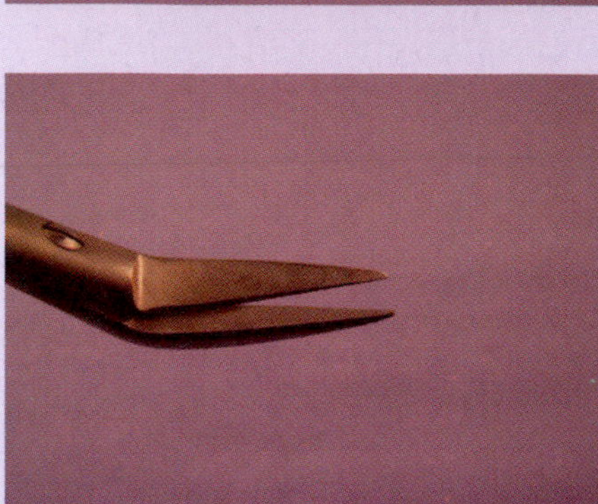

Name: wire cutter

Alias: none

Category: cutting

Use: cutting soft wires

Length: 7"

Additional Information: double action

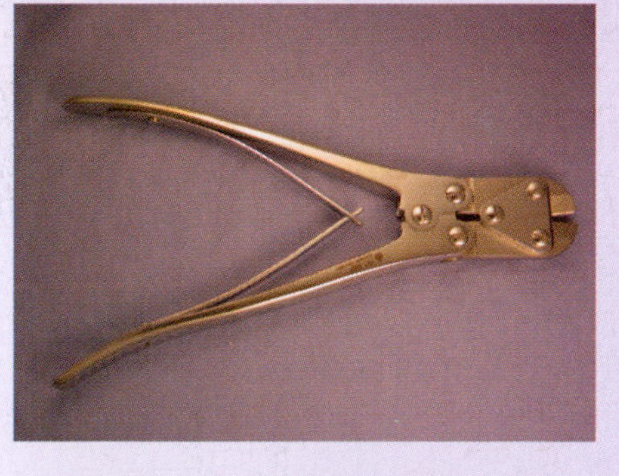

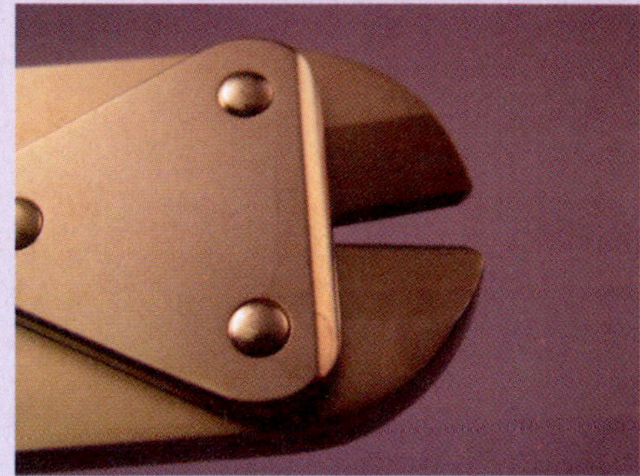

Name: Castroviejo locking forceps

Alias: none

Category: grasping

Use: grasping screws or other small objects

Length: 4.75"

Additional Information: has locking mechanism to hold object in place

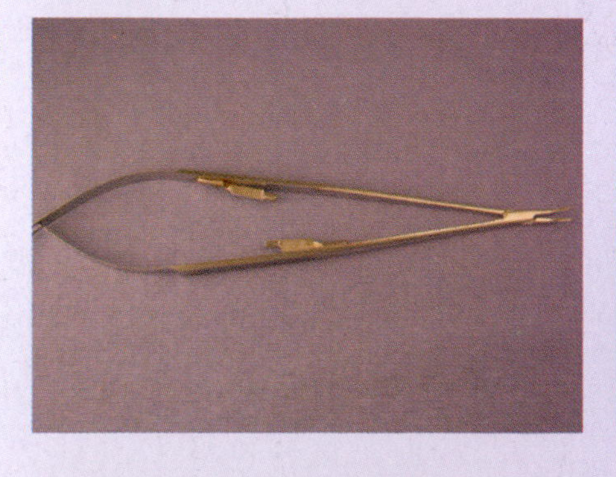

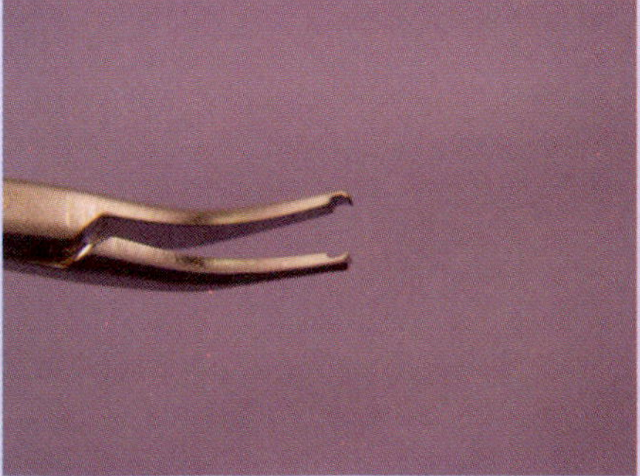

Name: 90-degree plate bender

Alias: none

Category: accessory

Use: contouring plates used to hold fractures in place

Length: n/a

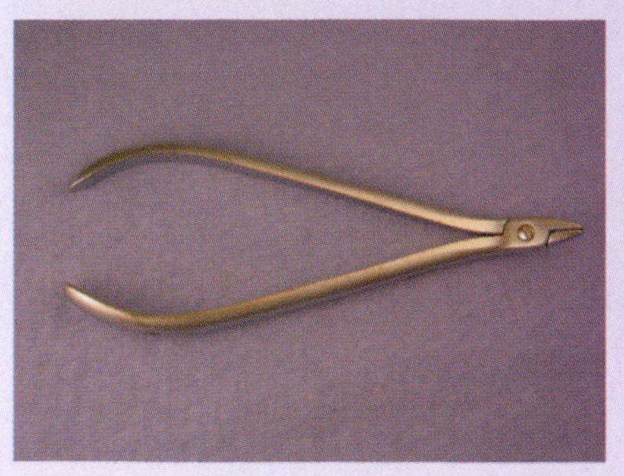

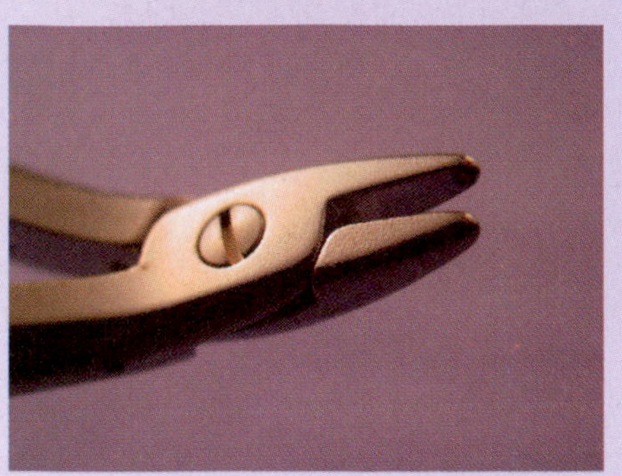

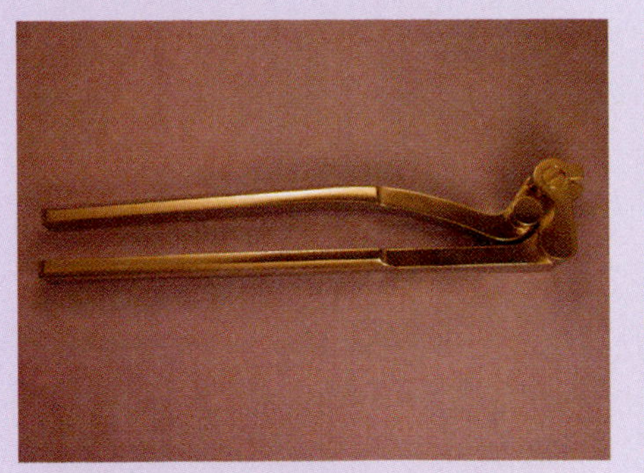

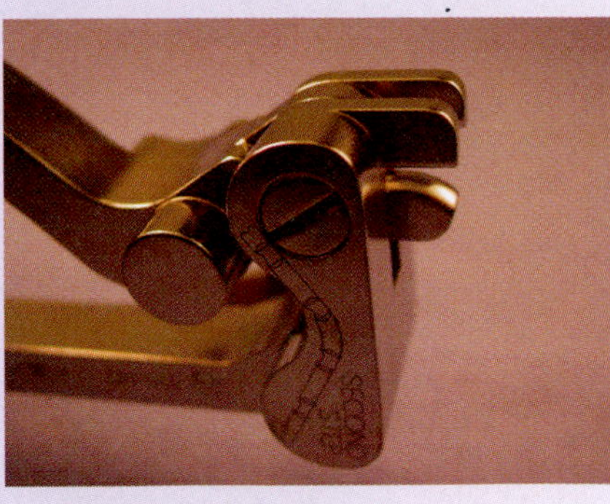

Name: combination plate bender

Alias: none

Category: accessory

Use: contouring plates used to hold fractures in place

Length: n/a

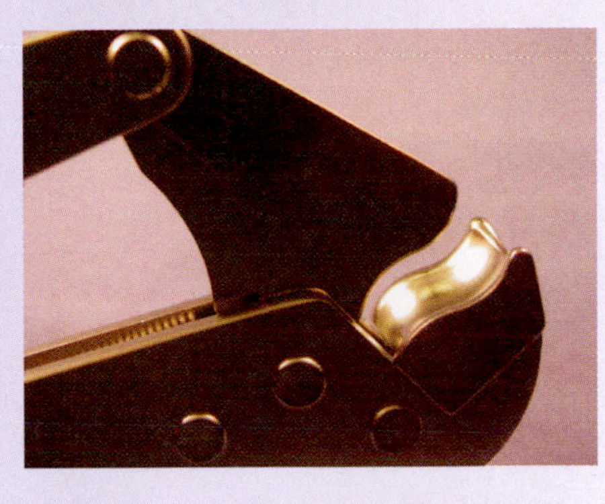

Name: large plate bender

Alias: none

Category: accessory

Use: contouring larger plates used to hold fractures in place

Length: n/a

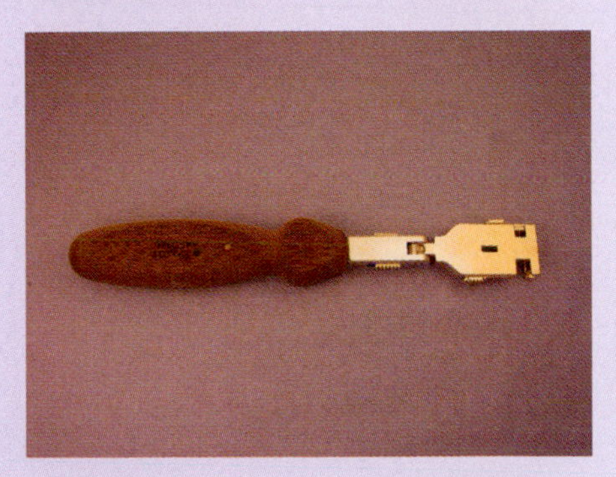

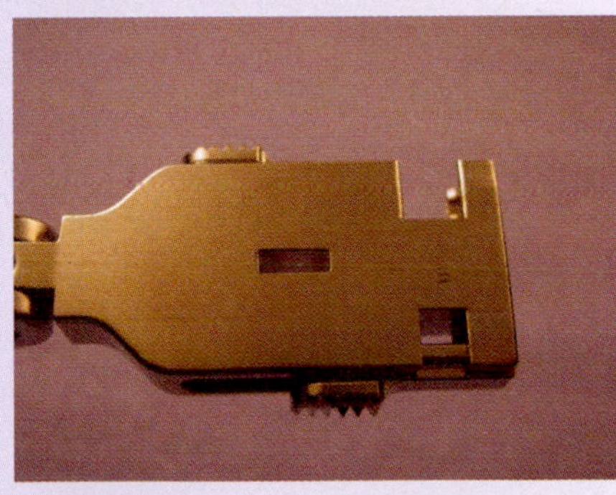

Name: plate bender

Alias: none

Category: accessory

Use: contouring plates used to hold fractures in place

Length: n/a

Additional Information: hinged head

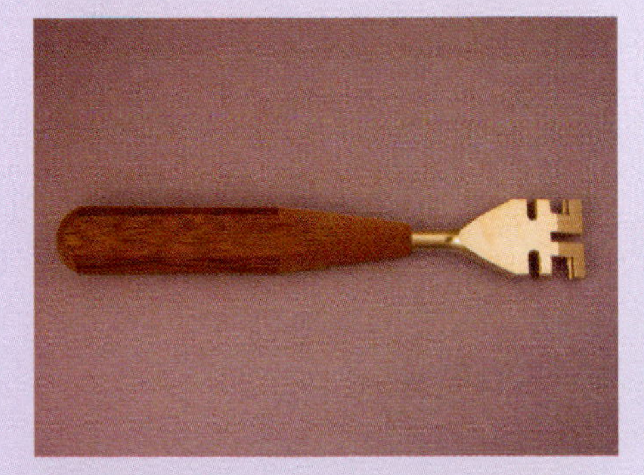

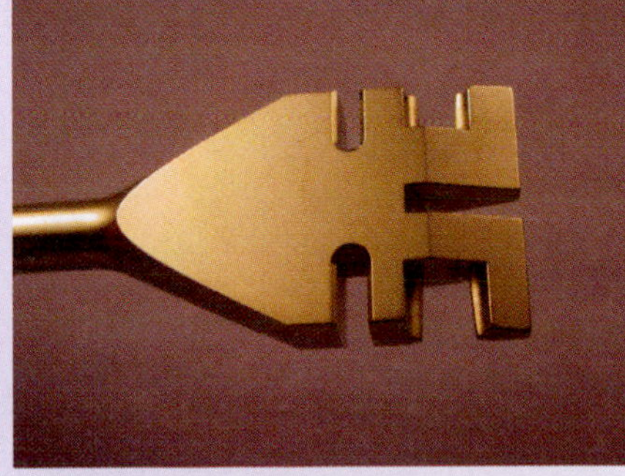

Name: bending iron

Alias: none

Category: accessory

Use: contouring plates used to hold fractures in place

Length: n/a

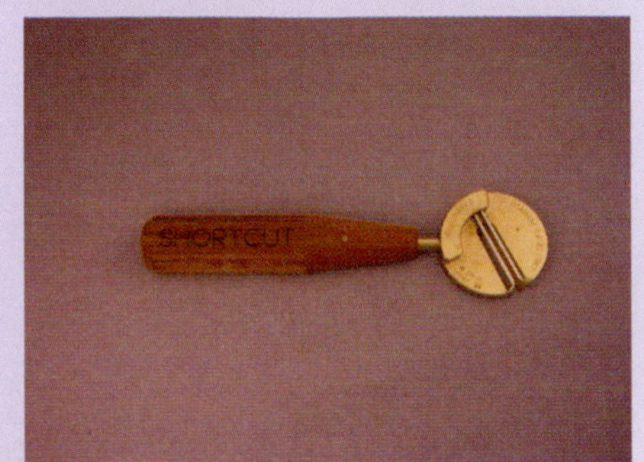

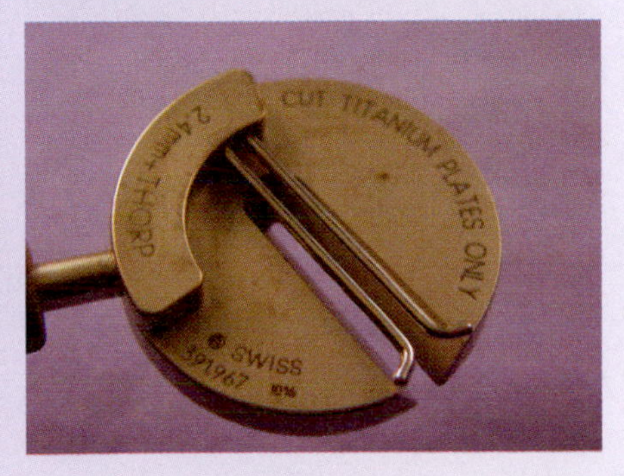

Name: titanium plate cutter

Alias: none

Category: cutting

Use: cutting titanium plates to the correct length to fit a fracture being repaired

Length: n/a

Additional Information: use on titanium plates only

Name: plate pliers

Alias: none

Category: accessory

Use: bending plates to fix a fracture site being repaired

Length: n/a

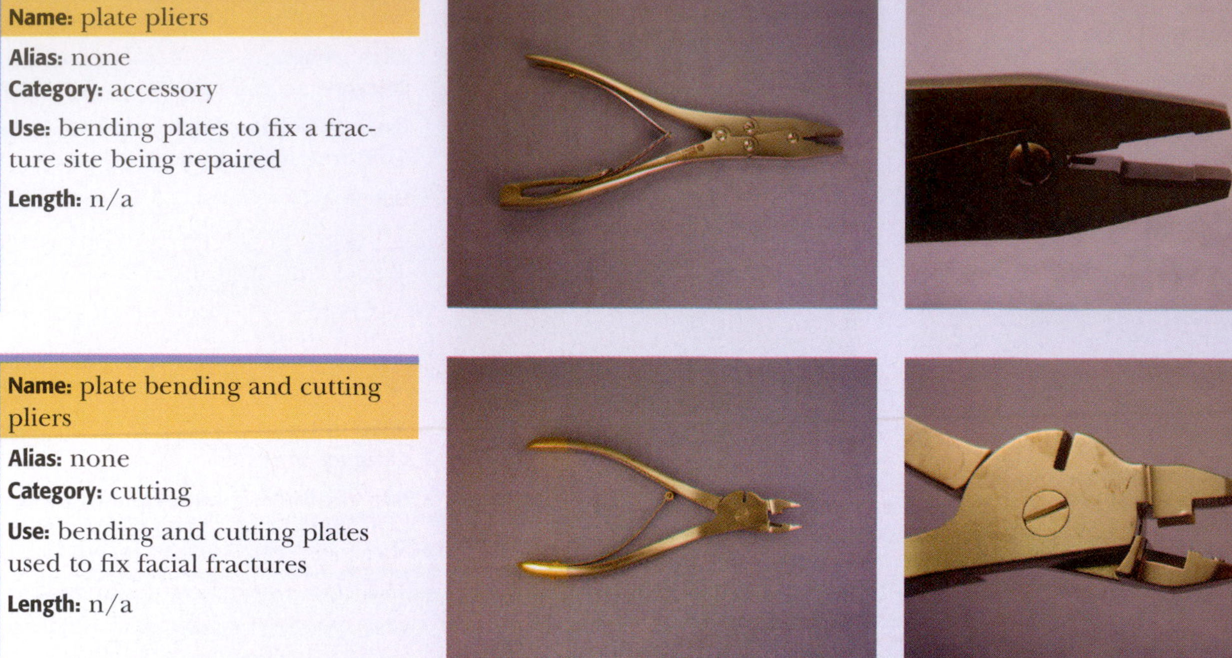

Name: plate bending and cutting pliers

Alias: none

Category: cutting

Use: bending and cutting plates used to fix facial fractures

Length: n/a

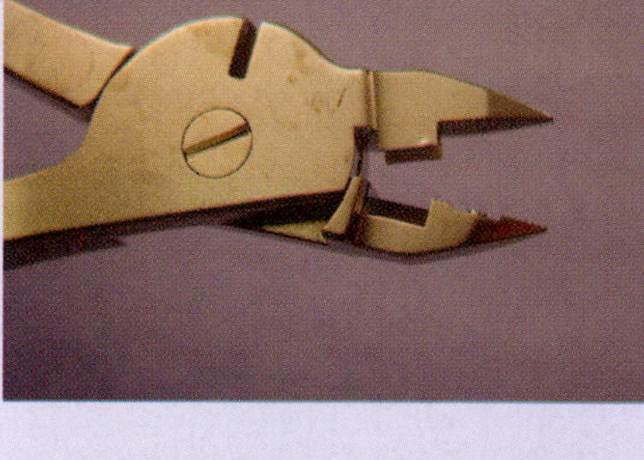

Name: screws and plates for facial fractures

Alias: none

Category: accessory

Use: repairing facial/mandibular fractures

Length: n/a

Additional Information: contain plates and screws of various sizes that can be contoured to repair most fractures

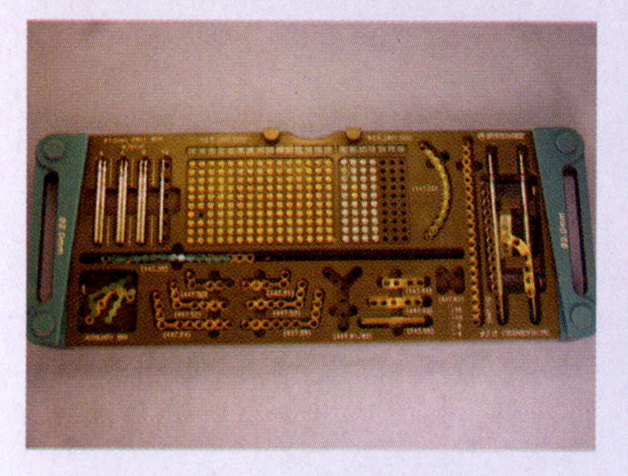

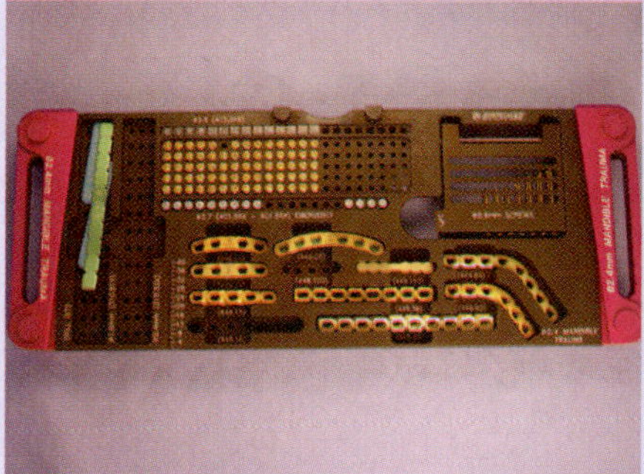

Name: drill guide

Alias: none

Category: accessory

Use: guiding drill bit

Length: n/a

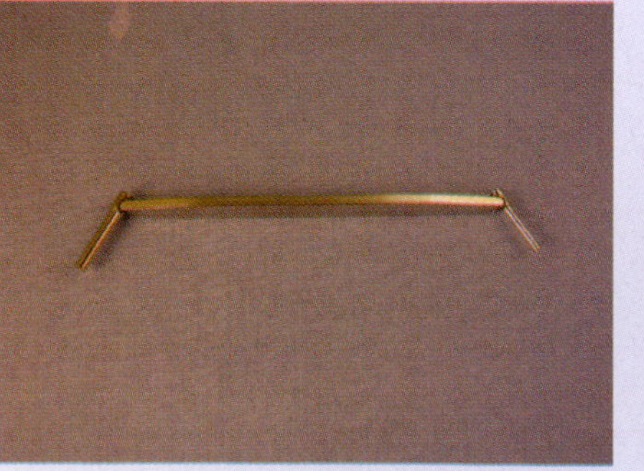

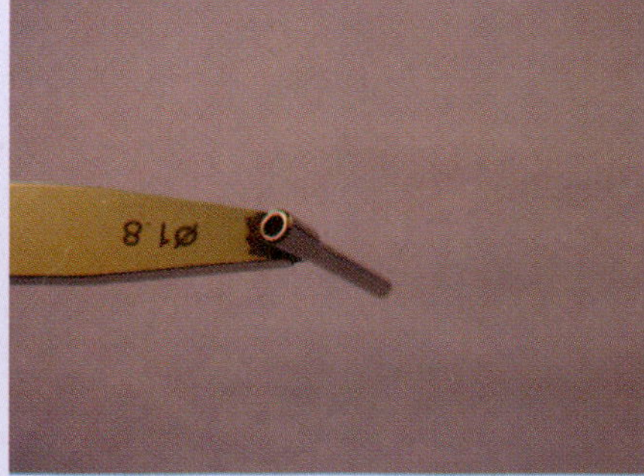

PLASTIC SURGERY INSTRUMENTS

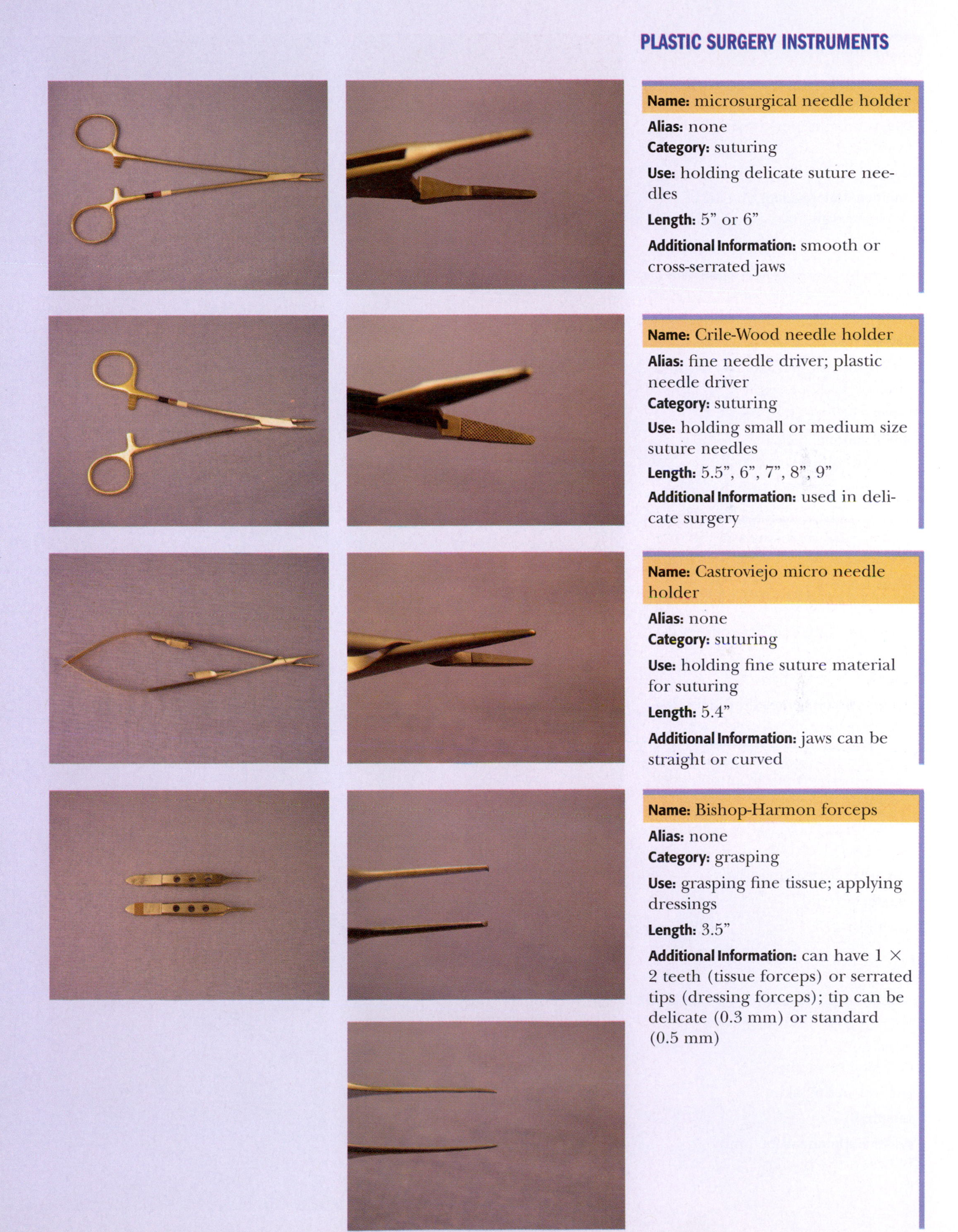

Name: microsurgical needle holder

Alias: none

Category: suturing

Use: holding delicate suture needles

Length: 5” or 6”

Additional Information: smooth or cross-serrated jaws

Name: Crile-Wood needle holder

Alias: fine needle driver; plastic needle driver

Category: suturing

Use: holding small or medium size suture needles

Length: 5.5”, 6”, 7”, 8”, 9”

Additional Information: used in delicate surgery

Name: Castroviejo micro needle holder

Alias: none

Category: suturing

Use: holding fine suture material for suturing

Length: 5.4”

Additional Information: jaws can be straight or curved

Name: Bishop-Harmon forceps

Alias: none

Category: grasping

Use: grasping fine tissue; applying dressings

Length: 3.5”

Additional Information: can have 1 × 2 teeth (tissue forceps) or serrated tips (dressing forceps); tip can be delicate (0.3 mm) or standard (0.5 mm)

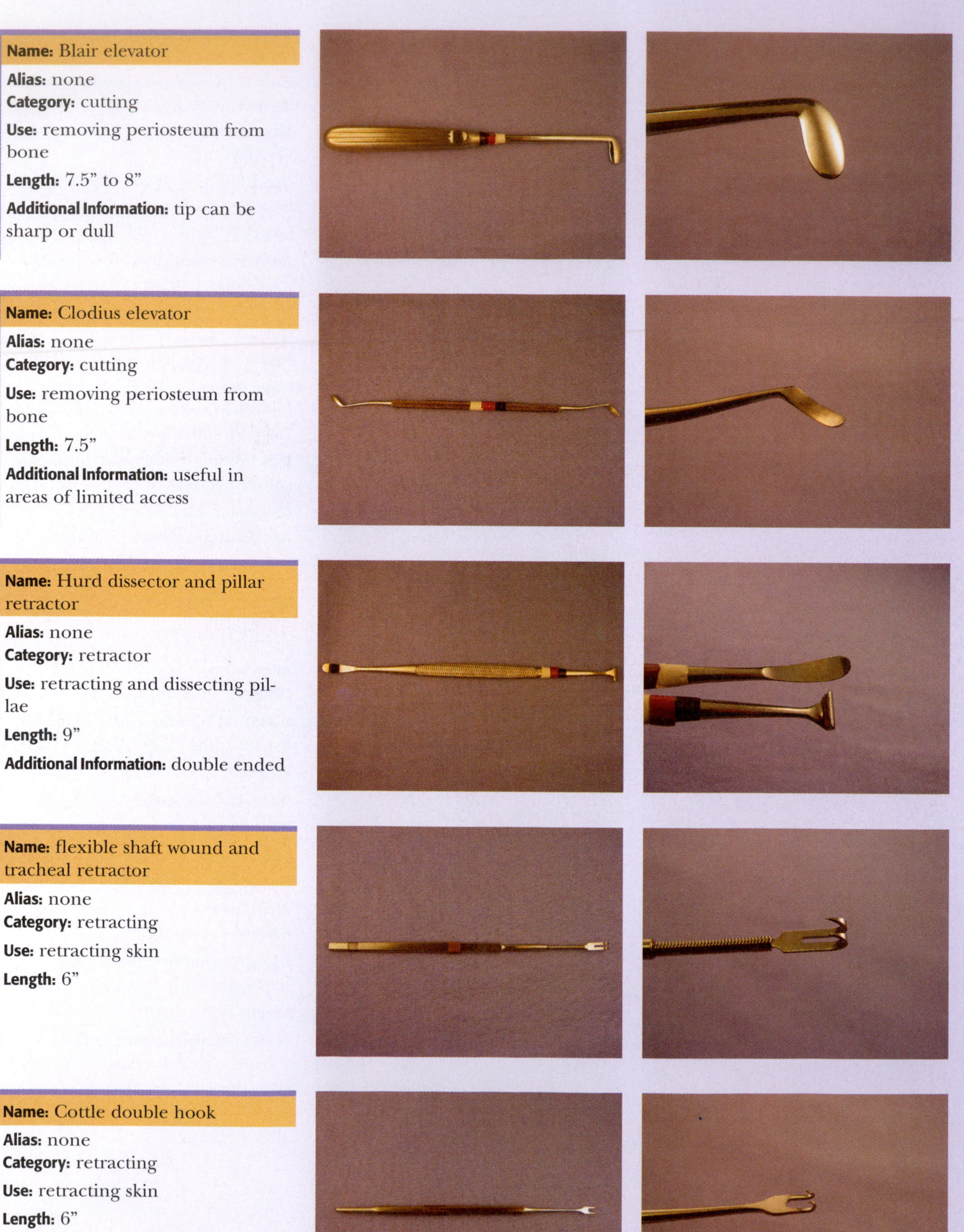

Name: Blair elevator

Alias: none

Category: cutting

Use: removing periosteum from bone

Length: 7.5" to 8"

Additional Information: tip can be sharp or dull

Name: Clodius elevator

Alias: none

Category: cutting

Use: removing periosteum from bone

Length: 7.5"

Additional Information: useful in areas of limited access

Name: Hurd dissector and pillar retractor

Alias: none

Category: retractor

Use: retracting and dissecting pillae

Length: 9"

Additional Information: double ended

Name: flexible shaft wound and tracheal retractor

Alias: none

Category: retracting

Use: retracting skin

Length: 6"

Name: Cottle double hook

Alias: none

Category: retracting

Use: retracting skin

Length: 6"

Additional Information: 3 mm between the prongs

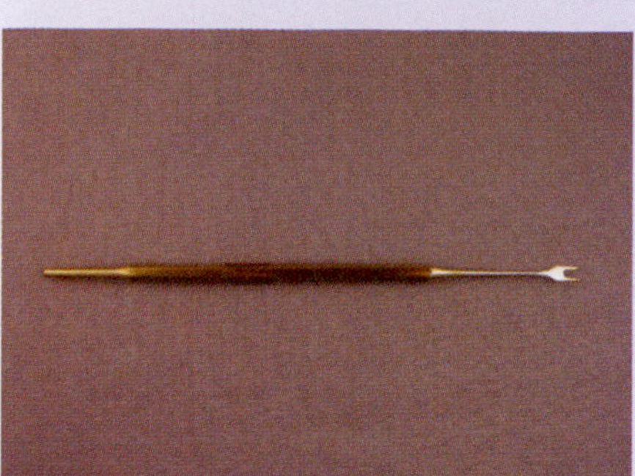

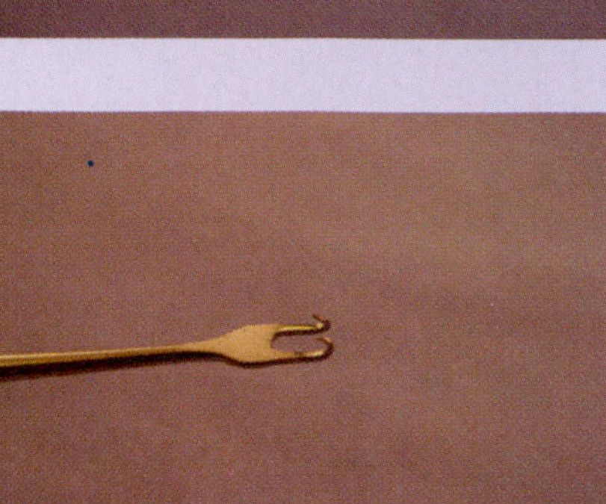

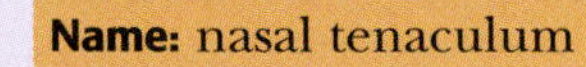

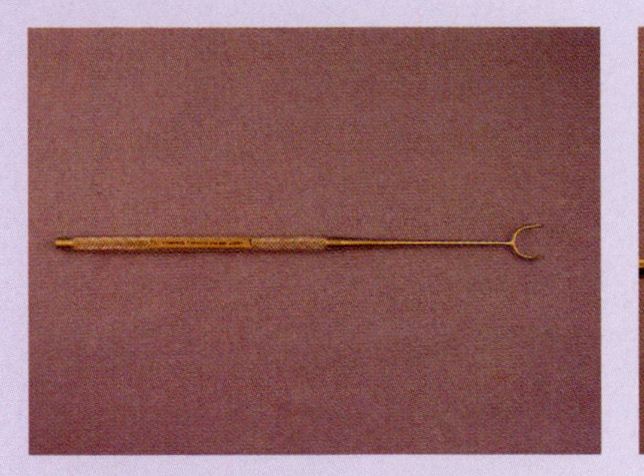

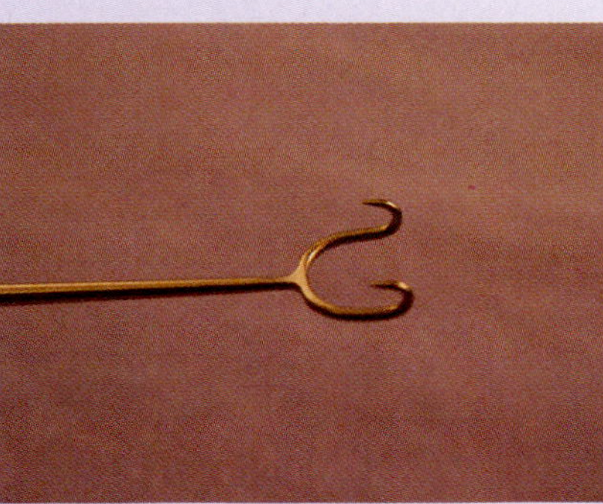

Name: nasal tenaculum

Alias: none

Category: retracting

Use: retracting nasal skin

Length: 6”

Additional Information: can have a single sharp hook or double sharp hooks; double hooks can have 2 mm to 10 mm between the prongs

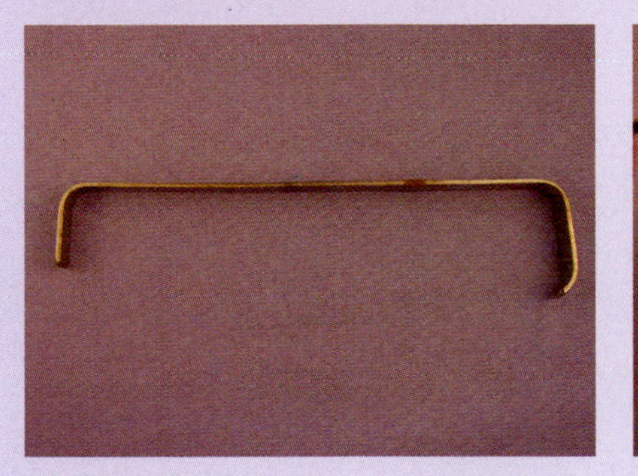

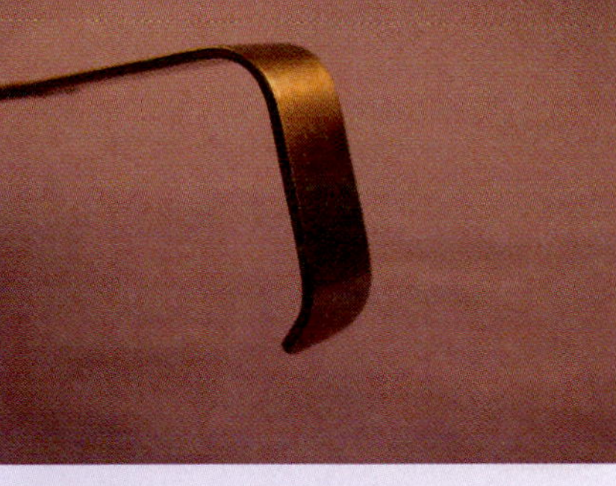

Name: Brewster phrenic retractor

Alias: none

Category: retracting

Use: retracting soft tissue

Length: 6”

Additional Information: blade can be 1.5” or 3/8” wide

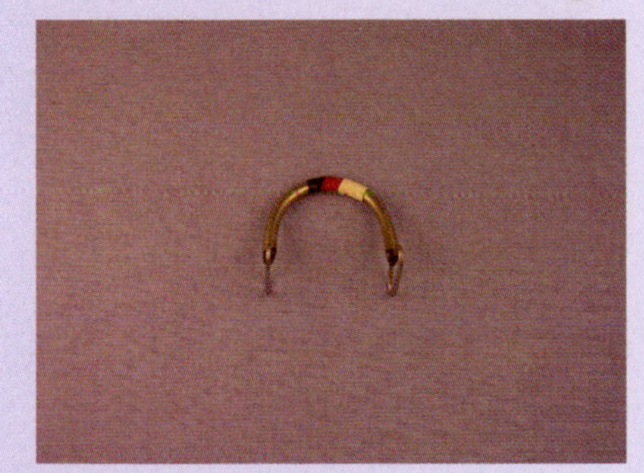

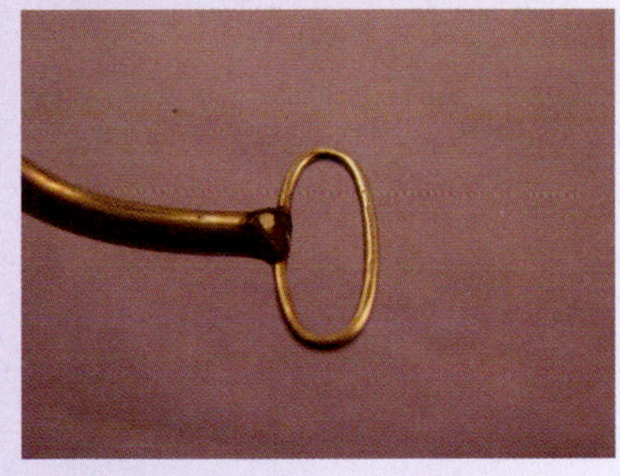

Name: lip traction bow

Alias: none

Category: accessory

Use: relieving suture line tension

Length: 1.5”

Additional Information: small, medium, and large sizes (spread is 2.8 cm to 3.5 cm)

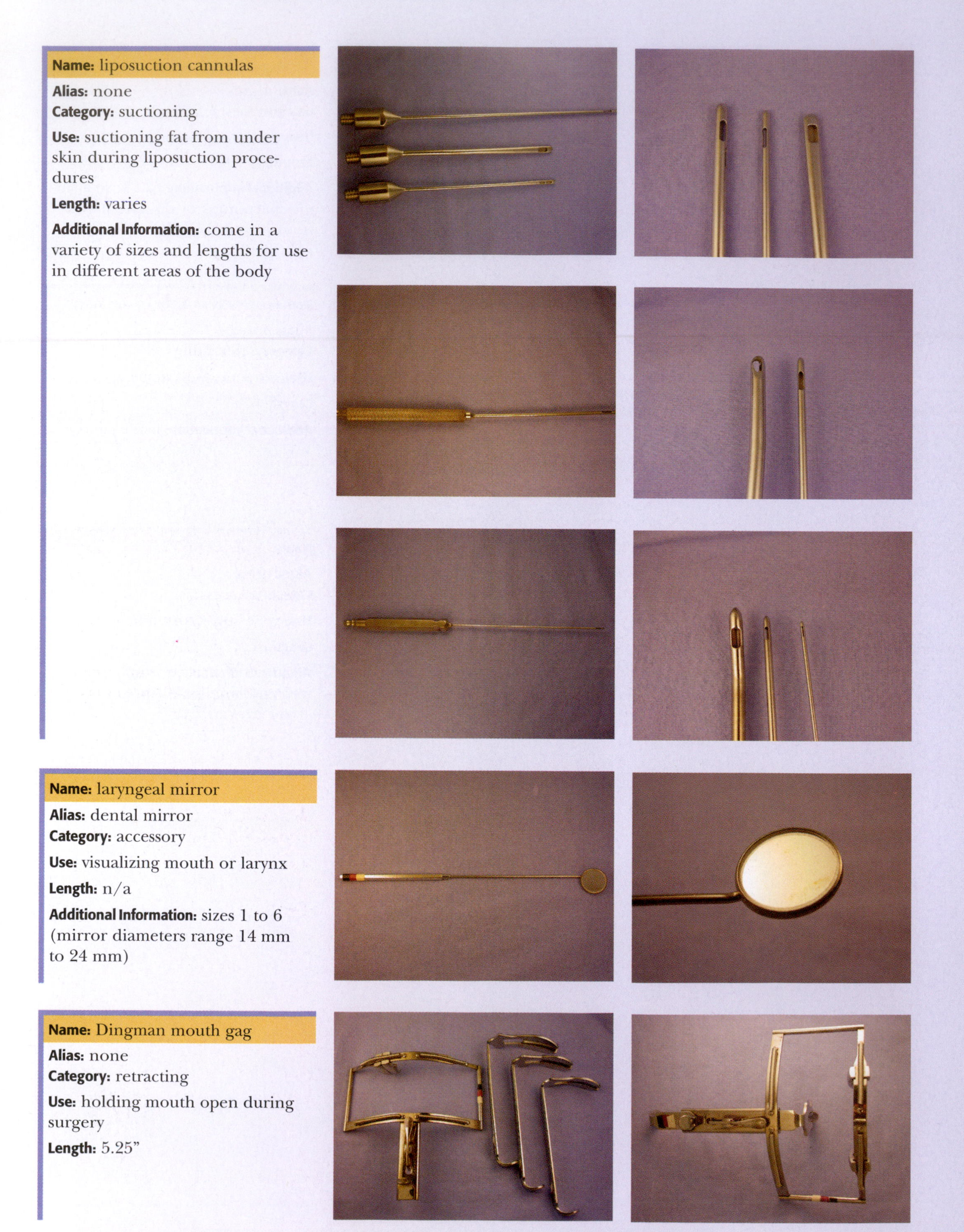

Name: liposuction cannulas

Alias: none

Category: suctioning

Use: suctioning fat from under skin during liposuction procedures

Length: varies

Additional Information: come in a variety of sizes and lengths for use in different areas of the body

Name: laryngeal mirror

Alias: dental mirror

Category: accessory

Use: visualizing mouth or larynx

Length: n/a

Additional Information: sizes 1 to 6 (mirror diameters range 14 mm to 24 mm)

Name: Dingman mouth gag

Alias: none

Category: retracting

Use: holding mouth open during surgery

Length: 5.25"

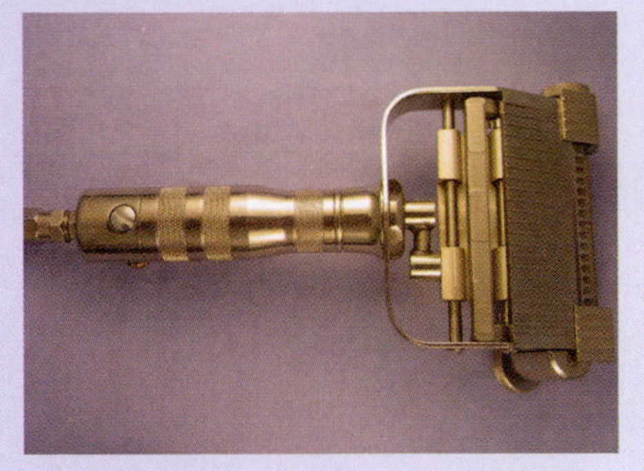

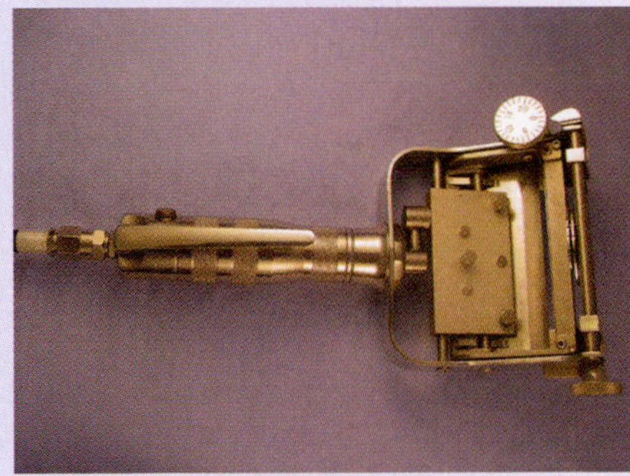

Name: Brown dermatome

Alias: none

Category: cutting

Use: cutting skin grafts of a uniform thickness

Length: n/a

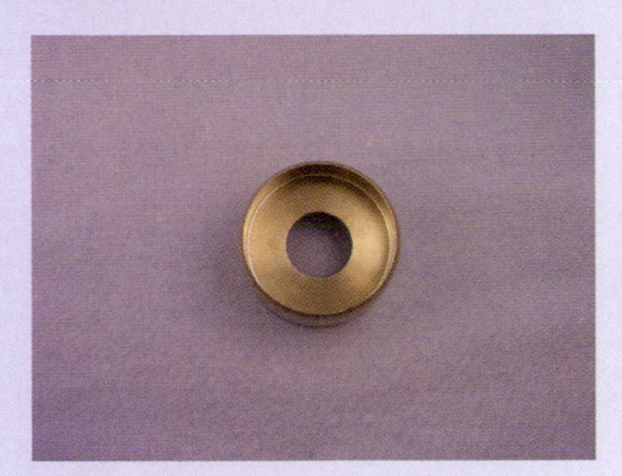

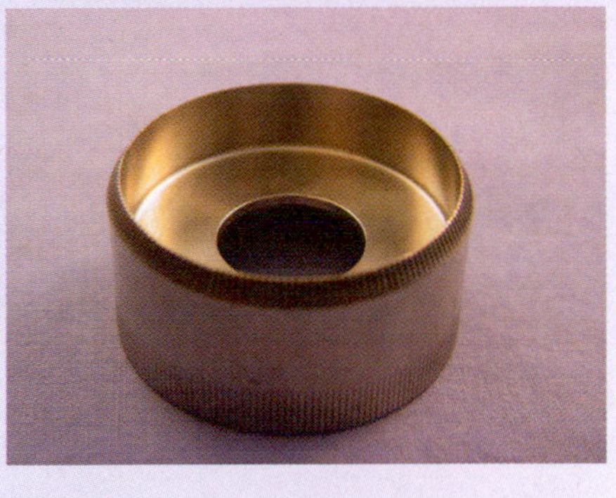

Name: circular marking template

Alias: cookie cutter, nipple washer

Category: accessory

Use: marking areola for breast surgery

Length: n/a

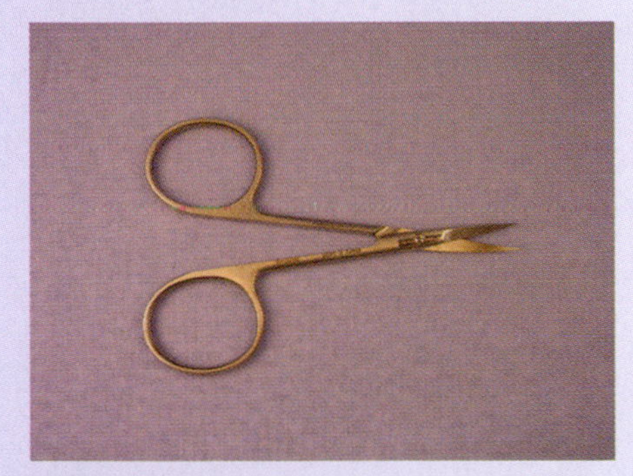

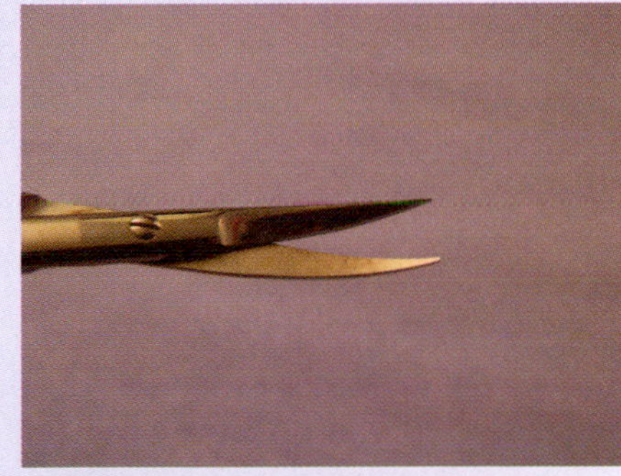

Name: Iris scissors

Alias: none

Category: cutting

Use: cutting fine tissue

Length: 3.5" or 4.5"

Additional Information: blades can be curved or straight; sharp points

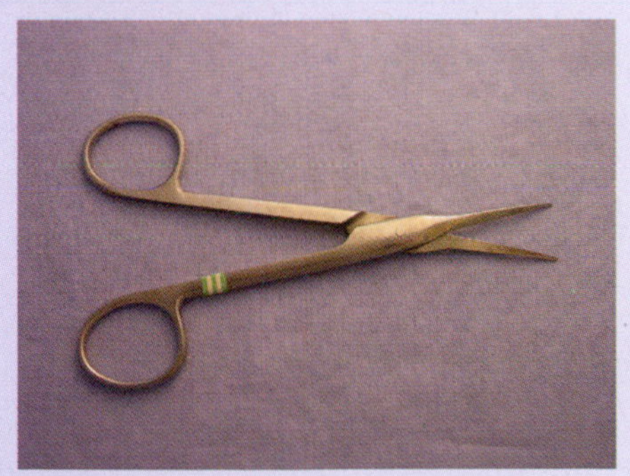

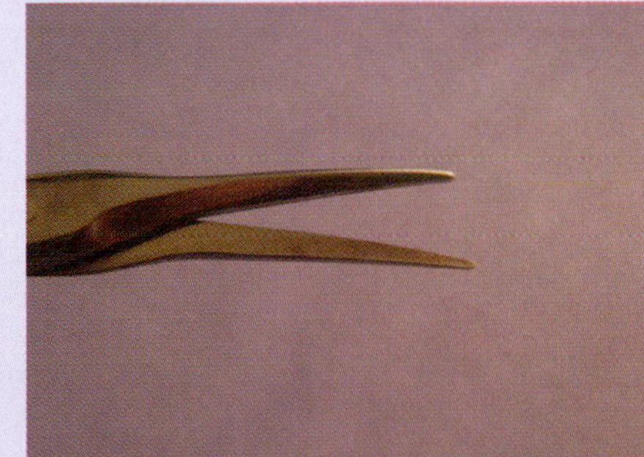

Name: Goldman-Fox scissors

Alias: face lift scissors

Category: cutting

Use: cutting and tissue dissection during face lifts

Length: 5"

Additional Information: curved blades

Q&A

Surgical Session—Dental, Plastic, and Maxillofacial Instruments

1) The surgeon requests an elevator. All of the following are elevators *except*:
   a. Cogswell
   b. Crane
   c. Lucas
   d. Sedillot
2) Extracting forceps are used to remove:
   a. periosteum
   b. teeth
   c. bone
   d. grafts
3) You hand the surgeon an osteotome. The next instrument to hand is a ________.
   a. Mead
   b. McKesson
   c. Crane
   d. Lucas
4) All of the following are types of double hook retractors *except*:
   a. Cottle
   b. nasal tenaculum
   c. Hurd
   d. flexible shaft wound/tracheal
5) At the beginning of breast reduction surgery the surgeon requests an instrument to mark the areola. You hand him/her a:
   a. Blair
   b. "cookie-cutter"
   c. Crile-Wood
   d. Clodius
6) A(n) ___________ is a phrenic retractor.
   a. Brewster
   b. Iris
   c. Sedillot
   d. Hurd
7) Which of the following is a type of suction?
   a. Mead
   b. McKesson
   c. Gillies
   d. Cottle
8) A ____________ is a type of self-retaining mouth gag.
   a. Cottle
   b. Blair
   c. Dingman
   d. Clodius
9) The surgeon requests a bone hook. You hand a ___________ to him/her.
   a. Mead
   b. Castroviejo
   c. Brown
   d. Gillies
10) You are scrubbed in on a skin graft. The surgeon is ready to cut the graft from the thigh. The instrument he/she may use is a:
   a. Lucas
   b. McKesson
   c. Brown dermatome
   d. Crane
11) Which of the following is TRUE about Bishop-Harmon tissue forceps?
   a. the tips have teeth
   b. the tips are serrated
   c. they are for use on heavy tissue
   d. tips are 1 mm in diameter
12) The surgeon needs to hold two fragments of a fracture together. The instrument used for this is a:
   a. rongeur
   b. bending iron
   c. tamp
   d. bone reduction forceps
13) The instrument used to measure the hole for screw length is a:
   a. tamp
   b. depth gauge
   c. trocar guide
   d. countersink

14) You are preparing to hand the surgeon a drill. What other instrument should you anticipate he/she might use with it?

a. tamp

b. depth gauge

c. drill guide

d. wire cutters

15) A variety of various size cannulas (depending on the body site) are used in what type of procedure?

a. skin graft

b. breast augmentation

c. liposuction

d. blepharoplasty

16) A ___________ is a type of rongeur.

a. Blair

b. Bane

c. Cogswell

d. Clodius

Appendix: Answers to Surgical Sessions Quizzes

Answers to Surgical Session—General Instruments

CHAPTER 1

1. d	2. c	3. a	4. c	5. b	6. c
7. b	8. c	9. d	10. b	11. c	12. c
13. c	14. d	15. b	16. a		

Answers to Surgical Session—OB-GYN Instruments

CHAPTER 2

1. b	2. c	3. b	4. d	5. a	6. b
7. b	8. c	9. b	10. a	11. b	12. c
13. a	14. c	15. d	16. b		

Answers to Surgical Session—Urology Instruments

CHAPTER 3

1. b	2. d	3. b	4. a	5. b	6. d
7. c	8. d	9. c	10. c	11. b	12. c
13. d	14. c	15. c	16. a		

Answers to Surgical Session—Orthopedic Instruments

CHAPTER 4

1. a	2. c	3. d	4. a	5. b	6. b
7. b	8. a	9. c	10. c	11. b	12. c
13. a	14. c	15. b	16. d		

Answers to Surgical Session—Neurosurgical Instruments

CHAPTER 5

1. b	2. b	3. c	4. b	5. d	6. d
7. c	8. b	9. d	10. a	11. b	12. a
13. c	14. d	15. a	16. b		

Answers to Surgical Session—Ear, Nose, and Throat Instruments

CHAPTER 6

1. a	2. b	3. d	4. d	5. c	6. c
7. a	8. d	9. b	10. a	11. d	12. c
13. b	14. a	15. b	16. c		

Answers to Surgical Session—Ophthalmologic Instruments

CHAPTER 7

1. c	2. a	3. b	4. a	5. d	6. d
7. a	8. c	9. b	10. b	11. a	12. d
13. b	14. a	15. c	16. b		

Answers to Surgical Session—Cardiothoracic and Vascular Instruments

CHAPTER 8

1. d	2. b	3. a	4. b	5. a	6. b
7. c	8. d	9. a	10. c	11. d	12. a
13. d	14. a	15. d	16. c		

Answers to Surgical Session—Dental, Plastic, and Maxillofacial Instruments

CHAPTER 9

1. c	2. b	3. a	4. c	5. b	6. a
7. b	8. c	9. d	10. c	11. a	12. d
13. b	14. c	15. c	16. b		

INDEX

I

J

K

L

M

N

O

P